Bladder Cancer

Bladder Cancer

Edited by

Ja Hyeon Ku
Seoul National University Hospital, Seoul, Korea

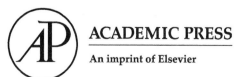

Academic Press is an imprint of Elsevier
125 London Wall, London EC2Y 5AS, United Kingdom
525 B Street, Suite 1800, San Diego, CA 92101-4495, United States
50 Hampshire Street, 5th Floor, Cambridge, MA 02139, United States
The Boulevard, Langford Lane, Kidlington, Oxford OX5 1GB, United Kingdom

Notices
Knowledge and best practice in this field are constantly changing. As new research and experience broaden
our understanding, changes in research methods, professional practices, or medical treatment may become
necessary.

Practitioners and researchers must always rely on their own experience and knowledge in evaluating and
using any information, methods, compounds, or experiments described herein. In using such information or
methods they should be mindful of their own safety and the safety of others, including parties for whom they
have a professional responsibility.

To the fullest extent of the law, neither the Publisher nor the authors, contributors, or editors, assume any
liability for any injury and/or damage to persons or property as a matter of products liability, negligence or
otherwise, or from any use or operation of any methods, products, instructions, or ideas contained in the
material herein.

British Library Cataloguing-in-Publication Data
A catalogue record for this book is available from the British Library

Library of Congress Cataloging-in-Publication Data
A catalog record for this book is available from the Library of Congress

ISBN: 978-0-12-809939-1

For Information on all Academic Press publications
visit our website at https://www.elsevier.com/books-and-journals

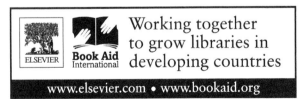

Working together
to grow libraries in
developing countries

www.elsevier.com • www.bookaid.org

Publisher: Mica Haley
Acquisition Editor: Tari K. Broderick
Editorial Project Manager: Fenton Coulthurst
Production Project Manager: Priya Kumaraguruparan
Cover Designer: Matthew Limbert

Typeset by MPS Limited, Chennai, India

Contents

Section I
Epidemiology, Etiology, and Pathophysiology

1. Epidemiology
Sue Kyung Park

2. Etiology (Risk Factors for Bladder Cancer)
Hyung Suk Kim

3. **Pathophysiology of Bladder Cancer**

Ju Hyun Shin, Jae Sung Lim and Byeong Hwa Jeon

Section II
Diagnosis

4. **Symptoms**

Min Soo Choo

5. **Physical Examination**

Kyungtae Ko

Section III
Pathology and Staging

Section IV
Treatment for Nonmuscle Invasive Bladder Cancer (NMIBC)

20. Immunotherapy: Bacille Calmette–Guérin

20.1 Indications for BCG

Sung Han Kim and Ho Kyung Seo

20.2 Optimal BCG Schedule

Sung Han Kim and Ho Kyung Seo

Section V
Treatment for Muscle-Invasive Bladder Cancer (MIBC)

Section VII
Follow-Up (Surveillance)

29. Surveillance for Non-Muscle-Invasive Bladder Cancer

Ji Sung Shim and Sung Gu Kang

30. The Surveillance for Muscle-Invasive Bladder Cancer (MIBC)

Yun-Sok Ha and Tae-Hwan Kim

31. ## Novel and Emerging Surveillance Markers for Bladder Cancer

Yang Hyun Cho, Seung Il Jung and Eu Chang Hwang

Section VIII
Future Perspective in Bladder Cancer

32. ## Microbiome

Malcolm Dewar, Jonathan Izawa, Fan Li, Ryan M. Chanyi, Gregor Reid and Jeremy P. Burton

List of Contributors

Jeremy P. Burton Schulich School of Medicine & Dentistry, London, ON, Canada; University of Western Ontario, London, ON, Canada; Canadian Centre for Human Microbiome and Probiotics Research, London, ON, Canada

Ryan M. Chanyi Schulich School of Medicine & Dentistry, London, ON, Canada; University of Western Ontario, London, ON, Canada; Canadian Centre for Human Microbiome and Probiotics Research, London, ON, Canada

Jeong Y. Cho Seoul National University Hospital, Seoul, South Korea

Kang Su Cho Yonsei University College of Medicine, Seoul, South Korea

Min Chul Cho Seoul Metropolitan Government − Seoul National University Borame Medical Center, Seoul, South Korea

Yang Hyun Cho Chonnam National University Medical School, Gwangju, South Korea

Min Soo Choo Hallym University College of Medicine, Chuncheon, South Korea

Seol Ho Choo Ajou University School of Medicine, Suwon, South Korea

Felix K.-H. Chun University Medical Center Hamburg-Eppendorf, Hamburg, Germany

Garrett M. Dancik Eastern Connecticut State University, Willimantic, CT, United States

Malcolm Dewar Schulich School of Medicine & Dentistry, London, ON, Canada

Margit Fisch University Medical Center Hamburg-Eppendorf, Hamburg, Germany

Hong Koo Ha Pusan National University Hospital, Busan, South Korea

Yun-Sok Ha Kyungpook National University, Daegu, South Korea

Jun Hyuk Hong University of Ulsan, Asan Medical Center, Seoul, South Korea

Sung-Hoo Hong Seoul St. Mary's Hospital, Seoul, South Korea

Eu Chang Hwang Chonnam National University Medical School, Gwangju, South Korea

Jonathan Izawa Schulich School of Medicine & Dentistry, London, ON, Canada

Byeong Hwa Jeon Chungnam National University, Daejeon, South Korea

Seung H. Jeon Kyung Hee University School of Medicine, Seoul, South Korea

Byong Chang Jeong Sungkyunkwan University, Seoul, South Korea

Chang Wook Jeong Seoul National University Hospital, Seoul, South Korea

Hyeon Jeong Seoul National University, Seoul, South Korea

Seung Il Jung Chonnam National University Medical School, Gwangju, South Korea

Ho-Won Kang Chungbuk National University, Cheongju, Republic of Korea

Minyong Kang Sungkyunkwan University School of Medicine, Seoul, South Korea

Seok H. Kang Korea University College of Medicine, Seoul, South Korea

Sung Gu Kang Korea University College of Medicine, Seoul, South Korea

Bhumsuk Keam Seoul National University Hospital, Seoul, Korea

Hyung Suk Kim Dongguk University Ilsan Medical Center, Goyang, South Korea

Jae Heon Kim Soonchunhyang University, Seoul, South Korea

Jeong Hyun Kim Kangwon National University School of Medicine, Chuncheon, South Korea

Soodong Kim Dong-A University Medical Center, Busan, South Korea

Sun Il Kim Ajou University School of Medicine, Suwon, South Korea

Sung Han Kim Research Institute and National Cancer Center, Goyang, South Korea

Tae-Hwan Kim Kyungpook National University, Daegu, South Korea

Young A. Kim Seoul Metropolitan Government Boramae Hospital, Seoul, South Korea

Luis A. Kluth University Medical Center Hamburg-Eppendorf, Hamburg, Germany

Kyungtae Ko Hallym University, Seoul, South Korea

Whi-An Kwon Wonkwang University Sanbon Hospital, Gunpo, South Korea

Jeong W. Lee Dongguk University Ilsan Hospital, Goyang, South Korea

Joo Yong Lee Yonsei University College of Medicine, Seoul, South Korea

Ok-Jun Lee Chungbuk National University, Cheongju, Republic of Korea

Richard J. Lee Harvard Medical School and Massachusetts General Hospital Cancer Center, Boston, MA, United States

Seung W. Lee Hanyang University Guri Hospital, Guri, South Korea

Fan Li Schulich School of Medicine & Dentistry, London, ON, Canada

Jae Sung Lim Chungnam National University, Daejeon, South Korea

Yuchen Liu Shenzhen Second People's Hospital, The First Affiliated Hospital of Shenzhen University, Shenzhen, P.R. China

Evangelina López de Maturana Spanish National Cancer Research Centre (CNIO), Madrid, Spain; Centro de Investigación Biomédica en red Cáncer (CIBERONC), Madrid, Spain

Núria Malats Spanish National Cancer Research Centre (CNIO), Madrid, Spain; Centro de Investigación Biomédica en red Cáncer (CIBERONC), Madrid, Spain

Gyeong E. Min Kyung Hee University School of Medicine, Seoul, South Korea

Kyung C. Moon Seoul National University College of Medicine, Seoul, South Korea

Jong Jin Oh Seoul National University Bundang Hospital, Seongnam, South Korea

Sunghyun Paick Konkuk University Medical Center, Seoul, South Korea

Jae Young Park Korea University Ansan Hospital, Ansan, South Korea

Jeong Hwan Park Seoul National University College of Medicine, Seoul, South Korea

Juhyun Park Seoul National University, Seoul, South Korea

Sue Kyung Park Seoul National University College of Medicine, Seoul, South Korea; Seoul National University, Seoul, South Korea

Jong H. Pyun Sungkyunkwan University School of Medicine, Seoul, South Korea

Gregor Reid Schulich School of Medicine & Dentistry, London, ON, Canada; University of Western Ontario, London, ON, Canada; Canadian Centre for Human Microbiome and Probiotics Research, London, ON, Canada

Victor M. Schüttfort University Medical Center Hamburg-Eppendorf, Hamburg, Germany

Ho Kyung Seo Research Institute and National Cancer Center, Goyang, South Korea

Ji Sung Shim Korea University College of Medicine, Seoul, South Korea

Ju Hyun Shin Chungnam National University, Daejeon, South Korea

Dan Theodorescu University of Colorado, Aurora, CO, United States

Sungmin Woo Seoul National University Hospital, Seoul, South Korea

Won Jae Yang Soonchunhyang University Hospital, Seoul, South Korea

Seok Joong Yun Chungbuk National University, Cheongju, Republic of Korea

About the Editor

Dr. Ja Hyeon Ku graduated from Soonchunhyang University School of Medicine, Korea, in 1995 and completed his Urology training at Soonchunhyang University Hospital in 2000. He completed fellowships at Seoul National University Hospital (2003−05) and subsequently obtained his PhD in Department of Urology, Seoul National University College of Medicine (2005).

He was appointed as a staff at Seoul Veterans Hospital, Korea (2005−07) and moved to Department of Urology, Seoul National Hospital, Korea, in 2007. He has studied bladder cancer as a Visiting Postdoc Fellow at Scott Department of Urology, Baylor College of Medicine, Houston, TX, United States under Dr. Seth P. Lerner (2011−12). He has been the faculty member since 2007 and is now a professor in Department of Urology, Seoul National University College of Medicine, Korea.

His clinical and research interests lie in the urologic cancers including urothelial carcinoma. He published more than 260 peer-reviewed journal articles and book chapters. He has also been active member of Korean Urological Association and board member of Korean Urological Oncology Society. He has been serving as an Editorial Board for the Investigative and Clinical Urology, Translational Cancer Research and Frontier in Oncology.

Preface

Bladder cancer is one of the most common cancers of the urinary tract. It is a highly fatal disease and has the highest recurrence rate of any solid tumor. Due to these factors, the per-patient cost of managing bladder cancer is among the highest for any cancer. Therefore there is a need for gaining an understanding of the exact pathophysiology of bladder cancer, as well as for developing new and effective treatment modalities.

This book is organized to give the investigators state-of-the art information on all aspects of bladder cancer. Authors provide insight into obstacles to improved survival, discuss methods to advance the field, and review the related supporting evidence. Each of the contributors has been extraordinarily generous with their time in making substantive contributions in the development of this book. I hope that this textbook will serve as an easy and complete guide for researchers, clinicians, individuals in training, allied health professionals, and medical students.

Finally, I am grateful to the authors for their contributions and commitment to the development and publication of this textbook. Organizing this book would not have been possible without the invaluable contributions of the authors of each chapter. I also appreciate the commitment of the outstanding staff at Elsevier. In particular, I thank Editorial Project Manager, Fenton Coulthurst, for managing the final editing and production of the text.

Ja Hyeon Ku MD, PhD
Department of Urology, Seoul National University Hospital, Seoul, Korea

Epidemiology, Etiology, and Pathophysiology

Chapter 1

Epidemiology

Sue Kyung Park[1,2]

[1]*Seoul National University College of Medicine, Seoul, South Korea,*
[2]*Seoul National University, Seoul, South Korea*

Chapter Outline

INTRODUCTION

Bladder cancer is the first leading malignancy presented in urinary system including kidney. In 2012, 429,000 new bladder cancer cases (330,000 men and 99,000 women) were diagnosed globally [1].

In global cancer incidence data in 2012, bladder cancer was listed as the ninth most common cancer, and according to sex, it is the 7th and the 19th common cancer in men and women, respectively [1].

Bladder Cancer. DOI: http://dx.doi.org/10.1016/B978-0-12-809939-1.00001-1

BLADDER CANCER INCIDENCE IS RELATED TO THE DEVELOPMENT LEVEL OF COUNTRY AND HUMAN

Worldwide incidence rates (IRs) of bladder cancer are 5.3 per 100,000 persons (Fig. 1.1). New cases of bladder cancer seem to be associated with the development level of the country. Bladder cancer ranks the third of cancers predominantly occurring in more developed countries among 15 highest cancers (prostate cancer: 2.1 times; kidney cancer: 1.5 times) (Fig. 1.2).

The number of new cases of bladder cancer in more developed countries ($N = 254,000$) is 1.4 times greater than that in less developed countries ($N = 176,000$), and of new cases of bladder cancer in 2012, about 60% was occurred in more developed regions [1]. Age-standardized incidence rates (ASIR) in more and less developed countries are 9.5 and 3.3 per 100,000, respectively (Fig. 1.1). Based on the IR, bladder cancer risk in more developed countries is 2.9-fold higher than that in less developed countries (rate ratio of ASIR = 2.9 = 9.5/3.3).

Bladder cancer incidence may also be associated with the development level of the human. The WHO classified countries with very high, high, medium, and low human development level by human development index, which is a composite index measuring average achievement of human development in three basic dimensions such as a long and healthy life, knowledge,

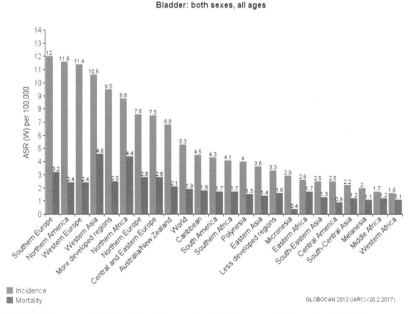

FIGURE 1.1 Age-standardized incidence rate (*ASR*) and mortality rate of bladder cancer according to world area (UN) (both sexes, all ages).

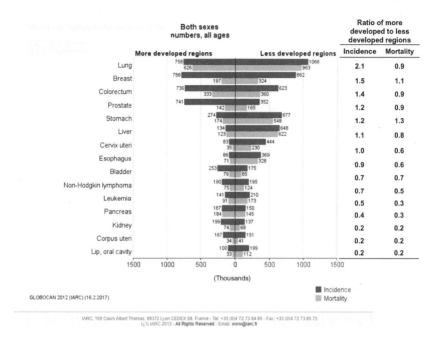

FIGURE 1.2   Number of incidence and death of 15 leading cancers in both sexes (Unit: ×1000).

and a decent standard of living (United Nations Development Programme) [2]. Based on WHO classification by human development level, a 72% of new bladder cancer cases occurred in countries with high and very high human development level ($N = 310,000$ for high and very high human development level vs $N = 119,000$ for low and medium human development level) [1]. Relative to low human developed countries (ASIR = 2.2 per 100,000), very high human developed countries (ASIR = 9.7 per 100,000) have 4.4-fold higher IR, and high (ASIR = 5.9 per 100,000) and medium human developed countries (ASIR = 2.9 per 100,000) have 2.7-fold and 1.3-fold higher IR, respectively [1].

GLOBAL IRs OF BLADDER CANCER IS DIFFERENT FROM THE DISTRIBUTION OF MAJOR RISK FACTORS

According to world countries, the highest IRs are seen in North America, South and West Europe, and Middle East and North Africa (MENA) (Egypt, Turkey, Lebanon, Israel, Armenia, Iraq, and Syria) and the lowest IRs are seen in Asia, including India, Vietnam, Philippines, Mongolia, and Africa, including Nigeria, Cameroon, Central African Republic, Uganda, and Kenya (Fig. 1.3). The top five countries with the highest incidence of bladder cancer

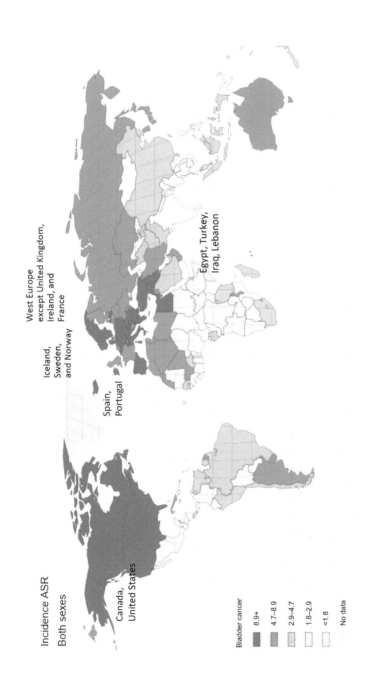

FIGURE 1.3 Geographical variation of bladder cancer incidence rates (Age-standardized incidence rate, *ASR*, both sexes).

Incidence ASR
Both sexes

West Europe
except United Kingdom,
Ireland, and
France

Iceland,
Sweden,
and Norway

Spain,
Portugal

Egypt, Turkey,
Iraq, Lebanon

Canada,
United States

Bladder cancer

8.9+

4.7–8.9

2.9–4.7

1.8–2.9

<1.8

No data

Source: GLOBOCAN 2012 (IARC)

Bladder: both sexes, all ages

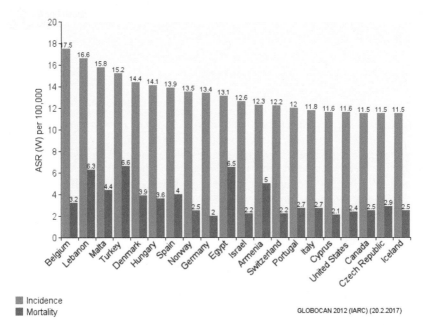

FIGURE 1.4   Age-standardized incidence rate (*ASR*) and mortality rate of top 20 countries with the highest incidence rates of bladder cancer (both sexes, all ages).

in 2012 are Belgium (17.5 per 100,000), Lebanon (16.6), Malta (15.8 per 100,000), Turkey (15.2 per 100,000), and Denmark (14.4 per 100,000) (Fig. 1.4). Among top 20 countries with the highest IRs of bladder cancer, 13 countries are included in South, West, and North Europe (Spain; Belgium, Malta), two countries are included in North America; and five countries are included in North America and the MENA regions (Lebanon, Turkey, Egypt, Israel, and Armenia) (Fig. 1.4).

The variability of IRs in bladder cancer depend on the accurate and reliable cancer registry and medical diagnosis system in each country, and the IRs are partly compatible with the distribution of major risk factors of bladder cancer. In developed regions such as North America and Europe, urothelial carcinoma of bladder cancer types is the most common (about 90%), whereas nonurothelial carcinoma such as primary squamous cell carcinoma is uncommon. In these developed countries, major risk factors are cigarette smoking and occupational exposure to industrial chemicals, such as 4-aminobiphenyl, 2-naphthylamine, benzidine, painting, and auramine, magenta, and rubber production [3]. In the other highest incidence area of bladder cancer including MENA regions, such as Egypt and Middle East, the *Schistosoma haematobium* is responsible for bladder cancer occurrence. It is an endemic area of the *S. haematobium* in MENA regions for a long time, and the link between bladder cancer and high prevalence of *S. haematobium* is evident [4]. In these endemic areas of *S. haematobium*, nonurothelial carcinoma, such as squamous cell carcinoma in the bladder, are the first common pathological type, and it is partly related to chronic infection of schistosomiasis and keratinization of squamous metaplasia in bladder mucosa.

LIFETIME CUMULATIVE RISK OF BLADDER CANCER IS 1 PER 100 MEN AND 1 PER 500 WOMEN GLOBALLY

Globally, lifetime cumulative risk of bladder cancer is 0.6% (1 per 170 persons), which is higher in men, i.e., 1% in men (1 per 100 men) and 0.24% in women (1 per 500 women) [1]. In the regions with the highest IRs of bladder cancer, i.e., Southern Europe, West Europe, the MENA, the lifetime probability of bladder cancer is 2.1%−2.5% in men [1] and, in other words, at least 1 of 50 men can develop bladder cancer during his lifetime, whereas about 1 of 200 women can develop bladder cancer in her lifetime (0.4%−0.6% in women). In contrast, in the regions with the lowest IRs, such as West African, Middle African, and South-Central Asia, about 1 of 400 men and 1 of 5000 women develops bladder cancer in their lifetime (0.25%−0.5% in men and 0.1%−0.2% in women) [1].

FOURFOLD HIGHER RISK IN MEN

The IRs of bladder cancer in men (9 per 100,000 men) are higher than those in women (2.2 per 100,000 women) [1]. According to sex, men are 4.1-fold more likely to get bladder cancer than women. Based on the number of new cases of bladder cancer, new cases in men ($N = 330,000$) occupy two-third of total bladder cancer in 2012 (women: $N = 99,000$) (Fig. 1.3).

Male dominance pattern in bladder cancer IRs is more strongly found in more developed countries (incidence rate ratio [IRR] of men relative to women = 4.6) than less developed countries (IRR = 3.5), and also in high and very high human developed countries (IRR = 4.3, for very high human developed countries, and IRR = 4.9, for high human developed countries) than low and medium human developed countries (IRR = 3.9, for medium human developed countries, and IRR = 2.2, for low human developed countries) (from calculation based on [1]).

VERY HIGH RISK AT VERY OLD AGED PEOPLE (70 YEARS OR OLDER)

According to age distribution, age increase is related to a steep increase in IRs of bladder cancer (Fig. 1.5). About 90% of bladder cancer occurs at age 55 years or older, and in particular, two-third of bladder cancer occurs at age

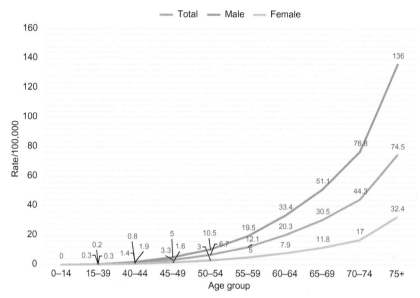

FIGURE 1.5   Age-specific incidence rates of bladder cancer in total men and women populations.

65 years or older; whereas only 1.8% of bladder cancer is developed at age younger than 40 years (Fig. 1.5). Relative to bladder cancer patients aged 40−44 years old, IRR was increased by age increase (IRR = 4.8 in age 50−54 years; 8.6 in 55−59 years; 14.5 in 60−64 years; 21.8 in 65−69 years; 31.6 in 70−74 years; and 53.2 in 75 years or older). In particular, IRRs in men are dramatically steeply increased by age increase (IRR = 5.5 in age 50−54 years; 10.3 in 55−59 years; 17.6 in 60−64 years; 26.9 in 65−69 years; 40.4 in 70−74 years; and 71.6 in 75 years or older), whereas IRRs in women are less strongly increased (IRR = 3.8 in age 50−54 years; 6.3 in 55−59 years; 9.9 in 60−64 years; 14.8 in 65−69 years; 21.3 in 70−74 years; and 40.5 in 75 years or older).

According to age increase, the gap of incidence between men and women is much more growing and thus male dominance in incidence relative to female is intensified. IRR of men relative to women is 1.5 at age 15−39 years, whereas that is 4.2 at age 75 years or older (Fig. 1.5).

STEEPLY INCREASING IRs BY AGE INCREASE, ESPECIALLY IN MORE DEVELOPED COUNTRIES

According to age, IRs of bladder cancer in more developed countries show a steep rise by the increase of age, whereas those in less developed countries are smoothly increasing but IRs has abruptly increased at very old age

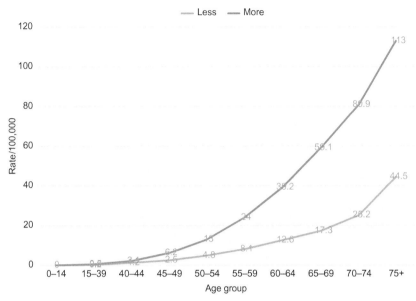

FIGURE 1.6 Age-specific incidence rates of bladder cancer between more and less developed countries.

(75 years or older) (Fig. 1.6). Relative to IRs in age 40−44 years, the IRR in each age group was 4.0 in age 50−54 years, 6.8 in 55−59 years, 10.5 in 60−64 years, 14.4 in 65−69 years, 21.0 in 70−74 years, and 37.1 in 75 years or older in less developed regions, whereas IRR was 6.2 in age 50−54 years, 11.4 in 55−59 years, 18.7 in 60−64 years, 28.1 in 65−69 years, 38.5 in 70−74 years, and 53.8 in 75 years or older in more developed regions. Therefore, the gap in IRs between more and less developed countries are larger with age increase.

Based on human development level, a dramatically steeply increasing pattern in age-specific IRs of bladder cancer is found in very high human developed countries by age increase; and the next higher age-specific IRs are showed in high human developed countries (Fig. 1.7). In medium and low human developed countries, age-specific IRs are lower and similar by age increase till 65−69 years, but the smaller gap in IRs between the two groups in older age group (70−74 years and 75 years or older) is observed. Relative to IRs in age 40−44 years, the higher rank of IRR is the order of IRR at very high, high, medium, and low human development level as following: IRR = 6.1, 4.9, 3.8, and 2.9 in age 50−54 years, respectively; 11.4, 8.7, 6.8, and 4.6 in age 55−59 years, respectively; 18.6, 13,5, 10.9, and 6.8 in age 60−64 years, respectively; 28.1, 19.0, 14.4, and 8.7 in age 65−69 years, respectively; and 40.1, 25.7, 21.1, and 10.7 in age 70−74 years, respectively. However, in the group of age 75 years or older, the rank of IRR in medium

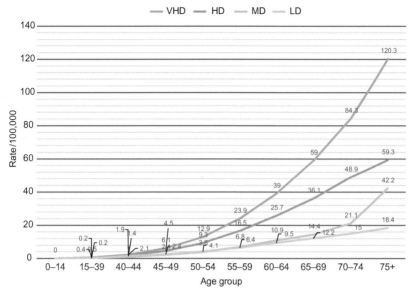

FIGURE 1.7 Age-specific incidence rates of bladder cancer according to human development level.

and high human development level is reversed, and IRR is 57.3 in high development level, 42.2 in medium development level, 31.2 in high development level, and 18.8 in low development level.

SMALLER GEOGRAPHICAL AND DEMOGRAPHICAL VARIATION IN MORTALITY OF BLADDER CANCER

Globally 165,000 patients having bladder cancer (123,000 men and 42,000 women) died in 2012 [1]. The mortality rates (MRs) in total bladder cancer patients are 4.5 per 100,000. Sex-specific ASRs are 3.2 per 100,000 in men and 0.9 per 100,000 in women, respectively [1], and the risk for death from bladder cancer in men is 3.6-fold higher that in women.

There are geographical variation in bladder cancer MRs between more to less developed regions, and very high and high to medium and low human developed area; the variation is not as large as that of bladder cancer IRs. A 48.5% of bladder cancer death occurs in more developed countries (vs a 59.1% of incidence occurs in more developed countries), and a 62.1% of death in high and very high human developed countries (vs a 72.3% of incidence occurs in high and very high human developed countries).

Moreover, a regional variation in MRs based on world area (UN) (Fig. 1.1) is smaller than the regional variation in IRs, and the mortality rate ratio (MRR) between the highest (4.6 per 100,000 in western Asian of the MENA) and the lowest MRs (0.9 per 100,000 in Central America; Micronesia was excluded due to small baseline population) among world regions by UN classification is 7.5-fold, whereas the IRR between the highest (12 per 100,000 in South Europe) and the lowest IRs (1.6 per 100,000 in West Africa) (Fig. 1.1). The reason for the smaller variability in MRs across countries is that the variation in definition and registration of high staged bladder cancer, which is highly responsible for death, is small among countries [5].

Among the 20 countries with the highest IRs of bladder cancer, 4 countries included in the MENA area, such as Lebanon, Turkey, Egypt, and Armenia, except Israel, show the highest MRs of bladder cancer (Turkey 6.6 per 100,000; Egypt 6.5 per 100,000; Lebanon 6.3 per 100,000; Armenia 5 per 100,000) (Fig. 1.4), whereas MRs in West and South Europe are lower than the countries included in the MENA but higher than countries with the lowest IRs such as most African and Asian countries (Fig. 1.1) because most death of bladder cancer patients is derived from higher incidence area with a lot of bladder cancer cases.

Although MRs in more developed regions (2.5 per 100,000) are higher than those in less developed regions (1.6 per 100,000) (Fig. 1.1), the gap of the two MRs between more and less developed regions is smaller (1.6-fold) than that of IRs between the two regions (2.9-fold between the two IRs such as 9.5 per 100,000 and 3.3 per 100,000) (Fig. 1.1). Also the gap in MRs across four human development levels is much smaller than that in IRs. Relative to low human developed countries (ASIR = 1.5 per 100,000), very high and high human developed countries (both ASIR = 2.4 per 100,000) have 1.6-fold higher IR, whereas medium human developed countries (ASIR = 1.4 per 100,000) have rather lower IR (0.9-fold) [1] (figure not shown).

DECREASING AGE-STANDARDIZED DEATH RATES BUT INCREASING NUMBER OF DEATH IN MOST COUNTRIES

In most countries in the world where the number of death from bladder cancer was reported to the WHO [6], the number of death from bladder cancers was increased but age-standardized death rates (ASDR) were decreased over the past 20 years. Among the 20 countries where the highest IRs of bladder cancer were observed, the largest death from bladder cancer around the world was occurred in the United States (annually 15,502 death between 2012 and 2013), and the number of death was increased by 43% over the past 20 years (annually 10,835 death between 1992 and 1993), whereas the ASDRs were decreased by 20% (ASDR = 3.3 in 1992−93 vs ASDR = 2.7 in 2012−13) (Fig. 1.8). In all European countries where high IRs are observed, the all ASDRs of bladder cancer are decreasing over the last two decades, but total number of death from bladder cancer vary by the country (50%− 60% increasing in Portugal and Spain; 20−30% increasing in Sweden,

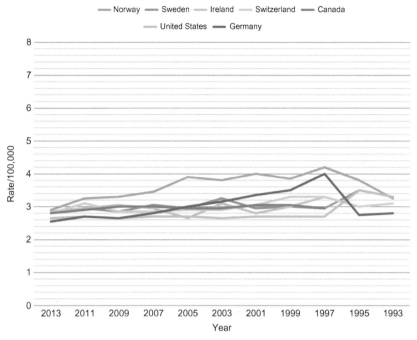

FIGURE 1.8   Age-standardized death rate in countries from North America and Europe.

Ireland, Switzerland, and Hungary; slightly decreasing within 10% in Norway and Belgium; decreasing over 10% in Germany and Denmark). In the MENA countries (Table 1.1), the ASDRs were changed dramatically over 20 years (from 1992−93 to 2012−13, 42% decreased in Turkey; in Egypt, 50% steeply increased between 1992−93 and 2004−05 and then, 62% decreased between 2004−05 and 2012−13) (Fig. 1.9).

MALE AND ELDERLY PEOPLES HAD HIGHER RISK FOR BLADDER CANCER DEATH

According to sex, male bladder cancer patients are 3.6-fold more likely to die than women (ASDR, 3.2 per 100,000 men; 0.9 per 100,000 women) [1], although male dominance in MRs is smaller than that in IRs.

Age-specific MRs are increasing by increase in patients' age. Over 50% of bladder cancer patients die at 75 years or older and about 80% of bladder cancer patients die at 65 years or older, whereas only 4% of bladder cancer patients die at younger than 50 years (Fig. 1.10). Relative to bladder cancer patients aged 40−44 years old, MRR was increased by increase in age (MRR = 3.8 in age 50−54 years; 7.3 in 55−59 years; 13.8 in 60−64 years; 23.3 in 65−69 years; 39.5 in 70−74 years; and 101 in age 75 years or older).

TABLE 1.1 Number of Bladder Cancer Death, Age-Standardized Death Rate (ASDR), and Changes in Number of Death (Ratio) or ASDR (Rate Ratio) Between 2012−13 and 1992−93 or 2002−03

| Countries | No of Death | | Change in No of Death Between | | ASDR | | ASDR Ratio | |
	12−13	92−93	Year 2012−13 and Year 1992−93	Year 2012−13 and Year 2002−03	2012−13	1992−93	Year 2012−13 and Year 1992−93	Year 2012−13 and Year 2002−03
United States	15,502	10,835	1.43	1.23	2.7	3.3	0.80	1.00
Canada	2010	1194	1.68	1.29	2.8		0.95	0.95
Sweden	679	570	1.19	1.01	2.9		0.81	0.88
Ireland	210	158	1.33	1.22	2.9	4.9	0.58	0.92
Switzerland	536		1.16	1.21	2.8	3.1	0.90	0.97
Hungary	941	789	1.19	1.14	4.7	5.3	0.89	1.02
Portugal	939	556	1.69	1.39	3.6	5.0	0.72	1.11
Spain	5203	3479	1.50	1.23	4.7		0.72	0.92

Italy	5727	5612	1.02	1.10	3.4		0.77	0.87
UK	5219	5513	0.95	1.06	3.6	4.6	0.77	0.89
Norway	325	325	1.00	0.88	2.9	3.3	0.89	0.76
Belgium	906	921	0.98	1.10	3.5	5.1	0.68	0.88
Germany	5687	6729	0.85	1.02	2.6	2.8	0.91	0.81
Denmark	502	502	0.82	0.93	4.1	4.9	0.84	0.79
Turkey	1827			1.31[a]	2.6	4.4	0.58	
Egypt	1653	1874	0.88	0.92	2.8	3.0	0.95	0.73
Israel	352	190	1.85	1.21	3.1	3.4	0.93	0.90
Korea	1251	436	2.87	1.33	1.7	1.4	1.26	0.77
S. Africa	540	355	1.52	1.18	1.5	1.5	1.00	0.79
Thailand	588	91	6.46	1.71	0.8	0.2	4.00	1.33

[a]Year 2012–13 vs year 2008–09.

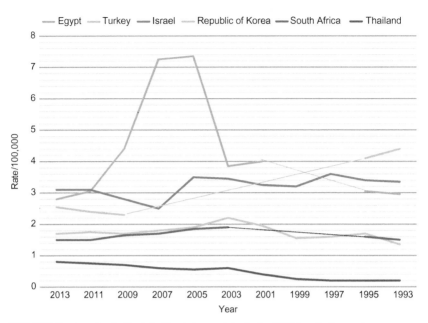

FIGURE 1.9   Age-standardized death rate in countries in the MENA and other regions.

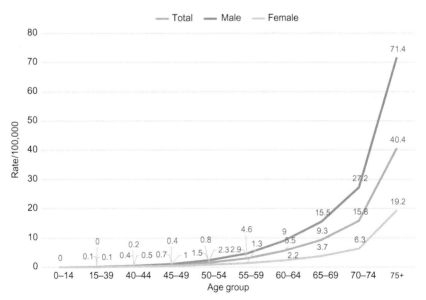

FIGURE 1.10   Age-specific death rates of bladder cancer according to total men and women population.

In particular, MRRs in men are dramatically steeply increased by increase in age (MRR = 4.6 in 50−54 years; 9.2 in 55−59 years; 18.0 in 60−64 years; 31.0 in 65−69 years; 54.4 in 70−74 years; and 142.8 in 75 years or older).

STEEPLY INCREASING MORTALITY WITH AGE INCREASE

MRs of bladder cancer in more developed countries and less developed countries show a steep rise with age increase, especially in age 75 years or older, and moreover, the increasing change of DRs by age increase is larger than that in IRs by age increase (Fig. 1.10). Relative to DRs in age 40−44 years, the DR ratio (DRR) in each age group was 3.5 in age 50−54 years, 6.3 in 55−59 years, 11.3 in 60−64 years, 19.3 in 65−69 years, 33.3 in 70−74 years, and 79.0 in 75 years or older in less developed regions, whereas IRR was 5.0 in age 50−54 years, 10.8 in 55−59 years, 19.8 in 60−64 years, 32.0 in 65−69 years, 51.8 in 70−74 years, and 129.0 in 75 years or older in more developed regions. Therefore, the gap in DRs between more and less developed countries is changed a little by age increase (Fig. 1.11).

The ranking of MRs of bladder cancer according to human development level changes by age group. In age younger than 50 years, the highest MR in low human developed level is observed, followed by high and very high development level, and the lowest mortality is observed in medium human development level, whereas in age between 50 and 74 years, the MR is observed in the order of high, very high, low, and medium human

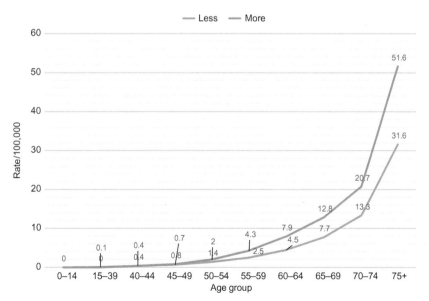

FIGURE 1.11   Age-specific death rates of bladder cancer according to more and less developed countries.

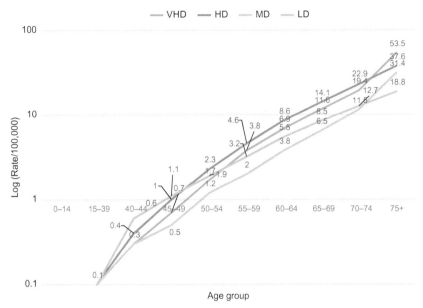

FIGURE 1.12   Age-specific death rates of bladder cancer according to human development level.

development level, and in age 75 years and more, the MR is observed in the order of very high, high, medium, and low human development level (Fig. 1.12), although the exact mechanisms is unclear.

PREVALENCE OF BLADDER CANCER

The GLOBOCAN estimates the number of 5-year prevalence of bladder cancer and globally 1.3 million people are living with bladder cancer in 2012 (about 1,000,000 men and 300,000 women) [1]. It is calculated as the sum of bladder cancer patients still alive between 2007 and 2012 and commonly neglected the time of diagnosis (onset time).

FUTURE CHANGE OF BLADDER CANCER RATES

Bladder cancer occurs in older aged people: about 90% of bladder cancer was occurred in peoples at age 55 years or older and two-third was observed in those at age 65 years or older.

Based on population forecasts of the United Nations and previous incidence and MRs, the number of new bladder cancer cases in 2035 will be 803,383 cases (623,263 men and 180,120 women cases) and 373,590 more cases will occur in 2035 than 2012. Relative to the number of new cases of bladder cancer in 2012, the number of new cases in 2035 will be increased by 87%.

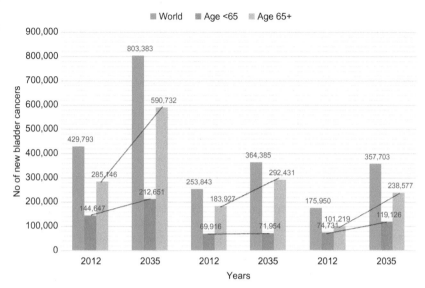

FIGURE 1.13   Number of bladder cancer cases in 2012 and 2035 (projection).

In addition, new bladder cancer incidence will increase by 107% in peoples aged 65 years or older but by 47% in those younger than 65 years (Fig. 1.13).

Less developed countries with a high birth rate will remain relatively young and increase rapidly, and also population aging will be exacerbated. Population growth rate in less developed countries is faster than more developed countries. Therefore, the number of new bladder cancer cases in 2035 will increase by 103% compared with 2012, especially by 136% in peoples aged 65 years or older but 59% in those younger than 65 years. However, in more developed countries, the number of new cases will increase by 44% in 2035 compared to 2012, with an increase of 59% in peoples aged 65 or older but only 3% in those younger than 65 years (Fig. 1.13).

For the results, in more developed countries the number of new bladder cases younger than 65 years is expected not to be changed and that of cases aged 65 years or older is expected to be slightly increased because whole population size remains unchanged. In contrast, the incidence of new bladder cancer in less developed countries will more than double than that in 2012. There will be a sharp increase in the age group of 65 years or older due to both effect of aging and population growth, and more than half of the world's bladder cancer patients younger than 65 years will be observed in less developed countries.

SUMMARY

The risk of bladder cancer is fourfold higher in men than women. In the lifetime, 1 in every 100 men and 1 in every 500 women can get bladder cancer.

Because the risk of bladder cancer and death increases, the risk of bladder cancer is higher in older age. The sex difference in incidence and death increases with age.

The disease burden from bladder cancer, based on the number of cases, IR, and MR, is higher in more developed countries than less developed countries. Also it is related to human development level, and the disease burden is higher in high and very high human development level than low and medium human development level. The relationship between bladder cancer burden and development level of country and human is partly compatible with the distribution of risk factors, such as industrial chemical exposure, and cigarette smoking. Specific countries with a high disease burden of bladder cancer are the MENA region, and these MENA countries are fairly consistent with the endemic area of *S. haematobium*.

With the increase in world population, the incidence of bladder cancer will also increase. Given the rapid population growth rate and the aging phenomenon, a high increase among people aged 65 years or older is expected in 2035, especially in less developed countries.

We anticipate that the development of bladder cancer in the future will be less than currently expected due to various global or national activities on cancer conquest, such as primary prevention of tobacco smoking, removal and blocking of propagation of *S. haematobium*, and control on carcinogen exposure in the workplace and general environment.

REFERENCES

[1] International Agency for Research on Cancer (IARC), World Health Organization (WHO). GLOBOCAN 2012: cancer incidence and mortality worldwide in 2012 [Internet]. Lyon, France: International Agency for Research on Cancer; 2014. Available from: http://globocan.iarc.fr [accessed on 01/02/2017].

[2] United Nations Development Programme. Human development reports. Human development index (HDI). Available from: http://hdr.undp.org/en; http://hdr.undp.org/en/indicators/137506 [accessed 01.02.17].

[3] International Agency for Research on Cancer (IARC), World Health Organization (WHO). List of classifications by cancer sites with sufficient or limited evidence in humans, IARC Monographs, Volumes 1 to 117* [Internet]. Lyon, France: International Agency for Research on Cancer; 2016. Available from: https://monographs.iarc.fr/ENG/Classification/Table4.pdf [accessed 01.02.17].

[4] Barakat R, Morshedy, HE, Farghaly A. Human schistosomiasis in the Middle East and North African region. McDowell MA, Rafati S, editors. Neglected tropical diseases—Middle East and North Africa, neglected tropical diseases, http://dx.doi.org/10.1007/978-3-7091-1613-5_2, Springer-Verlag Wien; 2014 file:///C:/Users/user/Downloads/9783709116128-c2.pdf [accessed 01.02.17].

[5] Ploeg M, Aben KK, Kiemeney LA. The present and future burden of urinary bladder cancer in the world. World J Urol 2009;27(3):289−93.

[6] World Health Organization (WHO). Health statistics and information systems, WHO Mortality Database; 2016. Available from: http://apps.who.int/healthinfo/statistics/mortality/whodpms/ [accessed 01.02.17].

Chapter 2

Etiology (Risk Factors for Bladder Cancer)

Hyung Suk Kim

Dongguk University Ilsan Medical Center, Goyang, South Korea

Chapter outline

GENETIC FACTORS

The genetic factors associated with bladder cancer development can be categorized into familial history, genetic polymorphism, phenotypes of acetyltransferase, activation and mutation of oncogenes and tumor suppressor genes (TSG), and chromosomal changes [1].

Oncogenes associated with bladder cancer include those of the *RAS* gene family, including the *p21 RAS* oncogene, which in some studies has been found to correlate with a higher histologic grade [2]. p21 is a guanosine triphosphatase and functions by transducing signals from the cell membrane to the nucleus, thus affecting cell proliferation and differentiation [3]. Although some reports have claimed that nearly 50% of UCs have *RAS* mutations, others have reported a far lower level [4]. Furthermore, overexpression of epidermal growth factor (EGF) receptor−related genes (*ERBB1*, *ERBB2*) correlates with higher grade bladder cancer development [5].

By using traditional molecular and cytogenetic methods, several TSGs have already been closely associated with bladder cancer. These include *p53* (on chromosome 17p); the retinoblastoma (*RB*) gene on chromosome 13q; genes on chromosome 9, at least one of which is likely to be on 9p in region 9p21 where the genes for the p19 and p16 proteins reside; and another on 9q

Bladder Cancer. DOI: http://dx.doi.org/10.1016/B978-0-12-809939-1.00002-3

in region 9q32-33 (and perhaps genes in other regions of 9q) [6−11]. Mutation of *p53* or the *RB* gene has been associated with the development of higher grade invasive bladder cancer [7,8,10]. In addition, loss of the 9q chromosome is related to the early development of lower grade noninvasive bladder cancer [6,11]. In addition, the mutation of several TSGs, such as EGFR3 and phosphoinositide 3-kinase (PI3K) genes, is known to be associated with the development of noninvasive bladder cancer [12].

The higher incidence of bladder cancer in white Americans than in African Americans may be due to genetic rather than environmental factors or related to differential susceptibility to carcinogens [13,14]. There are several polymorphisms that are associated with the formation of bladder cancer, in particular susceptibility to environmental carcinogens. *N*-acetyltransferase (NAT) detoxifies nitrosamines, which are well-known bladder carcinogens. In particular, NAT-2 regulates the rate of acetylation of compounds, such as caffeine, which are related to bladder cancer formation [15,16]. The slow acetylation*NAT2* polymorphism correlates with bladder cancer development with an odds ratio of 1.4 compared to the fast acetylation polymorphism [17−19]. Glutathione-S-transferase 1 (GSTM1) conjugates several reactive chemical carcinogens, such as arylamines and nitrosamines. The null *GSTM1* polymorphism is related to an increased bladder cancer risk with a relative risk of 1.5 [20,21]. Null *GSTM1* and slow acetylation *NAT2* induce high levels of 3-aminobiphenyl and a higher risk of bladder cancer formation [18,21]. These polymorphisms are found in 27% of white Americans, 15% of African Americans, and 3% of Asian men, thus partially demonstrating the different bladder cancer incidence rates among ethnic groups [13]. In addition, the polymorphisms of excision repair cross-complementing 2 (ERCC2), nibrin (NBN), and xeroderma pigmentosum complementation group C (XPC) gene, which correlated with DNA repairing mechanisms, have been reported in association with the development of bladder cancer [22−25]. In particular, the degree of NBN gene mutation is closely related to the amount and duration of smoking [25].

Hereditary evidence suggests that first-degree relatives of bladder cancer patients have a twofold increased risk of developing bladder cancer themselves, but whole families at high risk of bladder cancer are relatively scarce [26,27]. However, there are no clear Mendelian inheritance patterns, making classic linkage studies very challenging. It is most likely that there are a number of low-penetrance genes that can be inherited to make a person more susceptible to carcinogen exposure, thus increasing the risk of bladder cancer development. Furthermore, it has been reported that Costello syndrome, known as autosomal-dominant hereditary disorder, is related to the risk of developing urothelial carcinoma (UC) of the bladder, but the association of UC of the bladder with MSH2-related hereditary nonpolyposis colorectal cancer has not been reached a conclusion thus far [28].

ENVIRONMENTAL RISK FACTORS

Occupational Carcinogens

The bladder is the major internal organ that is affected by occupational carcinogens. Occupations related to increased risk of bladder cancer include that of an autoworker, painter, truck driver, drill press operator, leather worker, metal worker, and machine operator, as well as jobs that involve organic chemicals, such as that of a dry cleaner, paper manufacturer, rope and twine maker, dental technician, barber or beautician, physician, worker in apparel manufacturing, and plumber [29,30].

Most bladder carcinogens are aromatic amines that bind to DNA [31]. Other chemicals known as bladder carcinogens include 2-naphthylamine, b-naphthylamine, 4-aminobiphenyl, 4-nitrobiphenyl, benzidine, polycyclic aromatic hydrocarbons, and diesel exhaust [30,32,33]. It is estimated that occupational exposure accounts for approximately 20% of bladder cancer cases in the United States, and these cases usually have long latency periods (i.e., 30−50 years) [29,32]. There is often a long latency period of 10−20 years between industrial exposure and the formation of bladder cancer. Therefore, it is difficult to prove definitive causative associations between occupational carcinogens and bladder cancer formation. However, there are many occupations statistically associated with bladder cancer formation, and all are industrial in nature [30,33].

Cigarette Smoking

According to epidemiologic studies, there is a close relationship between smoking and the development of UC. Smoking is the most important single risk factor for the development and progression of UC of the bladder, and accounts for 60% and 30% of all UCs in men and women, respectively [34−36]. Overall, the relative risk of developing UC shows a fourfold (two to six times) increase in smokers (25 years or more of smoking) than in non-smokers [1,37]. This risk correlates with the number of cigarettes smoked, the duration of smoking, and the degree of inhalation of smoke [1,37]. This relative risk according to smoking status has been observed in both sexes. The relative risk of developing UC from smoking is 2.8 and 2.73 in men and women, respectively [35]. Moreover, compared with nonsmokers, patients with a history of smoking showed a higher proportion of invasive bladder cancer and a poorer prognosis in cases of recurrent bladder cancer [38]. In contrast, former cigarette smokers (who are currently nonsmokers) have a decreased incidence of bladder cancer compared to active smokers [35]. However, the reduction of this risk down to baseline level takes more than 20 years after smoking cessation, a period far longer than that for the reduction of the risk of cardiovascular disease and lung cancer [35,39]. The exposure to other types of tobacco is associated with only a slightly higher risk of bladder cancer [37]. Although several chemical carcinogens, including nitro-samines, 2-naphthylamine, and 4-aminobiphenyl, are known to be present and urinary tryptophan metabolites have also been demonstrated in cigarette smokers, the exact mechanism regarding the development of bladder cancer in relation to cigarette smoking has not been established [40,41]. The evidence with regard to increased bladder cancer risk from exposure to "second-hand" smoke is not clear. Such a risk was recently suggested based on an epigenetic study evaluating the degree of DNA methylation in a secondhand smoking population [42]. In contrast, several studies reported that the risk was not statistically different from the risk for nonsmokers [42,43]. Smoking is responsible for 30% of all deaths from bladder cancer in men and accounts for 46% of all bladder cancer–related deaths in high-income countries and 28% in low- to middle-income countries [39].

Nutrition

Most nutrients and other metabolites are excreted in the urine and have long contact with the urothelium, particularly in the bladder. Therefore, nutritional factors play a role in bladder UC formation [44,45]. There are inconsistent reports with respect to the exact fruits and vegetables that are beneficial for the prevention of UC formation [44–48]. Both fruits and vegetables, including apples, berries, tomatoes, carrots, and cruciferous vegetables, contain several active components that are crucial in detoxification. Micronutrients with and effect on the prevention of UC formation are usually antioxidants, such as vitamins A, C, and E, selenium, and zinc [44–46,48]. Rice, fish, and cereals are not likely to have a protective or detrimental role in UC formation [49]. The risk of developing UC is usually higher in coffee and caffein-ated tea drinkers [50–52]. However, these results may be compounded by smoking and other dietary factors related to people who drink coffee and tea [53]. Furthermore, unlike smoking, there is no clear association between quantity or duration of coffee and tea consumption and bladder cancer risk, suggesting an indirect causative effect [54]. In conclusion, there are inconsis-tencies with regard to nutritional factors associated with UC formation, in part owing to confounding effects and associations, including coffee con-sumption and smoking, consumption of fruits and vegetables without the involvement of smoking, and epidemiologic factors.

Artificial Sweeteners

Some animal studies have shown that large doses of artificial sweeteners, including saccharin and cyclamates, may have an impact on the development of bladder cancer [55]. These studies are controversial because extremely high doses of sweeteners were administered to the animals. As a result, urinary pH was markedly affected by the dose and electrolyte composition of the saccharin administered, which in turn influenced susceptibility to carcinogenesis [55]. In contrast, several epidemiologic studies conducted in humans consistently show no evidence for increased risk of bladder cancer among consumers of artificial sweeteners [56−59].

Analgesics

Consumption of large quantities (5−15 kg during a 10-year period) of analgesic combinations containing acetaminophen and phenacetin is associated with an increased risk of UC of the renal pelvis and bladder, especially in middle-aged women [60,61]. The latency period is longer for bladder tumors than for renal pelvic tumors, whose latency period may be as long as 25 years [62]. A relationship between the use of other analgesics and bladder cancer risk has been investigated but is yet not clear [63−65].

Infection and Inflammation

Chronic inflammation in the presence of indwelling catheters or calculi is associated with an increased risk of squamous cell carcinoma (SqCC) of the bladder [66]. About 2%−10% of paraplegic patients with long-term indwelling catheters develop bladder cancer, 80% of which is SqCC [67,68]. Through reducing the use of chronic indwelling catheters, the incidence of bladder cancer and the preponderance of SqCCs seems to be decreasing. Despite these favorable trends, well over half of all patients have muscle-invasive cancers at diagnosis [67]. Although they have a high risk of bladder cancer, periodic screening with cystoscopy and/or cytology for patients with chronic indwelling catheters is not strongly supported [69].

Likewise, *Schistosoma haematobium*−induced cystitis appears to be causally related to the development of SqCC of the bladder [70,71]. In Egypt, where schistosomiasis is endemic among men, SqCC of the bladder (bilharzial bladder cancer) is the most common malignancy [70]. Cystitis-induced bladder cancer from all causes is usually associated with severe, long-term infections. The mechanisms of carcinogenesis are not fully understood but may involve the formation of nitrite and *N*-nitroso compounds in the bladder, presumably from parasitic or microbial metabolism of normal urinary constituents [72].

There is a possible correlation between human papilloma virus (HPV) and UC formation [73]. The role of exposure to HPV in bladder cancer has been evaluated by several groups with widely divergent findings [74−80]. Reports have demonstrated that from as few as 2% to as many as 35% of human bladder cancers are contaminated with HPV DNA [74−76]. The reasons for these disparate results are not clear although it was concluded that the virus was more likely to play a role in transitional cell tumorigenesis in immunocompromised hosts than in cancers arising in immunologically competent individuals [73]. A recent meta-analysis supports a possible association between HPV infection and bladder cancer risk, reporting a 2.84 odds ratio with a 95% confidence interval of 1.39–5.80 [77].

Pelvic Irradiation

Women treated with pelvic radiation for carcinoma of the uterine cervix or ovary have a two to four times increased risk of subsequently developing bladder cancer compared to women only undergoing surgery [81,82]. The risk of bladder cancer secondary to radiation rises further when chemotherapeutic agents are administered, including thiotepa, melphalan, and cyclophosphamide [82]. The risks in all groups continued to rise after 10 years [82]. The majority of these tumors are poorly differentiated and locally advanced at the time of diagnosis [83]. UC formation after radiation exposure is not age-related, but the latency period spans 15–30 years. There is further evidence that radiation increases the risk of secondary bladder cancer in patients with prostate cancer who were treated with radiation therapy [84].

Chemotherapy

The only chemotherapeutic agent that has been proven to induce bladder cancer is cyclophosphamide [85–88]. Patients treated with cyclophosphamide have an approximately ninefold increased risk of developing bladder cancer [86]. The risk of bladder cancer formation is directly associated with the duration and dose of cyclophosphamide treatment, indicating a causative role. The majority of these tumors are high grade and muscle-invasive at the time of diagnosis, occur in patients younger than those with sporadic UC, and have an equal incidence in both sexes [87,88]. A urinary metabolite of cyclophosphamide, acrolein, is considered responsible for both hemorrhagic cystitis and bladder cancer [89]. However, the development of hemorrhagic cystitis does not necessarily correlate with the development of bladder cancer [90]. The latency period for cyclophosphamide-induced bladder cancer is relatively short, ranging from 6 to 13 years.

Other Environmental Risk Factors

Blackfoot disease is endemic in South Taiwan and is usually related to vascular and cardiac disease and with the development of numerous malignancies, including transitional cell carcinoma of the bladder [91]. This condition seems to be associated with ingestion of large amount of arsenic in artesian well water. Similar endemic pockets of bladder cancer are found in other regions with high arsenic concentrations in drinking water [92]. In a nested case–control study, specific cytogenetic abnormalities, including chromosome-type breaks, gaps, exchanges, and other aberrations, were more frequent in peripheral blood cells of exposed patients who ultimately developed cancer over a 4-year period of observation compared with exposed individuals who did not [93].

Aristolochic acid is an ingredient of Chinese herb (containing *Stephania tetrandra* and *Magnolia officinalis*) that was imported into Belgium as a popular weight-reduction aid primarily used by women and is responsible for an epidemic of interstitial nephropathy [94]. Subsequently, patients with Chinese herb nephropathy have been reported to have a higher risk for developing UC, primarily of the upper urinary tract but also of the bladder [95,96]. A major mechanism in this condition appears to be the development of aristolochic acid—related DNA adducts in the urothelium of both the upper tract and bladder [97].

Other potential risk factors include being a renal transplant recipient [98,99] and having a chronically low quantity of fluid ingestion [100—102]. Renal transplant recipients are known to have a higher risk for developing numerous tumors, presumably because of prolonged immunosuppression [99,103]. Likewise, if certain chemicals are responsible for initiating mutational events, long-term exposure to higher concentrations of them appears to be more mutagenic/carcinogenic than exposure to lower concentrations.

REFERENCES

[1] Morrison AS. Advances in the etiology of urothelial cancer. Urol Clin North Am 1984;11:557—66.

[2] Czerniak B, Chaturvedi V, Li L, Hodges S, Johnston D, Roy JY, et al. Superimposed histologic and genetic mapping of chromosome 9 in progression of human urinary bladder neoplasia: implications for a genetic model of multistep urothelial carcinogenesis and early detection of urinary bladder cancer. Oncogene 1999;18:1185—96.

[3] Cote RJ, Chatterjee SJ. Molecular determinants of outcome in bladder cancer. Cancer J Sci Am 1999;5:2—15.

[4] Knowles MA, Elder PA, Williamson M, Cairns JP, Shaw ME, Law MG. Allelotype of human bladder cancer. Cancer Res 1994;54:531—8.

[5] Messing EM. Clinical implications of the expression of epidermal growth factor receptors in human transitional cell carcinoma. Cancer Res 1990;50:2530—7.

[6] Tsai YC, Nichols PW, Hiti AL, Williams Z, Skinner DG, Jones PA. Allelic losses of chromosomes 9, 11, and 17 in human bladder cancer. Cancer Res 1990;50:44—7.

[7] Cairns P, Proctor AJ, Knowles MA. Loss of heterozygosity at the RB locus is frequent and correlates with muscle invasion in bladder carcinoma. Oncogene 1991;6: 2305—23059.

[8] Esrig D, Elmajian D, Groshen S, Freeman JA, Stein JP, Chen SC, et al. Accumulation of nuclear p53 and tumor progression in bladder cancer. N Engl J Med 1994;331:1259—64.

[9] Chang F, Syrjanen S, Syrjanen K. Implications of the p53 tumor-suppressor gene in clinical oncology. J Clin Oncol 1995;13:1009—22.

[10] Cote RJ, Dunn MD, Chatterjee SJ, Stein JP, Shi SR, Tran QC, et al. Elevated and absent pRb expression is associated with bladder cancer progression and has cooperative effects with p53. Cancer Res 1998;58:1090—4.

[11] Simoneau M, Aboulkassim TO, La Rue H, Rousseau F, Fradet Y. Four tumor suppressor loci on chromosome 9q in bladder cancer: evidence for two novel candidate regions at 9q22.3 and 9q31. Oncogene 1999;18:157−63.

[12] Castillo-Martin M, Domingo-Domenech J, Karni-Schmidt O, Matos T, Cordon-Cardo C. Molecular pathways of urothelial development and bladder tumorigenesis. Urol Oncol 2010;28:401−8.

[13] Schairer C, Hartge P, Hoover RN, Silverman DT. Racial differences in bladder cancer risk: a case-control study. Am J Epidemiol 1988;128:1027−37.

[14] Madeb R, Messing EM. Gender, racial and age differences in bladder cancer incidence and mortality. Urol Oncol 2004;22:86−92.

[15] Hosen MB, Islam J, Salam MA, Islam MF, Hawlader MZ, Kabir Y. N-acetyltransferase 2 gene polymorphism as a biomarker for susceptibility to bladder cancer in Bangladeshi population. Asia Pac J Clin Oncol 2015;11:78−84.

[16] Frederickson SM, Messing EM, Reznikoff CA, Swaminathan S. Relationship between in vivo acetylator phenotypes and cytosolic N-acetyltransferase and O-acetyltransferase activities in human uroepithelial cells. Cancer Epidemiol Biomarkers Prev 1994;3: 25−32.

[17] Okkels H, Sigsgaard T, Wolf H, Autrup H. Arylamine N-acetyltransferase 1 (NAT1) and 2 (NAT2) polymorphisms in susceptibility to bladder cancer: the influence of smoking. Cancer Epidemiol Biomarkers Prev 1997;6:225−31.

[18] Gu J, Liang D, Wang Y, Lu C, Wu X. Effects of N-acetyl transferase 1 and 2 polymorphisms on bladder cancer risk in caucasians. Mutat Res 2005;581:97−104.

[19] Risch A, Wallace DM, Bathers S, Sim E. Slow N-acetylation genotype is a susceptibility factor in occupational and smoking related bladder cancer. Hum Mol Genet 1995;4: 231−6.

[20] Gong M, Dong W, An R. Glutathione S-transferase T1 polymorphism contributes to bladder cancer risk: a meta-analysis involving 50 studies. DNA Cell Biol 2012;31:1187−97.

[21] Kang HW, Song PH, Ha YS, Kim WT, Kim YJ, Yun SJ, et al. Glutathione S-transferase M1 and T1 polymorphisms: susceptibility and outcomes in muscle invasive bladder cancer patients. Eur J Cancer 2013;49:3010−19.

[22] Corral R, Lewinger JP, Van Den Berg D, Joshi AD, Yuan JM, Gago-Dominguez M, et al. Comprehensive analyses of DNA repair pathways, smoking and bladder cancer risk in Los Angeles and Shanghai. Int J cancer 2014;135:335−47.

[23] Wang Y, Li Z, Liu N, Zhang G. Association between CCND1 and XPC polymorphisms and bladder cancer risk: a meta-analysis based on 15 case-control studies. Tumour Biol 2014;35:3155−65.

[24] Wu Y, Yang Y. Complex association between ERCC2 gene polymorphisms, gender, smoking and the susceptibility to bladder cancer: a meta-analysis. Tumour Biol 2014;35: 5245−57.

[25] Stern MC, Lin J, Figueroa JD, Kelsey KT, Kiltie AE, Yuan JM, et al. Polymorphisms in DNA repair genes, smoking, and bladder cancer risk: findings from the international consortium of bladder cancer. Cancer Res 2009;69:6857−64.

[26] Murta-Nascimento C, Silverman DT, Kogevinas M, Garcia-Closas M, Rothman N, Tardon A, et al. Risk of bladder cancer associated with family history of cancer: do low-penetrance polymorphisms account for the increase in risk? Cancer Epidemiol Biomarkers Prev 2007;16:1595−600.

[27] Kiemeney LA, Grotenhuis AJ, Vermeulen SH, Wu X. Genome-wide association studies in bladder cancer: first results and potential relevance. Curr Opin Urol 2009;19:540−6.

[28] Mueller CM, Caporaso N, Greene MH. Familial and genetic risk of transitional cell carcinoma of the urinary tract. Urol Oncol 2008;26:451−64.

[29] Morrison AS, Cole P. Epidemiology of bladder cancer. Urol Clin North Am 1976;3: 13−29.

[30] Colt JS, Karagas MR, Schwenn M, Baris D, Johnson A, Stewart P, et al. Occupation and bladder cancer in a population-based case-control study in Northern New England. Occup Environ Med 2011;68:239−49.

[31] Schulte PA, Ringen K, Hemstreet GP, Altekruse EB, Gullen WH, Tillett S, et al. Risk factors for bladder cancer in a cohort exposed to aromatic amines. Cancer 1986;58:2156−62.

[32] Steineck G, Plato N, Norell SE, Hogstedt C. Urothelial cancer and some industry-related chemicals: an evaluation of the epidemiologic literature. Am J Ind Med 1990;17:371−91.

[33] Cumberbatch MG, Cox A, Teare D, Catto JW. Contemporary occupational carcinogen exposure and bladder cancer: a systematic review and meta-analysis. JAMA Oncol 2015;1:1282−90.

[34] Howe GR, Burch JD, Miller AB, Cook GM, Esteve J, Morrison B, et al. Tobacco use, occupation, coffee, various nutrients, and bladder cancer. J Natl Cancer Inst 1980;64: 701−13.

[35] Augustine A, Hebert JR, Kabat GC, Wynder EL. Bladder cancer in relation to cigarette smoking. Cancer Res 1988;48:4405−8.

[36] Tao L, Xiang YB, Wang R, Nelson HH, Gao YT, Chan KK, et al. Environmental tobacco smoke in relation to bladder cancer risk—the Shanghai bladder cancer study. Cancer Epidemiol Biomarkers Prev 2010;19:3087−95.

[37] Burch JD, Rohan TE, Howe GR, Risch HA, Hill GB, Steele R, et al. Risk of bladder cancer by source and type of tobacco exposure: a case-control study. Int J Cancer 1989;44:622−8.

[38] Grotenhuis AJ, Ebben CW, Aben KK, Witjes JA, Vrieling A, Vermeulen SH, et al. The effect of smoking and timing of smoking cessation on clinical outcome in non-muscle-invasive bladder cancer. Urol Oncol 2015;33(65):e9−e17.

[39] van Osch FH, Jochems SH, van Schooten FJ, Bryan RT, Zeegers MP. Significant role of lifetime cigarette smoking in worsening bladder cancer and upper tract urothelial carcinoma prognosis: a meta-analysis. J Urol 2016;195:872−9.

[40] Hoffman D, Masuda Y, Wynder EL. Alpha-naphthylamine and beta-naphthylamine in cigarette smoke. Nature 1969;221:255−6.

[41] Van Hemelrijck MJ, Michaud DS, Connolly GN, Kabir Z. Secondhand smoking, 4-aminobiphenyl, and bladder cancer: two meta-analyses. Cancer Epidemiol Biomarkers Prev 2009;18:1312−20.

[42] Wilhelm-Benartzi CS, Christensen BC, Koestler DC, Houseman EA, Schned AR, Karagas MR, et al. Association of secondhand smoke exposures with DNA methylation in bladder carcinomas. Cancer Causes Control 2011;22:1205−13.

[43] Alberg AJ, Kouzis A, Genkinger JM, Gallicchio L, Burke AE, Hoffman SC, et al. A prospective cohort study of bladder cancer risk in relation to active cigarette smoking and household exposure to secondhand cigarette smoke. Am J Epidemiol 2007;165:660−6.

[44] Brinkman M, Zeegers MP. Nutrition, total fluid and bladder cancer. Scand J Urol 2008;25−36.

[45] Steinmaus CM, Nunez S, Smith AH. Diet and bladder cancer: a meta-analysis of six dietary variables. Am J Epidemiol 2000;151:693−702.

[46] Zeegers MP, Goldbohm RA, Bode P, van den Brandt PA. Prediagnostic toenail selenium and risk of bladder cancer. Cancer Epidemiol Biomarkers Prev 2002;11:1292−7.

[47] Schabath MB, Spitz MR, Lerner SP, Pillow PC, Hernandez LM, Delclos GL, et al. Case-control analysis of dietary folate and risk of bladder cancer. Nutr Cancer 2005;53: 144−51.

[48] Bradbury KE, Appleby PN, Key TJ. Fruit, vegetable, and fiber intake in relation to cancer risk: findings from the European Prospective Investigation into Cancer and Nutrition (EPIC). Am J Clin Nutr 2014;100(Suppl 1):394s−8s.

[49] Radosavljevic V, Ilic M, Jankovic S, Djokic M. Diet in bladder cancer ethiopathogenesis. ActaChir Iugosl 2005;52:77−82.

[50] D'Avanzo B, La Vecchia C, Franceschi S, Negri E, Talamini R, Buttino I. Coffee consumption and bladder cancer risk. Eur J Cancer 1992;28a:1480−4.

[51] Lu CM, Lan SJ, Lee YH, Huang JK, Huang CH, Hsieh CC. Tea consumption: fluid intake and bladder cancer risk in Southern Taiwan. Urology 1999;54:823−8.

[52] Zeegers MP, Dorant E, Goldbohm RA, van den Brandt PA. Are coffee, tea, and total fluid consumption associated with bladder cancer risk? Results from the Netherlands Cohort Study. Cancer Causes Control 2001;12:231−8.

[53] Morgan RW, Jain MG. Bladder cancer: smoking, beverages and artificial sweeteners. Can Med Assoc J 1974;111:1067−70.

[54] Turati F, Bosetti C, Polesel J, Zucchetto A, Serraino D, Montella M, et al. Coffee, tea, cola, and bladder cancer risk: dose and time relationships. Urology 2015;86:1179−84.

[55] Sontag JM. Experimental identification of genitourinary carcinogens. Urol Clin North Am 1980;7:803−14.

[56] Morrison AS, Buring JE. Artificial sweeteners and cancer of the lower urinary tract. N Engl J Med 1980;302:537−41.

[57] Morrison AS, Verhoek WG, Leck I, Aoki K, Ohno Y, Obata K. Artificial sweeteners and bladder cancer in Manchester, U.K., and Nagoya, Japan. Br J Cancer 1982;45:332−6.

[58] Moller-Jensen O, Knudsen JB, Sorensen BL, Clemmesen J. Artificial sweeteners and absence of bladder cancer risk in Copenhagen. Int J Cancer 1983;32:577−82.

[59] Morgan RW, Wong O. A review of epidemiological studies on artificial sweeteners and bladder cancer. Food Chem Toxicol 1985;23:529−33.

[60] Piper JM, Tonascia J, Matanoski GM. Heavy phenacetin use and bladder cancer in women aged 20 to 49 years. N Engl J Med 1985;313:292−5.

[61] McCredie M, Stewart JH, Ford JM, MacLennan RA. Phenacetin-containing analgesics and cancer of the bladder or renal pelvis in women. Br J Cancer 1983;55:220−4.

[62] Steffens J, Nagel R. Tumours of the renal pelvis and ureter. Observations in 170 patients. Br J Urol 1988;61:277−83.

[63] Castelao J, Yuan J, Gago-Dominguez M, Yu M, Ross R. Non-steroidal anti-inflammatory drugs and bladder cancer prevention. Br J Cancer 2000;82:1364.

[64] Fortuny J, Kogevinas M, Garcia-Closas M, Real FX, Tardón A, Garcia-Closas R, et al. Use of analgesics and nonsteroidal anti-inflammatory drugs, genetic predisposition, and bladder cancer risk in Spain. Cancer Epidemiol Biomarkers Prev 2006;15:1696−702.

[65] Fortuny J, Kogevinas M, Zens MS, Schned A, Andrew AS, Heaney J, et al. Analgesic and anti-inflammatory drug use and risk of bladder cancer: a population based case control study. BMC Urol 2007;7:1−9.

[66] Michaud DS. Chronic inflammation and bladder cancer. Urol Oncol 2007;25:260−8.

[67] Pannek J. Transitional cell carcinoma in patients with spinal cord injury: a high risk malignancy? Urology 2002;59:240−4.

[68] Hess MJ, Zhan EH, Foo DK, Yalla SV. Bladder cancer in patients with spinal cord injury. J Spinal Cord Med 2003;26:335−8.

[69] Hamid R, Bycroft J, Arya M, Shah PJ. Screening cystoscopy and biopsy in patients with neuropathic bladder and chronic suprapubic indwelling catheters: is it valid? J Urol 2003;170:425−7.

[70] Bedwani R, Renganathan E, El Kwhsky F, Braga C, Abu Seif HH, AbulAzm T, et al. Schistosomiasis and the risk of bladder cancer in Alexandria, Egypt. Br J Cancer 1998;77:1186−9.

[71] Rambau PF, Chalya PL, Jackson K. Schistosomiasis and urinary bladder cancer in North Western Tanzania: a retrospective review of 185 patients. Infect Agent Cancer 2013;8:19.

[72] Tricker AR, Mostafa MH, Spiegelhalder B, Preussmann R. Urinary excretion of nitrate, nitrite and N-nitroso compounds in Schistosomiasis and bilharzia bladder cancer patients. Carcinogenesis 1989;10:547−52.

[73] Griffiths TR, Mellon JK. Human papillomavirus and urological tumours: II. Role in bladder, prostate, renal and testicular cancer. BJU Int 2000;85:211−17.

[74] Maloney KE, Wiener JS, Walther PJ. Oncogenic human papillomaviruses are rarely associated with squamous cell carcinoma of the bladder: evaluation by differential polymerase chain reaction. J Urol 1994;151:360−4.

[75] LaRue H, Simoneau M, Fradet Y. Human papillomavirus in transitional cell carcinoma of the urinary bladder. Clin Cancer Res 1995;1:435−40.

[76] Aynaud O, Tranbaloc P, Orth G. Lack of evidence for a role of human papillomaviruses in transitional cell carcinoma of the bladder. J Urol 1998;159:86−9.

[77] Li N, Yang L, Zhang Y, Zhao P, Zheng T, Dai M. Human papillomavirus infection and bladder cancer risk: a meta-analysis. J Infect Dis 2011;204:217−23.

[78] Polesel J, Gheit T, Talamini R, Shahzad N, Lenardon O, Sylla B, et al. Urinary human polyomavirus and papillomavirus infection and bladder cancer risk. Br J Cancer 2012;106:222−6.

[79] Shaker OG, Hammam OA, Wishahi MM. Is there a correlation between HPV and urinary bladder carcinoma? Biomed Pharmacother 2013;67:183−91.

[80] Shigehara K, Kawaguchi S, Sasagawa T, Nakashima K, Nakashima T, Shimamura M, et al. Etiological correlation of human papillomavirus infection in the development of female bladder tumor. APMIS 2013;121:1169−76.

[81] Duncan RE, Bennett DW, Evans AT, Aron BS, Schellhas HF. Radiation-induced bladder tumors. J Urol 1977;118:43−5.

[82] Kaldor JM, Day NE, Kittelmann B, Pettersson F, Langmark F, Pedersen D, et al. Bladder tumours following chemotherapy and radiotherapy for ovarian cancer: a case-control study. Int J Cancer 1995;63:1−6.

[83] Quilty PM, Kerr GR. Bladder cancer following low or high dose pelvic irradiation. Clin Radiol 1987;38:583−5.

[84] Stokkevag CH, Engeseth GM, Hysing LB, Ytre-Hauge KS, Ekanger C, Muren LP. Risk of radiation-induced secondary rectal and bladder cancer following radiotherapy of prostate cancer. Acta Oncol 2015;54:1317−25.

[85] Pearson RM, Soloway MS. Does cyclophosphamide induce bladder cancer? Urology 1978;11:437−47.

[86] Fairchild WV, Spence CR, Solomon HD, Gangai MP. The incidence of bladder cancer after cyclophosphamide therapy. J Urol 1979;122:163−4.

[87] Fernandes ET, Manivel JC, Reddy PK, Ercole CJ. Cyclophosphamide associated bladder cancer−a highly aggressive disease: analysis of 12 cases. J Urol 1996;156:1931−3.

[88] Vlaovic P, Jewett MA. Cyclophosphamide-induced bladder cancer. Can J Urol 1999;6:745–8.

[89] Cohen SM, Garland EM, St John M, Okamura T, Smith RA. Acrolein initiates rat urinary bladder carcinogenesis. Cancer Res 1992;52:3577–81.

[90] Pedersen-Bjergaard J, Ersboll J, Hansen VL, Sorensen BL, Christoffersen K, Hou-Jensen K, et al. Carcinoma of the urinary bladder after treatment with cyclophosphamide for non-Hodgkin's lymphoma. N Engl J Med 1988;318:1028–32.

[91] Tan LB, Chen KT, Guo HR. Clinical and epidemiological features of patients with genitourinary tract tumour in a blackfoot disease endemic area of Taiwan. BJU Int 2008;102:48–54.

[92] Mendez Jr. WM, Eftim S, Cohen J, Warren I, Cowden J, Lee JS, et al. Relationships between arsenic concentrations in drinking water and lung and bladder cancer incidence in U.S. counties. J Expo Sci Environ Epidemiol 2017;27:235–43. Available from: http://dx.doi.org/10.1038/jes.2016.58.

[93] Liou SH, Lung JC, Chen YH, Yang T, Hsieh LL, Chen CJ, et al. Increased chromosome-type chromosome aberration frequencies as biomarkers of cancer risk in a blackfoot endemic area. Cancer Res 1999;59:1481–4.

[94] Li J, Zhang L, Jiang Z, He X, Zhang L, Xu M. Expression of renal aquaporins in aristolochicacid I and aristolactam I-induced nephrotoxicity. Nephron 2016;133:213–21.

[95] Chen CH, Dickman KG, Huang CY, Moriya M, Shun CT, Tai HC, et al. Aristolochic acid-induced upper tract urothelial carcinoma in Taiwan: clinical characteristics and outcomes. Int J Cancer 2013;133:14–20.

[96] Clyne M. Bladder cancer: aristolochic acid—one of the most potent carcinogens known to man. Nat Rev Urol 2013;10:552.

[97] Nortier JL, Martinez MC, Schmeiser HH, Arlt VM, Bieler CA, Petein M, et al. Urothelial carcinoma associated with the use of a Chinese herb (Aristolochia fangchi). N Engl J Med 2000;342:1686–92.

[98] Buzzeo BD, Heisey DM, Messing EM. Bladder cancer in renal transplant recipients. Urology 1997;50:525–8.

[99] Pendon-Ruiz de Mier V, Navarro Cabello MD, Martinez Vaquera S, Lopez-Andreu M, Aguera Morales ML, Rodriguez-Benot A, et al. Incidence and long-term prognosis of cancer after kidney transplantation. Transplant P 2015;47:2618–21.

[100] Bai Y, Yuan H, Li J, Tang Y, Pu C, Han P. Relationship between bladder cancer and total fluid intake: a meta-analysis of epidemiological evidence. World J Surg Oncol 2014;12:223.

[101] Zhou J, Kelsey KT, Giovannucci E, Michaud DS. Fluid intake and risk of bladder cancer in the nurses' health studies. Int J Cancer 2014;135:1229–37.

[102] Di Maso M, Bosetti C, Taborelli M, Montella M, Libra M, Zucchetto A, et al. Dietary water intake and bladder cancer risk: an Italian case-control study. Cancer Epidemiol 2016;45:151–6.

[103] Demir T, Ozel L, Gokce AM, Ata P, Kara M, Eris C, et al. Cancer screening of renal transplant patients undergoing long-term immunosuppressive therapy. Transplant P 2015;47:1413–17.

Chapter 3

Pathophysiology of Bladder Cancer

Ju Hyun Shin, Jae Sung Lim and Byeong Hwa Jeon
Chungnam National University, Daejeon, South Korea

Chapter Outline

Numerous molecular factors are involved in the development of urothelial cell cancers. Tumorigenesis is a complex process with multiple phases that reflect underlying molecular changes. Multiple steps of alterations modify different cellular functions, leading to self-sufficient growth, evasion of apoptosis, insensitivity to anti-growth signals, unlimited self-replications, sustained angiogenesis, and eventually the invasion of adjacent organs and distant metastasis [1]. The deletion of chromosome fragments, epigenetic alterations, gene mutations, as well as the more recently reported miRNA alterations are among the most common factors associated with carcinogenesis. These alterations further affect downstream pathways through loss of cell cycle control, telomere dysfunction, genomic instability, and growth advantages [2]. Low-grade non-muscle-invasive bladder cancer (NMIBC) and high-grade muscle-invasive bladder cancer (MIBC) are two types of bladder cancers that are divided into different pathogenetic pathways (Fig. 3.1). Well-differentiated, noninvasive papillary urothelial cancers are derived from

Bladder Cancer. DOI: http://dx.doi.org/10.1016/B978-0-12-809939-1.00003-5

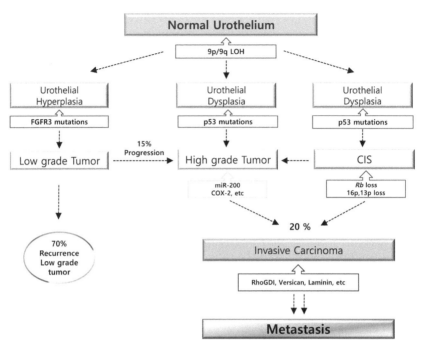

FIGURE 3.1   Putative molecular pathways of oncogenesis in low- and high-grade urothelial carcinoma of the urinary bladder. Genetic alterations are depicted in key stages of disease progression.

benign lesions through a process called urothelial hyperplasia, whereas poorly differentiated muscle-invasive cancers are derived from carcinoma in situ (CIS), urothelial dysplasia, or high-grade papillary bladder lesions.

GENETIC ALTERATIONS

Numerical chromosomal alterations cause changes in copy numbers at various genetic regions. The accumulation of sequential genetic changes results in the progressive disruption of the regulatory circuits controlling normal proliferation and differentiation [1]. Progression from superficial to muscle-invasive tumors occurs in a relatively small fraction of noninvasive lesions. Genetic instability is an important factor in the accumulation of genetic alterations required for such progression [3,4]. Muscle-invasive high-grade tumors alter the oncogenes and tumor suppressors, such as p53, retinoblastoma (*Rb*), and the phosphatase and tensin homolog (*PTEN*) tumor suppressor gene. CIS is a distinct entity, that although confined to the urothelium, exists as a flat, nonpapillary, poorly differentiated lesion displaying genetic alterations characteristic of both papillary and muscle-invasive tumors [5]. The presence of CIS correlates strongly with the risk of invasive disease, demonstrating the close association between loss of urothelial differentiation and the ultimate development of MIBC.

MOLECULAR PATHWAYS TO UROTHELIAL CARCINOMA OF THE URINARY BLADDER

Genes Involved in the Initiation of Urothelial Hyperplasia and Progression to Dysplasia and CIS

The first step of structural and numerical chromosome changes in normal urothelium involves loss of heterozygosity (LOH) on chromosome 9 [6]. LOH causes inactivation of the tumor suppressor gene, resulting in cell transformation. The loss of the long arm of chromosome 9 (9q) is not only involved in urothelial hyperplasia but also in dysplasia and CIS [7–9]. Deletions on chromosome 9p (short arm) are also known to induce dysplasia and CIS, which are both regarded as precursors of MIBC [7]. A complex genomic region at 9p21 (INK4A-ARF-INK4B locus) encodes p14ARF, p15, and p16 proteins, which all act as negative cell cycle regulators and are considered as potential tumor suppressor genes [10]. Homozygous deletion appears to be the common mechanism of inactivating the entire locus in transitional cell carcinoma (TCC) [11,12]. Such a deletion will commonly remove all three 9p21 tumor suppressor genes [13].

Genetic Alterations Related to Urothelial Hyperplasia and Low-Grade Noninvasive Bladder Tumor

Fibroblast growth factor receptor 3 (FGFR3) mutations occur mainly in low-grade noninvasive papillary urothelial tumors. FGFR3, a tyrosine kinase receptor gene, is located at chromosome 4p16.3 and is composed of 19 exons [14]. The extracellular portion can bind with fibroblast growth factors, initiating cascades of downstream signals that ultimately influence cell growth, migration, angiogenesis, and differentiation [14]. The presence of FGFR3 mutations has been associated with genetic instability and aneuploidy [15]. More than 75% of stage Ta tumors have FGFR3 mutations, whereas alterations of the FGFR3 gene have not been found in invasive CIS tumors, suggesting that FGFR3 mutations are characterized to low-grade noninvasive tumors, which have a favorable clinical outcomes [16–18]. Van Rhijn et al. [19] conducted a study where 72 patients with bladder cancer were separated according to different stage and grade, revealing that out of 53 Ta bladder cancers between Grades 1 and 2, 34 had FGFR3 mutations. Meanwhile, all 19 patients with higher stage tumor tested negative for any FGFR3 mutations. A 12-month follow-up study on 57 patients with Ta bladder cancer revealed that 61% of the patients in the wild-type GFR3 group developed recurrence, compared with only 20% of patients who had FGFR3 mutations.

The recurrence rate per year was 4.7-fold lower for tumors that contained the FGFR3 mutation than that for tumors with the wild-type gene [19]. This suggests that mutation of FGFR3 is closely related with low recurrence rates in noninvasive bladder cancers.

Genes Associated With Urothelial Dysplasia Progression and CIS

The transcription factor p53 controls the expression of multiple apoptosis regulatory genes that participate in the mitochondrial or intrinsic pathway, as well as the death-inducing signaling complex receptors, which form part of the extrinsic apoptotic pathway. Transcriptional targets of p53 include intrinsic apoptotic regulators such as Bax, Noxa, and p53 upregulated modulator of apoptosis [20,21]. New insights into the noncanonical role of p53 in apoptosis have been reported, which reveal that p53 can trigger apoptosis in a transcription-independent manner. Primary DNA structure is altered by cellular metabolites and DNA-damaging agents. These modifications may cause simple base changes or more complex alterations, such as deletions and translocations [22]. Ataxia telangiectasia mutated and checkpoint kinase 2 act as sensors and transducers of DNA damage, subsequently activating p53 to produce cycle arrest. This then allows DNA repair to occur, but if repair cannot be achieved, then p53 activates cell death. Alterations of these checkpoint genes have been associated with failure of apoptosis and are thought to be causal events in the development of human cancer [23].

Genes Involved in CIS and Their Progression to T1 Bladder Tumors

The *Rb* susceptibility gene encodes a 110-kDa nuclear phosphoprotein, which functions as a negative cell cycle regulator by sequestering members of the E2F family of transcription factors. Rb is phosphorylated by certain cyclin-dependent kinases (CDKs) and is dephosphorylated by protein phosphatase 1, and it has been postulated that Rb is phosphorylated, becomes inactive and allows cell cycle progression. A concentrated and homogeneous nuclear immunoreactivity pattern displayed by certain tumors corresponds to the accumulation of the inactive and hyperphosphorylated form of pRB, which mostly results from either cyclin D1 overexpression or p16 deletions [24]. Like p53, Rb is thought to play an important role in bladder cancer progression. *Rb* gene mutations are noted in 25–30% of bladder tumors [25], and LOH at the *Rb* locus (13q) is strongly associated with the absence of Rb protein expression in invasive bladder cancers [26].

Genes Associated With Invasive Bladder Tumors and Metastasis

Invasive tumors are genetically unstable and accumulate many genomic alterations. Metastasis of NMIBC is rare, whereas half of all MIBCs metastasize [27]. The finding of a subtype of invasive carcinomas with FGFR3 mutation and loss of cyclin-dependent kinase inhibitor 2A (CDKN2A) may suggest a route by which low-grade noninvasive papillary tumors can progress to muscle invasion. Epithelial–mesenchymal transition (EMT) is mediated by zinc-finger E-box binding homeobox 1 (ZEB1), ZEB2, TWIST, SNAIL (also known as SNAI1), and SLUG (also known as SNAI2), which transcriptionally repress epithelial markers. ZEB1 and ZEB2 are regulated by members of the miR-200 family and miR-205 [28]. miR-200 is downregulated in bladder cancer cell lines with mesenchymal phenotype, and epigenetic silencing is reported in MIBC [29]. These miRNAs also regulate ERBB receptor feedback inhibitor 1 (*ERRFI1*), and their silencing confers resistance to EGFR in mesenchymal bladder cancer cells that can be reversed by the expression of miR-200. FGFR1 signaling and subsequent COX2 upregulation can induce EMT in bladder cancer cells. In an animal model of bladder cancer metastasis using an FGFR1-dependent cell line, FGFR inhibition reduced the development of circulating tumor cells and metastasis but not primary tumor growth.

In addition to genes involved in EMT, preclinical studies suggest that Rho GDP dissociation inhibitor 2 (RhoGDI2), the activity of which is regulated by Src, is a metastasis suppressor in MIBC [30,31]. In contrast to most tumor types, the expression and activation of Src is highest in NMIBC [31–33], which is consistent with the activity of RhoGDI2 in these tumors. Further work on the consequences of loss of RhoGDI2 expression is associated with metastasis of MIBC. Versican, a structural protein of extracellular matrix, is closely related with invasive or metastasis of tumors. Reduced expression of RhoGDI2 is associated with upregulated versican expression, and functional blockade of chemokine C-C motif 2 and its receptor binding axis or macrophage depletion inhibits versican-mediated metastasis [34,35], suggesting the functional crosstalk of RhoGDI2, versican, and inflammatory environments in MIBC.

Pathophysiology and Clinical Significance of Genetic Aberrations as Diagnostic Markers

Several chromosomal structural alterations involve segmental gains and losses, complex rearrangements, and translocations. These aberrations can be assessed by FISH (multicolor interphase fluorescence in situ hybridization), microsatellite analysis, SNP (single-nucleotide polymorphism) analysis, and CGH (comparative genomic hybridization). The most commonly observed chromosomal aberrations have been identified as deletion on chromosome

9p21 [36]. The chromosomal alterations are commercially available and FISH-based urine cytogenetic assays are commonly used for diagnosis of TCC. The 3q, 7p, and 17q chromosome gains are other common genetic alterations [37], which can be the target for diagnostic assays.

The DNA repair function of a cell is vital in maintaining genome integrity. A mutation or loss of function of DNA repair genes is thought to play an important role in tumorigenesis. Genomic instability participates in the pathogenesis of malignancy transformation, and deficiencies in DNA repair arise either by mutations in DNA repair enzymes or due to epigenetic reduction in expression of the DNA repair enzymes [38]. Apurinic/apyrimidinic (AP) sites in DNA can be formed by spontaneous hydrolysis, by DNA damaging agents or ionizing radiation, or by DNA glycosylases that remove specific abnormal bases. Apurinic/apyrimidinic endonuclease 1/redox factor-1 (APE1/Ref-1) functions as an apurinic/apyrimidinic endonuclease in the DNA base repair pathway and as a redox modulator for several transcriptional factors including AP-1 and nuclear factor kappa B [39]. The human *APE1/Ref-1* gene is approximately 3 kb in length; it consists of four introns and five exons and is located on chromosome 14q11.2−12 [40]. There is accumulating evidence suggesting that the alteration of APE1/Ref-1 may be related to an increased risk of cancer or cancer etiology. Especially since APE1/Ref-1 regulates genomic stability against oxidative stress, any mutations in APE1/Ref-1 would be expected to contribute to carcinogenesis [41]. SNP analyses show that APE1/Ref-1 polymorphisms may specifically contribute to an increased risk of bladder cancer [42,43]. The most common of *APE1/Ref-1* mutation was identified as Asp/Glu at codon 148 (D148E), which is found in approximately 60% of patients with bladder cancer [44]. Additionally, the secretory activity of D148E mutant APE1/Ref-1 was significantly increased compared to that of wild-type APE1/Ref-1. Interestingly, plasma and urine APE1/Ref-1 levels were significantly increased in patients with bladder cancer, which can be a useful marker for clinical diagnosis of bladder cancer [45,46]. Although the exact mechanism of association between *APE1/Ref-1* mutations and bladder cancer is not fully understood, there is ample evidence that dysregulation of the base excision repair system may promote bladder carcinogenesis. Therefore, further studies focusing on the *APE1/Ref-1* gene comprise a definitive step forward in bladder cancer research.

CONCLUSIONS

Unraveling the complex molecular mechanisms involved in bladder cancer development is impacting our approach to diagnosis and management of bladder cancer. With accumulating molecular genetic insights of bladder cancer, its evaluation of target molecules could contribute to establish molecular markers to predict the risk of tumor recurrence and progression.

REFERENCES

[1] Hanahan D, Weinberg RA. The hallmarks of cancer. Cell 2000;100(1):57−70.

[2] Cheng L, Zhang S, MacLennan GT, Williamson SR, Lopez-Beltran A, Montironi R. Bladder cancer: translating molecular genetic insights into clinical practice. Hum Pathol 2011;42(4):455−81.

[3] Mitra AP, Cote RJ. Molecular screening for bladder cancer: progress and potential. Nat Rev Urol 2010;7(1):11−20.

[4] Mitra AP, Cote RJ. Molecular pathogenesis and diagnostics of bladder cancer. Annu Rev Pathol 2009;4:251−85.

[5] Goebell PJ, Knowles MA. Bladder cancer or bladder cancers? Genetically distinct malignant conditions of the urothelium. Urol Oncol 2010;28(4):409−28.

[6] Droller MJ. Biological considerations in the assessment of urothelial cancer: a retrospective. Urology 2005;66(5 Suppl):66−75.

[7] Hartmann A, Schlake G, Zaak D, Hungerhuber E, Hofstetter A, Hofstaedter F, et al. Occurrence of chromosome 9 and p53 alterations in multifocal dysplasia and carcinoma in situ of human urinary bladder. Cancer Res 2002;62(3):809−18.

[8] Spruck 3rd CH, Ohneseit PF, Gonzalez-Zulueta M, Esrig D, Miyao N, Tsai YC, et al. Two molecular pathways to transitional cell carcinoma of the bladder. Cancer Res 1994;54(3):784−8.

[9] Hopman AH, Kamps MA, Speel EJ, Schapers RF, Sauter G, Ramaekers FC. Identification of chromosome 9 alterations and p53 accumulation in isolated carcinoma in situ of the urinary bladder versus carcinoma in situ associated with carcinoma. Am J Pathol 2002;161(4):1119−25.

[10] Knowles MA. The genetics of transitional cell carcinoma: progress and potential clinical application. BJU Int 1999;84(4):412−27.

[11] Orlow I, Lacombe L, Hannon GJ, Serrano M, Pellicer I, Dalbagni G, et al. Deletion of the p16 and p15 genes in human bladder tumors. J Natl Cancer Inst 1995;87(20):1524−9.

[12] Packenham JP, Taylor JA, Anna CH, White CM, Devereux TR. Homozygous deletions but no sequence mutations in coding regions of p15 or p16 in human primary bladder tumors. Mol Carcinog 1995;14(3):147−51.

[13] Williams SV, Sibley KD, Davies AM, Nishiyama H, Hornigold N, Coulter J, et al. Molecular genetic analysis of chromosome 9 candidate tumor-suppressor loci in bladder cancer cell lines. Genes Chromosomes Cancer 2002;34(1):86−96.

[14] Jaye M, Schlessinger J, Dionne CA. Fibroblast growth factor receptor tyrosine kinases: molecular analysis and signal transduction. Biochim Biophys Acta 1992;1135(2):185−99.

[15] Junker K, van Oers JM, Zwarthoff EC, Kania I, Schubert J, Hartmann A. Fibroblast growth factor receptor 3 mutations in bladder tumors correlate with low frequency of chromosome alterations. Neoplasia 2008;10(1):1−7.

[16] Zieger K, Dyrskjot L, Wiuf C, Jensen JL, Andersen CL, Jensen KM, et al. Role of activating fibroblast growth factor receptor 3 mutations in the development of bladder tumors. Clin Cancer Res 2005;11(21):7709−19.

[17] Hernandez S, Lopez-Knowles E, Lloreta J, Kogevinas M, Amoros A, Tardon A, et al. Prospective study of FGFR3 mutations as a prognostic factor in nonmuscle invasive urothelial bladder carcinomas. J Clin Oncol 2006;24(22):3664−71.

[18] Kompier LC, van der Aa MN, Lurkin I, Vermeij M, Kirkels WJ, Bangma CH, et al. The development of multiple bladder tumour recurrences in relation to the FGFR3 mutation status of the primary tumour. J Pathol 2009;218(1):104−12.

[19]   van Rhijn BW, Lurkin I, Radvanyi F, Kirkels WJ, van der Kwast TH, Zwarthoff EC. The fibroblast growth factor receptor 3 (FGFR3) mutation is a strong indicator of superficial bladder cancer with low recurrence rate. Cancer Res 2001;61(4):1265−8.

[20]   Levine AJ. p53, the cellular gatekeeper for growth and division. Cell 1997;88(3):323−31.

[21]   Giaccia AJ, Kastan MB. The complexity of p53 modulation: emerging patterns from divergent signals. Genes Dev 1998;12(19):2973−83.

[22]   Castillo-Martin M, Domingo-Domenech J, Karni-Schmidt O, Matos T, Cordon-Cardo C. Molecular pathways of urothelial development and bladder tumorigenesis. Urol Oncol 2010;28(4):401−8.

[23]   Cordon-Cardo C. Molecular alterations associated with bladder cancer initiation and progression. Scand J Urol Nephrol Suppl 2008;(218):154−65.

[24]   Chatterjee SJ, George B, Goebell PJ, Alavi-Tafreshi M, Shi SR, Fung YK, et al. Hyperphosphorylation of pRb: a mechanism for RB tumour suppressor pathway inactivation in bladder cancer. J Pathol 2004;203(3):762−70.

[25]   Cordon-Cardo C, Wartinger D, Petrylak D, Dalbagni G, Fair WR, Fuks Z, et al. Altered expression of the retinoblastoma gene product: prognostic indicator in bladder cancer. J Natl Cancer Inst 1992;84(16):1251−6.

[26]   Xu HJ, Cairns P, Hu SX, Knowles MA, Benedict WF. Loss of RB protein expression in primary bladder cancer correlates with loss of heterozygosity at the RB locus and tumor progression. Int J Cancer 1993;53(5):781−4.

[27]   Knowles MA, Hurst CD. Molecular biology of bladder cancer: new insights into pathogenesis and clinical diversity. Nat Rev Cancer 2015;15(1):25−41.

[28]   Lamouille S, Subramanyam D, Blelloch R, Derynck R. Regulation of epithelial-mesenchymal and mesenchymal-epithelial transitions by microRNAs. Curr Opin Cell Biol 2013;25(2):200−7.

[29]   Wiklund ED, Bramsen JB, Hulf T, Dyrskjot L, Ramanathan R, Hansen TB, et al. Coordinated epigenetic repression of the miR-200 family and miR-205 in invasive bladder cancer. Int J Cancer 2011;128(6):1327−34.

[30]   Griner EM, Theodorescu D. The faces and friends of RhoGDI2. Cancer Metastasis Rev 2012;31(3-4):519−28.

[31]   Wu Y, Moissoglu K, Wang H, Wang X, Frierson HF, Schwartz MA, et al. Src phosphorylation of RhoGDI2 regulates its metastasis suppressor function. Proc Natl Acad Sci USA 2009;106(14):5807−12.

[32]   Fanning P, Bulovas K, Saini KS, Libertino JA, Joyce AD, Summerhayes IC. Elevated expression of pp60c-src in low grade human bladder carcinoma. Cancer Res 1992;52 (6):1457−62.

[33]   Qayyum T, Fyffe G, Duncan M, McArdle PA, Hilmy M, Orange C, et al. The interrelationships between Src, Cav-1 and RhoGDI2 in transitional cell carcinoma of the bladder. Br J Cancer 2012;106(6):1187−95.

[34]   Said N, Sanchez-Carbayo M, Smith SC, Theodorescu D. RhoGDI2 suppresses lung metastasis in mice by reducing tumor versican expression and macrophage infiltration. J Clin Invest 2012;122(4):1503−18.

[35]   Said N, Theodorescu D. RhoGDI2 suppresses bladder cancer metastasis via reduction of inflammation in the tumor microenvironment. Oncoimmunology 2012;1(7):1175−7.

[36]   Kawauchi S, Sakai H, Ikemoto K, Eguchi S, Nakao M, Takihara H, et al. 9p21 index as estimated by dual-color fluorescence in situ hybridization is useful to predict urothelial carcinoma recurrence in bladder washing cytology. Hum Pathol 2009;40(12):1783−9.

[37] Netto GJ. Molecular genetics and genomics progress in urothelial bladder cancer. Semin Diagn Pathol 2013;30(4):313−20.

[38] Corcos D. Unbalanced replication as a major source of genetic instability in cancer cells. Am J Blood Res 2012;2(3):160−9.

[39] Xanthoudakis S, Curran T. Identification and characterization of Ref-1, a nuclear protein that facilitates AP-1 DNA-binding activity. EMBO J 1992;11(2):653−65.

[40] Harrison L, Ascione G, Menninger JC, Ward DC, Demple B. Human apurinic endonuclease gene (APE): structure and genomic mapping (chromosome 14q11.2-12). Hum Mol Genet 1992;1(9):677−80.

[41] Choi S, Joo HK, Jeon BH. Dynamic regulation of APE1/Ref-1 as a therapeutic target protein. Chonnam Med J 2016;52(2):75−80.

[42] Wang M, Qin C, Zhu J, Yuan L, Fu G, Zhang Z, et al. Genetic variants of XRCC1, APE1, and ADPRT genes and risk of bladder cancer. DNA Cell Biol 2010;29(6):303−11.

[43] Huang M, Dinney CP, Lin X, Lin J, Grossman HB, Wu X. High-order interactions among genetic variants in DNA base excision repair pathway genes and smoking in bladder cancer susceptibility. Cancer Epidemiol Biomarkers Prev 2007;16(1):84−91.

[44] Lee YR, Lim JS, Shin JH, Choi S, Joo HK, Jeon BH. Altered secretory activity of APE1/Ref-1 D148E variants identified in human patients with bladder cancer. Int Neurourol J 2016;20(Suppl 1):S30−7.

[45] Choi S, Shin JH, Lee YR, Joo HK, Song KH, Na YG, et al. Urinary APE1/Ref-1: a potential bladder cancer biomarker. Dis Markers 2016;2016:7276502.

[46] Shin JH, Choi S, Lee YR, Park MS, Na YG, Irani K, et al. APE1/Ref-1 as a serological biomarker for the detection of bladder cancer. Cancer Res Treat 2015;47(4):823−33.

Section II

Diagnosis

Chapter 4

Symptoms

Min Soo Choo

Hallym University College of Medicine, Chuncheon, South Korea

Chapter Outline

INTRODUCTION

A symptom is the subjective experience that is reported by the patient. Physicians should be able to transform these subjective symptoms into objective signs that indicate some medical disease. Symptoms occur in clusters and form a pattern, with the aggregate of such symptoms suggesting a particular disease.

Cancer is a group of diseases that can produce almost any signs or symptoms. The signs and symptoms depend on location, size, invasiveness, and metastasis. However, early stage cancers generally do not cause specific symptoms. In the case of bladder cancer, some symptoms can be detected early, if enough attention is paid to the patient. Fortunately, approximately 70% of bladder cancers are detected and are nonmuscle invasive upon presentation [1]. Early detection of cancer improves the chances of curing it successfully.

In this chapter, we review the presenting symptoms of bladder cancer that are identifiable, thereby offering the best chance for early diagnosis and successful treatment.

HEMATURIA

The most common presenting symptom of bladder cancer is hematuria. Hematuria is defined as blood in the urine that is detected by performing either gross or microscopic examination [2].

Bladder Cancer. DOI: http://dx.doi.org/10.1016/B978-0-12-809939-1.00004-7
45

GROSS HEMATURIA

Gross hematuria is defined as a single observation of visible urine discoloration due to the presence of blood [2]. Approximately 80%−90% of patients with bladder cancer present with painless gross hematuria [3]. The prevalence of gross hematuria is approximately 2.5% in adults [4]. In previous studies, 10%−28% of all patients and 10% of patients younger than 40 years of age were found to have bladder cancer [3,5]. In an analysis of 1000 consecutive patients who were evaluated for painless total gross hematuria, 15% were found to have bladder cancer [3].

History taking, physical examination, and a review of systems can provide important clues to narrow the differential diagnosis in patients with hematuria. A thorough health history that includes medical and surgical history, family history, social history, recreational and occupational information, radiation exposure, and medication use, often provides insight into the etiology of hematuria.

One of the most important considerations is age since the causes of hematuria in children may be greatly different from those in adults. For example, hypercalciuria is a common cause of hematuria in children, but is rare in adults [6].

The urine color of patients with gross hematuria usually ranges from pink or bright red to dark brown, resembling "tea" or "Coca-Cola." Patients who have vascular bleeding or lower urinary tract bleeding often describe the urine as bright red or cherry-colored [7]. The color is not indicative of the concentration of red blood cells (RBCs) because as little as 1 mL of whole blood per liter of urine can produce a visible color change [8]. It is important to note that the degree of hematuria is not related to the aggressiveness of disease or to the stage or grade of the tumor, and that hematuria may be intermittent, even in patients with bladder cancer [3].

Total gross hematuria throughout voiding is common. In the case of initial gross hematuria (i.e., at the beginning of voiding), anterior urethral lesions are considered first. Terminal gross hematuria (i.e., at the termination of voiding) suggests the presence of a lesion at the prostate or bladder neck.

Asymptomatic, painless gross hematuria is common. However, irritative voiding symptoms, such as frequency, urgency, and dysuria, can be accompanied by carcinoma in situ (CIS). When there are associated symptoms, other causes are considered first. Dysuria may suggest urinary tract infection (UTI) or inflammation, such as urethritis or cystitis. Colicky flank pain suggests urolithiasis. The presence of lower urinary tract symptoms, such as slow stream, hesitancy, and intermittency, is associated with bladder outlet obstruction that is usually due to benign prostatic hyperplasia. The present of blood clots almost never indicates glomerular bleeding, but rather suggests a postrenal source in the urinary tract.

A history of recent upper respiratory or skin infection in a patient with hematuria may suggest postinfectious glomerulonephritis or IgA nephropathy [8]. The presence of a concurrent rash and arthritis suggests lupus erythematosus. Rash, arthritis, and gastro intestinal symptoms suggest Henoch–schönlein purpura [2]. Hemoptysis indicates Wegener or Goodpasture syndrome [7]. Cyclical hematuria in women can be indicative of endometriosis in patients with implants in their ureters, or vesicouterine fistulas [8].

Several classes of medications have been implicated in causing hematuria. Most notable are the chemotherapeutic agents, cyclophosphamide, and mitotane, which may induce hemorrhagic cystitis [9]. Papillary necrosis and the resultant hematuria have been reported to be due to chronic ingestion of nonsteroidal antiinflammatory agents, particularly phenacetin, the use of which has also been implicated in the malignant transformation of the urothelium [10]. Finally, many drugs may cause allergic interstitial nephritis, including penicillin and cephalosporin groups [11]. Quinine, nonsteroidal antiinflammatory drugs, and some antibiotics are a few of the medications that can cause acute interstitial nephritis with microscopic hematuria [8] (Table 4.1).

TABLE 4.1 Causes of Hematuria [9]

Urinary tract	Medical or renal disease
Urinary tract infection	Glomerulonephritis
Urinary calculi	Interstitial nephritis
Urinary tract malignancy	Papillary necrosis
Urothelial cancer	Alport syndrome
Renal cancer	Renal artery stenosis
Prostate cancer	Metabolic disorders
Benign prostatic hyperplasia	Hypercalciuria
Radiation cystitis and/or nephritis	Hyperuricosuria
Endometriosis	Coagulation abnormalities
Anatomic abnormalities	Miscellaneous
Arteriovenous malformation	Trauma
Urothelial stricture disease	Exercise-induced hematuria
Ureteropelvic junction obstruction	Benign familial hematuria
Vesicoureteral reflux	Loin pain–hematuria syndrome
Nutcracker syndrome	

TABLE 4.2 Common Risk Factors for Urinary Tract Malignancy in Patients With Hematuria [14]

Male gender

Age (>35 years)

Past or current smoking

Occupational or other exposure to chemicals or dyes (benzenes or aromatic amines)

Analgesic abuse

History of any of following:

  Gross hematuria

  Urologic disorder or disease

  Irritative voiding symptoms

  Pelvic irradiation

  Chronic UTI

  Exposure to known carcinogenic agents or chemotherapy such as alkylating agents

  Chronic indwelling foreign body

Cigarette smoking is a known risk factor for transitional cell carcinoma of the bladder, conferring a three- to fivefold increased risk [12]. Occupational exposure to aromatic amines and amides, such as 4-aminobiphenyl, benzidine, and 2-naphthylamine, may occur in occupations related to leather and rubber manufacturing. Particularly worrisome is exposure during work in factories that produce aniline dyes [13] (Table 4.2).

Recent menstruation, vigorous exercise, or sexual activities may produce transient hematuria in otherwise healthy patients. After boxing or football, direct trauma is responsible for hematuria. In a long-distance runner, hematuria is usually due to the trauma caused by the up and down movement of the bladder. In 30% of cases of transient hematuria in runners, the presence of dysmorphic RBCs and RBC casts suggests that hematuria could originate from the glomerulus. Regardless of cause, exercise-induced hematuria carries a benign prognosis.

A positive family history of polycystic kidney disease, hereditary nephritis, and other renal diseases can provide clues to a genetic diagnosis. A history of travel to areas with endemic schistosomiasis, malaria, or tuberculosis may be additional important clues to the cause of hematuria [15]. Hematuria in an otherwise healthy, young African-American should lead the clinician to also consider the presence of a sickle cell phenotype or hemoglobin sickle cell disease [6].

In addition to medical history, the physical examination often provides insight into the etiology of hematuria. Peripheral edema is associated with nephrotic syndrome. Cardiac abnormalities, such as atrial fibrillation, predispose patients to renal artery embolism. Examination of the abdomen may reveal a flank mass, bruit, or a pulsatile aortic aneurysm. Costovertebral angle tenderness suggests nephrolithiasis, ureteropelvic junction obstruction, or pyelonephritis. Genital and rectal examination can provide evidence of prostatitis, prostate cancer, epididymitis, or meatal stenosis in men. In women, urethral and vaginal examinations are necessary to exclude any local causes of microscopic hematuria [9].

The presence of red urine does not always indicate gross hematuria and so it is necessary to consider a differential diagnosis. When grossly red urine is centrifuged, there are RBC-containing sediment and a clear supernatant in the urine of patients with true hematuria. However, pseudohematuria exhibits a red supernatant that is negative for hemoglobin. There are a number of pharmacologic, dietary, and metabolic factors that can produce a pink or reddish supernatant of urine, thereby giving the impression of gross hematuria [2,15]. A supernatant that is red and tests positive for hemoglobin can be due to hemoglobinuria or myoglobinuria [8] (Table 4.3).

Asymptomatic gross hematuria in patients on anticoagulants therapy also requires a complete urologic evaluation, regardless of the type or level of anticoagulant therapy [17]. Anticoagulant therapy dose not induce hematuria de novo. It may influence the duration and severity of hematuria from another cause. Patients on anticoagulation therapy with undiagnosed urologic pathology may actually present earlier in their disease process, and may represent a population more likely to benefit from prompt investigation and treatment. Indeed, a significant urologic condition was identified in 13%−45% of this cohort in a published case series review [9].

ASYMPTOMATIC MICROSCOPIC HEMATURIA

Asymptomatic microscopic hematuria (AMH) is a much more common presenting symptom in patients with bladder cancer than is gross hematuria [3].

Healthy individuals may excrete blood in the urine, with microscopic hematuria being detected in at least 9%−18% of groups tested; however, the threshold below which hematuria is considered normal has not been established. Several reports have suggested that the upper limit of normal RBC excretion is 500,000−600,000 RBCs per 12 hours, with a urine volume of 300 mL [9]. Two RBCs per high-powered microscopy field (HPF) are roughly equivalent to the threshold of 500,000 RBCs per 12 hours [9].

In most guidelines, AMH is defined as three or more RBCs per HPF on a properly collected urinary specimen in the absence of obvious benign causes, such as infection, vigorous exercise, menstruation, viral illness, trauma, medical renal disease, or recent urological procedures [14]. Canadian guidelines state that significant AMH is defined as more than two RBCs per HPF, as indicated on two separate microscopic urinalyses [18].

TABLE 4.3 Causes of Red Urine Without Hematuria [16]

Pharmacologic	Dietary	Metabolic
Antibiotics	Beets	Bile pigments
Metronidazole	Blackberries	Homogentisic acid
Nitrofurantoin	Food coloring	Melanin
Rifampicin	Rhubarb	Methemoglobin
Sulfonamides	Blueberries	Porphyrin
Antipyretics	Paprika	Tyrosine
Ibuprofen	Fava beans	Urates
Salicylates		
Anticonvulsants		
Phenytoin		
Phenothiazine		
Prochlorperazine		
Laxatives		
Phenolphthalein		
Antimalarial agents		
Chloroquine		
Quinine		
Miscellaneous agents		
Phenazopyridine		
Levodopa		
Methyldopa		
Adriamycin		
Desferoxamine		
Iron sorbitol		

The positive rate of AMH in the general population is 1.7%−21.1% in Europe and the United States, 3.9%−16.0% in Asia, and, in Africa, 0.55% for pediatrics and 17.7% for adults [19]. Hematuria also has been found in up to 13% of postmenopausal women [6]. A long-term observational study of AMH showed that hematuria disappeared in approximately 45% of subjects [19].

Previous studies have shown that between 2% and 22% of patients with AMH will be found to experience a malignancy. In 17 screening studies, including 3762 individuals with AMH, an overall rate of urinary tract malignancy was 2.6% [14]. In 32 studies that conducted initial work-ups of 9206 AMH patients, the overall rate of malignancy was found to be 4.0% [14]. In older patients with transient hematuria, 2.4% of these patients had urinary tract malignancy, and 20% had renal stone or glomerular or interstitial renal diseases [20].

In previous the diagnosis of AMH in adults required that two of the three properly collected samples be positive on microscopy. The American Urology Association (AUA) 2012 guidelines note that this requires only a single positive urinalysis verified by microscopy, for the following three reasons [14].

First, AMH that is caused by a serious underlying condition, such as a malignancy, can have a highly intermittent nature. Therefore, requiring multiple positive samples may result in an undetermined risk of missing a fatal malignancy. Second, patient work-up in response to one positive sample resulted in the detection of a significant number of life-threatening conditions. A meta-analysis revealed a pooled urinary tract malignancy rate of 3.6% in patients with one positive sample. Third, possible underlying malignancies as well as other conditions that may not be life threatening, but that would benefit from active clinical management and/or follow-up, are frequently revealed during the AMH work-up. These conditions include medical renal disease, calculous disease, benign prostatic enlargement, and urethral stricture [14].

Urine specimens should be 10 mL in volume and obtained using a freshly voided clean-catch midstream format, without instrumentation, in a sterile collection device and should be evaluated within 1 hour of collection [9,14]. If a delay in transport to the laboratory or in time to microscopic analysis is anticipated, the specimen should be refrigerated [9]. If a clean-catch specimen cannot be obtained reliably (e.g., obese patient, phimosis), then a catheterized urinary specimen can be indicated [9].

Urine specimens collected immediately after prolonged recumbence (first void in morning) or the first voiding after vigorous physical or sexual activity should not be examined to assess for microscopic hematuria [14,21]. In schoolchildren, the Japanese guidelines indicate the collection of early morning first-void urine to avoid hematuria caused by physical exercise [19]. While in the Canadian guidelines, a repeat microscopic exam should be done once the contributing factor has ceased in patients with a history of recent exercise, menses, sexual activity, or urethral trauma/instrumentation [18]. Under these guidelines, if the subsequent exam is negative, then further work-up is not required [18]. It should also be noted that in dilute urine, usually below an osmolality of 308 mOsm, most RBCs lyse; therefore, the number of RBCs per HPF may be artificially reduced [14].

Patients with hematuria and evidence of a UTI should be rechecked 6 weeks after antibiotic therapy. Patients whose hematuria has resolved require only consideration of the factors that predisposed the patient to infection [9].

The urine dipstick test uses a chemical reagent strip on which the peroxidase-like activity of hemoglobin catalyzes the oxidation of a chromogen indicator [9]. The result of 1 + of a urine blood reagent strip corresponds to approximately five RBCs per HPF. Dipsticks detect one to two RBCs per high-power field and are, therefore, at least as sensitive as microscopic examination of the urine sediment [15]. This method is 91%−100% sensitive for the detection of microscopic hematuria when there are more than three RBCs per HPF [9].

However, a positive dipstick does not define AMH because of a specificity of 65%−99% [9]. The AUA guideline recommends that the evaluation of hematuria should be based solely on findings from microscopic examination of urinary sediment and not on a dipstick reading. A positive dipstick reading merits microscopic examination to confirm or refute the diagnosis of AMH [14]. Conversely, the British Association of Urological Surgeons and Renal Association (BAUS) guideline recommends that urine dipstick of a freshly voided urine sample that contains no preservatives is considered to be a sensitive means of detecting the presence of hematuria. The BAUS guideline also comments that routine microscopy for confirmation of dipstick hematuria is not necessary since it is laborious in nature and adds little to establishing the diagnosis of hematuria [22].

False positives may be observed in the presence of myoglobin, free hemoglobin, semen, highly alkaline (pH >9) or concentrated urine, and antiseptic solutions, such as povidone-iodine [9]. However, false negatives rarely occur. Negative dipstick reliably excludes hematuria. Ascorbic acid, also known as vitamin C, has been shown to cause false negative results on dipstick testing because of its reducing properties [17].

Patients who screen positive for hematuria with a dipstick test, but have a negative follow-up microscopic urinalysis, should undergo three additional microscopic examinations to rule out AMH. If one of these repeat microscopic urinalyses is positive, the patient is considered to have AMH. If all three specimens are negative upon microscopy, the patient does not require further evaluation for AMH, and other causes of a positive dipstick test result, such as hemoglobinuria and myoglobinuria, should be considered [17].

If a potential benign cause is identified, including infection, menstruation, vigorous exercise, viral illness, exposure to trauma, or recent urologic procedures (e.g., catheterization), the insult should be removed or treated appropriately, and the urine should be retested after at least 48 hours [9]. Persistent hematuria warrants a full work-up. Patients with AMH in the presence of pyuria or bacteriuria should be rechecked 6 weeks after culture-directed antibiotic therapy. If hematuria persists, diagnostic evaluation should commence [17].

The presence of other signs, including significant proteinuria, various form of casts, dysmorphic RBCs, or renal insufficiency, is suggestive of a glomerular hematuria, and such patients should undergo an evaluation for potential underlying renal parenchymal disease [19]. Dysmorphic RBCs, which involve various erythrocyte morphologies, such as doughnut shapes with a hump or a target shape, can be caused by changes in pH and osmolality while RBCs travel through distal tubules of nephrons, or by mechanical deformation from extravasation gaps of the basement membrane of glomerular vessels [23,24]. The presence of acanthocytes may provide greater evidence of a glomerular etiology [9].

IRRITATIVE VOIDING SYMPTOMS

Bladder cancer also can cause irritative voiding symptoms, including dysuria, frequency, nocturia, urgency, and/or feeling of incomplete emptying, and is particularly associated with CIS or muscle invasive bladder cancer. There is a report that 80% of patients with CIS experienced irritative symptoms upon presentation [25]. In addition, patients with CIS may present with irritative voiding symptoms without AMH [26].

In advanced tumors, symptoms-related urinary tract obstruction or reduced bladder capacity also may occur [27,28]. Although these symptoms are more likely to be caused by benign conditions, such as a UTI, bladder stones, an overactive bladder, or a benign prostatic enlargement, if there is no other definitive cause, a diagnostic work-up for bladder cancer should be considered in patients with irritative voiding symptoms. Bacteriuria occurs in approximately 50% of patients with squamous cell carcinoma of the bladder. According to the National Institute of Health and Care Excellence (NICE) guideline, patients who complain of dysuria with unexplained nonvisible hematuria and at least 60 years of age are recommended to be referred for cancer work-up within 2 weeks [29]. The NICE guidelines also recommend a possible nonurgent referral for bladder cancer in people who are at least 60 years of age and experience recurrent or persistent unexplained UTI [29].

OTHER SYMPTOMS

Patients with large-volume or invasive tumors may be found to have bladder wall thickening or a palpable mass that may be detected during a careful bimanual examination under anesthesia. An immobile bladder is suggestive of tumor fixation to adjacent structures after direct invasion.

If patients have already been experiencing invasion or metastasis when the first symptoms appear, various symptoms can occur depending on where the cancer has spread. The patient may complain of bone pain due to bone metastases, flank pain due to retroperitoneal metastases, or ureteral obstruction as the first symptom of advanced bladder cancer. Lung metastasis may cause coughing or shortness of breath, while liver metastasis may cause abdominal pain or jaundice.

Patients may present with nonspecific general symptoms, such as a loss of appetite, weight loss, and fatigue [29,30].

Hepatomegaly and supraclavicular lymphadenopathy may be signs of metastatic disease. Lymphedema from occlusive pelvic lymphadenopathy may occasionally be observed. On rare occasions, patients can experience unusual metastases, such as to the skin, whereby patients present with painful nodules and ulcerations [31].

CONCLUSION

Painless gross or microscopic hematuria is the most common presenting symptom of bladder cancer. Since hematuria has a highly intermittent nature, and can cause serious medical conditions, a single positive urinalysis on microscopy must prompt further evaluation for bladder cancer. The usefulness of dipstick urine test is limited due to its low specificity. Since there are many other medical conditions that cause hematuria, clinicians must obtain a differential diagnosis through history taking, physical examination, and systemic review.

Unexplained irritative voiding symptoms may be a sign of bladder cancer, particularly of CIS. In advanced bladder cancer, obstructive voiding symptoms are also present. Metastatic bladder cancer upon presentation also indicates various symptoms according to the location of metastasis. Weight loss or fatigue may also be seen in advanced bladder cancer.

REFERENCES

[1] Ro JY, Staerkel GA, Ayala AG. Cytologic and histologic features of superficial bladder cancer. Urol Clin North Am 1992;19(3):435−53.

[2] Tu WH, Shortliffe LD. Evaluation of asymptomatic, atraumatic hematuria in children and adults. Nat Rev Urol 2010;7(4):189−94.

[3] Amling CL. Diagnosis and management of superficial bladder cancer. Curr Probl Cancer 2001;25(4):219−78.

[4] Khadra MH, Pickard RS, Charlton M, Powell PH, Neal DE. A prospective analysis of 1,930 patients with hematuria to evaluate current diagnostic practice. J Urol 2000;163 (2):524−7.

[5] van der Molen AJ, Hovius MC. Hematuria: a problem-based imaging algorithm illustrating the recent Dutch guidelines on hematuria. Am J Roentgenol 2012;198(6):1256−65.

[6] Ahmed Z, Lee J. Asymptomatic urinary abnormalities. Hematuria and proteinuria. Med Clin North Am 1997;81(3):641−52.

[7] Pan CG. Evaluation of gross hematuria. Pediatr Clin North Am 2006;53(3):401−12.

[8] Sandhu KS, LaCombe JA, Fleischmann N, Greston WM, Lazarou G, Mikhail MS. Gross and microscopic hematuria: guidelines for obstetricians and gynecologists. Obstet Gynecol Surv 2009;64(1):39−49.

[9] Yun EJ, Meng MV, Carroll PR. Evaluation of the patient with hematuria. Med Clin North Am 2004;88(2):329−43.

[10] Gonwa TA, Corbett WT, Schey HM, Buckalew Jr. VM. Analgesic-associated nephropathy and transitional cell carcinoma of the urinary tract. Ann Intern Med 1980;93(2):249−52.

[11] Roxe DM. Toxic nephropathy from diagnostic and therapeutic agents. Review and commentary. Am J Med 1980;69(5):759–66.

[12] Silverman DT, Hartge P, Morrison AS, Devesa SS. Epidemiology of bladder cancer. Hematol Oncol Clin North Am 1992;6(1):1–30.

[13] Cohen SM, Shirai T, Steineck G. Epidemiology and etiology of premalignant and malignant urothelial changes. Scand J Urol Nephrol Suppl 2000;(205):105–15.

[14] Davis R, Jones JS, Barocas DA, Castle EP, Lang EK, Leveillee RJ, et al. Diagnosis, evaluation and follow-up of asymptomatic microhematuria (AMH) in adults: AUA guideline. J Urol 2012;188(6 Suppl):2473–81.

[15] Margulis V, Sagalowsky AI. Assessment of hematuria. Med Clin North Am 2011;95 (1):153–9.

[16] Bryant JS, Gausche-Hill M. When is red urine not hematuria?: a case report. J Emerg Med 2007;32(1):55–7.

[17] Sharp VJ, Barnes KT, Erickson BA. Assessment of asymptomatic microscopic hematuria in adults. Am Fam Physic 2013;88(11):747–54.

[18] Wollin T, Laroche B, Psooy K. Canadian guidelines for the management of asymptomatic microscopic hematuria in adults. Can Urol Assoc J 2009;3(1):77–80.

[19] Horie S, Ito S, Okada H, Kikuchi H, Narita I, Nishiyama T, et al. Japanese guidelines of the management of hematuria 2013. Clin Exp Nephrol 2014;18(5):679–89.

[20] Murakami S, Igarashi T, Hara S, Shimazaki J. Strategies for asymptomatic microscopic hematuria: a prospective study of 1,034 patients. J Urol 1990;144(1):99–101.

[21] Harris NM, Yardley I, Basketter V, Holmes SA. Is sexual intercourse a significant cause of haematuria? BJU Int 2002;89(4):344–6.

[22] Fawcett D, Kelly J, Goldberg L, Anderson J, Feehally J, MacTier R, on behalf of the Renal Association and British Association of Urological Surgeons. Joint consensus statement on the initial assessment of haematuria. <www.renal.org/docs/default-source/what-we-do/RA-BAUS_Haematuria_Consensus_Guidelines.pdf?sfvrsn=0>; 2008 [accessed 21.01.17].

[23] Kazi SN, Benz RL. Work-up of hematuria. Prim Care 2014;41(4):737–48.

[24] Sokolosky MC. Hematuria. Emerg Med Clin North Am 2001;19(3):621–32.

[25] Mohr DN, Offord KP, Owen RA, Melton III LJ. Asymptomatic microhematuria and urologic disease. A population-based study. JAMA 1986;256(2):224–9.

[26] Tissot WD, Diokno AC, Peters KM. A referral center's experience with transitional cell carcinoma misdiagnosed as interstitial cystitis. J Urol 2004;172(2):478–80.

[27] Witjes JA, Comperat E, Cowan NC, De Santis M, Gakis G, Lebret T, et al. EAU guidelines on muscle-invasive and metastatic bladder cancer: summary of the 2013 guidelines. Eur Urol 2014;65(4):778–92.

[28] Clark PE, Agarwal N, Biagioli MC, Eisenberger MA, Greenberg RE, Herr HW, et al. Bladder cancer. J Natl Compr Canc Netw 2013;11(4):446–75.

[29] National Institute for Health and Care Excellence. Suspected cancer: recognition and referral. NICE guideline. London: National Institute for Health and Care Excellence; 2015. <www.nice.org.uk/guidance/ng12/resources/suspected-cancer-recognition-and-referral-1837268071621> [accessed 21.01.17].

[30] Kirkali Z, Chan T, Manoharan M, Algaba F, Busch C, Cheng L, et al. Bladder cancer: epidemiology, staging and grading, and diagnosis. Urology 2005;66(6 Suppl 1):4–34.

[31] Block CA, Dahmoush L, Konety BR. Cutaneous metastases from transitional cell carcinoma of the bladder. Urology 2006;67(4):846.e15-7.

Chapter 5

Physical Examination

Kyungtae Ko

Hallym University, Seoul, South Korea

Chapter Outline

Improvements in the quality of radiology diagnostic equipment, such as those for ultrasonography, computed tomography (CT), and magnetic resonance image (MRI), as well as the popularization of regular medical checkups, have decreased the dependency on physical examination for diagnostic purposes. In particular, high-definition CT and 3 T MRI provide highly accurate anatomical images of neighboring organs, eliminating the need for clinicians to perform bimanual pelvic examination for diagnosis of prostate cancer and bladder cancer [1,2]. However, as in all other medical fields, detailed history taking and thorough physical examination are critical for the diagnosis and treatment of bladder cancer. A complete physical examination is not performed merely to observe the extent of a particular disease. It provides dynamic component information, which cannot be obtained through radiological equipment such as CT or MRI, at no additional cost. If the bladder is fixed to the surrounding organs, the lesion may be at an advanced stage and this information would help in the interpretation of CT or MRI findings. Furthermore, clinicians can quickly judge the patient's general medical condition through a complete physical examination. It enables efficient use of medical resources by preventing redundant tests and also enables the clinician to appropriately select additional testing methods depending on the patient's condition [3].

The patient's nutritional status can be predicted based on the skin condition. For instance, a cachexic general appearance is frequently observed in many types of cancer. A soft oval mass that is palpable immediately above the symphysis pubis may indicate a distended bladder caused by bladder outlet obstruction, and edema limited to the external genitalia or lower extremities may suspect an obstruction of pelvic lymphatic channel. In male

Bladder Cancer. DOI: http://dx.doi.org/10.1016/B978-0-12-809939-1.00005-9

57

patients, the size of the prostate that is palpated during digital rectal examination (DRE) is important for selecting appropriate drug therapy, and palpation of a stony hard nodule could indicate prostate cancer. Urethral caruncles, which are seen in women, may induce hematuria and recurrent cystitis. Finally, thorough physical examinations are important because clinicians must treat people, not diseases. Physical examinations impart a sense of comfort and trust to patients, allowing clinicians to build trust, based on which clinicians can help their patients make better decisions.

The bladder is a half retroperitoneal organ, and the top of the dome and the posterior bladder walls are enveloped by the peritoneum [4]. The peritoneum that coats the bladder runs dorsally, forming the rectovesical pouch (Douglas pouch, Fig. 5.1) in men and the vesicouterine pouch and rectouterine pouch (cul-de-sac, Fig. 5.2) in women. After a full voiding, a normal bladder is tucked under the pelvis, and thus is not palpable during physical examination. However, owing to its high elasticity, a bladder filled with 300−400 mL of urine is visible as a small lump in the lower abdomen in a thin person in the supine position. Although it is not visible to the eye in relatively obese people, a distended bladder can be diagnosed based on a dull percussion sound.

DRE must be used for screening in men aged 55 years or greater or men aged 40 or greater with an immediate family history of prostate cancer, and it must be performed regardless of age in all male patients who have urological disorders, including lower urinary tract symptoms [5]. Most cases of prostate cancer that are identified through DRE are at clinical stage II or lower, which can be completely cured [6]. In addition, one-fourth of all

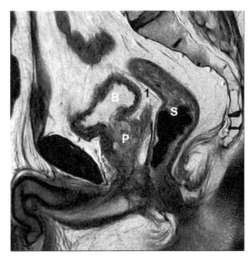

FIGURE 5.1 The male pelvis. The bladder is a half retroperitoneal organ (B, bladder; P, prostate; S, sigmoid colon; 1, rectovesical pouch).

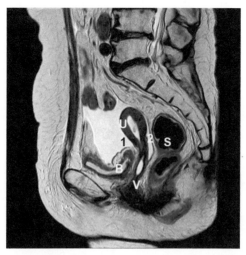

FIGURE 5.2 The female pelvis. The bladder is a half retroperitoneal organ (B, bladder; U, uterus; V, vagina; S, sigmoid colon; 1, vesicouterine pouch; 2, rectouterine pouch (cul-de-sac)).

colorectal cancer cases can be diagnosed using DRE. In general, DRE is a final procedure during a physical examination. First, in an upright position, the patient leans his upper body on the examination table in a 90-degree angle (Fig. 5.3A). If the patient cannot take this position because of a physical impairment, DRE can also be performed with the patient lying in a lateral position with knees bent toward the chest or in a supine position (Fig. 5.3B, C). Physicians must provide adequate explanation regarding the purpose and method of DRE to the patients. Letting the patient know when beginning the examination and comforting the patient by saying things such as the examination will be performed gently can help tremendously while performing the examination. Furthermore, laying one hand on the patient's body may also be comforting for the patient. DRE procedures are as follows. First, the clinician instructs the patient to take a deep breath and gently inserts a gloved, well-lubricated index finger through the external anal sphincter. The clinician checks if the anal sphincter tone is normal. The external anal sphincter tone reflects the external urethral sphincter tone; an abnormal tone indicates an abnormal neurologic component, and helps in performing a differential diagnosis of the neurologic disease. After the external anal sphincter is adequately relaxed, the clinician inserts the index finger deeply to feel the entire posterior surface of the prostate. The average size of the prostate is about two top segments of the index finger, and has the consistency of a rubber eraser. By gently feeling the prostate surface, the clinician can check for any irregularity, nodularity, tenderness, and local heating sensation which are felt in acute prostatitis, and whether the prostate is fixed or movable. Then, the clinician puts his or her left hand on the patient's lower abdomen and inserts

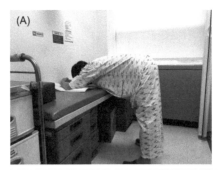

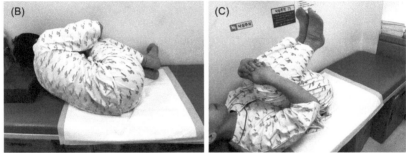

FIGURE 5.3 Digital rectal examination. (A) Standing position, (B) lateral knee-chest position, and (C) supine knee-chest position.

his index finger as deeply as possible to check whether the boundary of the bladder and prostate is felt and whether the prostate is fixed to the bladder neck. Finally, the clinician sends the fecal residue on the glove to the laboratory for a fecal occult blood test [7]. After DRE is concluded, the clinician must step away to give sufficient time for the patient to tidy himself up. Consultation regarding the results of the physical examination should be performed after the patient is dressed and ready.

Pelvic examination for a female patient must be performed in the presence of a female nurse or female physical assistant. In addition, the clinician must explain each step of the procedure before performing them. Even a minor behavior of a male physician may cause misunderstandings by female patients, which may cause great humiliation. Even worse, the patient's pelvic muscles will become strained if the patient is tense, hindering a complete physical examination. Although patients are sometimes examined with a full bladder depending on the purpose of the examination, such as urinary incontinence, in general, patients are examined after they completely empty their bladder. The patient changes into a gown in a private space and lies in the lithotomy position with assistance from a female nurse. Then, a drape should be placed near the navel such that the patient and the physician cannot see each other (Fig. 5.4). As in other examinations, less uncomfortable examinations should be performed first, such as observation of the external genitalia for any anomalies.

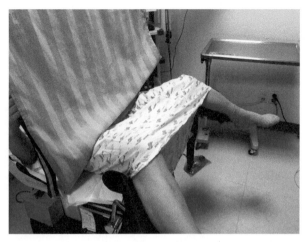

FIGURE 5.4   Female pelvic examination. Place a drape so that the physician and the patient cannot see each other during the examination.

First, mucosal erosion change or ulcer change in the labium major or minor may indicate viral infections, such as sexually transmitted diseases, or autoimmune disease, such as Bechet disease. In addition, vaginal atrophic changes in accordance with estrogen hormonal changes may be observed in menopausal women. Purulent vaginal discharge is commonly observed in microbacterial infection, such as *Gardnerellavaginalis* infection. All of these lesions may induce voiding symptoms, such as hematuria or painful urination. Urethral caruncle, which exhibits spots of blood after urination, or urethral prolapse may show in the urethral meatus. The clinician must carefully inspect whether there is pain or induration in the urethra while palpating the anterior vaginal wall. If urethral diverticulum is present, remnant urine or purulent discharge that is pooled within the diverticulum may ooze out through the urethral meatus. For patients with bladder cancer, the clinician must carefully inspect whether any mass is present in the urethra and whether the bladder neck and urethra are well fixed. The physician should instruct the patient to do a Valsalva maneuver, in which the patient takes a deep breath and tries to breath out while covering up her mouth and nostrils, to examine the presence of pelvic organ prolapse and its grade. For patients who complain of abnormal urine leakage, instruct them to cough to check for stress urinary incontinence.

To perform a bimanual pelvic examination, the physician stands in between the patient's legs, who is in the lithotomy position. Insert the right index and middle fingers into the vagina (anus for men), and press the patient's lower abdomen with the left hand with adequate force to allow the two right fingers to better palpate the abdominal organs. Through bimanual pelvic examination, the physician should gather the following information: (1) the presence of a mass in the bladder, (2) mobility of the bladder,

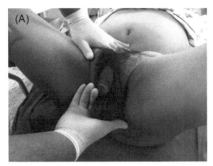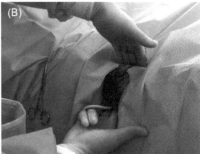

FIGURE 5.5 Bimanual pelvic examination. (A) Male patient, preoperation and (B) female patient, postoperation.

(3) fixation of the bladder to the cervix or surrounding organs, and (4) the presence of a mass outside the bladder, such as an ovarian tumor. Even though bimanual pelvic examination is an important procedure that offers much important information, it is a rather difficult examination for both men and women. It should never be forced on patients who complain of severe discomfort or pain. The best time to perform the examination is when the patient is under anesthesia, such as prior to or after TUR-B (Fig. 5.5A, B).

The pathological stage of muscle invasive bladder cancer can be determined after radical cystectomy is performed. Thus, the clinical stage identified prior to the operation procedure is important in predicting patient prognosis and preparing an appropriate treatment plan [8]. Based on clinical stage, clinicians decide on a specific technique for the surgical procedure and whether neoadjuvant chemotherapy should be given to the patient. For accurate clinical staging, clinicians need to determine the extent of tumor invasion to the bladder muscle layers after transurethral resection of the bladder (TUR-B). Second, images of the upper urinary tract and pelvic organs are obtained by using urography CT. Finally, bimanual pelvic examination is performed under anesthesia before and after TUR-B [9]. Clinical staging after bimanual pelvic examination was first introduced by Marshall et al. Later, clinical staging according to tumor status before and after TUR-B was introduced by Ploeg et al. (Table 5.1) [10,11]. However, some discrepancy existed between clinical and pathologic stages. Previous reports indicated that less than 20% of clinical stage T2 bladder cancer cases were down-staged in the pathological staging and 53.8% were up-staged. By contrast, 60% of clinical stage T3 bladder cancer cases remained the same in the pathological staging (i.e., T3 pathologic stage), while 20% were up-staged and another 20% were down-staged [12]. According to the 2007 American Urology Association guideline, the role of bimanual physical examination is not clear in nonmuscle invasive bladder cancer, but it is helpful for clinical staging of muscle invasive bladder cancer during TUR-B [9]. Similarly, the

TABLE 5.1 Clinical Stage

	Marshall [10]	Ploeg and Witjes [11]
cT1		No mass felt on bimanual examination
cT2a	Nonpalpable	Mobile mass felt only before TURBT
cT2b	Induration but no three-dimensional mass	
cT3	Three-dimensional mass that is mobile	Mobile mass felt before and after TURBT
cT4a	Invading adjacent structures; prostate, vagina, rectum	Immobile mass
cT4b	Fixed to pelvic sidewall and not mobile	

Bimanual examination should be performed before and after transurethral resection of bladder (TUR-B).

2016 American Urology Association nonmuscle invasive bladder cancer guideline also states that bimanual pelvic examination performed under anesthesia after complete resection of tumor via TUR-B is helpful for clinical staging [13].

The 2013 European Urology Association guideline for nonmuscle invasive bladder cancer recommends bimanual pelvic examination be conducted under anesthesia prior to TUR-B (grade of recommendation: C), but it also recommends bimanual pelvic examination be performed after TUR-B [14]. The 2014 European Urology Association guideline for muscle invasive bladder cancer also recommends bimanual pelvic examination be performed even if there is a discrepancy between bimanual pelvic examination and pathologic T stage [15,16]. Literature on this discrepancy has suggested that 11% of bladder cancer was overstaged while 31% was understaged, indicating that bimanual pelvic examination bladder cancer staging is relatively more associated with clinical understaging. Even if there is a 42% discrepancy between bimanual pelvic examination and pathologic staging, a surgeon could anticipate difficulty in dissection of the bladder during radical cystectomy regardless of the pathologic results if the bladder is fixed to surrounding tissues. Even highly experienced surgeons believe that a bladder fixed to the pelvic wall or surrounding organs, as discovered through a bimanual pelvic examination, is a contraindication to robot-assisted laparoscopic radical cystectomy [17]. In addition, bimanual pelvic examination also provides information regarding the exact extent of urethral invasion of bladder cancer, which is an important piece of information for determination of the operation plan, such as ileal conduit or neobladder.

Despite advances in radiology diagnostic equipment have provided access to accurate static anatomical images, a complete physical examination including the bimanual pelvic examination is still a critical procedure for patients with bladder cancer.

REFERENCES

[1] Patel U, Dasgupta P, Challacombe B, Cahill D, Brown C, Patel R, et al. Pre-biopsy 3T MRI and targeted biopsy of the index prostate cancer—correlation with robot assisted radical prostatectomy. BJU Int 2017;119:82–90.

[2] Rajesh A, Sokhi HK, Fung R, Mulcahy KA, Bankart MJ. Bladder cancer: evaluation of staging accuracy using dynamic MRI. Clin Radiol 2011;66:1140–5.

[3] Glenn SG, Charles BB. History, physical examination, and urinalysis. In: Wein AJ, Kavoussi LR, Partin AW, Peters CA, editors. Campbell-Walsh urology. 11th ed. Philadelphia: Elsevier; 2016. p. 1–25.

[4] Clinton WC, Adam PK. Anatomy of the bladder. In: Keane TE, Graham Jr. SD, editors. Glenn's urologic surgery. 8th ed. Philadelphia: Wolters Kluwer; 2016. p. 138–45.

[5] Carter HB, Albertsen PC, Barry MJ, Etzioni R, Freedland SJ, Greene KL, et al. Early detection of prostate cancer: AUA Guideline. J Urol 2013;190:419–26.

[6] Kibel AS, Ciezki JP, Klein EA, Reddy CA, Lubahn JD, Haslag-Minoff J, et al. Survival among men with clinically localized prostate cancer treated with radical prostatectomy or radiation therapy in the prostate specific antigen era. J Urol 2012;187:1259–65.

[7] Bond JH. Fecal occult blood tests in occult gastrointestinal bleeding. Semin Gastrointest Dis 1999;10:48–52.

[8] Rozanski AT, Benson CR, McCoy JA, Green C, Grossman HB, Svatek RS, et al. Is exam under anesthesia still necessary for the staging of bladder cancer in the era of modern imaging? Baldder Cancer 2015;1:91–6.

[9] Hall MC, Chang SS, Dalbagni G, Pruthi RS, Schellhammer PF, Seigne JD, et al. Guideline for the management of nonmuscle invasive bladder cancer: stages Ta, T1 and Tis: Update (2007). J Urol 2007;178:2314–30.

[10] Marshall VF. The relation of the preoperative estimate to the pathologic demonstration of the extent of vesical neoplasms. J Urol 1952;68:714–23.

[11] Ploeg M, Witjes JA. Bladder cancer diagnosis and detection: current status. In: Lokeshwar VB, Merseburger AS, Hautmann SH, editors. Bladder tumors. New York: Humana Press; 2010. p. 68.

[12] Svatek RS, Shariat SF, Novara G, Skinner EC, Fradet Y, Bastian PJ, et al. Discrepancy between clinical and pathological stage: external validation of the impact on prognosis in an international radical cystectomy cohort. BJU Int 2011;107:898–904.

[13] Chang SS, Boorjian SA, Chou R, Clark PE, Daneshmand S, Konety BR, et al. Diagnosis and treatment of non-muscle invasice bladder cancer: AUA/SUO guideline. American Urological Association (AUA) guideline. J Urol 2016;196:1021–9.

[14] Babjuk M, Burger M, Zigeuner R, Shariat SF, van Rhijn BW, Comperat E, et al. EAU guidelines on non-muscle-invasive urothelial carcinoma of the bladder: update 2013. Eur Urol 2013;64:639–53.

[15] Ploeg M, Kiemeney LA, Smits GA, Vergunst H, Viddeleer AC, Geboers AD, et al. Discrepancy between clinical staging through bimanual palpation and pathological staging after cystectomy. Urol Oncol 2012;30:247–51.

[16] Witjes JA, Comperat E, Cowan NC, De Santis M, Gakis G, Lebret T, et al. EAU guidelines on muscle-invasive and metastatic bladder cancer: summary of the 2013 guidelines. Eur Urol 2014;65:778−92.

[17] Andre LCA, Sameer C, Inderbir SG. Minimally invasice bladder procedures: radical cystectomy, partial cystectomy, urachal excision, diverticulectomy. In: Keane TE, Graham Jr. SD, editors. Glenn's urologic surgery. 8th ed. Philadelphia: Wolters Kluwer; 2016. p. 230−44.

Chapter 6

Urine Cytology and Urinary Biomarkers

Ok-Jun Lee, Ho-Won Kang and Seok Joong Yun
Chungbuk National University, Cheongju, Republic of Korea

Chapter Outline

INTRODUCTION

Diagnosis of bladder cancer currently depends on urine cytology and cystoscopy. Cystoscopy is the gold-standard method for diagnosis, but ideally most of patients would be preferable to avoid cystoscopy because of its invasive nature. The contact between bladder tumors and urine suggests that urine should be a valuable source of biomarkers for diagnosis of bladder cancer. However, although urinary cytology is an established diagnostic tool, only a limited number of biomarkers have yet been used in clinical practice, and it remains a challenge to urologists to develop convenient and accurate assays for measurement of biomarkers in urine.

Urinary biomarkers could have a role in detection of bladder cancer, which is generally diagnosed following presentation with hematuria or voiding symptoms. Cystoscopy remains the standard tool for diagnosis of bladder cancer, but identification of urinary biomarkers with high negative-predictive value would be helpful to reduce the need for cystoscopy. Urinary biomarkers with high positive-predictive values could also be used for follow-up of patients with bladder cancer for accurate and early diagnosis of cancer recurrence or progression.

Many reports have been published on experimental assessment of tumor DNA, RNA, microRNA, methylation, and proteins as urinary biomarkers for

Bladder Cancer. DOI: http://dx.doi.org/10.1016/B978-0-12-809939-1.00006-0
67

bladder cancer. However, only a few markers have progressed to clinical trials. In general, these experimental urinary markers are not close to clinical application. We therefore describe here existing urinary markers and tests, including urinary cytology, nuclear matrix protein-22 (NMP22), bladder tumor antigen (BTA), and BCLA-4.

URINE CYTOLOGY

Urine cytology is an important noninvasive approach for the detection of urothelial carcinoma. The combined use of urine cytology with cystoscopic biopsy has a major role in the diagnosis of urothelial carcinoma. Despite many attempts to develop tests with better diagnostic accuracy, urine cytology remains one of the best ways to diagnose a variety of cancers of the urinary tract.

Conventional urine smear has been popular as a diagnostic procedure since the 1940s [1]. An improved technique, liquid-based cytology (LBC), was developed in the 1990s as an alternative to conventional cytology for processing gynecological specimens [2]. LBC proceeds via cell enrichment to reduce levels of background inflammatory cells and blood cells, after which a uniform layer of cells is deposited on a microscope slide by an automated process, facilitating the identification of malignant cells. LBC has now become the preferred method for urine diagnosis, but differences with conventional cytology have been reported [3–5]. Although differences occur according to the LBC method that is adopted, results suggest that LBC and conventional cytology are comparable for the morphological assessment of tumor cells, and no significant improvement in sensitivity is observed with LBC [6,7]. However, the automation and excellent slide quality associated with LBC techniques are notable advantages of this approach. Regardless of the difference between conventional smear and LBC preparations, it should be noted that urine cytological diagnosis is very effective in high-grade urothelial carcinomas, but less effective in low-grade urothelial tumors. The mean sensitivity of urine cytology is ∼50% for detecting urothelial carcinoma (∼80% in high-grade carcinomas and ∼25% in low-grade lesions) [8]. To make any cytological diagnosis, it is necessary to differentiate between urothelial cancer cells and detached, normal urothelial cells, which requires an understanding of the cytological differences between these cell types.

Normal Cytology

The two types of urine specimen are voided urine and instrumented urine [9]. Instrumented samples are generated from cystoscopy, bladder wash-outs, catheterization, and direct brushing (Figs. 6.1 and 6.2). Voided and instrumented samples, as well as samples that are not suitable for diagnostic purposes, have the following cytological characteristics:

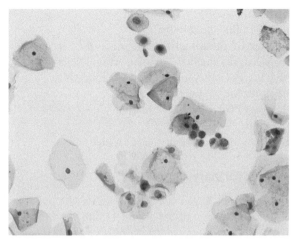

FIGURE 6.1   Normal (noncancerous) voided-urine liquid-based cytology. Most voided-urine samples reveal a mixture of urothelial cells and squamous cells. Most of the urothelial cells are basal or intermediate.

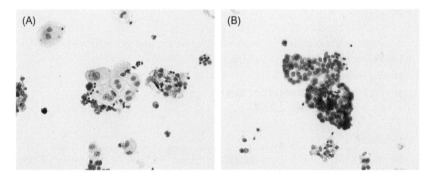

FIGURE 6.2   Liquid-based cytology of a sample prepared by bladder washing. (A) Superficial umbrella cells are large and have abundant cytoplasm and prominent nucleoli. Binucleation and multinucleation are common. (B) Basal urothelial cells are tightly clustered. These cells show round nuclei with evenly distributed granular chromatin.

1. Voided-urine samples
   - Samples have variable cellularity and are often sparsely cellular
   - Usually consist of isolated individual cells; tight clusters of urothelial cells are uncommon
   - Contain intermediate and superficial (umbrella) cells
   - Contain bland urothelial cells with homogeneous, granular, or finely vacuolated cytoplasm, round nuclei, and small nucleoli
   - Contain squamous cells
   - Contain epithelial cells of the prostate or seminal vesicles in men (rare)

2. Instrumented samples
   - Samples have high cellularity
   - Contain clusters of urothelial cells, often quite large
   - Contain basal, intermediate, and superficial cells
3. Samples that are not suitable for diagnostic purposes
   - Samples with low cellularity
   - Samples with obscuring inflammation
   - Samples consisting of blood only
   - Samples with marked degenerative changes

Neoplasms of the Urinary Bladder

Multiple grading schemes have been used to define urothelial neoplasms, but the 2004 classification system of the World Health Organization (WHO) and the International Society of Urological Pathology (ISUP) is now widely accepted [10,11]. Cytological diagnoses based on the WHO/ISUP 2004 classification can be divided into two groups: low-grade urothelial lesions and high-grade urothelial carcinomas.

Cytological diagnosis according to the WHO/ISUP 2004 classification system defines the following types of urothelial neoplasm:

1. Low-grade urothelial lesions
   - Papillary urothelial neoplasm of low malignant potential (PUNLMP)
   - Papillary carcinoma, low grade
2. High-grade urothelial lesions
   - Papillary carcinoma, high grade
   - Carcinoma *in situ* (CIS)

Low-Grade Urothelial Lesions

In the WHO/ISUP 2004 classification system, a PUNLMP consists of delicate papillae with little or no fusion, and its covering urothelium is usually thickening but shows minimal. Nuclei are normal in size or slightly enlarged, without notable nuclear atypia. Low-grade papillary urothelial carcinoma shows papillae that are mostly delicate and separate, with some fusion. The nuclei tend to be uniformly enlarged, with mild atypia (Fig. 6.3). The cytological features of these lesions are similar, but PUNLMPs are more difficult to recognize cytologically than low-grade carcinomas because PUNLMPs have less atypia. Diagnosis of low-grade urothelial lesions is made by the following cytological criteria:

1. Papillary fragments with fibrovascular cores rarely identified
2. Cytological features that suggest underlying tumors
   - Increased homogeneity of urothelial cytoplasm
   - Mild increase in nuclear-to-cytoplasmic ratio
   - Irregular nuclear membranes

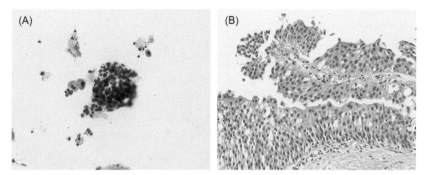

FIGURE 6.3 Features of a low-grade urothelial lesion. (A) Voided-urine liquid-based cytology shows an increased nuclear-to-cytoplasmic ratio compared with noncancerous samples and irregular nuclear outlines, but these changes are subtle. (B) Subsequent histology of a low-grade papillary urothelial carcinoma from the same patient.

High-Grade Urothelial Lesions

Histologically, high-grade urothelial carcinoma is defined as a tumor with moderate-to-marked cytological atypia and disordered growth. Urothelial CIS is most often seen in association with high-grade papillary carcinoma or invasive urothelial carcinoma. De novo CIS accounts for only 1%−3% of newly diagnosed cases of bladder cancer [12,13]. Urothelial CIS is a flat and noninvasive lesion that is confined to the epithelium and shows marked cytological atypia. The cytological distinction between high-grade urothelial carcinoma and CIS is very difficult to determine, and they are considered together in the following description of cytological diagnostic features (Figs. 6.4 and 6.5):

1. Increased cellularity
2. Individual cells and cohesive groups
3. Enlarged nuclei with marked hyperchromasia
4. High nuclear-to-cytoplasmic ratio
5. Irregular nuclear outlines
6. Coarsely granular chromatin
7. Necrosis and/or red blood cells in the background

Other Malignant Lesions

Other primary cancers of the urinary tract include squamous-cell carcinoma, adenocarcinoma, urachal carcinoma, and small-cell carcinoma. The limited diagnostic accuracy of urinary cytology, and the infrequent occurrence of these tumors, means that accurate diagnosis is challenging, and they are likely to be interpreted as urothelial carcinomas. Despite these limitations, urinary cytology is valuable for diagnosis of rare tumors when combined with histological confirmation.

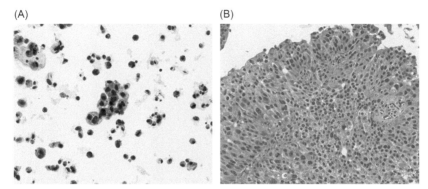

FIGURE 6.4 Features of high-grade urothelial carcinoma. (A) Voided-urine liquid-based cytology shows loosely cohesive clusters and individually dispersed cells with enlarged nuclei with marked hyperchromasia. Irregular nuclear outlines are evident. (B) Histology of a high-grade papillary urothelial carcinoma from the same patient.

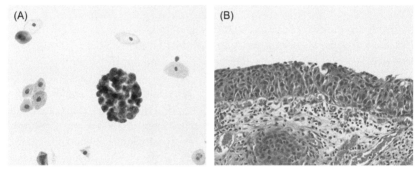

FIGURE 6.5 Features of urothelial carcinoma *in situ*. (A) Voided-urine, liquid-based cytology shows loosely cohesive urothelial cells with enlarged nuclei with coarsely granular chromatin, high nuclear-to-cytoplasmic ratios, and irregular nuclear outlines. Based on cytological features, high-grade urothelial carcinoma and carcinoma in situ are indistinguishable. (B) Histological features of carcinoma in situ from the same patient.

URINARY BIOMARKERS

Urinary biomarkers have been investigated for roles as potential alternatives or adjuncts to standard tests for the initial diagnosis of bladder cancer or the identification of recurrent disease. The FDA has approved qualitative BTA *Stat* (Polymedco, Cortland, NY, USA), quantitative BTA TRAK (Polymedco), quantitative NMP22 (Alere, Waltham, MA, USA), qualitative NMP22 BladderChek Test (Alere), and UroVysion (Abbot Laboratoris, Abbott Park, IL, USA) for diagnosis and follow-up, whereas ImmunoCyt/UCyt (DiagnoCure, Québec, Canada) is approved for follow-up [14,15]. The qualitative NMP22 and BTA tests can be performed as point-of-care tests, whereas the others are performed in a laboratory. These biomarker tests are summarized in Table 6.1.

TABLE 6.1 Currently Available Urinary Biomarker Assays

Urinary Biomarker	Assay Type	Sensitivity Mean (Range)	Specificity Mean (Range)	Advantages	Disadvantages
NMP22	Immunochromatic assay or sandwich ELISA	67.5% (31.0%–91.7%)	74.4% (5.1%–94.3%)	Unaffected by BCG, detects low-grade tumors	High false-positive rate, no clearly defined cutoff value
BTA *stat* (complement factor H-related protein)	Dipstick immunoassay	68.7% (52.8%–89.0%)	73.7% (54.0%–93.0%)	Sensitivity and specificity	Influenced by benign genitourinary conditions
BTA TRAK	Sandwich ELISA	62.0% (17.0%–77.5%)	73.6% (50.5%–95.0%)		
BLCA-4	ELISA	93% (90%–95%)	97% (95%–98%)	Sensitivity and specificity	Needs further study
UroVysion (chromosomal aneuploidy)	Multicolor, multiprobe FISH	77% (73%–81%)	98% (96%–100%)	Unaffected by BCG	Labor-intensive and expensive
ImmunoCyt	Immunocytochemistry	58.2% (38.5%–86.1%)	78.8% (73.0%–83.9%)		High interobserver variability
Survivin	Bio-dot test, ELISA	64% (35%–83%)	93% (88%–93%)	Sensitivity and specificity	Needs further study
UBC (cytokeratins)	Sandwich ELISA or point-of-care test	60.7% (48.7%–70.0%)	83.8% (72.0%–95.0%)		Influenced by benign genitourinary conditions and vesical instillations
CYFRA 21-1 (cytokeratin fragment)	Immunoradiometric assay or electrochemiluminescent immunoassay	74.2% (69.0%–79.3%)	91.3% (88.6%–94.0%)		

Soluble Urinary Biomarkers

Nuclear Matrix Protein-22

Nuclear matrix proteins (NMPs) form part of the internal structural framework of the cell nucleus. This nonchromatin structure supports the nuclear shape, organizes DNA, and has important roles in DNA replication, transcription, and gene expression. NMP22 is a nuclear mitotic protein that is involved in the proper distribution of chromatin to daughter cells during cellular replication [14]. Healthy individuals have low levels of urinary NMP22, whereas patients with bladder cancer may have levels that are 25-fold higher. Urinary elevation of the ubiquitous cellular protein NMP22 is associated with increased cell death [16,17].

The standard test for NMP22 is a quantitative microtiter sandwich ELISA that uses two antibodies, each of which recognizes a different epitope of the protein. This assay should be carried out in a laboratory by trained personnel, so it is not a point-of-care test. Because the NMP22 test is quantitative, it is important to note the cutoff value that is used in any particular study. Although the manufacturer's recommended cutoff value is 10 U/mL, variable limits ranging from 3.6 U/mL to 27 U/mL have been applied, depending on the optimum sensitivity and specificity determined by the receiver operating curve. A qualitative point-of-care NMP22 assay has now become available, which involves addition of four drops of urine to a proprietary immunochromatographic-assay device; the results can be read 30–50 minutes later [18–20].

Results from various studies have demonstrated that the sensitivity of the NMP22 ELISA ranges from 47% to 100%, and is typically 60%–70%. Notably, these studies mostly involved patients without a history of bladder cancer. The sensitivity of the NMP22 assay increases with tumor size, grade, and stage. NMP22 measurement has a lower sensitivity to detect recurrent tumors than primary tumors because recurrent tumors often are smaller. The reported specificity of the ELISA assay is between 60% and 90%, depending on the cutoff value used. The NMP22 test has higher false-positive rates (33%–50%) in patients with urolithiasis, inflammation, benign prostatic hyperplasia, or urinary tract infections. Because of the high false-positive rate, the assay cannot be recommended without cystoscopy [15,21–23].

Both tests for NMP22 have been approved by the FDA for surveillance of bladder cancer, and BladderChek test is also approved for diagnosis in high-risk patients.

Bladder Tumor Antigen

BTA is also known as human complement factor H-related protein [24,25]. The BTA TRAK and BTA *stat* assays both measure levels of the protein in urine. BTA *stat* is a qualitative immunoassay that can be performed at the point-of-care within several minutes. BTA TRAK is a quantitative test that is performed in a laboratory [20]. The sensitivity of both the BTA *stat* and BTA TRAK tests varies with tumor grade and stage and the cutoff limit used on the test. The specificity of BTA *stat* and BTA TRAK tests in healthy individuals is ≥90%. However, these tests have lower specificity in patients with urinary tract infections, urinary calculi, nephritis, renal stones, cystitis, benign prostatic hyperplasia, hematuria, or proteinuria. Complement factor H is present in human serum at high concentrations (0.5 mg/mL), so the BTA *stat* test might give false-positive results in many benign conditions that cause hematuria. The manufacturer recommends that the BTA *stat* and BTA TRAK tests should only be used when information is available for the clinical evaluation of the patient and alongside other diagnostic procedures, and that the tests should not be used for screening [14,18,22,26,27].

The FDA has approved both BTA *stat* and BTA TRAK tests for use in the management of bladder cancer in combination with cystoscopy.

BLCA-4

Six NMPs that are specifically expressed in bladder cancer have been identified, including BLCA-4. Overexpression of BLCA-4 seems to increase the cellular growth rate and also causes cells to express a more tumorigenic phenotype [28]. Urinary levels of BLCA-4 are analyzed by ELISA, which has a reported sensitivity of 89%−96.4% and specificity of 95%−100%. These levels of sensitivity and specificity for detecting bladder cancer are promising but should be confirmed in a larger trial. In addition to BCLA-4, BLCA-1 is a potentially useful marker for bladder cancer that is currently under investigation [27,29,30].

Cytokeratins

Cytokeratins are proteins of cytoskeletal intermediate filaments, and their main function is to enable cells to withstand mechanical stress. In humans, 20 different cytokeratin isotypes have been identified. Cytokeratins 8, 18, 19, and 20 have been associated with bladder [31].

Cytokeratin fragment 21-1 (CYFRA 21-1) is a soluble fragment of cytokeratin 19 that can currently be measured either by a solid-phase sandwich immunoradiometric assay or an electrochemiluminescent immunoassay. On the basis of a limited number of studies, these CYFRA 21-1 assays have been estimated to have sensitivities of 75%−97% and specificities of 67%− 71% for the detection of bladder cancer [18]. Although CYFRA 21-1 seems to be the best cytokeratin-associated antigen for use as a urinary biomarker for bladder cancer, it does not perform well as a marker for low-stage bladder cancer, and urinary CYFRA21-1 levels are strongly influenced by benign urological diseases and therapeutic intravesical instillations [32].

The urinary bladder cancer tests UBC Rapid (Concile, Freiburg, Germany) and UBC-ELISA detects fragments of cytokeratins 8 and 18 in urine. UBC

Rapid is a point-of-care test, whereas UBC-ELISA is a 2 hour sandwich ELISA test. The results of several retrospective cohort and case–control studies have demonstrated that the sensitivities of UBC tests for detection of bladder cancer (both primary and recurrent) are between 35% and 79%. In addition to low overall sensitivity, these tests have especially low sensitivity for detection of both low-grade and low-stage tumors [33,34].

Survivin

Survivin is a member of a family of proteins that regulate cell death, known as the inhibitor of apoptosis family [35]. Overexpression of survivin inhibits extrinsic and intrinsic pathways of apoptosis. In bladder cancer, survivin is expressed in urine, and its expression is associated with disease recurrence, stage, progression, and mortality [32,35]. Immunohistochemical studies have shown that survivin expression is elevated in bladder cancer tissues, and that nuclear localization of survivin may be related to disease-free survival. The survivin levels in urine have been measured by immunoblotting with the BioDot microfiltration detection system, in which urine samples are blotted as dots on nitrocellulose membranes, and survivin present in the samples is detected using a rabbit polyclonal antisurvivin antibody and standard dot-blot detection reagents. In studies with limited numbers of patients with bladder cancer, the survivin dot-blot assay had 100% sensitivity. Its specificities among healthy individuals and patients with benign genitourinary conditions were 100% and 87%, respectively. Results from a limited number of studies have shown that survivin may be a useful marker for the detection of bladder cancer. However, more cohort studies are needed to evaluate this marker [18,35,36].

HA–HAase Test

The HA–HAase test is a combination of two tests that measure urinary levels of hyaluronic acid (HA) and hyaluronidase (HAase) [37]. HA is a glycosaminoglycan that promotes tumor metastasis, and its concentration is elevated in several tumors. Small, angiogenic fragments of HA are generated when HAase degrades HA. HYAL1-type HAase is the major tumor-derived HAase secreted by tumor cells, and a molecular determinant of bladder tumor growth and invasion. The HA test is an ELISA-like assay based on the competitive-binding principle that measures urinary HA levels (ng/mL), which are then normalized to total urinary protein (mg/mL). Urinary HA levels ≥ 500 ng/mg total protein (cutoff limit) constitute a positive HA test result. The HAase test is also an ELISA-like assay that measures urinary HAase activity (mU/mL), which is normalized to total urinary protein. Urinary HAase levels ≥ 10 mU/mg total protein constitute a positive HAase test result. The HA test detects bladder cancer, regardless of the tumor grade, whereas the HAase test preferentially detects bladder tumors of grades G2 and G3. The HA−HAase test is a combination of the HA and HAase tests. For a positive HA−HAase test result, either or both individual tests must be positive [18,37].

In case−control and cohort studies, the sensitivity of the HA−HAase test varies between 83% and 94% for detection of both primary and recurrent bladder tumors. The sensitivities of the test for detection of G1, G2, and G3 tumors are 75%−90%, 84%−100%, and 92%−100%, respectively. The overall specificity of the HA−HAase test in healthy individuals, patients with benign genitourinary conditions, and patients with a history of bladder cancer varies between 77% and 84%. This test may also be useful in screening a high-risk population for bladder cancer. However, the test is not commercially available [14,18,23,29].

Cell-Based Markers

uCyt

Immunocytology is based on the visualization of tumor-associated antigens in urothelial carcinoma cells via binding of labeled monoclonal antibodies [38]. uCyt, formerly known as ImmunoCyt, is a commercially available immunocytological assay that detects bladder cancer cells through the use of fluorescein-labeled monoclonal antibodies M344 and LDQ10 that are directed against sulfated-mucin glycoproteins, and a Texas red-linked monoclonal antibody 19A211 against glycosylated forms of high-molecular-weight carcinoembryonic antigens [34]. The sensitivity of uCyt varies from 38% to 100%, and the specificity ranges from 75% to 90%. The uCyt assay is sensitive and reasonably specific, and is suitable for use in combination with voided-urine cytology. However, issues associated with a steep learning curve, observer-dependent inference, and quality control should be addressed to improve the general acceptability of this test [18,28]. The assay has been approved by the FDA for surveillance of patients with a history of bladder cancer.

DD23

DD23 is a monoclonal antibody that detects a protein dimer expressed on bladder cancer cells [39]. This immunoglobulin G1 murine monoclonal antibody resulted from the immunization of a BALB/c mouse with fresh human bladder cancer. The DD23 antibody is used in an alkaline phosphatase-conjugated immunohistochemical assay and to visualize tumor cells in urine specimens. In a case−control study, the sensitivity for detection of bladder cancer was 85%, with a specificity of 95% [14,18,40].

UroVysion

UroVysion is a multitarget, multicolor fluorescence *in situ* hybridization (FISH) assay that involves staining of exfoliated cells in urine with four denatured, fluorescent, centromeric chromosome-enumeration probes [41]. These probes detect chromosome 3, chromosome 7, chromosome 17, and the chromosome 9p21 locus. After staining, cells are observed under a fluorescence microscope. The criteria for detection of bladder cancer by the UroVysion test are observation of five or more cells with a gain of two or more chromosomes, ≥10 cells with a gain of one chromosome, or ≥20% of cells with a loss of the 9p21 locus. Currently, however, no universally accepted criteria exist to determine the positivity of a FISH test. In case−control studies, the sensitivity of the UroVysion test ranges from 69% to 87%. The test has a high sensitivity to detect high-grade and high-stage tumors (83%−97%) and also to detect CIS (∼100%). The specificity of the UroVysion test, as reported in various studies, is high (89%−96%) in patients with a variety of benign genitourinary conditions. A potential advantage of a FISH-based method is the ability to detect occult disease not visible on urethrocystoscopy. A false-positive FISH test result can predict future recurrence within 3−12 months in 41%−89% of patients. Another advantage of FISH is that it is unaffected by Bacillus Calmette-Guérin (BCG) therapy and can be used for surveillance in patients who have been treated with intravesical BCG instillation. A disadvantage is that this test is labor-intensive and has a learning curve for reliable operation [18,29,35,42].

The UroVysion test has been approved by the FDA both for monitoring patients with a history of bladder cancer and for detection of bladder cancer in patients with hematuria.

CONCLUSIONS

Urinary cytology is undoubtedly effective for the detection of urothelial carcinomas, especially in high-grade cancer. Although technological improvements have been introduced to the process, urinary cytology has so far been limited to a mean sensitivity of ∼50% for the detection of urothelial carcinoma. Urinary biomarker assays that can be carried out in the clinic or laboratory each have strengths and weaknesses, and further validation studies or development of new assays will be needed before they can replace or fully complement urinary cytology. For routine use, these assays should reach quality criteria established by guidelines for the development of accurate biomarker tests [43]. Therefore urologists and scientists should contribute to the standardization of detection techniques and conduct prospective randomized trials to determine the most appropriate urinary biomarkers for the detection of bladder cancer.

REFERENCES

[1] Papanicolaou GN, Marshall VF. Urine sediment smears as a diagnostic procedure in cancers of the urinary tract. Science 1945;101:519−20.
[2] Hutchinson ML, Agarwal P, Denault T, Berger B, Cibas ES. A new look at cervical cytology. ThinPrep multicenter trial results. Acta Cytol 1992;36:499−504.

[3] Granados R, Butron M, Santonja C, Rodriguez JM, Martin A, Duarte J, et al. Increased risk of malignancy for non-atypical urothelial cell groups compared to negative cytology in voided urine. Morphological changes with LBC. Diagn Cytopathol 2016;44:582−90.

[4] Son SM, Koo JH, Choi SY, Lee HC, Lee YM, Song HG, et al. Evaluation of urine cytology in urothelial carcinoma patients: a comparison of cellprepplus(r) liquid-based cytology and conventional smear. Korean J Pathol 2012;46:68−74.

[5] Lu DY, Nassar A, Siddiqui MT. High-grade urothelial carcinoma: comparison of SurePath liquid-based processing with cytospin processing. Diagn Cytopathol 2009;37: 16−20.

[6] Straccia P, Bizzarro T, Fadda G, Pierconti F. Comparison between cytospin and liquid-based cytology in urine specimens classified according to the Paris system for reporting urinary cytology. Cancer Cytopathol 2016;124:519−23.

[7] Luo Y, She DL, Xiong H, Yang L, Fu SJ. Diagnostic value of liquid-based cytology in urothelial carcinoma diagnosis: a systematic review and meta-analysis. PLoS One 2015;10:e0134940.

[8] Bastacky S, Ibrahim S, Wilczynski SP, Murphy WM. The accuracy of urinary cytology in daily practice. Cancer 1999;87:118−28.

[9] Kocjan G, Gray W, Levine T, Kardum-Skein I, Vielh P. Diagnostic cytopathology essentials. Edinburgh: Churchill Livingstone Press; 2013.

[10] Eble JN, Sauter G, Epstein JI, Sesterhenn IA. World Health Organization pathology and genetics of tumours of the urinary system and male genital organs. Lyon: IARC Press; 2004.

[11] Grignon DJ. The current classification of urothelial neoplasms. Mod Pathol 2009;22 (Suppl 2):S60−9.

[12] O'Flanagan SJ, Fulton G, O'Beirne J, McElwain JP. Operative fixation of unstable pelvic ring injuries in polytrauma patients. Ir J Med Sci 1992;161:39−41.

[13] Orozco RE, Martin AA, Murphy WM. Carcinoma *in situ* of the urinary bladder. Clues to host involvement in human carcinogenesis. Cancer 1994;74:115−22.

[14] Mbeutcha A, Lucca I, Mathieu R, Lotan Y, Shariat SF. Current status of urinary biomarkers for detection and surveillance of bladder cancer. Urol Clin North Am 2016;43: 47−62.

[15] Chou R, Gore JL, Buckley D, Fu R, Gustafson K, Griffin JC, et al. Urinary biomarkers for diagnosis of bladder cancer: a systematic review and meta-analysis. Ann Intern Med 2015;163:922−31.

[16] Kumar A, Kumar R, Gupta NP. Comparison of NMP22 BladderChek test and urine cytology for the detection of recurrent bladder cancer. Jpn J Clin Oncol 2006;36:172−5.

[17] Chang Y-H, Wu C-H, Lee Y-L, Huang P-H, Kao Y-L, Shiau M-Y. Evaluation of nuclear matrix protein-22 as a clinical diagnostic marker for bladder cancer. Urology 2004;64:687−92.

[18] Lokeshwar VB, Habuchi T, Grossman HB, Murphy WM, Hautmann SH, Hemstreet GP, et al. Bladder tumor markers beyond cytology: international consensus panel on bladder tumor markers. Urology 2005;66:35−63.

[19] Dey P. Urinary markers of bladder carcinoma. Clin Chim Acta 2004;340:57−65.

[20] Glas AS, Roos D, Deutekom M, Zwinderman AH, Bossuyt PM, Kurth KH. Tumor markers in the diagnosis of primary bladder cancer. A systematic review. J Urol 2003; 169:1975−82.

[21] Shariat SF, Karam JA, Lotan Y, Karakiewizc PI. Critical evaluation of urinary markers for bladder cancer detection and monitoring. Rev Urol 2008;10:120−35.

[22] Miremami J, Kyprianou N. The promise of novel molecular markers in bladder cancer. Int J Mol Sci 2014;15:23897−908.

[23] Tilki D, Burger M, Dalbagni G, Grossman HB, Hakenberg OW, Palou J, et al. Urine markers for detection and surveillance of non−muscle-invasive bladder cancer. Eur Urol 2011;60:484−92.

[24] Raitanen M, Kaasinen E, Rintala E, Hansson E, Nieminen P, Aine R, et al. Prognostic utility of human complement factor H related protein test (the BTA stat® Test). Br J Cancer 2001;85:552.

[25] D'Hallewin M-A, Baert L. Initial evaluation of the bladder tumor antigen test in superficial bladder cancer. J Urol 1996;155:475−6.

[26] Van Rhijn BW, Van der Poel HG, van Der Kwast TH. Urine markers for bladder cancer surveillance: a systematic review. Eur Urol 2005;47:736−48.

[27] Van Tilborg AA, Bangma CH, Zwarthoff EC. Bladder cancer biomarkers and their role in surveillance and screening. Int J Urol 2009;16:23−30.

[28] Konety BR, Nguyen T-ST, Dhir R, Day RS, Becich MJ, Stadler WM, et al. Detection of bladder cancer using a novel nuclear matrix protein, BLCA-4. Clin Cancer Res 2000;6: 2618−25.

[29] Vrooman OP, Witjes JA. Molecular markers for detection, surveillance and prognostication of bladder cancer. Int J Urol 2009;16:234−43.

[30] van Rhijn BW, van der Poel HG, van der Kwast TH. Cytology and urinary markers for the diagnosis of bladder cancer. Eur Urol Suppl 2009;8:536−41.

[31] Buchumensky V, Klein A, Zemer R, Kessler O, Zimlichman S, Nissenkorn I. Cytokeratin 20: a new marker for early detection of bladder cell carcinoma. J Urol 1998;160:1971−4.

[32] Vrooman OP, Witjes JA. Urinary markers in bladder cancer. Eur Urol 2008;53:909−16.

[33] Sullivan PS, Chan JB, Levin MR, Rao J. Urine cytology and adjunct markers for detection and surveillance of bladder cancer. Am J Transl Res 2010;2:412.

[34] Konety BR. Molecular markers in bladder cancer: a critical appraisal. Urol Oncol 2006;326−37.

[35] Smith SD, Wheeler MA, Plescia J, Colberg JW, Weiss RM, Altieri DC. Urine detection of survivin and diagnosis of bladder cancer. JAMA 2001;285:324−8.

[36] Shariat SF, Ashfaq R, Karakiewicz PI, Saeedi O, Sagalowsky AI, Lotan Y. Survivin expression is associated with bladder cancer presence, stage, progression, and mortality. Cancer 2007;109:1106−13.

[37] Hautmann SH, Lokeshwar VB, Schroeder GL, Civantos F, Duncan RC, Gnann R, et al. Elevated tissue expression of hyaluronic acid and hyaluronidase validates the HA-HAase urine test for bladder cancer. J Urol 2001;165:2068−74.

[38] Olsson H, Zackrisson B. ImmunoCytTM a useful method in the follow-up protocol for patients with urinary bladder carcinoma. Scand J Urol Nephrol 2001;35:280−2.

[39] Bonner RB, Liebert M, Hurst RE, Grossman HB, Bane BL, Hemstreet GP. Characterization of the DD23 tumor-associated antigen for bladder cancer detection and recurrence monitoring. Marker Network for Bladder Cancer. Cancer Epidemiol Biomarkers Prev 1996;5:971−8.

[40] Gilbert SM, Veltri RW, Sawczuk A, Shabsigh A, Knowles DR, Bright S, et al. Evaluation of DD23 as a marker for detection of recurrent transitional cell carcinoma of the bladder in patients with a history of bladder cancer. Urology 2003;61:539−43.

[41] Sarosdy MF, Schellhammer P, Bokinsky G, Kahn P, Chao R, Yore L, et al. Clinical evaluation of a multi-target fluorescent *in situ* hybridization assay for detection of bladder cancer. J Urol 2002;168:1950−4.

[42] Lokeshwar VB, Selzer MG. Urinary bladder tumor markers. Urol Oncol 2006;528−37.

[43] Shariat SF, Lotan Y, Vickers A, Karakiewicz PI, Schmitz-Drager BJ, Goebell PJ, et al. Statistical consideration for clinical biomarker research in bladder cancer. Urol Oncol 2010;28:389−400.

Chapter 7

Cystoscopy

Jeong W. Lee
Dongguk University Ilsan Hospital, Goyang, South Korea

Chapter Outline

The cystoscopy has currently remained the major technique for detection and surveillance of the bladder cancer with technical advancements in endoscopes and instruments. White light cystoscopy with rigid rod-lens systems is usually performed in the outpatient setting and offers excellent visualization of the whole mucosa of the bladder, in addition to the anterior and prostatic urethra. On the basis of the presence of visible change of the smooth urothelium, physicians can readily suspect and identified the site and characteristics of the most tumors. Macroscopic papillary tumors are relatively easy to visualize but dysplasia and carcinoma in situ (CIS) can be overlooked. Random biopsy of normal-appearing areas rarely results in the identification of unsuspected neoplasms, usually CIS. And it may increase tumor seeding. Riedl and colleagues demonstrated that 37% of the biopsies performed on the basis of suspicious cystoscopic findings results in a false-negative biopsy (Fig. 7.1).

Since white light cystoscopy can fail to detect many bladder lesions, such as CIS, there have been efforts to improve detection. Recent studies demonstrated that porphyrin-based fluorescence cystoscopy may improve the endoscopic detection of bladder tumors. This technique involves inspecting the bladder mucosa with blue light following the instillation of a precursor of a photoactive porphyrin, such as hexaminolevulinate (HAL). Photoactive porphyrins accumulate preferentially in neoplastic tissue and under blue light they emit red fluorescence, which can help in the diagnosis of premalignant and malignant lesions. Topical application of 5-aminolevulinic acid (5-ALA), a precursor of photoactive porphyrin, has improved the detection of bladder tumors with avoidance of systemic photosensitization but chemical modification of 5-ALA may be improved accumulation in tumor cells with deeper tissue penetration. HAL, a lipophilic ester of 5-ALA, was

Bladder Cancer. DOI: http://dx.doi.org/10.1016/B978-0-12-809939-1.00007-2

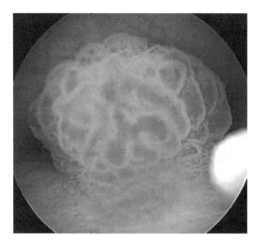

FIGURE 7.1 Papillary bladder tumor under white light cystoscopy.

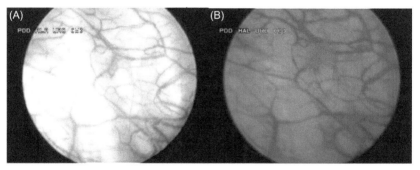

FIGURE 7.2 Small micropapillary tumor. (A) under white light cystoscopy and (B) under HAL fluorescence cystoscopy [1].

developed for fluorescence diagnosis of bladder cancer under blue light illumination. In a study of 52 patients with bladder cancer the sensitivity of HAL fluorescence cystoscopy was 96% and was 73% for white light cystoscopy. Two multicenter, phase 3 trials for the detection of bladder cancer presented that detection rates for Ta tumors were 95% for HAL cystoscopy and 83% for white light cystoscopy. Detection rates were 95% and 86%, respectively, for T1 tumors. At the biopsy level the mean detection rate for CIS lesions was 92% with HAL cystoscopy compared with only 68% for white light cystoscopy. The mean false-positive detection rate for HAL cystoscopy was higher than that for white light cystoscopy (39% vs 31%). Jocham and colleagues demonstrated that HAL cystoscopy improved detection of overall tumor, including dysplasia, CIS, and superficial papillary tumors. Of all tumors 96% were detected with HAL cystoscopy compared with 77% using white light cystoscopy. This difference was particularly noticeable for dysplasia (93% vs 48%), CIS (95% vs 68%), and superficial papillary tumors (96% vs 85%) (Fig. 7.2).

Flexible fiberoptic cystoscopy is almost as effective and cause markedly less pain than rigid cystoscopy in men, although there is no clear advantage to their use in women. HAL fluorescence flexible cystoscopy compared to HAL rigid cystoscopy is almost equivalent results in detecting papillary and flat lesion in bladder cancer patients. Both procedures were superior to standard white light flexible cystoscopy.

REFERENCE

[1] Jocham D, Witjes F, Wagner S, Zeylemaker B, van Moorselaar J, Grimm MO, et al. Improved detection and treatment of bladder cancer using hexaminolevulinate imaging: a prospective, phase III multicenter study. J Urol 2005;174:862−6.

FURTHER READING

van der Meijden A, Oosterlinck W, Brausi M, Kurth KH, Sylvester R, de Balincourt C. Significance of bladder biopsies in Ta, T1 bladder tumors: a report from the EORTC Genito-Urinary Tract Cancer Cooperative Group. EORTC-GU Group Superficial Bladder Committe. Eur Urol 1999;35:267−71.

Riedl CR, Daniltchenko D, Koenig F, Simak R, Loening SA, Pflueger H. Fluorescence endoscopy with 5-aminolevulinic acid reduces early recurrence rate in superficial bladder cancer. J Urol 2001;165:1121−3.

Jichlinski P, Guillou L, Karlsen SJ, Malmstrom PU, Jocham D, Brennhovd B, et al. Hexyl aminolevulinate fluorescece cystoscopy: new diagnostic tool for photodiagnosis of superficial bladder cancer—a multicenter study. J Urol 2003;170:226−9.

Zaak D, Hungerhuber E, Schneede P, Stepp H, Frimberger D, Corvin S, et al. Role of 5-aminolevulinic acid in the detection of urothelial premalignant lesions. Cancer 2002;95:1234−8.

Schmidbauer J, Witjes F, Schmeller N, Donat R, Susani M, Marberger M. Improved detection of urothelial carcinoma in situ with hexaminolevulinate fluorescence cystoscopy. J Urol 2004;171:135−8.

Koenig F, McGovern FJ, Larne R, Enquist H, Schomacker KT, Deutsch TF. Diagnosis of bladder carcinoma using protoporphyrin IX fluorescence indeced by 5-aminolaevulinic acid. BJU Int 1999;83:129−35.

Grossman HB, Gomella L, Fradet Y, Morales A, Presti J, Ritenour C, et al. A phase III, multicenter comparison of hexaminolevulinate fluorescence cystoscopy and white light cystoscopy for the detection of superficial papillary lesions in patients with bladder cancer. J Urol 2007;178:62−7.

Fradet Y, Grossman HB, Gomella L, Lerner S, Cookson M, Albala D, et al. A comparison of hexaminolenulinate fluorescence cystoscopy and white light cystoscopy for the detection of carcinoma in situ in patients with bladder cancer: a phase III, multicenter study. J Urol 2007;178:68−73.

Clayman RV, Reddy P, Lange PH. Flexible fiberoptic and rigid-rod lens endoscopy of the lower urinary tract: a prospective controlled comparison. J Urol 1984;131:715−16.

Walker L, Liston TG, Lloyd-Davies RW. Does flexible cystoscopy miss more tumours than rod-lens examinations? Br J Urol 1993;72:449−50.

Seklehner S, Remzi M, Fajkovic H, Saratlija-Novakovic Z, Skopek M, Resch I, et al. Prospective multi-institutional study analyzing pain perception of flexible and rigid cystoscopy in men. Urology 2015;85:737−41.

Loidl W, Schmidbauer J, Susani M, Marberger M. Flexible cystoscopy assisted by hexaminolevulinate induced fluorescence: a new approach for bladder cancer detection and surveillance? Eur Urol 2005;47:323−6.

Chapter 8

Bladder Cancer: Imaging

Sungmin Woo and Jeong Y. Cho
Seoul National University Hospital, Seoul, South Korea

Chapter Outline

INTRODUCTION

Bladder cancer is the fifth most commonly diagnosed cancer in the United States with estimated 76,960 new cases and 16,390 cancer-related deaths in 2016 [1]. The incidence is greater in men and increased with age, peaking in the 60s and 70s. About 90% of all bladder tumors originate from the urothelium, and hence are called transitional cell carcinoma (TCC) [2]. Bladder TCC is commonly staged according to the tumor, nodes, metastases (TNM) staging system [3]. While T stage is categorized according to the degree of invasion of the bladder wall, bladder TCC is largely divided into nonmuscle-invasive bladder cancer (NMIBC) and MIBC, which account for approximately 80%−85% and 20%−25%, respectively [4].

Determination of the correct TNM staging category is important in patients with bladder cancer, because it directly associated with treatment planning, prediction of treatment success and prognosis. For example, NMIBC may be solely treated with transurethral resection (TUR), while MIBC will require

Bladder Cancer. DOI: http://dx.doi.org/10.1016/B978-0-12-809939-1.00008-4
87

cystectomy or even adjuvant treatment. Unfortunately, preoperative clinical staging by clinical examination, cystoscopic biopsy, and imaging is often discrepant from final pathologic staging. Currently, preoperative imaging is mainly based on conventional anatomical imaging using computed tomography (CT) or magnetic resonance imaging (MRI). They are in widely used in this clinical setting and have replaced the more traditional intravenous pyelography [5]. However, there is still concern with regard to their ability to detect small tumors, accurately stage local invasion, and identify metastatic lymph nodes. Recent advances in MRI technology show promising results and there is cumulating evidence for them to be used for bladder cancer assessment.

In this chapter, we discuss several aspects of imaging used for diagnosis and staging of bladder cancer. Especially, the role of each imaging modality including their strengths and limitations is described. As CT and MRI are currently the most commonly used imaging techniques for assessment of the bladder, common imaging findings and differential imaging features between stages is focused on those acquired with CT and MRI. Furthermore, the potential of advanced MRI techniques as imaging biomarkers with predictive and prognostic value is discussed. In addition, although most of the chapters will deal with bladder TCC, a brief summary of the imaging findings of rare nonurothelial tumors is also provided.

DIAGNOSIS

Brief Introduction of Imaging Modalities

The role of imaging in patients with diagnosed or presumed TCC of the bladder differs according to the modality of imaging used. This depends on several factors such as the inherent spatial and contrast (soft tissue) resolution of each modality, which significantly affect the efficacy in detecting small-sized tumors and differentiating between the tumor and layers of the bladder wall for accurate staging. Therefore it is important to understand the inherent ability and limitation of each modality in order to apply them in the appropriate clinical setting, and to accurately interpret them.

Currently, CT urography is considered the imaging modality of choice when investigating hematuria and radiologically staging known bladder cancer patients [6]. With contemporary scanners (64-slice multidetector CT), high spatial resolution is guaranteed, enabling high detection rates of even small tumors. However, the most important disadvantage of CT is that it cannot distinguish the layers of the bladder [7]. In addition, another major problem with using CT urography is the high radiation dose. Some experts recommend modalities other than CT be used in patients who are unlikely to harbor urothelial cancer or are radiosensitive [8].

MRI is another important imaging modality in bladder cancer management. While conventional MRI sequences, that is, T1-weighted imaging

(T1WI) and T2-weighted imaging (T2WI), which are used for morphological assessment, are already implemented in clinical practice, relatively new functional MRI sequences such as diffusion-weighted imaging (DWI), dynamic contrast-enhanced MRI (DCE-MRI), and lymphotrophic nanoparticle-enhanced MRI are being investigated with promising preliminary results [9]. Compared with CT, MRI demonstrates better soft tissue contrast and provides a multiparametric approach using various MRI sequences, potentially offering better detection and staging ability. For instance, on T1WI, urine shows low signal intensity (SI), while both the bladder tumor and detrusor muscle demonstrate intermediate SI. On the contrary, perivesical fat shows high SI [9]. On T2WI, urine shows very high SI (commonly referred to as fluid SI), while bladder tumors demonstrate high SI and the detrusor muscle exhibits prominent low SI [9]. Fig. 8.1 shows the differentiation of normal layers of the bladder wall with relationship with bladder tumor on T2WI of MRI. How such information can be used for local staging will be dealt with in more depth in the section describing TNM staging of bladder tumors.

Ultrasound is widely used for evaluating patients with hematuria. This is mainly due to its ability to detect renal masses and hydronephrosis. However, it is not included in most staging algorithms or guidelines for diagnosis of bladder cancer due to several limitations. Transabdominal sonography shows poor sensitivity in detecting bladder tumors. Imaging efficacy can be improved using transvaginal or transrectal approaches, but only in specific areas of the bladder. However, local staging cannot be done accurately as the

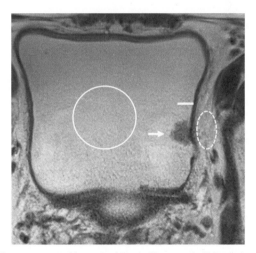

FIGURE 8.1 Fifty-seven-year-old man with papillary urothelial carcinoma demonstrating normal differentiation of layers of the bladder wall on axial T2WI of MRI. Bladder tumor (*arrow*) on left lateral wall of bladder shows high SI between that of urine (*circle*) and detrusor muscle of bladder wall (*line*) showing prominently low SI. Adjacent perivesical fat shows high SI (*dotted circle*) and can be differentiated from tumor and bladder wall.

normal layers of the bladder wall cannot be distinguished and extravesical structures are poorly visualized on ultrasound [10]. Nevertheless, there have been recent improvements in ultrasound technology, including three-dimensional ultrasound, contrast-enhanced ultrasound using microbubbles, and cystoscopic intravesical ultrasound with potential to increase the accuracy of detection and staging of bladder cancer (Fig. 8.2) [11,12]. Still, compared with CT and MRI, ultrasonography is subjective, and dependent on the experience of the examiner [13].

Virtual cystoscopy is a technique, which reconstructs a three-dimensional model from cross-sectional imaging data [5]. While it can be rendered from any of the modalities of ultrasound, CT or MRI, one of several methods is utilized in order for better visualization of bladder wall abnormalities: using catheterization to drain residual urine followed by insufflation with air or carbon dioxide [14]; without catheterization but delayed bladder filling with

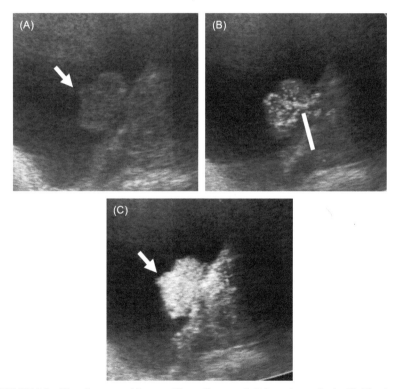

FIGURE 8.2 Sixty-four-year-old man with papillary urothelial carcinoma in the bladder demonstrated on contrast-enhanced ultrasound. (A) Papillary mass (*arrow*) on bladder wall protruding into lumen is seen on gray-scale ultrasound. (B,C) After intravenous injection with microbubble contrast agent, flow of microbubbles via the stalk into tumor (*line*) is initially detected (B), followed by homogeneous bright enhancement (*arrow*) of whole tumor (C). TUR of bladder revealed grade II Ta stage urothelial carcinoma.

intravenous contrast media [15]; direct contrast media administration into the bladder via catheterization [16]; oral hydration [17]; or without any preparative measures other than simply "not emptying the bladder for at least 1 hour" [18]. According to the literature, virtual cystoscopy using three-dimensional ultrasound showed greater sensitivity than transabdominal ultrasound (Fig. 8.2) [19]. In addition, when comparing between modalities, virtual cystoscopy using CT was more sensitive (94% vs 91%) and specific (98% vs 95%) than that using MRI in a recent meta-analysis [20]. Despite these reported high diagnostic accuracies, there are a few obstacles for virtual cystoscopy to be used routinely. First, flat lesions cannot be detected because virtual cystoscopy can only visualize the morphology of the intraluminal surface but not discoloration; second, small lesions may be obscured in dependent areas due to pooled urine or contrast media; third, it is relatively more invasive compared with CT urography or MRI, especially when catheterization is performed for bladder filling with air or contrast media [21].

When evaluating the bladder using CT or MRI, contrast media administration is frequently performed for two reasons. First, contrast media excreted in the urinary tract improve distension of the upper urinary tract (in order to evaluate the presence of coexistent upper urinary tract TCC) and of the bladder. In case of the bladder, underdistention causes diffuse wall thickening, which hinders detection of small bladder TCCs. Furthermore, it can be mistaken for diffuse TCC [22]. Although several contrast agents including air and carbon dioxide insufflation have been tested for this rationale [23], currently iodinated contrast media for CT and gadolinium-based contrast media for MRI are regarded as the standard. High attenuation or SI on CT and MRI, respectively, of the contrast media filling the bladder lumen renders not only bladder distension but also enhanced differentiation between the intraluminal space and the tumor. Along with contrast media administration, several other ancillary techniques can be applied when performing CT and MRI for bladder distension: oral hydration, intravenous (IV) hydration with saline, and IV diuretics administration [24]. Second, there is increasing evidence that early phase enhanced images, whether arterial or venous, can increase lesion conspicuity, or even increase the sensitivity of bladder TCC detection [24,25]. Although TCC has been regarded as hypovascular, they show considerable early enhancement (at approximately 60 seconds) followed by washout compared with the bladder wall, therefore making them more conspicuous in early enhanced phases. Regarding the use of contrast media, caution is required in a certain subgroup of patients. Iodinated contrast media should be carefully administered if the patient has previously experienced allergic or adverse reactions. Guidelines recommend hydration, discontinuation of nephrotoxic drugs, premedication with appropriate drugs (i.e., corticosteroids), and prompt treatment in case of adverse reactions [26]. In case of gadolinium-based contrast media, those with severe renal insufficiency (glomerular filtration rate <30 mL/min/1.73 m^2) should be cautioned of the increased risk of nephrogenic systemic fibrosis [27].

In order to optimally assess CT urography and MRI for detecting and staging bladder TCC, several important approaches are needed. First, image review should be done in at least two planes (axial, coronal, or sagittal) as smaller tumors are better visualized in certain planes [28]. For example, lesions in the lateral wall and dome of the bladder are better demonstrated on coronal planes, while those in the anterior or posterior wall are optimally visualized in the sagittal planes [9]. On CT, the window width should be adjusted to both narrow and wide settings in order to enhance detection of small lesions in the early enhanced and excretory phases. Using a too narrow window width setting (soft tissue window) in the excretory phase will hinder detection of small filling defects.

Imaging Findings of Bladder Cancer (Including Detection Rate)

Typical Imaging Features

Bladder cancer can manifest with diverse imaging findings. It can appear as wall thickening, nodule or mass, abnormal urothelial enhancement, or calcification.

Wall thickening associated with bladder TCC is usually nodular or irregular (Fig. 8.3) [24]. On the other hand, diffuse wall thickening is generally

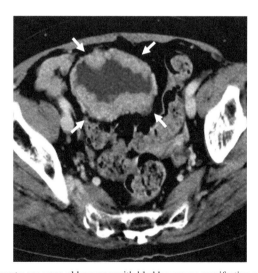

FIGURE 8.3   Seventy-one-year-old woman with bladder cancer manifesting with diffuse irregular bladder wall thickening. Axial contrast-enhanced CT scan shows diffuse, nodular, and irregular wall thickening involving whole bladder (*arrows*). Radical cystectomy revealed T2b stage high-grade papillary urothelial carcinoma.

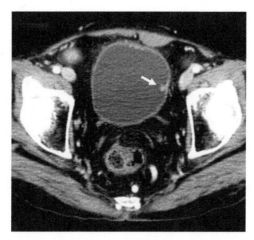

FIGURE 8.4 Sixty-nine-year-old man with small bladder cancer appearing as small nodule. Axial contrast-enhanced CT scan shows small nodule on left lateral wall of bladder. TUR of bladder revealed Ta stage grade II papillary urothelial carcinoma.

found in benign conditions, such as cystitis. Furthermore, in a nondistended bladder, the bladder wall (especially anterior) could normally look thickened, and should be interpreted with caution [22].

Bladder nodules or masses should always raise the suspicion for bladder TCC (Fig. 8.4). On CT urography, they can be found as early enhancing nodules or masses surrounded by low-density water attenuation urine, or as filling defects surrounded by the high-attenuating contrast media on excretory phases. On MRI, the nodule or mass shows intermediate SI on T1WI and high SI on T2WI [29]. Compared with TCC, the bladder wall shows similar SI on T1WI and lower SI on T2WI (especially low SI of the detrusor muscle), and urine shows lower SI on T1WI and higher SI on T2WI, allowing for detection of the urothelial nodule or mass. Early contrast-enhanced images and excretory phases on MRI can also be used similarly to CT urography for clearer demonstration of the nodule or mass [30].

Abnormal urothelial enhancement, especially associated with bladder wall thickening or nodule/mass, is another suspicious finding for bladder TCC (Fig. 8.5). Due to increased vascular density and also the increased diameter and permeability of vessels in the tumor, bladder TCC shows earlier and stronger enhancement (at about 1 minute after contrast administration) on CT and MRI, compared with the bladder muscle layer, which remains relatively poorly enhanced [9,31,32].

Calcification can also be seen in bladder TCC (Fig. 8.6) [22]. Although it is more frequently encountered after previously treated infection or malignancy or after intravesical *Bacille Calmette Guérin* therapy, when calcification is found in areas of bladder wall thickening or nodule/mass, the patient should be further evaluated for the presence of TCC.

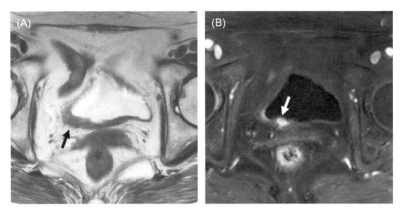

FIGURE 8.5   Seventy-nine-year-old woman with bladder tumor manifesting with abnormal urothelial enhancement on MRI. (A) On axial T2-weighted image, tumor is difficult to recognize because diffuse bladder wall thickening from previous procedures is seen in right posterior bladder wall. (B) On axial contrast-enhanced MRI, focal nodular enhancement of the urothelium is demonstrated within the diffuse wall thickening. TUR of bladder revealed high-grade papillary urothelial carcinoma with proper muscle invasion.

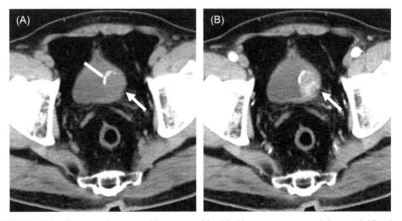

FIGURE 8.6   Seventy-nine-year-old man with bladder cancer containing calcification. (A) Axial unenhanced CT demonstrates mass (*arrow*) at left posterolateral bladder wall showing surface calcification (*line*). (B) Axial contrast-enhanced CT shows irregular enhancement in the solid portion of mass (*arrow*). Radical cystectomy revealed T2 stage high-grade urothelial carcinoma.

DWI is useful for identifying bladder TCC. DWI is a functional MRI sequence, which measures Brownian motion, or in other words, the random movement of water molecules [33]. In tumorous conditions, such as bladder TCC, increased cellularity and the resultant loss of extracellular space inhibit this random motion, causing "diffusion restriction," which is demonstrated as high SI on DWI (Fig. 8.7). In contrast, normal tissue (i.e., bladder wall

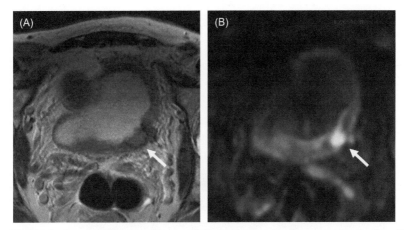

FIGURE 8.7 Seventy-three-year-old man with bladder cancer showing better visualization with DWI. (A) Axial T2WI shows focal nodular lesion (*arrow*) on left posterolateral bladder with slightly higher SI than bladder wall. (B) On axial DWI tumor is better localized due to suppression of background signal, highlighting area with tumor (*arrow*). Radical cystectomy revealed T3b stage high-grade papillary urothelial carcinoma.

not involved with cancer) and the background tissues are suppressed [34]. Not only does bladder TCC manifest with high SI lesions on DWI, but also quantitatively measured apparent diffusion coefficients (ADCs) of bladder TCC are reported to be significantly lower than those measured in urine and normal bladder wall: 1.18, 3.28, and 2.27×10^{-3} mm^2/s for bladder TCC, urine and normal bladder wall, respectively [35].

Bladder TCC is sometimes seen in diverticula. Bladder diverticula are outpouching of the urothelial lining via a defect or thinning in the muscle layer. As diverticula are lined with urothelium and urinary stasis with subsequent chronic infection/inflammation leads to metaplasia, bladder TCC can form within the diverticula [36]. The imaging findings of diverticular bladder cancer are not significantly different from that of nondiverticular tumors, other than the fact that they are located within the diverticulum (Fig. 8.8). However, the presence of TCC in diverticula should be carefully evaluated on imaging, because cystoscopic approach may be limited and because diverticular TCC poses a higher risk for extravesical spread due to the lack or thinning of muscle layer [37].

Diagnostic Efficacy of Detecting Bladder TCC Using Imaging

Currently, cystoscopy is the reference standard for diagnosing bladder TCC. However, recent advances in CT and MRI have significantly increased the ability to detect and localize bladder cancer.

In the era of MDCT, CT urography has shown relatively good efficacy for detecting bladder TCC. In contemporary studies that have comprehensively

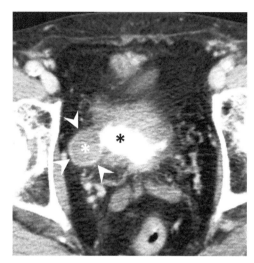

FIGURE 8.8 Seventy-two-year-old man with diverticular bladder cancer. On axial excretory phase contrast-enhanced CT, outpouching of bladder wall representing diverticulum (*arrowheads*) is seen on right upper lateral bladder wall. Lumen of diverticulum contains enhancing soft tissue (*white asterisk*) without filling of contrast material is bladder lumen elsewhere (*black asterisk*). Radical cystectomy revealed T3a stage grade II papillary urothelial carcinoma originating from diverticulum.

analyzed the efficacy of CT urography, the sensitivity, specificity, positive predictive value (PPV), and negative predictive value (NPV) ranged from 79% to 93%, 94% to 99%, 75% to 98%, and 95% to 97%, respectively [38,39]. There is increasing evidence that the addition of early contrast-enhanced phases (which include arterial, portal venous, or corticomedullary phases) may increase the detection rate (89%−97%) [25,32,40].

MRI using only conventional sequences (i.e., T2WI) has shown moderate efficacy for detecting bladder cancer. In a study by Nguyen et al. [41], T2WI yielded a sensitivity, specificity, and accuracy of 81%, 63%, and 77%, respectively, for detecting bladder cancer based on cystectomy as the reference standard. Using functional MRI sequences of DWI and DCE-MRI solely or as an adjunct to conventional MRI is considered to enhance bladder cancer detection. Investigators have reported sensitivity of 83%−100%, specificity of 75%−100%, PPV of 89%−100%, NPV of 91%−92%, and overall accuracies of 78%−98% for bladder cancer detection [42−44]. Other investigators found that DCE-MRI can help identify bladder TCC with sensitivity of 90%−92%, specificity of 63%−92%, PPV of 98%, NPV of 69%, and overall accuracy of 86%−90% [41,45]. Although DWI and DCE-MRI may add incremental value for detection of bladder TCC, it is recommended that they be used in conjunction with conventional sequences (i.e., T2WI), especially in the case of DWI, as the poorer spatial resolution of functional MRI sequence limits accurate anatomical evaluation.

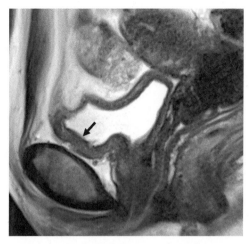

FIGURE 8.9   Pseudothickening of bladder wall due to underdistention in 45-year-old woman who underwent MRI for evaluation of uterine fibroids. On sagittal T2WI, bladder is diffusely thickened, especially at the anterior wall (*arrow*). This is not pathological finding but commonly encountered pseudothickening in bladder with underdistention.

As such, CT urography and MRI have shown remarkable improvement in the detection of bladder TCC. However, the most important limitation of CT and MRI is that they have limited ability in detecting small (<1 cm) or flat tumors [28,46]. Wang et al. [46] found that approximately two-thirds of tumors smaller than 1 cm were undetectable on CT urography. Especially, the fact that CT and MRI cannot detect flat tumors is problematic in that they will not be able to detect carcinoma in situ (CIS), a high-grade flat bladder TCC, which is known to harbor greater risk of recurrence after treatment and progression into MIBC compared with papillary tumors [4]. CIS is easily identified at cystoscopy with a "velvety" appearance (Fig. 8.9). Therefore CT and MRI cannot be replaced the role of cystoscopy as the reference standard for initial detection of bladder cancer. Yet, there are some instances in which CT and MRI can identify tumors that may be missed using cystoscopy. One example would be detection of bladder TCC in a diverticula, where cystoscopic approach may not be possible.

STAGING

Current guidelines recommend some form of radiological assessment for staging after the diagnosis of bladder cancer [47]. CT or MRI is one of the most frequently used modalities for staging of sessile or high-grade NMIBC and MIBC. However, despite the remarkable technological improvements in CT and MRI, they perform relatively poorly, especially with high rates of understaging (up to 42%) in MIBC and only moderate sensitivity and specificity in identifying metastatic lymph nodes. Therefore the T staging is initially performed using cystoscopy with deep biopsy. The following section describes the imaging findings of bladder TCC according to TNM staging, and the diagnostic efficacy of CT and MRI for staging.

T Stage

Before assessing the T stage of bladder TCC, it is important to assess the degree of bladder distension. When underdistended, the normal bladder wall may appear thickened and mistakenly considered to be tumor (Fig. 8.9); on the other hand, when overdistended, small tumors may become flattened and missed, and therefore hindering accurate assessment of T stage [48].

According to the literature, CT and MRI perform relatively poorly in determining the primary stage of bladder TCC. The reported sensitivity, specificity, and accuracy for overall T staging are 93%−95%, 28%−71%, and 35%−55% for CT and 80%−100%, 78%−91%, and 62%−85% for MRI, respectively [49−56]. Especially, CT is prone to poor differentiation between T1, T2, and T3 bladder TCCs, because of its lack of ability to identify the layers of the normal bladder wall. As a result, CT cannot be used to differentiate between NMIBC and MIBC. Compared with CT, MRI offers significantly better soft tissue resolution and therefore can potentially improve the assessment of the depth of tumor invasion [55]. On T2WI the tumor shows high SI compared to low SI of the detrusor muscle. As a result, in certain cases, non-MIBC can be accurately diagnosed if the low SI layer (detrusor muscle) is preserved [29]. Even with the advantage of greater soft tissue resolution, the diagnostic accuracy for staging of MRI has not been significant superior to CT during the past few decades. Nevertheless, with recent implementation of functional MRI sequences, initial reports show promising results using DWI and DCE-MRI for improved staging accuracy of the primary tumor.

The following are representative imaging features for each T stage according to the TNM staging system [3]. However, the reader must keep in mind they are not specific for each stage. In addition, as CT cannot distinguish between the normal anatomical layers of the bladder wall, differentiation between T1 through T3 tumors are limited. Therefore the described imaging findings for each stage are focused on MRI.

Tis (Carcinoma In Situ)

By definition, Tis tumors are invisible on CT and MRI [34]. The spatial resolution of these imaging modalities is unable to depict the flat cancerous changes in the urothelium.

Ta-T1

Stage Ta or T1 tumors appear as a papillary or sessile mass. Papillary tumors characteristically have a stalk, which consists of submucosal edema and fibrosis [57]. This stalk usually shows low SI on T2WI compared with the high SI of the tumor itself, therefore resembling an "inchworm." However, the T2WI SI of the stalk can sometimes be variable (higher, similar, and lower SI compared with the muscle in 14%, 56%, and 30%, respectively). If the SI of the stalk is similar to the tumor, the tumor may be misinterpreted as a sessile mass. Even in such cases, DWI be of added value as the stalk will almost always show low SI (Fig. 8.10) [34]. In sessile tumors, thickening of the submucosa due to inflammation or fibrosis can mimic muscle invasion from the tumor on T2WI. In T1 or lower tumors, this submucosal area shows lower SI than that of the tumor, which shows high SI on DWI [58]. On DCE-MRI the tumor, mucosa, and submucosa enhance earlier than the muscle layer. Therefore the presence of submucosal linear enhancement under the tumor base at early enhanced phases indicates stage T1 or lower (Fig. 8.11) [52]. When the stalk and submucosal linear enhancement are comprehensively used together, the ability of differentiating stage T1 or lower from T2 cancers can be enhanced [59].

T2

T2 tumors consist of T2a and T2b tumors according to the depth of muscle invasion (less than half and more than half, respectively). However, they cannot be accurately discriminated using MRI. On T2WI the low SI line

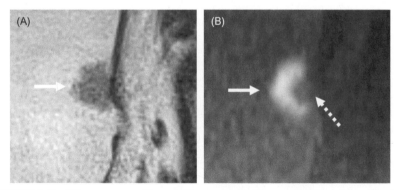

FIGURE 8.10 Fifty-seven-year-old man with stage Ta papillary urothelial carcinoma showing stalk on MRI. (A) Axial T2-weighted image shows papillary mass (*arrow*) on left lateral bladder wall. Stalk is not well visualized as it shows similar SI with mass. (B) On axial diffusion-weighted image, mass (*arrow*) shows high SI while stalk (*dotted arrow*) demonstrates low SI. TUR of bladder revealed Ta stage low-grade papillary urothelial carcinoma. Stalk can show variable SI with regard to bladder wall, sometimes leading to misinterpretation as sessile mass, but use of DWI can help identify stalk.

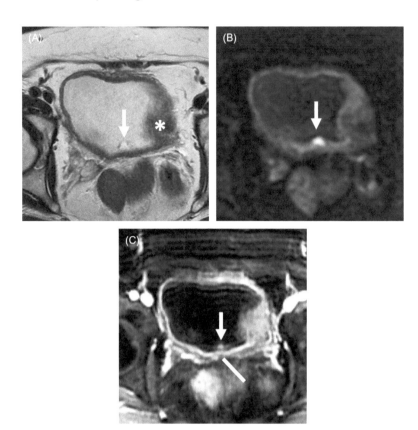

FIGURE 8.11 Seventy-one-year-old woman with T1 stage papillary urothelial carcinoma showing submucosal linear enhancement on MRI. (A) Axial T2WI shows nodular lesion (*arrow*) at posterior bladder wall showing high SI. Note that left lateral wall appears falsely thickened due to partial volume artifact (*asterisk*). (B) On axial DWI, nodule (*arrow*) shows bright SI, indicating tumor. (C) On contrast-enhanced MRI, submucosal linear enhancement (*line*) is seen just beneath tumor (*arrow*) indicating T1 or lower stage. Radical cystectomy revealed T1 stage high-grade urothelial carcinoma.

beneath the tumor, which is representative of the muscle layer, is focally disrupted (Fig. 8.12) [60]. In sessile tumors, when thickening of the submucosal layer is seen on T2WI, shows high SI similar to the tumor, but does not extend into the perivesical fat, and shows a smooth outer margin, it can be considered to be stage T2 [58]. Occasionally, retraction of the bladder wall can be associated with the bladder tumor. When such imaging finding is present, it provides indirect evidence of muscle invasion (stage T2) [29].

T3

T3 tumors are defined as tumors invading the perivesical tissue, which is mainly composed of fat. They are subclassified into T3a (microscopic

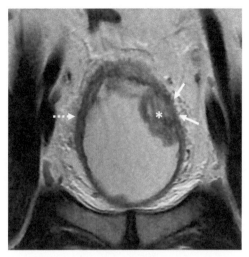

FIGURE 8.12 Forty-seven-year-old man with T2 stage papillary urothelial carcinoma. Coronal T2-weighted image shows papillary mass (*asterisk*) on left lateral wall of bladder. Compared with contralateral bladder wall (*dotted arrow*) showing normal low SI characteristics, there is disruption of bladder wall adjacent to tumor (*arrows*) suggestive of muscle invasion. Radical cystectomy revealed T2a stage high-grade papillary urothelial carcinoma.

invasion) and T3b (macroscopic invasion). The spatial resolution of CT and MRI is not sufficient to detect microscopic invasion into the perivesical tissue, and therefore, T3a tumors cannot be distinguished from T2b tumors. T3b tumors show perivesical stranding or extension of the tumor into the perivesical fat with irregular margin or nodularity (Fig. 8.13) [28,48,58]. MRI tends to show better sensitivity for detecting T3 disease compared with CT. However, this increased sensitivity is provided at the cost of lower specificity: it is not uncommon for MRI to overstage T2 tumors with perivesical inflammation as T3, especially if imaging is performed after TUR [32,61].

T4

Stage T4 is defined as invasion of the bladder tumor into adjacent organs. T4 is subcategorized into T4a, which includes invasion of the prostate, uterus, or vagina, and T4b, which includes invasion into the pelvic or abdominal wall. Imaging findings of T4 bladder tumors are relatively straightforward. CT and MRI can both be used to identify invasion of adjacent organs (Fig. 8.14). Although functional MRI sequences (especially DWI) assist in depicting the tumor extent, there is yet no evidence that using them have added value to conventional MRI sequences for identifying T4 disease [34].

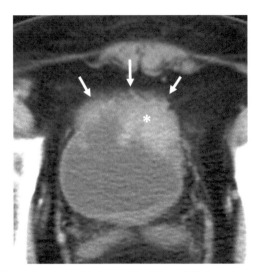

FIGURE 8.13 Seventy-one-year-old man with T3 urothelial carcinoma. Axial contrast-enhanced CT shows irregular wall thickening at anterior bladder wall (*asterisk*). Irregular and nodular outer contour (*arrows*) of bladder wall suggests perivesical fat invasion. Radical cystectomy revealed T3 stage high-grade urothelial carcinoma.

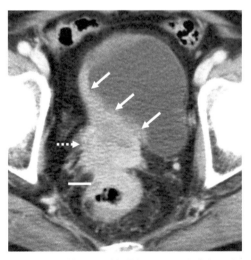

FIGURE 8.14 Eighty-two-year-old man with T4 stage urothelial carcinoma. Axial contrast-enhanced CT demonstrates enhancing mass-like wall thickening (*arrows*) in the left lateral and posterior bladder wall. This lesion is continuous with enhancing soft tissue extending via uterus (*dotted arrow*) to rectum (*line*). Pelvic exenteration revealed grade II urothelial carcinoma with invasion of uterine corpus and rectal submucosa (T4b stage).

N Stage

Detection of regional lymph node metastasis is important because the presence or absence of metastatic nodes will significantly alter treatment planning. Regional lymph nodes of bladder cancer include, perivesical, sacral and presacral, hypogastric, obturator, and external iliac stations [48]. Metastasis to further stations (common iliac and paraaortic) are regarded as distant metastasis. Conventional CT and MRI are limited in detecting metastatic lymph nodes, because it only provides anatomical and morphological information, as compared with positron-emission tomography (PET), which offers functional information (i.e., glucose metabolism in ^{18}F-fluorodeoxyglucose-PET). However, recent advances in technology, especially functional MRI techniques, have shown promising initial results and possibly will be implemented as routine imaging with further validation.

The conventional method to assess nodal metastasis is based on size criteria. Although several cut-off values have been used, contemporary studies suggest that nodes with a short diameter greater than 8 or 10 mm be considered as metastases [62]. However, this methodology is inherently faulty as small-sized lymph nodes can harbor micrometastatic deposits, and also because lymph nodes can be enlarged due to inflammatory reactive changes [49]. The reported accuracy of CT and conventional MRI for detecting metastatic lymph nodes are as follows: sensitivity, specificity, and overall accuracy of 85%, 67%−91%, and 54%−97% for CT and 76%−83%, 89%−98%, and 73%−98% for MRI, respectively [13,63−65].

In order to increase the accuracy of differentiating between metastatic and reactive lymph nodes, several measures can be taken. First, the shape of the lymph node may be useful in determining the metastatic status. Round nodes, that is, relatively similar dimensions of the short and long axes, have a greater chance of being metastases compared with ovoid nodes [66]. Furthermore, pelvic lymph nodes with irregular or ill-defined borders and SI lower than muscle or groin lymph nodes on T2WI are suggestive of metastasis [67]. On the contrary, bilateral symmetric appearance of the nodes and the presence of eccentrically located fat within the node indicate benignity. Fig. 8.15 shows a representative case demonstrating differential imaging points between benign and metastatic lymph nodes.

Advanced MRI techniques have been tested for their potential to increase the yield of detecting metastatic lymph nodes. These techniques include DCE-MRI, DWI, and nanoparticle-enhanced MRI. Regarding DCE-MRI the results have been controversial: some investigators argue that metastatic nodes show more rapid contrast agent uptake compared with benign nodes [66]; others report that the sensitivity of DCE-MRI is too low with a high false-negative rate [68]. DWI shows some promise in improving metastatic lymph node detection. First of all, DWI more clearly visualizes all lymph nodes, whether benign or metastatic (Fig. 8.16). Second, metastatic lymph

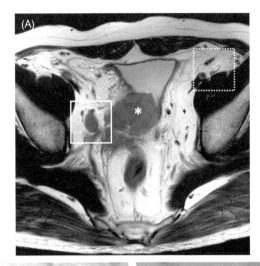

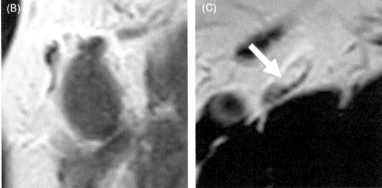

FIGURE 8.15 MRI of normal and metastatic lymph nodes in 62-year-old man with muscle-invasive high-grade urothelial carcinoma and metastatic lymphadenopathy. (A) Axial T2-weighted image shows irregular mass with high SI at posterior bladder wall (*asterisk*) suggestive of bladder cancer. Note right high obturator (*square*) and left external iliac lymph node (*dotted square*). (B) Right high obturator lymph node is enlarged and measures 1.2 cm in short axis (>8 or 10 mm) suggestive of metastasis. Also note its relatively round shape and loss of normal fatty hilum. (C) Left external iliac lymph node is small measuring 0.3 cm in short diameter. It is relatively flat-shaped with preserved fatty hilum (*arrow*). TUR of bladder revealed grade III muscle-invasive urothelial carcinoma. No histolopathology was acquired for lymph nodes, but after chemotherapy with gemcitabine-cisplatin size of right high obturator lymph node was significantly decreased suggestive of metastasis. Stability in size and initial imaging characteristics presume left external iliac lymph node to be benign.

nodes tend to show lower ADC values than benign nodes. In a study by Papalia et al. [64], metastatic and nonmetastatic lymph nodes were differentiated with a sensitivity and specificity of 76% and 89%, respectively, using a criteria of $<0.86 \times 10^{-3}$ mm^2/s for metastatic nodes. Still, there are conflicting results from other authors, suggesting that there are no significant

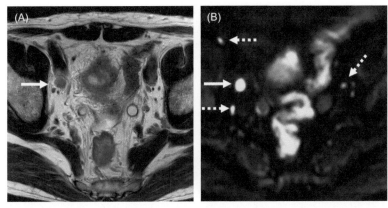

FIGURE 8.16 MRI of 73-year-old man with urothelial carcinoma and metastatic lymph nodes demonstrating usefulness of DWI for identifying lymph nodes. (A) Axial T2-weighted image above level of bladder shows enlarged right external iliac lymph node (*arrow*) suggestive of metastasis. Multiple enhancing polypoid lesions were present along bladder wall (not shown). (B) Axial DWI shows not only metastatic right external iliac lymph node (*arrow*), but also numerous smaller lymph nodes (*lines*) that were difficult to appreciate on T2-weighted image alone. Radical cystectomy with pelvic lymphadenectomy revealed multifocal T3a stage high-grade urothelial carcinoma and multiple metastatic lymph nodes only in the right external iliac, right common iliac, and right obturator stations. In clinical practice, it is useful to first use DWI to identify all nodes (whether benign or metastatic), and then characterize the nodes (size, shape, fatty hilum, etc.) on T1WI or T2WI.

differences in the ADC values between the two entities, and further investigation is warranted [67]. Among the several advanced MRI sequences, nanoparticle-enhanced MRI is the most promising. In nanoparticle-enhanced MRI, ultrasmall superparamagnetic particles of iron oxide (USPIO), a lymphotrophic agent, is intravenously administered. USPIO is taken up by lymphatics and phagocytosed by macrophages in benign lymph nodes. This causes SI drop in T2WI or T2*WI, allowing for identification of normal lymph nodes. However, metastatic nodes are infiltrated with tumor cells, and therefore do not take up USPIO—therefore showing no SI loss on T2WI [6]. Using USPIO, Deserno et al. [69] found that metastatic lymph nodes can be diagnosed with a sensitivity, specificity, and overall accuracy of 96%, 95%, and 95%, respectively. Nanoparticle-enhanced MRI can also be used in conjunction with DWI, in order to achieve shorter time required for image interpretation [70,71]. Yet the degree of SI loss is correlated with the tumor burden within the lymph node. Therefore the diagnostic yield can be lower in normal-sized ($\leq$5 mm) or micrometastatic lymph nodes [72,73].

M Stage

Bladder TCC can also metastasize hematogenously with increased risk in tumors with higher T and N stages. Well-known sites of distant metastasis

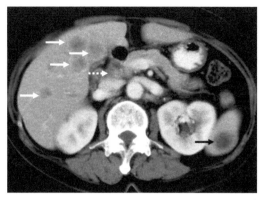

FIGURE 8.17 Fifty-nine-year-old woman with liver, spleen, and portocaval lymph node metastases from invasive urothelial carcinoma. Patient underwent radical cystectomy due to bladder wall thickening suspicious for malignancy (not shown) and was diagnosed with T2a stage grade III urothelial carcinoma. At axial contrast-enhanced CT performed 7 months after surgery, newly appeared rim-enhancing nodules and masses in the liver parenchyma (*white arrows*) and spleen (*black arrow*), and enlarged lymph nodes in left external iliac, paraaortic, aortocaval, and portocaval (*dotted arrow*) were demonstrated. Imaging characteristics and interval appearance on follow-up imaging indicate that these lesions are distant metastases (M1 stage).

include liver, bones, and lungs [74]. American Urological Association and National Comprehensive Cancer Network guidelines recommend that CT or MRI be used for assessment of the abdomen and pelvis, and that a simple radiograph or nonenhanced CT be acquired to evaluate lung metastasis in patients with MIBC (Fig. 8.17) [47,75]. Bone scintigraphy can be used to detect skeletal metastasis, when the patient experiences symptoms or signs suspicious for metastasis, or when alkaline phosphatase levels are elevated.

IMAGING BIOMARKERS WITH PROGNOSTIC AND PREDICTIVE VALUE

Tumor Grade

Tumor grade is an important prognostic factor. It is well known that high-grade tumors have a higher risk of progression and a less favorable prognosis [76]. Among several imaging modalities, DWI has the potential to aid in the differentiation between high- and low-grade tumors. Several investigators have assessed the association between ADC derived from DWI, and have found that high-grade tumors have lower ADC value (Fig. 8.18) [44,57,77]. For instance, Avcu et al. [77] reported that ADC values were 0.92 ± 0.20 and $1.28 \pm 0.18 \times 10^{-3}$ mm^2/s in high- and low-grade bladder TCCs, respectively. Higher grade TCC has increased cellularity compared with lower grade TCC. This is reflected by the more impeded random movement of water molecules within the tumor, leading to greater diffusion restriction, and in turn, lower

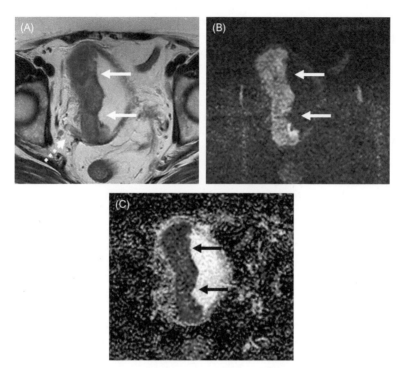

FIGURE 8.18 Sixty-eight-year-old woman with high-grade urothelial carcinoma showing strong diffusion restriction on DWI. (A) Axial T2WI shows large mass-like wall thickening (*arrows*) in right lateral bladder wall involving right ureterovesical junction (*dotted arrow*). Not only is normal low SI line disrupted, but also slightly irregular infiltration into perivesical fat is suspicious, indicating high-grade and stage bladder cancer. (B) On axial DWI (*b*-value = 800 s/mm^2), mass (*arrows*) demonstrates high SI. (C) On ADC map derived from DWI (*b*-values = 0, 800 s/mm^2), mass (*arrows*) shoes very low SI, that is strong "diffusion restriction." Using region of interest measurement, ADC of tumor was measured as 0.864×10^{-3} mm^2/s. Radical cystectomy revealed T3 stage high-grade urothelial carcinoma.

ADC value. However, there is still overlap between the ADC values between each grade, and ADC values are known to vary according to technical factors (such as magnet strength and vendor of the scanner). Therefore specific cutoff values cannot be provided for clinical practice. Furthermore, information regarding the grade of the tumor is often already known by cystoscopic biopsy or TUR. Determining the grade of bladder TCC using DWI still requires validation regarding reproducibility and practicality.

Prediction of Sensitivity and Monitoring Response to Chemotherapy and Chemoradiation

Although the standard treatment for MIBC is radical cystectomy with pelvic lymph node dissection, high-risk patients are often offered neoadjuvant or adjuvant chemotherapy in order to control occult micrometastatic disease

[75]. Furthermore, when considering bladder-sparing strategies, chemoradiation is included in the majority of the protocols [78]. Accurate prediction of the sensitivity to chemotherapy- or chemoradiation therapy prior to or during treatment would optimize patient management, applying treatment to sensitive patients while changing the regimen and avoiding unnecessary adverse reactions in resistant patients.

Conventional CT and MRI are not adequate for predicting the sensitivity or monitoring the response to chemotherapy and chemoradiation therapy. Posttreatment changes after TUR (which is performed prior to therapy for debulking purposes and acquisition of pathological information) and chemotherapy induce fibrosis and inflammatory changes, resulting in bladder wall thickening [79]. This prohibits accurate assessment of the tumor, often with overestimation [78]. Functional MRI techniques including DCE-MRI and DWI have the potential to predict sensitivity to treatment. Not only do information acquired from functional MRI reflect the pathological changes earlier than conventional imaging (which is based on simply measuring the size of the tumor), they can partially overcome the confusion rendered by posttreatment changes.

ADC values derived from DWI have been shown to have an inverse correlation with sensitivity to chemoradiation. In the study by Yoshida et al. [80], in which MIBC patients underwent neoadjuvant chemoradiation prior to cystectomy, tumors with pathologically complete response demonstrated lower ADC than those with residual tumor on pretreatment MRI. Using a criteria of ADC $<0.74 \times 10^{-3}$ mm^2/s, the sensitivity, specificity, and accuracy were 92%, 90%, and 91%, respectively, for predicting complete response after neoadjuvant chemoradiation (Fig. 8.19). Since ADC value of bladder TCC is also inversely correlated with Ki-67 labeling index, tumors with lower ADC may be more sensitive to chemoradiation due to their higher proliferative activity [81].

DCE-MRI has been used to distinguish between responders and nonresponders after chemotherapy. Schrier et al. [82] used DCE-MRI and compared the time to enhancement during the course of chemotherapy in tumor tissue in patients with clinical N1 and N2 disease. They found that in nonresponders, tumors persistently demonstrated early enhancement, while in responders, previous areas involved with bladder TCC showed late enhancement, at more than 10 seconds after aortic enhancement. Not only this method was accurate (sensitivity, specificity, and accuracy of 91%, 93%, and 92%, respectively), but also these imaging findings showed correlation with median disease-specific survival (12 and 42 months in radiological nonresponders and responders, respectively). Other studies report that quantitative analysis of DCE-MRI parameters (relative SI and plasma perfusion) has potential to differentiate residual tumor from therapy-related hemorrhage and inflammation in MIBC treated with neoadjuvant chemotherapy [83].

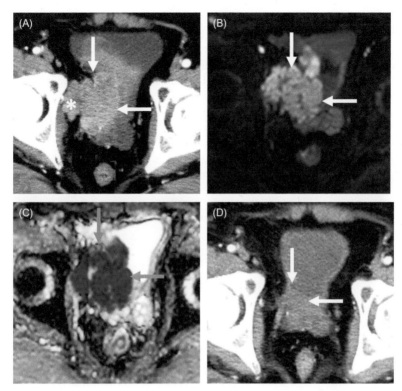

FIGURE 8.19 Sixty-two-year-old man with muscle-invasive high-grade urothelial carcinoma showing partial response to chemotherapy. (A) Initial axial contrast-enhanced CT shows about 6-cm-sized lobulating mass (*arrows*) in right bladder wall. Mass shows locally advanced features of gross extravesical infiltration (*asterisk*), seminal vesical and prostate invasion (not shown), and right ureterovesical junction involvement causing hydronephrosis (not shown). TUR of bladder revealed grade III muscle-invasive urothelial carcinoma. (B,C) On MRI, mass shows high SI on (B) axial DWI (b-value = 1000 s/mm^2) and very dark SI on (C) ADC map (b-values = 0, 1000 s/mm^2), signifying strong diffusion restriction. Measured ADC of mass was 0.627×10^{-3} mm^2/s. (D) Follow-up axial contrast-enhanced CT after one cycle of chemotherapy using gemcitabine and cisplatin, size of bladder mass is significantly reduced (about 1.5 cm).

As such, more and more data are accumulating to support the use of advanced MRI techniques to predict the sensitivity and monitor the response to adjuvant treatment. Nevertheless, even with promising results, when and exactly how to utilize this information is not yet established and warrants further studies for them to be implemented into routine clinical practice.

Posttransurethral Resection Imaging

Imaging bladder cancer after TUR can be problematic because post-TUR inflammatory changes can be difficult to be differentiated from recurrence.

Especially, TUR-induced inflammation and fibrosis manifest with thickening of the bladder wall on conventional CT and MRI. These changes related with TUR can last up to several years, even on DCE-MRI, potentially causing false positive results for recurrent or residual cancer [84−86]. However, DWI is gaining attention as a potential imaging modality for follow-up of patients with bladder TCC treated with TUR. In recent studies, DWI was able to differentiate between recurrent bladder tumor and post-TUR inflammation and fibrosis with sensitivities, specificities, and accuracies of 91.6%−100%, 81.8%−91.3%, and 91.5%−92.6%, respectively, showing very high agreement with cystoscopy [87,88]. Fig. 8.20

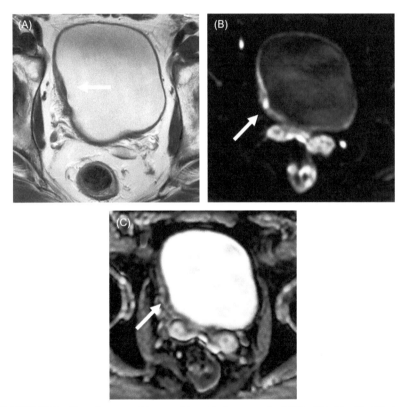

FIGURE 8.20 Forty-five-year-old man with residual cancer after TUR of bladder identified on DWI. (A) Axial T2WI shows diffuse bladder wall thickening on right lateral wall. It is difficult to determine whether this is solely due to postprocedural changes due to TUR or if residual tumor is present. (B) On axial DWI (b-value = 1000 s/mm^2), focal high SI (*arrow*) is noted within diffuse wall thickening suspicious for residual tumor. (C) ADC map (b-values = 0, 1000 s/mm^2) demonstrating lesion (*arrow*) detected on DWI shows diffusion restriction. TUR of bladder prior to MRI found high-grade invasive urothelial carcinoma with proper muscle invasion. Radical cystectomy followed by MRI revealed residual urothelial carcinoma invading subepithelial connective tissue (T1 stage) at right bladder wall.

shows a representative case in which DWI was helpful for identifying residual cancer after TUR.

RARE TUMORS (OTHER THAN TCC)

As up to 90% of bladder cancers are urothelial (transitional cell) carcinoma, nonurothelial cancers are very rare in the bladder [2]. Among these rare non-urothelial bladder cancers, squamous cell carcinoma, adenocarcinoma, small cell tumor, and lymphoma are relatively common entities. Other tumors arising from mesenchymal origin include benign tumors such as leiomyoma, paraganglioma, fibroma, plasmacytoma, neurofibroma, and lipoma, and malignant tumors including rhabdomyosarcoma, leiomyosarcoma, and osteosarcoma. Benign mesenchymal tumors are usually seen as smooth intramural lesions located in the submucosal layer. However, such tumors with mesenchymal origin are very rare, and therefore we will deal with the relatively more common tumors (squamous cell carcinoma, adenocarcinoma, small cell tumor, and lymphoma) in this section. Most of these tumors are relatively more aggressive than TCC and show nonspecific findings. Furthermore, due to their rare incidence, specific imaging findings have not been established. However, some tumors, such as urachal adenocarcinoma, show characteristics findings.

Squamous Cell Carcinoma

Squamous cell carcinoma is the most common nonurothelial cancer in the bladder, consisting of less than 5% [2]. They manifest with nonspecific imaging features, such as focal or diffuse wall thickening of the bladder or a bladder mass showing contrast enhancement (Fig. 8.21) [89]. Most of the time, they are solitary and large at initial detection [90]. The location of wall thickening or mass can be helpful in suggesting the diagnosis of squamous cell carcinoma. They commonly are found in the trigone, lateral wall, or in a diverticulum [91]. In contrast to bladder TCC, which can appear as papillary or sessile lesions, squamous cell carcinomas usually are sessile, unless found in diverticula, which commonly manifests as soft tissue mass [91]. Calcification can be present, either within the wall thickening or mass, or along the surface in diverticular squamous cell carcinoma. Due to their higher grade and aggressive pathological nature, muscle invasion, extensive extravesical extension, and nodal and distant metastasis can be found at the time of diagnosis [90,92].

Adenocarcinoma

Adenocarcinoma is the second most common nonurothelial bladder cancer. It is known to constitute about 2% of bladder cancers [2]. Primary

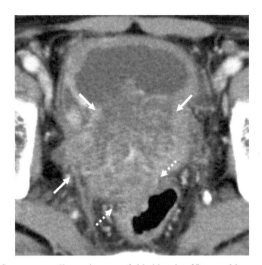

FIGURE 8.21 Squamous cell carcinoma of bladder in 65-year-old man. Axial contrast-enhanced CT shows large heterogeneous solid and cystic mass (*arrows*) in posterior wall of bladder. Mass shows gross extravesical infiltration with wide abutment to anterior rectal wall suggestive of rectal invasion (*dotted arrows*). Several enlarged lymph nodes were seen in iliac, paraaortic, and aortocaval stations indicating metastatic lymphadenopathy (not shown). Distant metastases to right kidney and lungs were also detected (not shown). Biopsy from mass revealed squamous cell carcinoma.

adenocarcinomas of the bladder can be found anywhere in the bladder, but is more common in the bladder base. However, it is important to understand that they can be associated with anomalies of the urachus, in which they are found in the bladder dome. Secondary adenocarcinomas are more common, and can be direct invasion from primary malignancy in the pelvis (colon, prostate, and rectum) or less commonly arise as hematogenous metastases from distant organs (stomach, breast, and lung) [93]. Because differentiation between primary and secondary adenocarcinomas of the bladder may be difficult even after obtaining pathological specimens, it is important to assess the presence of primary malignancy in other organs on imaging [93]. Because of the rarity of this disease, only scattered reports of small number of patients have been published in the literature. In a small case series of eight patients of nonurachal adenocarcinomas of the bladder by Hughes et al. [94], they demonstrated diffuse (75%−100%) and circumferential thickening of the bladder wall on CT and MRI in all patients (Fig. 8.22). Perivesical fat stranding was also a common imaging feature, seen in 88%. Other less common findings included abdominal wall invasion (25%), nodal metastasis (25%), peritoneal deposits (25%), and distant metastasis to the lungs (12.5%) [94]. Urachal adenocarcinomas appear as large (average size of 6 cm) mixed cystic solid lesions or less commonly as solid masses in the midline antero-superior bladder dome (Fig. 8.23) [95]. Cystic components are composed of

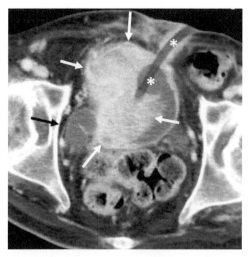

FIGURE 8.22   Nonurachal adenocarcinoma in 61-year-old man with indwelling foley catheter. On axial contrast-enhanced CT, large enhancing mass-like wall thickening (*white arrows*) originating from right bladder wall is nearly replacing bladder. Mass involves right ureterovesical junction causing hydronephrosis (*black arrow*). Note indwelling foley catheter via suprapubic cystostomy tract (*asterisks*) due to paraplegia and neurogenic bladder from previous spinal injury. Prior to CT, which was performed for evaluation of hematuria, patient has history of stone removal. Cystoscopic biopsy revealed adenocarcinoma of bladder.

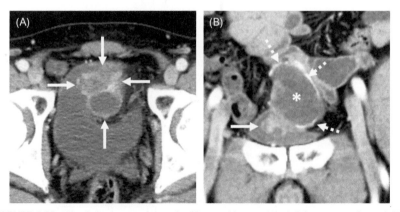

FIGURE 8.23   Urachal adenocarcinoma in 55-year-old man. (A) Axial contrast-enhanced CT shows $5.6 \times 5.5 \times 8.5$ cm-sized lobulated solid and cystic mass (*arrows*) at anterosuperior wall of bladder. (b) Coronal contrast-enhanced CT better demonstrates entire cranio-caudal extent of mass with solid component caudally (*arrow*) and predominantly cystic portion (*asterisk*) cranially, with rim-like calcification (*dotted arrows*) along the cyst wall. Radical cystectomy revealed urachal mucin-producing moderately differentiated adenocarcinoma.

mucin and therefore show low attenuation on CT and high SI on T2WI [96]. Common features include calcifications (either peripheral, central, or both) in 72%, invasion of the bladder wall in 92%, extravesical extension (extravesical portion greater than intraluminal) in 88%, and metastasis to various locations in 48% [95].

Small Cell Tumors

Small cell tumors of the bladder are very rare tumor, consisting approximately 0.5% of bladder tumors [97,98]. Small cell bladder tumors are typically large (3−8 cm) ill-defined and well enhancing broad-based polypoid intramural masses (Fig. 8.24) [99]. They may have ulcerated surfaces [100]. Unlike TCC, small cell tumors show patchy enhancement [101]. Posterior and trigonal location are common. Cystic change may be identified in half of the patients. However, unlike squamous cell carcinoma and adenocarcinoma, calcification is rare. Interestingly, the solid portion of the mass shows low SI on both T1WI and T2WI [99]. They show aggressive behavior with an extensive degree of invasion to adjacent organs, including the seminal vesicles, ureters, vagina, and abdominal wall. Lymph node metastases is

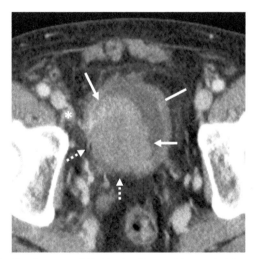

FIGURE 8.24 Small cell tumor of bladder in 69-year-old man. Axial contrast-enhanced CT shows 5-cm-sized enhancing mass (*arrows*) in right posterolateral bladder wall. Mass invades prostate (not shown) and subtle perivesicular stranding is seen in bladder wall underlying mass (*dotted arrows*). Also note diffuse bladder wall thickening (*line*), probably due to obstructive uropathy. Multiple enlarged lymph nodes were seen in right external iliac (*asterisk*), common iliac, and paraaortic stations, suggestive of metastases (not shown). Cystoscopic tumor resection revealed small cell bladder cancer. After several cycles of chemotherapy, distant metastases to liver and left supraclavicular lymph nodes were detected (not shown).

frequently found (66%) and distant metastases has been reported in the liver, bone, lung, and brain [99,100].

Lymphoma

Lymphomas involving the bladder are more commonly secondary rather than primary. Secondary lymphoma is found in 10%−25% of all lymphoma patients, and is relatively easier to differentiate from TCC [102]. The presence of enlarged lymph nodes in the abdomen and pelvis is an important clue to diagnosing secondary lymphoma. However, primary lymphoma of the bladder is not only very rare, but also cannot be differentiated from primary TCC of the bladder [103]. Therefore differentiation is mainly based on cystoscopic biopsy. The most common type of primary bladder lymphoma is a low-grade B-cell mucosa-associated lymphoid tissue lymphoma [104]. The reported imaging findings of primary bladder lymphoma have been variable, including the following in decreasing frequency [105]: sessile and solitary mass (66%), multiple sessile masses (14%), polypoid mass (10%), and diffuse bladder wall thickening (10%) (Fig. 8.25). An even more erratic finding of eccentric lateral wall thickening showing heterogeneous enhancement and presence of dense calcification has been reported [106]. Although the differentiation between primary bladder lymphoma and TCC may be difficult, some differential points have been suggested. Since primary bladder lymphoma does not usually involve the whole bladder or urethral orifices, hydronephrosis is not common.

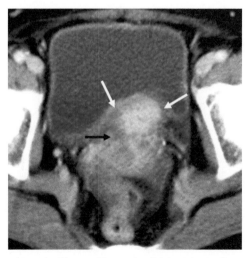

FIGURE 8.25 Lymphoma in 74-year-old woman. Axial contrast-enhanced CT shows 3-cm-sized submucosal mass (*white arrows*) with homogeneous enhancement at posterior bladder wall. Suspicious involvement (*black arrow*) of anterior uterus is seen. Cystoscopic biopsy revealed diffuse large B-cell lymphoma.

Furthermore, primary lymphoma does not commonly show extravesical spread even when it manifests as a large mass [103].

REFERENCES

[1] National Cancer Institute. Surveillance, epidemiology, and end results program (SEER) fact sheet, <www.seer.cancer.gov > ; 2016 [accessed 09.07.16].

[2] Murphy WM, Grignon D, Perman EJ. Tumors of the kidney, bladder, and related urinary structures. Washington, DC: American Registry of Pathology; 2004. p. 394.

[3] Sobin L. International Union Against Cancer (UICC). TNM classification of malignant tumors. New York, NY: Wiley; 2002.

[4] Pashos CL, Botteman MF, Laskin BL, Redaelli A. Bladder cancer: epidemiology, diagnosis, and management. Cancer Pract 2002;10:311−22.

[5] Moses KA, Zhang J, Hricak H, Bochner BH. Bladder cancer imaging: an update. Curr Opin Urol 2011;21:393−7.

[6] Hafeez S, Huddart R. Advances in bladder cancer imaging. BMC Med 2013;11:104.

[7] Tritschler S, Mosler C, Tilki D, Buchner A, Stief C, Graser A. Interobserver variability limits exact preoperative staging by computed tomography in bladder cancer. Urology 2012;79:1317−21.

[8] Van Der Molen AJ, Cowan NC, Mueller-Lisse UG, Nolte-Ernsting CC, Takahashi S, Cohan RH, et al. CT urography: definition, indications and techniques. A guideline for clinical practice. Eur Radiol 2008;18:4−17.

[9] de Haas RJ, Steyvers MJ, Futterer JJ. Multiparametric MRI of the bladder: ready for clinical routine? Am J Roetgenol 2014;202:1187−95.

[10] Dershaw DD, Scher HI. Sonography in evaluation of carcinoma of bladder. Urology 1987;29:454−7.

[11] Li QY, Tang J, He EH, Li YM, Zhou Y, Zhang X, et al. Clinical utility of three-dimensional contrast-enhanced ultrasound in the differentiation between noninvasive and invasive neoplasms of urinary bladder. Eur J Radiol 2012;81:2936−42.

[12] Xu C, Zhang Z, Wang H, Song Q, Wei R, Yu Y, et al. A new tool for distinguishing muscle invasive and non-muscle invasive bladder cancer: the initial application of flexible ultrasound bronchoscope in bladder tumor staging. PLoS One 2014;9:e92385.

[13] McKibben MJ, Woods ME. Preoperative imaging for staging bladder cancer. Curr Urol Rep 2015;16:22.

[14] Bernhardt TM, Schmidl H, Philipp C, Allhoff EP, Rapp-Bernhardt U. Diagnostic potential of virtual cystoscopy of the bladder: MRI vs CT. Preliminary report. Eur Radiol 2003;13:305−12.

[15] Kawai N, Mimura T, Nagata D, Tozawa K, Kohri K. Intravenous urography-virtual cystoscopy is a better preliminary examination than air virtual cystoscopy. BJU Int 2004;94:832−6.

[16] Panebianco V, Pavone P, Laghi A. MR virtual cystoscopy: preliminary results [abstract]. Eur Radiol 2000;10(suppl 1):143.

[17] Kocakoc E, Kiris A, Orhan I, Poyraz AK, Artas H, Firdolas F. Detection of bladder tumors with 3-dimensional sonography and virtual sonographic cystoscopy. J Ultrasound Med 2008;27:45−53.

[18] Beer A, Saar B, Zantl N, Link TM, Roggel R, Hwang SL, et al. MR cystography for bladder tumor detection. Eur Radiol 2004;14:2311−19.

[19] Moon MH, Kim SH, Lee YH, Cho JY, Jung SI, Park SH, et al. Diagnostic potential of three-dimensional ultrasound-based virtual cystoscopy: an experimental study using pig bladders. Invest Radiol 2006;41:883−9.

[20] Qu X, Huang X, Wu L, Huang G, Ping X, Yan W. Comparison of virtual cystoscopy and ultrasonography for bladder cancer detection: a meta-analysis. Eur J Radiol 2011;80: 188−97.

[21] Bernhardt TM, Rapp-Bernhardt U. Virtual cystoscopy of the bladder based on CT and MRI data. Abdom Imaging 2001;26:325−32.

[22] Shinagare AB, Sadow CA, Sahni VA, Silverman SG. Urinary bladder: normal appearance and mimics of malignancy at CT urography. Cancer Imaging 2011;11:100−8.

[23] Caterino M, Giunta S, Finocchi V, Giglio L, Mainiero G, Carpanese L, et al. Primary cancer of the urinary bladder: CT evaluation of the T parameter with different techniques. Abdom Imaging 2001;26:433−8.

[24] Raman SP, Fishman EK. Bladder malignancies on CT: the underrated role of CT in diagnosis. Am J Roentgenol 2014;203:347−54.

[25] Helenius M, Dahlman P, Lonnemark M, Brekkan E, Wernroth L, Magnusson A. Comparison of post contrast CT urography phases in bladder cancer detection. Eur Radiol 2016;26:585−91.

[26] Bush WH, Swanson DP. Acute reactions to intravascular contrast media: types, risk factors, recognition, and specific treatment. Am J Roentgenol 1991;157:1153−61.

[27] Thomsen HS, Morcos SK, Almen T, Bellin MF, Bertolotto M, Bongartz G, et al. Nephrogenic systemic fibrosis and gadolinium-based contrast media: updated ESUR Contrast Medium Safety Committee guidelines. Eur Radiol 2013;23:307−18.

[28] Cohan RH, Caoili EM, Cowan NC, Weizer AZ, Ellis JH. MDCT urography: exploring a new paradigm for imaging of bladder cancer. Am J Roentgenol 2009;192:1501−8.

[29] Ng CS. Radiologic diagnosis and staging of renal and bladder cancer. Sem Roentgenol 2006;41:121−38.

[30] Verma S, Rajesh A, Prasad SR, Gaitonde K, Lall CG, Mouraviev V, et al. Urinary bladder cancer: role of MR imaging. Radiographics 2012;32:371−87.

[31] Tuncbilek N, Kaplan M, Altaner S, Atakan IH, Süt N, Inci O, et al. Value of dynamic contrast-enhanced MRI and correlation with tumor angiogenesis in bladder cancer. Am J Roentgenol 2009;192:949−55.

[32] Kim JK, Park SY, Ahn HJ, Kim CS, Cho KS. Bladder cancer: analysis of multi-detector row helical CT enhancement pattern and accuracy in tumor detection and perivesical staging. Radiology 2004;231:725−31.

[33] Koh DM, Collins DJ. Diffusion-weighted MRI in the body: applications and challenges in oncology. Am J Roentgenol 2007;188:1622−35.

[34] Takeuchi M, Sasaki S, Naiki T, Kawai N, Kohri K, Hara M, et al. MR imaging of urinary bladder cancer for T-staging: a review and a pictorial essay of diffusion-weighted imaging. J Magn Reson Imaging 2013;38:1299−309.

[35] Matsuki M, Inada Y, Tatsugami F, Tanikake M, Narabayashi I, Katsuoka Y. Diffusion-weighted MR imaging for urinary bladder carcinoma: initial results. Eur Radiol 2007;17: 201−4.

[36] Di Paolo PL, Vargas HA, Karlo CA, Lakhman Y, Zheng J, Moskowitz CS, et al. Intradiverticular bladder cancer: CT imaging features and their association with clinical outcomes. Clin Imaging 2015;39:94−8.

[37] Golijanin D, Yossepowitch O, Beck SD, Sogani P, Dalbagni G. Carcinoma in a bladder diverticulum: presentation and treatment outcome. J Urol 2003;170:1761−4.

[38] Turney BW, Willatt JM, Nixon D, Crew JP, Cowan NC. Computed tomography urography for diagnosing bladder cancer. BJU Int 2006;98:345−8.

[39] Sadow CA, Silverman SG, O'Leary MP, Signorovitch JE. Bladder cancer detection with CT urography in an Academic Medical Center. Radiology 2008;249:195−202.

[40] Park SB, Kim JK, Lee HJ, Choi HJ, Cho KS. Hematuria: portal venous phase multi detector row CT of the bladder—a prospective study. Radiology 2007;245:798−805.

[41] Nguyen HT, Pohar KS, Jia G, Shah ZK, Mortazavi A, Zynger DL, et al. Improving bladder cancer imaging using 3-T functional dynamic contrast-enhanced magnetic resonance imaging. Invest Radiol 2014;49:390−5.

[42] Abou-El-Ghar ME, El-Assmy A, Refaie HF, El-Diasty T. Bladder cancer: diagnosis with diffusion-weighted MR imaging in patients with gross hematuria. Radiology 2009;251: 415−21.

[43] Halefoglu AM, Sen EY, Tanriverdi O, Yilmaz F. Utility of diffusion-weighted MRI in the diagnosis of bladder carcinoma. Clin Imaging 2013;37:1077−83.

[44] Kobayashi S, Koga F, Yoshida S, Masuda H, Ishii C, Tanaka H, et al. Diagnostic performance of diffusion-weighted magnetic resonance imaging in bladder cancer: potential utility of apparent diffusion coefficient values as a biomarker to predict clinical aggressiveness. Eur Radiol 2011;21:2178−86.

[45] Barentsz JO, Jager GJ, van Vierzen PB, et al. Staging urinary bladder cancer after transurethral biopsy: value of fast dynamic contrast-enhanced MR imaging. Radiology 1996;201:185−93.

[46] Wang LJ, Wong YC, Ng KF, Chuang CK, Lee SY, Wan YL. Tumor characteristics of urothelial carcinoma on multidetector computerized tomography urography. J Urol 2010;183:2154−60.

[47] Clark P. NCCN clinical practice guidelines in oncology: bladder cancer, version 2. Fort Washington, PA: NCCN; 2014.

[48] Vikram R, Sandler CM, Ng CS. Imaging and staging of transitional cell carcinoma: part 1, lower urinary tract. Am J Roentgenol 2009;192:1481−7.

[49] Paik ML, Scolieri MJ, Brown SL, Spirnak JP, Resnick MI. Limitations of computerized tomography in staging invasive bladder cancer before radical cystectomy. J Urol 2000;163:1693−6.

[50] Tanimoto A, Yuasa Y, Imai Y, Izutsu M, Hiramatsu K, Tachibana M, et al. Bladder tumor staging: comparison of conventional and gadolinium-enhanced dynamic MR imaging and CT. Radiology 1992;185:741−7.

[51] Yaman O, Baltaci S, Arikan N, Yilmaz E, Gogus O. Staging with computed tomography, transrectal ultrasonography and transurethral resection of bladder tumour: comparison with final pathological stage in invasive bladder carcinoma. Br J Urol 1996;78:197−200.

[52] Hayashi N, Tochigi H, Shiraishi T, Takeda K, Kawamura J. A new staging criterion for bladder carcinoma using gadolinium-enhanced magnetic resonance imaging with an endorectal surface coil: a comparison with ultrasonography. BJU Int 2000;85:32−6.

[53] Kim B, Semelka RC, Ascher SM, Chalpin DB, Carroll PR, Hricak H. Bladder tumor staging: comparison of contrast-enhanced CT, T1- and T2-weighted MR imaging, dynamic gadolinium-enhanced imaging, and late gadolinium-enhanced imaging. Radiology 1994; 193:239−45.

[54] Watanabe H, Kanematsu M, Kondo H, Goshima S, Tsuge Y, Onozuka M, et al. Preoperative T staging of urinary bladder cancer: does diffusion-weighted MRI have supplementary value? Am J Roentgenol 2009;192:1361−6.

[55] Tekes A, Kamel I, Imam K, Szarf G, Schoenberg M, Nasir K, et al. Dynamic MRI of bladder cancer: evaluation of staging accuracy. Am J Roentgenol 2005;184:121−7.

[56] Liedberg F, Bendahl PO, Davidsson T, Gudjonsson S, Holmer M, Månsson W, et al. Preoperative staging of locally advanced bladder cancer before radical cystectomy using 3 tesla magnetic resonance imaging with a standardized protocol. Scand J Urol 2013;47: 108−12.

[57] Takeuchi M, Sasaki S, Ito M, Okada S, Takahashi S, Kawai T, et al. Urinary bladder cancer: diffusion-weighted MR imaging—accuracy for diagnosing T stage and estimating histologic grade. Radiology 2009;251:112−21.

[58] Wu LM, Chen XX, Xu JR, Zhang XF, Suo ST, Yao QY, et al. Clinical value of T2-weighted imaging combined with diffusion-weighted imaging in preoperative T staging of urinary bladder cancer: a large-scale, multiobserver prospective study on 3.0-T MRI. Acad Radiol 2013;20:939−46.

[59] Wang HJ, Pui MH, Guan J, Li SR, Lin JH, Pan B, et al. Comparison of early submucosal enhancement and tumor stalk in staging bladder urothelial carcinoma. Am J Roentgenol 2016;1−7.

[60] Rholl KS, Lee JK, Heiken JP, Ling D, Glazer HS. Primary bladder carcinoma: evaluation with MR imaging. Radiology 1987;163:117−21.

[61] El-Assmy A, Abou-El-Ghar ME, Mosbah A, El-Nahas AR, Refaie HF, Hekal IA, et al. Bladder tumour staging: comparison of diffusion- and T2-weighted MR imaging. Eur Radiol 2009;19:1575−81.

[62] Barentsz JO, Engelbrecht MR, Witjes JA, de la Rosette JJ, van der Graaf M. MR imaging of the male pelvis. Eur Radiol 1999;9:1722−36.

[63] Tritschler S, Mosler C, Straub J, Buchner A, Karl A, Graser A, et al. Staging of muscle-invasive bladder cancer: can computerized tomography help us to decide on local treatment? World J Urol 2012;30:827−31.

[64] Papalia R, Simone G, Grasso R, Augelli R, Faiella E, Guaglianone S, et al. Diffusion-weighted magnetic resonance imaging in patients selected for radical cystectomy: detection rate of pelvic lymph node metastases. BJU Int 2012;109:1031−6.

[65] Bostrom PJ, van Rhijn B, Fleshner N, Finelli A, Jewett M, Thoms J, et al. Staging and staging errors in bladder cancer. Eur Urol Suppl 2010;9:2−9.

[66] Jager GJ, Barentsz JO, Oosterhof GO, Witjes JA, Ruijs SJ. Pelvic adenopathy in prostatic and urinary bladder carcinoma: MR imaging with a three-dimensional TI-weighted magnetization-prepared-rapid gradient-echo sequence. Am J Roentgenol 1996;167: 1503−7.

[67] Thoeny HC, Froehlich JM, Triantafyllou M, Huesler J, Bains LJ, Vermathen P, et al. Metastases in normal-sized pelvic lymph nodes: detection with diffusion-weighted MR imaging. Radiology 2014;273:125−35.

[68] Daneshmand S, Ahmadi H, Huynh LN, Dobos N. Preoperative staging of invasive bladder cancer with dynamic gadolinium-enhanced magnetic resonance imaging: results from a prospective study. Urology 2012;80:1313−18.

[69] Deserno WM, Harisinghani MG, Taupitz M, Jager GJ, Witjes JA, Mulders PF, et al. Urinary bladder cancer: preoperative nodal staging with ferumoxtran-10-enhanced MR imaging. Radiology 2004;233:449−56.

[70] Birkhauser FD, Studer UE, Froehlich JM, Triantafyllou M, Bains LJ, Petralia G, et al. Combined ultrasmall superparamagnetic particles of iron oxide-enhanced and diffusion-weighted magnetic resonance imaging facilitates detection of metastases in

normal-sized pelvic lymph nodes of patients with bladder and prostate cancer. Eur Urol 2013;64:953−60.

[71] Thoeny HC, Triantafyllou M, Birkhaeuser FD, Froehlich JM, Tshering DW, Binser T, et al. Combined ultrasmall superparamagnetic particles of iron oxide-enhanced and diffusion-weighted magnetic resonance imaging reliably detect pelvic lymph node metastases in normal-sized nodes of bladder and prostate cancer patients. Eur Urol 2009;55:761−9.

[72] Triantafyllou M, Studer UE, Birkhauser FD, Fleischmann A, Bains LJ, Petralia G, et al. Ultrasmall superparamagnetic particles of iron oxide allow for the detection of metastases in normal sized pelvic lymph nodes of patients with bladder and/or prostate cancer. Eur J Cancer 2013;49:616−24.

[73] Green DA, Durand M, Gumpeni N, Rink M, Cha EK, Karakiewicz PI, et al. Role of magnetic resonance imaging in bladder cancer: current status and emerging techniques. BJU Int 2012;110:1463−70.

[74] Knap MM, Lundbeck F, Overgaard J. Prognostic factors, pattern of recurrence and survival in a Danish bladder cancer cohort treated with radical cystectomy. Acta Oncol 2003;42:160−8.

[75] Witjes JA, Comperat E, Cowan NC, De Santis M, Gakis G, Lebret T, et al. EAU guidelines on muscle-invasive and metastatic bladder cancer: summary of the 2013 guidelines. Eur Urol 2014;65:778−92.

[76] Kim HS, Ku JH, Kim SJ, Hong SJ, Hong SH, Kim HS, et al. Prognostic factors for recurrence and progression in Korean non-muscle-invasive bladder cancer patients: a retrospective, multi-institutional study. Yonsei Med J 2016;57:855−64.

[77] Avcu S, Koseoglu MN, Ceylan K, Bulut MD, Unal O. The value of diffusion-weighted MRI in the diagnosis of malignant and benign urinary bladder lesions. Br J Radiol 2011;84:875−82.

[78] Yoshida S, Koga F, Kobayashi S, Tanaka H, Satoh S, Fujii Y, et al. Diffusion-weighted magnetic resonance imaging in management of bladder cancer, particularly with multimodal bladder-sparing strategy. World J Radiol 2014;6:344−54.

[79] Raza SA, Jhaveri KS. MR imaging of urinary bladder carcinoma and beyond. Radiol Clin North Am 2012;50:1085−110.

[80] Yoshida S, Koga F, Kobayashi S, Ishii C, Tanaka H, Tanaka H, et al. Role of diffusion-weighted magnetic resonance imaging in predicting sensitivity to chemoradiotherapy in muscle-invasive bladder cancer. Int J Radiat Oncol Biol Phys 2012;83:e21−27.

[81] Kobayashi S, Koga F, Kajino K, Yoshita S, Ishii C, Tanaka H, et al. Apparent diffusion coefficient value reflects invasive and proliferative potential of bladder cancer. J Magn Reson Imaging 2014;39:172−8.

[82] Schrier BP, Peters M, Barentsz JO, Witjes JA. Evaluation of chemotherapy with magnetic resonance imaging in patients with regionally metastatic or unresectable bladder cancer. Eur Urol 2006;49:698−703.

[83] Donaldson SB, Bonington SC, Kershaw LE, Cowan R, Lyons J, Elliott T, et al. Dynamic contrast-enhanced MRI in patients with muscle-invasive transitional cell carcinoma of the bladder can distinguish between residual tumour and post-chemotherapy effect. Eur J Radiol 2013;82:2161−8.

[84] Johnson RJ, Carrington BM, Jenkins JP, Barnard RJ, Read G, Isherwood I. Accuracy in staging carcinoma of the bladder by magnetic resonance imaging. Clin Radiol 1990;41:258−63.

[85] Therasse P, Arbuck SG, Eisenhauer EA, Wanders J, Kaplan RS, Rubinstein L, et al. New guidelines to evaluate the response to treatment in solid tumors. European Organization for Research and Treatment of Cancer, National Cancer Institute of the United States, National Cancer Institute of Canada. J Natl Cancer Inst 2000;92:205−16.

[86] Yoshida S, Koga F, Masuda H, Fujii Y, Kihara K. Role of diffusion-weighted magnetic resonance imaging as an imaging biomarker of urothelial carcinoma. Int J Urol 2014;21:1190−200.

[87] El-Assmy A, Abou-El-Ghar ME, Refaie HF, Mosbah A, El-Diasty T. Diffusion-weighted magnetic resonance imaging in follow-up of superficial urinary bladder carcinoma after transurethral resection: initial experience. BJU Int 2012;110:E622−627.

[88] Wang HJ, Pui MH, Guo Y, Yang D, Pan BT, Zhou XH. Diffusion-weighted MRI in bladder carcinoma: the differentiation between tumor recurrence and benign changes after resection. Abdom Imaging 2014;39:135−41.

[89] Wong JT, Wasserman NF, Padurean AM. Bladder squamous cell carcinoma. Radiographics 2004;24:855−60.

[90] Tekes A, Kamel IR, Chan TY, Schoenberg MP, Bluemke DA. MR imaging features of non-transitional cell carcinoma of the urinary bladder with pathologic correlation. Am J Roentgenol 2003;180:779−84.

[91] Dondalski M, White EM, Ghahremani GG, Patel SK. Carcinoma arising in urinary bladder diverticula: imaging findings in six patients. Am J Roentgenol 1993;161: 817−20.

[92] Serretta V, Pomara G, Piazza F, Gange E. Pure squamous cell carcinoma of the bladder in Western countries. Report on 19 consecutive cases. Eur Urol 2000;37:85−9.

[93] Bates AW, Baithun SI. Secondary neoplasms of the bladder are histological mimics of nontransitional cell primary tumours: clinicopathological and histological features of 282 cases. Histopathology 2000;36:32−40.

[94] Hughes MJ, Fisher C, Sohaib SA. Imaging features of primary nonurachal adenocarcinoma of the bladder. Am J Roentgenol 2004;183:1397−401.

[95] Thali-Schwab CM, Woodward PJ, Wagner BJ. Computed tomographic appearance of urachal adenocarcinomas: review of 25 cases. Eur Radiol 2005;15:79−84.

[96] Brick SH, Friedman AC, Pollack HM, Fishman EK, Radecki PD, Siegelbaum MH, et al. Urachal carcinoma: CT findings. Radiology 1988;169:377−81.

[97] Cheng L, Pan CX, Yang XJ, Lopez-Beltran A, MacLennan GT, Lin H, et al. Small cell carcinoma of the urinary bladder: a clinicopathologic analysis of 64 patients. Cancer 2004;101:957−62.

[98] Sved P, Gomez P, Manoharan M, Civantos F, Soloway MS. Small cell carcinoma of the bladder. BJU Int 2004;94:12−17.

[99] Kim JC, Kim KH, Jung S. Small cell carcinoma of the urinary bladder: CT and MR imaging findings. Korean J Radiol 2003;4:130−5.

[100] Wong-You-Cheong JJ, Woodward PJ, Manning MA, Sesterhenn IA. From the archives of the AFIP: neoplasms of the urinary bladder: radiologic-pathologic correlation. Radiographics 2006;26:553−80.

[101] Kim JC. CT features of bladder small cell carcinoma. Clin Imaging 2004;28:201−5.

[102] Bates AW, Norton AJ, Baithun SI. Malignant lymphoma of the urinary bladder: a clinicopathological study of 11 cases. J Clin Pathol 2000;53:458−61.

[103] Yeoman LJ, Mason MD, Olliff JF. Non-Hodgkin's lymphoma of the bladder—CT and MRI appearances. Clin Radiol 1991;44:389−92.

[104] Maninderpal KG, Amir FH, Azad HA, Mun KS. Imaging findings of a primary bladder maltoma. Br J Radiol 2011;84:e186–190.

[105] Tasu JP, Geffroy D, Rocher L, Eschwege P, Strohl D, Benoit G, et al. Primary malignant lymphoma of the urinary bladder: report of three cases and review of the literature. Eur Radiol 2000;10:1261–4.

[106] Choi JH, Jeong YY, Shin SS, Lim HS, Kang HK. Primary calcified T-cell lymphoma of the urinary bladder: a case report. Korean J Radiol 2003;4:252–4.

Chapter 9

Transurethral Resection of Bladder Tumors

Minyong Kang
Sungkyunkwan University School of Medicine, Seoul, South Korea

Chapter Outline

INTRODUCTION OF TURBT

Bladder cancer is the ninth most common malignant disease worldwide, and the most common cancer involving the urinary tract [1]. The American Cancer Society estimated that in 2015 in the United States, there were approximately 74,000 new cases of bladder cancer (with a 3:1 concerning males versus females) and about 16,000 deaths from bladder cancer [2]. Approximately 90% of cancer in the urinary bladder is pathologically diagnosed with urothelial carcinoma (UC) [3]. At the time of initial diagnosis, approximately 70% of UC of the urinary bladder is nonmuscle invasive bladder cancer (NMIBC), including Ta, carcinoma in situ (CIS), and T1 tumors [4].

Over a century ago, Edwin Beer first showed that papillary bladder tumors could be endoscopically treated using electrocautery [5]. Stern and McCarthy invented the practical cutting loop resectoscope. Thereafter, transurethral resection of bladder tumor (TURBT) has become the gold standard for initial diagnosis and definitive treatments of choice for NMIBC (Fig. 9.1) [6].

Two critical goals of TURBT are to eradicate any visible tumors and to take tissue specimens with adequate depth of resection for the accurate determination of the pathologic stage and tumor grade [7]. If the initial resection is incomplete, repeat-TUR (or second-TUR) should be conducted to obtain

Bladder Cancer. DOI: http://dx.doi.org/10.1016/B978-0-12-809939-1.00009-6
123

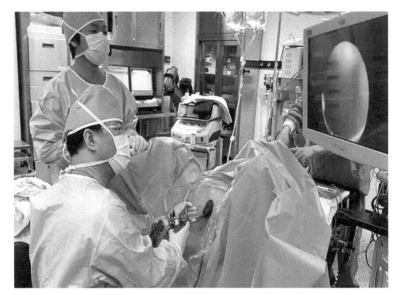

FIGURE 9.1   Depiction of TURBT.

deeper tissue samples including proper muscle layers [8]. Although advancements in endoscopic instruments, such as video imaging systems and electrocautery devices, have improved the efficacy and safety of TURBT, the procedure is still considered one of the most fundamental and challenging techniques for urologists to master.

Here, we describe the key steps and principles of current TURBT techniques, the role of random biopsies, TURBT-related complications, and recent en-bloc techniques using laser devices.

KEY STEPS AND PRINCIPLES OF TURBT

Complete TURBT is the most important step for treating NMIBC [4]. There are four basic surgical principles of complete TURBT. First is the resection of all visible tumors. Second is the resection of normal urothelium on the border of the visible tumors. Third is the resection of the muscle layer at the tumor bed until normal muscle fibers are observed. Fourth is the random biopsy of apparently normal mucosa of the bladder wall and both sides of the prostatic urethra, particularly in high-risk patients [9,10].

The patient is positioned in dorsal lithotomy under general anesthesia rather than a spinal anesthesia in order to minimize the risk of obturator nerve stimulation and resulting abrupt adduction of the thigh muscles. Tumor resection is carried out using a 24F to 28F continuous flow resectoscope with a 12°, 30°, or 70° lens and wire cutting loop. A continuous flow sheath is valuable to achieve a clear resection field, to prevent bladder

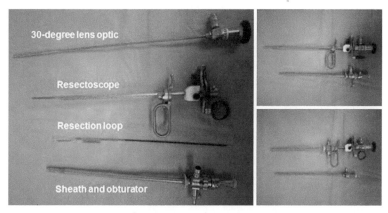

FIGURE 9.2   Basic equipment for TURBT.

overdistension and perforation, and to avoid obturator nerve stimulation [11]. It is important that the bladder is kept partially distended status throughout the procedure. The basic equipment for TURBT is shown in Fig. 9.2.

Resection with a cutting loop should be carried out in a systematic, piece-meal fashion. Practically, resection should begin superficially and advance toward the deeper layers of the tumor with appropriate bleeding control. Also, resection should be performed from one end of the tumor toward the other end. The tumor is resected by precise movements of a cutting loop at a speed that is appropriate to ensure sufficient depth to acquire proper muscle layers for accurate diagnosis without bladder perforation. After most tumor lesions have been removed, the tumor stalk should be resected, which makes it easier by maintaining counteraction of the resected lesions. Once the tumor is resected, the resection bed should be either biopsied by using cold-cup biopsy forceps or further resected using a resection loop to achieve good sampling of the detrusor muscle, which is separately sent for pathologic review. Furthermore, because bladder cancers usually sprout beyond the visible boundary of the tumor, surgeons should more widely resect the lesion even include the normal-appearing mucosa near the tumor margin (Fig. 9.3).

Some authors suggest that small and easily accessible tumors should be resected first, with subsequent treatment of tumors located in the anterior bladder neck and dome [11]. Conversely, others recommend that tumors located in poorly accessible sites should be resected early because the surgical field of view is still fine [11]. Tumors located in a diverticulum should be managed by simple fulguration or open resection, such as partial cystectomy, due to the risk of perforation [12].

Achieving complete hemostasis is also critical step at the time of TURBT. Any bleeding vessels should be meticulously coagulated throughout the resection to prevent hemorrhage after surgery. Moreover, the tumor resection bed and a surrounding edge should be carefully examined for

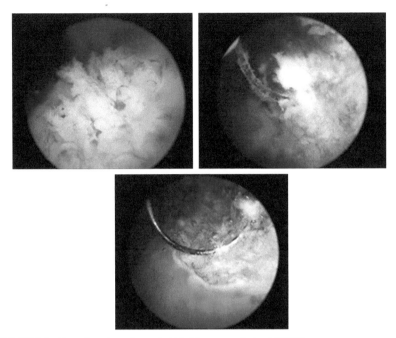

FIGURE 9.3   Operative view of resected bladder cancer during TURBT.

complete hemostasis at the end of the procedures. To finally ensure complete hemostasis before terminating surgery, the bladder should be reexamined in the emptying status. Rarely, postoperative bleeding may occur and require adjunctive procedures, such as an insertion of large-bore catheter with manual irrigation, clot evacuation using the Ellik or Toomey evacuators or transurethral coagulation at the operating room.

Although the value of bimanual examination appears to be limited with accurate staging in the era of modern imaging, it can be still valuable for urologists to perform bimanual examination for appropriate staging and to acquire additional information before and after procedures [13]. Fixation or persistence of a palpable mass after tumor resection suggests the presence of clinical T3b disease. Rozanski et al. [13] recently examined 414 of the 1898 patients from the radical cystectomy database of the University of Texas MD Anderson Cancer Center to explore the role of exam under anesthesia (EUA) in predicting the tumor extension at least pathological T3 (pT3) stage. The authors reported that 128 patients (30.9%) had findings suggestive of pT3 stage on EAU, while 119 patients (28.7%) had radiologic findings suggestive of pT3 disease. Notably, multivariate analysis identified EUA as an independent predictor of pT3 disease [odds ratio (OR), 2.22; 95% confidence interval (CI), 1.34−3.69] in addition to imaging modalities (OR, 2.18; 95% CI, 1.33−3.58). Thus a bimanual examination under anesthesia should be

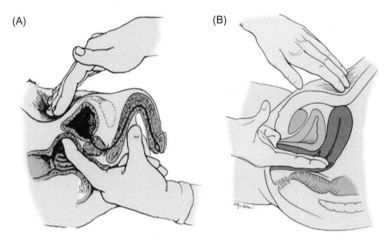

FIGURE 9.4   Bimanual examination for bladder tumors in (A) male and (B) female patients. *The use of these figures is permitted by Elsevier.*

performed in the bladder emptying state before and after complete resection of tumors (Fig. 9.4).

SECOND TURBT

In order to achieve better oncologic outcomes, correct and complete resection of tumors should be guaranteed, including suspicious areas suggestive of CIS. While small papillary tumors (<1 cm) can be resected with mucosal and submucosal layers around tumors, larger tumors require deep resection up to the detrusor muscle of bladder for accurate tumor staging.

In this context, TURBT can be conducted as the one-stage or two-stage resection according to the operative condition, such as tumor burden. In the one-stage resection the surgeon completely resects tumor lesions and the remained tissue at the tumor resection bed as the superficial layer of detrusor muscle. One-stage resection is usually used for a small tumor. Two-stage resection should be performed when the initial resection is insufficient, such as for multiple, large tumors, and when the initial TUR specimen does not contain proper muscle layers, particularly in T1 tumors. Technically the two-stage resection includes the initial resection for tumor removal at the lower level of the mucosa and the second resection for tissue sampling at the superficial muscle layer for accurate cancer staging.

More importantly, more than 40% of cases are identified as residual tumors when resecting the initial TUR sites, and repeat-TUR produces a poor prognostic outcomes in up to 25% of specimens [14,15]. Divrik et al. [16] first reported the results of a randomized controlled trial in which repeat-TUR significantly improved the recurrence-free survival in patients

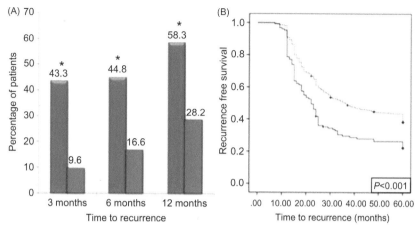

FIGURE 9.5   (A) Recurrence rates in patients treated with single (blue bars) or restaging (red bars) TUR. (B) Kaplan−Meier survival curves in high-risk NMIBC patients who underwent a single TUR (*solid curve*) versus restaging TUR (*dashed curve*). *The use of these figures is permitted by Elsevier.*

with T1 tumors. Sfakianos et al. [17] recently demonstrated that treatment with a single TUR was associated with a higher recurrence rate and shorter time to recurrence than restaging TUR in patients with high-risk NMIBC who received intravesical bacillus Calmette-Guérin (BCG) (Fig. 9.5). They suggested that restaging resection should be conducted before initiating intra-vesical BCG instillation in all individuals with high-risk NMIBC.

A second TURBT should be considered 2−6 weeks after primary TUR if T1 or high-grade diseases are evident at initial TURBT, if muscle layers were not included in TUR specimens, and in cases of previous incomplete resection due to situations like excessive tumor burden, inapproachable location of tumor, or higher risk of bladder perforation. In these situations, complete tumor removal may not be possible at the initial resection [18].

ROLE OF RANDOM BIOPSIES

Additional targeted biopsies of any suspicious lesions of CIS, such as a velvet-like and reddish mucosa, are critical in managing bladder cancer patients. Random biopsies are usually performed to obtain tissues from normal-looking mucosa in patients with persistent positive urine cytology and in the absence of visible tumors, in patients at risk of high-grade tumors [18]. Recommended sites of random biopsies are the trigone, bladder dome, right and left anterior and posterior walls of bladder, and the prostatic urethra in male patients [18]. The rate of positive findings in random biopsy has varied from 8% to 23% [19]. Although some studies have suggested the prognostic significance of additional biopsies of normal appearing or any suspicious mucosa during TURBT, it is still debatable whether a random biopsy can influence the pathological staging and oncologic prognosis. An additional random biopsy during the initial resection may not improve the diagnostic accuracy and therefore, and so should not influence therapeutic decision-making.

The current consensus is that random biopsies are not recommend for low-risk patients based on the International Bladder Cancer Group risk classification, that is, those with low-grade papillary tumors and negative urine cytology [18]. Random biopsy should be carried out in select patients with multiple tumors and repeatedly positive urine cytology. The EAU guideline also recommends that random biopsies should only be performed in patients with suspicious CIS lesions or patients with persistent positive cytology without visible tumors as follows: "In patients with positive cytology, but negative cystoscopy, exclude a upper tract urothelial carcinoma, carcinoma in situ in the bladder (random biopsies or photodynamic diagnosis targeted biopsies) and tumor in prostatic urethra (prostatic urethra biopsy) (Grade of evidence is C)" [4].

In patients with suspicious CIS, random biopsies can be unreliable for accurately detecting CIS in bladder mucosa. So, negative findings should be interpreted with caution. Gudjonsson et al. [20] reported that sensitivity and specificity rates of cold-cup biopsies of 46% and 89%, respectively, for CIS lesions in the bladder. Taken together, random biopsies are not routinely recommended in patients judged to be low risk, such as those with no visible tumor or low-grade papillary tumor with negative urine cytology. For patients with multiple, high-grade cancer or persistent positive cytology, even in the absence of suspicious lesions, random biopsies should be performed for normal-looking mucosa, including the bladder and prostatic urethra.

ROLE OF PROSTATIC URETHRAL BIOPSIES

The incidence of prostatic urothelial involvement in patients with bladder UC reportedly ranges from 15% to 57% [21–24]. Nixon et al. [22] showed that prostatic urethral involvement was found in 15.6% of radical cystectomy specimens (30/192 cases). Of note, 31.3% of patients with bladder CIS had concomitant prostatic urethral involvement, while only 4.5% of patients without bladder CIS had UC in prostatic urethra. Shen et al. [21] also reported prostatic involvement in 30 of 214 (32%) radical cystoprostatectomy specimens. Particularly, bladder CIS was detected in 43% of patients, indicating that the presence of bladder CIS is a significant predictor of prostatic urethral involvement of bladder cancer. Thus prostatic urethral biopsy is currently recommended in patients with bladder CIS during TURB.

Prostatic urethra biopsy is crucial to determine clinical staging and surgical plan in patients undergoing radical cystoprostatectomy, even in the presence of normal-looking mucosa [24]. According to the 2010 American Joint Committee on Cancer staging system, UC in urinary bladder with concomitant prostatic stromal involvement is classified as pathologic T4a [4,25]. In this regard, prostatic urethra biopsy can be useful to identify patients with T4a disease who may benefit from neoadjuvant systemic chemotherapy before surgery [24]. In addition, prostatic urethra biopsy can offer the proper guidance in deciding the most favorable type of urinary diversion, particularly for the patients undergoing orthotopic neobladder formation [24].

COMPLICATIONS OF TURBT

After TURBT, common adverse effects are urethral pain, irritation during micturition, and gross hematuria during early postoperative time. Bladder perforation is one of the most common and significant complications following TURBT, occurring in approximately 5% of cases [26]. Key signs of bladder perforation include reduced drainage volume of irrigation fluid, abdominal distension, and tachycardia. Moreover, using endoscopy surgeons can directly observe a yellowish perivesical fat or a dark cavity between detrusor muscles, indicating bladder perforation [11]. Particularly, large and bulky mass or tumors at bladder dome are at more risk for perforation during surgery.

To avoid bladder perforation, continuous irrigation is recommended without over distention of bladder wall as much as possible. Moreover, delicate movement of the cutting loop and sheath is required to follow the curve of the bladder when resecting, with resection depth adjusted appropriately. Most perforations occur at extraperitoneal sites, while intraperitoneal rupture is relatively rare [26,27]. Extraperitoneal perforation is usually resolved by a longer period of indwelling urethral catheter [28,29]. However, intraperitoneal perforation requires surgical exploration and repair by suturing a perforated lesion [28,29]. To prevent bladder perforation in patients with huge and invasive masses, a staged resection is a good technical approach because repeated resection can remove residual tumors in a safer manner.

TUR syndrome due to the large amount of fluid absorption is common following transurethral resection of the prostate. Still, it is a concern and requires early detection and appropriate management. Clinicians should be very concerned about the possibility of TUR syndrome when confronted by abnormal clinical findings including acutely reduced consciousness, severe hyponatremia and hyperkalemia, and reduced platelet counts [30]. Supportive management is sufficient to manage TUR syndrome if early diagnosis and interventions are made prior to systemic development of serious complications [31].

When tumors are located near the ureteral orifice, unexpected thermal injury to the orifice can occur [32]. Pure cutting current should be applied to reduce the risk of ureteral orifice stenosis. When the orifice is injured by electrocautery and the injury is not detected, asymptomatic or symptomatic ureteral obstruction may develop postoperatively. In order to determine the presence of an obstruction immediately after injury, urine efflux should be checked by cystoscopy after intravenous injection of indigo carmine. Alternately, retrograde ureteropyelography can be performed. In the case of moderate to severe thermal orifice injury, scarring of injured sites can be treated most often by balloon dilation or endoscopic incision, and rarely by ureteral reimplantation [33]. Although postoperative obstruction rarely occurs, since the ureteral orifice is resected by pure cutting current, it may result in vesicoureteral reflux with the potential risk of infection or upper tract seeding [34–36].

RECENT TECHNICAL ADVANCES OF TURBT

Although conventional TURBT is the diagnostic and therapeutic standard for NMIBC, it has various pitfalls, including risk of TUR syndrome, obturator nerve stimulation, tumor fragmentation during resection, and thermal damage of the surgical specimens. These may lead to misclassification of pathologic findings. In this regard, tumor vaporization (TV) or en-bloc resection of bladder tumors (ERBT) using Holmium (Ho):YAG and Thulium (Tm):YAG lasers has been recognized as potentially useful alternatives to conventional TURBT for select patients with NMIBC (Figs. 9.6 and 9.7) [37]. Kramer et al. [37] recently reviewed 18 publications comprising 800 NMIBC patients, and recommended TV for recurrent, small NMIBC in the office-based setting. ERBT can achieve more accurate staging in primary tumors with lesser second-TUR.

The Ho:YAG laser has a depth of penetration of only 3–4 mm, which makes the risk of bladder perforation very low [38]. Although perforation can develop in cases of repeated TUR or irradiation, bladder injury has rarely been reported during laser resection [39]. In addition, less discomfort, better hemostasis capacity, and resection in saline as continuous irrigant are major advantages of laser device [39]. Thus it can be a good option for resecting bladder tumors. In one study, while there was no statistical difference of operative time between these two techniques, laser TURBT showed lower perioperative complications including obturator nerve reflex, bladder

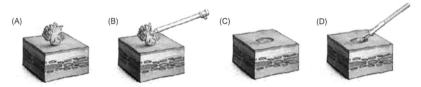

FIGURE 9.6 Stepwise procedures of bladder TV using laser devices. (A) After tumor identification, (B) the tumor can be vaporized as the distal tip of the laser fiber is held 3 mm away from the tumor. (C) Adequate laser vaporization should result in complete visible shrinkage of tumor tissue. (D) Tumor biopsy can be taken from the tumor bed after complete laser ablation of tumor. *The use of these figures is permitted by Elsevier.*

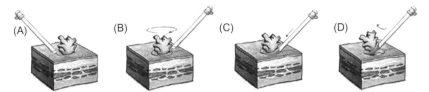

FIGURE 9.7 Stepwise procedures of ERBT using laser devices. (A and B) Circular incision is first performed around the tumor with a distance of approximately 3–5 mm. (C) The tumor is finally extracted by blunt dissection along this circular marking line. (D) The adequate depth of tumor resection is determined when detrusor muscle fibers are observed. *The use of these figures is permitted by Elsevier.*

perforation, and catheter indwelling time compared to conventional TURBT, in a recent meta-analysis [40].

In terms of oncologic outcomes, there was a trend toward decreased recurrence rates after laser TURBT (24%–31%) compared to conventional TURBT (30%–45%). However, no significant differences in oncological outcomes have been clearly demonstrated between laser TURBT and conventional TURBT, particularly in well-designed randomized clinical trials [41].

CONCLUSION

TURBT is the current gold standard for the initial diagnosis, staging, and grading of all bladder cancer. Two primary goals of TURBT are the pathologic confirmation, such as histology and stage of tumors, and eradication of visible tumors. Particularly, complete TURBT is the most important step for treating NMIBC. The basic surgical principles of TURBT are resection of all visible tumors, resection of normal urothelium on the border of the visible tumors, resection of the muscle layer at the tumor bed until normal muscle fibers are observed, and random biopsy of apparently normal mucosa of the bladder wall and both sides of the prostatic urethra, particularly in high-risk patients.

REFERENCES

[1] Ferlay J, Soerjomataram I, Dikshit R, Eser S, Mathers C, Rebelo M, et al. Cancer incidence and mortality worldwide: sources, methods and major patterns in GLOBOCAN 2012. Int J Cancer 2015;136:E359–86.

[2] Siegel RL, Miller KD, Jemal A. Cancer statistics, 2015. CA Cancer J Clin 2015;65:5–29.

[3] Burger M, Catto JWF, Dalbagni G, Grossman HB, Herr H, Karakiewicz P, et al. Epidemiology and risk factors of urothelial bladder cancer. Eur Urol 2013;63:234–41.

[4] Babjuk M, Bohle A, Burger M, Capoun O, Cohen D, Comperat EM, et al. EAU guidelines on non-muscle-invasive urothelial carcinoma of the bladder: update 2016. Eur Urol 2016. Available from: http://dx.doi.org/10.1016/j.eururo.2016.05.041.

[5] Herr HW. Legacy of Edwin Beer: fulguration of papillary bladder tumors. J Urol 2005;173:1087–9.

[6] Reuter MA, Reuter HJ. The development of urological endoscopy in America. World J Urol 1999;17:176–83.

[7] Holzbeierlein JM, Smith Jr. JA. Surgical management of noninvasive bladder cancer (stages Ta/T1/CIS). Urol Clin North Am 2000;27:15–24.

[8] Herr HW. Role of re-resection in non-muscle-invasive bladder cancer. SciWorld J 2011;11:283–8.

[9] Babjuk M. Transurethral resection of non-muscle-invasive bladder cancer. Eur Urol Suppl 2009;8:542–8.

[10] Furuse H, Ozono S. Transurethral resection of the bladder tumour (TURBT) for non-muscle invasive bladder cancer: basic skills. Int J Urol 2010;17:698–9.

[11] Traxer O, Pasqui F, Gattegno B, Pearle MS. Technique and complications of transurethral surgery for bladder tumours. BJU Int 2004;94:492–6.

[12] Yu CC, Huang JK, Lee YH, Chen KK, Chen MT, Chang LS. Intradiverticular tumors of the bladder: surgical implications—an eleven-year review. Eur Urol 1993;24:190–6.

[13] Rozanski A, McCoy JA, Benson CR, Green C, Grossman HB, Svatek R, et al. Is exam under anesthesia still necessary for the staging of bladder cancer in the ERA of modern imaging? J Urol 2014;191:E692.

[14] Miladi M, Peyromaure M, Zerbib M, Saighi D, Debre B. The value of a second transurethral resection in evaluating patients with bladder tumours. Eur Urol 2003;43:241–5.

[15] Schwaibold HE, Sivalingam S, May F, Hartung R. The value of a second transurethral resection for T1 bladder cancer. BJU Int 2006;97:1199–201.

[16] Divrik RT, Yildirim U, Zorlu F, Ozen H. The effect of repeat transurethral resection on recurrence and progression rates in patients with T1 tumors of the bladder who received intravesical mitomycin: a prospective, randomized clinical trial. J Urol 2006;175:1641–4.

[17] Sfakianos JP, Kim PH, Hakimi AA, Herr HW. The effect of restaging transurethral resection on recurrence and progression rates in patients with nonmuscle invasive bladder cancer treated with intravesical bacillus Calmette-Guerin. J Urol 2014;191:341–5.

[18] Anastasiadis A, de Reijke TM. Best practice in the treatment of nonmuscle invasive bladder cancer. Ther Adv Urol 2012;4:13–32.

[19] Librenjak D, Novakovic ZS, Situm M, Milostic K, Duvnjak M. Biopsies of the normal-appearing urothelium in primary bladder cancer. Urol Ann 2010;2:71–5.

[20] Gudjonsson S, Blackberg M, Chebil G, Jahnson S, Olsson H, Bendahl PO, et al. The value of bladder mapping and prostatic urethra biopsies for detection of carcinoma in situ (CIS). BJU Int 2012;110:E41–5.

[21] Shen SS, Lerner SP, Muezzinoglu B, Truong LD, Amiel G, Wheeler TM. Prostatic involvement by transitional cell carcinoma in patients with bladder cancer and its prognostic significance. Hum Pathol 2006;37:726–34.

[22] Nixon RG, Chang SS, Lafleur BJ, Smith JJ, Cookson MS. Carcinoma in situ and tumor multifocality predict the risk of prostatic urethral involvement at radical cystectomy in men with transitional cell carcinoma of the bladder. J Urol 2002;167:502–5.

[23] Njinou Ngninkeu B, Lorge F, Moulin P, Jamart J, Van Cangh PJ. Transitional cell carcinoma involving the prostate: a clinicopathological retrospective study of 76 cases. J Urol 2003;169:149–52.

[24] von Rundstedt FC, Lerner SP, Godoy G, Amiel G, Wheeler TM, Truong LD, et al. Usefulness of transurethral biopsy for staging the prostatic urethra before radical cystectomy. J Urol 2015;193:58–63.

[25] Edge SB, Compton CC. The American Joint Committee on Cancer: the 7th edition of the AJCC cancer staging manual and the future of TNM. Ann Surg Oncol 2010;17:1471–4.

[26] Collado A, Chechile GE, Salvador J, Vicente J. Early complications of endoscopic treatment for superficial bladder tumors. J Urol 2000;164:1529–32.

[27] Balbay MD, Cimentepe E, Unsal A, Bayrak O, Koc A, Akbulut Z. The actual incidence of bladder perforation following transurethral bladder surgery. J Urol 2005;174:2260–2.

[28] Lynch TH, Martinez-Pineiro L, Plas E, Serafetinides E, Turkeri L, Santucci RA, et al. EAU guidelines on urological trauma. Eur Urol 2005;47:1–15.

[29] Summerton DJ, Kitrey ND, Lumen N, Serafetinidis E, Djakovic N, et al. EAU guidelines on iatrogenic trauma. Eur Urol 2012;62:628–39.

[30] Hahn RG. Transurethral resection syndrome from extravascular absorption of irrigating fluid. Scand J Urol Nephrol 1993;27:387–94.

[31] Hahn RG. Transurethral resection syndrome after transurethral resection of bladder tumours. Can J Anaesth 1995;42:69–72.

[32] Mano R, Shoshany O, Baniel J, Yossepowitch O. Resection of ureteral orifice during transurethral resection of bladder tumor: functional and oncologic implications. J Urol 2012;188:2129–33.

[33] Corcoran AT, Smaldone MC, Ricchiuti DD, Averch TD. Management of benign ureteral strictures in the endoscopic era. J Endourol 2009;23:1909–12.

[34] Goldwasser B, Bogokowsky B, Nativ O, Sidi AA, Jonas P, Many M. Urinary infections following transurethral resection of bladder tumors—rate and source. J Urol 1983;129:1123–4.

[35] De Torres Mateos JA, Banus Gassol JM, Palou Redorta J, Morote Robles J. Vesicorenal reflux and upper urinary tract transitional cell carcinoma after transurethral resection of recurrent superficial bladder carcinoma. J Urol 1987;138:49–51.

[36] Palou J, Salvador J, Millan F, Collado A, Algaba F, Vicente J. Management of superficial transitional cell carcinoma in the intramural ureter: what to do? J Urol 2000;163:744–7.

[37] Kramer MW, Wolters M, Cash H, Jutzi S, Imkamp F, Kuczyk MA, et al. Current evidence of transurethral Ho:YAG and Tm:YAG treatment of bladder cancer: update 2014. World J Urol 2015;33:571–9.

[38] Zarrabi A, Gross AJ. The evolution of lasers in urology. Ther Adv Urol 2011;3:81–9.

[39] Kramer MW, Abdelkawi IF, Wolters M, Bach T, Gross AJ, Nagele U, et al. Current evidence for transurethral en bloc resection of non-muscle-invasive bladder cancer. Minim Invasive Ther Allied Technol 2014;23:206–13.

[40] Bai YJ, Liu L, Yuan HC, Li JH, Tang Y, Pu CX, et al. Safety and efficacy of transurethral laser therapy for bladder cancer: a systematic review and meta-analysis. World J Surg Oncol 2014;12:301.

[41] Karl A, Herrmann TRW. En bloc resection of urothelial cancer within the urinary bladder: the upcoming gold standard? Re: Kramer MW, Wolters M, Cash H, Jutzi S, Imkamp F, Kuczyk MA, Merseburger AS, Herrmann TR. Current evidence of transurethral Ho:YAG and Tm:YAG treatment of bladder cancer: update 2014. World J Urol 2015;33:581–2.

Chapter 10

Recent Technological Advances in Cystoscopy for the Detection of Bladder Cancer

Byong Chang Jeong
Sungkyunkwan University, Seoul, South Korea

Chapter Outline

INTRODUCTION

Bladder cancer is the most common type of malignancy in the urinary tract showcasing a high recurrence rate and aggressive feature [1]. Most patients with bladder cancer are pathologically diagnosed with urothelial carcinoma [2,3]. Approximately 70% of patients with urothelial carcinoma in the urinary bladder have a superficial or non-muscle invasive tumor confined to mucosa or submucosa layers of the wall [2,3].

Since the 1930s, cystoscopy has been regarded as a fundamental diagnostic tool for detecting bladder cancer [4]. However, conventional cystoscopy such as the white light imaging system has a critical drawback when detecting small papillary tumors or carcinoma *in situ* (CIS) [5]. Actually, white light cystoscopy shows the 10%−20% of missing rates of these ill-defined lesions of bladder tumors. In this regard, non-muscle-invasive bladder cancers (NMIBC) show an early and high recurrence rate [3].

To overcome this limitation, technological advancements in endoscopic visualization of bladder cancers, such as narrow band imaging (NBI), fluorescence

Bladder Cancer. DOI: http://dx.doi.org/10.1016/B978-0-12-809939-1.00010-2
135

cystoscopy, and optical coherence, have been achieved [6]. Here, the clinical evidence supporting the use of these specific technologies are reviewed.

VARIOUS CYSTOSCOPIC FINDINGS OF BLADDER TUMOR

Various cystoscopic findings of bladder tumor are illustrated in Figs. 10.1–10.5.

NARROW BAND IMAGING

NBI, developed in 2005, is a high-resolution endoscopic optical image enhancement technology [7]. This novel tool can improve the visibility of microvasculatures or capillary networks [8]. NBI utilizes the light of two

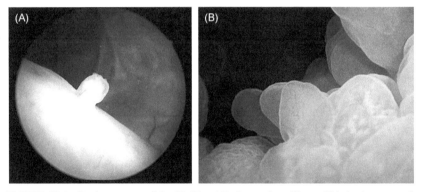

FIGURE 10.1 Benign tumors of the bladder. (A). Inverted papilloma. This benign tumor is typically a pedunculated or sessile polypoid lesion usually <30 mm in size, with a smooth or nodular mucosal surface. (B). Cystitis glandularis. It is a common finding in normal bladder and most often found in the trigone area. These benign tumors are usually present as cystic nests.

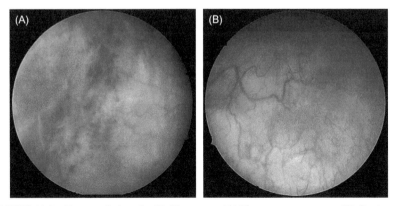

FIGURE 10.2 Non-muscle invasive bladder cancer. (A) Flat tumor appearance. (B) Carcinoma in situ. Carcinoma in situ is a high-grade, flat (velvety patch or moss-like growth) malignancy confined to the urothelium.

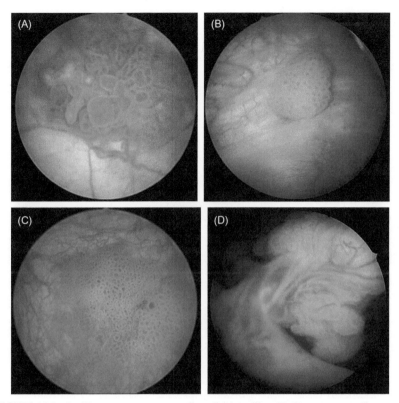

FIGURE 10.3   Papillary tumor appearance. Superficial papillary bladder tumors usually appear as small mushrooms growing out of the bladder wall (Ta low-grade tumor) (A, B). Flat (sessile) papillary bladder tumors (Ta high-grade tumor) (C). Small papillary tumor on a stalk (Ta low grade tumor) (D).

distinct wavelengths, blue (415 nm) and green (540 nm), both of which are well absorbed by hemoglobin [8]. The blue and green lights focus the capillary networks and subepithelial blood vessels, respectively [9]. Thus, blood vessels are shown in brown or green colors compared to the surrounding mucosa in NBI system, enhancing its visibility. Therefore, it is very useful in differentiating normal tissue from a more vascularized malignant tissue [9].

Since the first utilization of the NBI system in 2007 [10], several reports have shown the advantage of this system in detecting bladder cancer compared to standard white light cystoscopy. Li et al. [11] conducted a meta-analysis from seven prospective studies encompassing 1040 patients with NMIBC. Here, NBI showed an additional 24% and 28% detection rate of papillary tumors and CIS, respectively, when compared to white light cystoscopy. Xiong and colleagues recently published a meta-analysis of 25 studies and revealed that NBI had higher detection rates in NMIBC than white light

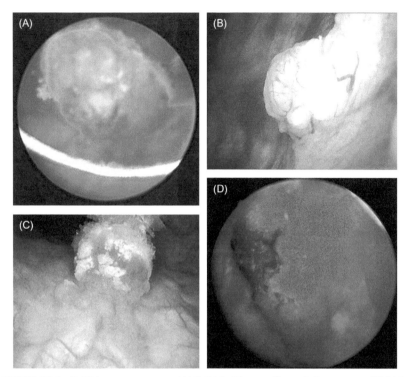

FIGURE 10.4 Solid tumor appearance. (A) Solid looking, small round shape tumors (T1 high-grade tumor). (B) Papillo-nodular tumors (T1 low-grade tumor). Papillary and sessile mixed, round tumors partly covered with calcification (C) and blood clot (D) (T1 high-grade tumor).

cystoscopy, and an additional 18.6% and 31.1% for superficial tumors and CIS lesion, respectively [12]. Furthermore, NBI significantly decreased the risk of the disease recurrence at 3 months [hazard ratio (HR) = 0.43, 95% confidence interval (CI) = 0.23−0.79] and 12 months (HR = 0.81, 95% CI = 0.69−0.95) after initial treatment.

However, the current limitation of NBI is the high frequency of false positives and subsequent negative biopsies [13]. In addition, the effects of NBI on oncological outcomes such as the progression and cancer-specific survival are still ill-defined [13]. Thus, further research is required to determine the routine use of the NBI system for endoscopic examination of bladder cancers (Fig. 10.6).

FLUORESCENCE CYSTOSCOPY

Fluorescent cystoscopy is a novel diagnostic tool using topical photosensitizers, 5-aminolevulinic acid (5-ALA), or hexyl-aminolevulinate (HAL), improving the ability in detecting bladder cancers, particularly small

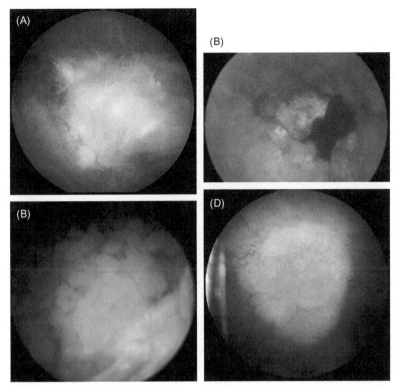

FIGURE 10.5 Invasive and metastatic bladder cancer. Muscle-invasive bladder cancer. Solid, infiltrating bladder tumor. (A) Its surface is wholly necrotic. (B) The normal vessel architecture has completely disappeared. (C) Large papillary bladder tumors. (D) Metastatic bladder tumor form gastric cancer.

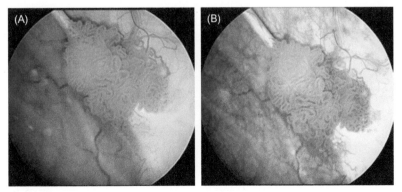

FIGURE 10.6 (A) White light cystoscopy image. (B) NBI image with enhanced contrast of vasculature.

papillary and CIS lesions [14]. After intravesical instillation of 5-ALA or HAL, there is a preferential uptake of these agents by precancerous and cancerous cells and they convert into photoactive porphyrin (protoporphyrin IX) [15]. When fluorescent blue light is illuminated on the urothelium of the urinary bladder, only red fluorescence is emitted from the abnormal urothelium [15]. This distinct feature allows the differentiation between normal and malignant tissue.

Many studies confirmed that fluorescent cystoscopy showed higher detection rates of bladder cancers when compared to the standard resulting in lower recurrence rates. Burger et al. [16] conducted a meta-analysis to clinically assess the ability of fluorescent cystoscopy to detect NMIBC and tumor recurrence. They showed that fluorescent cystoscopy significantly increased the detection rates and reduced the risk of recurrence at 9−12 months. More importantly, Chou et al. [17] investigated the comparative effectiveness of fluorescent cystoscopy and white light cystoscopy on oncological outcomes in patients with NMIBC. Notably, the authors reported that fluorescent cystoscopy was significantly associated with a risk reduction of disease recurrence at short-term [relative risk (RR) = 0.59], intermediate-term (RR = 0.70), and long-term follow-up periods (RR = 0.81). However, there were no significant differences of the disease progression rates and survival estimates between the two techniques.

Current evidence indicates that fluorescent cystoscopy can improve the detection rate of bladder cancer and reduce the recurrence compared to white light cystoscopy. However, further clinical trials are required to confirm its effects on the disease progression and survival outcome among bladder cancer patients (Fig. 10.7).

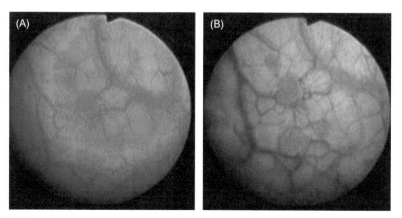

FIGURE 10.7 (A) White light cystoscopy alone. (B) Blue light cystoscopy as an adjunct to white light.

OPTICAL COHERENCE TOMOGRAPHY

Optical coherence tomography (OCT) is an emerging minimally invasive imaging technology using a near-infrared light to obtain cross-sectional images of the tissue [18]. In contrast to the low spatial resolution (70−1000 μm) of conventional noninvasive imaging tools such as ultrasonography or computed tomography, OCT produces higher resolution images using 10−20 μm of spatial resolution and 2−3 mm of imaging depths by calculating the magnitude and echo time delay of the unique backscattered light. [19]. Interestingly, OCT has been widely used in ophthalmology to examine the retina and has recently gained interest in the field of urology [19,20]. By inserting the probe via the working channel of a cystoscope, this attractive real-time imaging method can significantly differentiate the cancerous mucosa from normal urothelium of the urinary bladder by performing functional and structural analysis of the images [21].

Several reports have shown the ability of OCT to distinguish cancerous lesions from normal mucosa of the urinary bladder. The prospective single-center study by Schmidbauer et al. [22] investigated whether targeted OCT for the suspicious lesions on the standard cystoscopy or fluorescent cystoscopy potentiated the diagnostic accuracy for bladder cancer. The authors studied 66 patients with 232 lesions of NMIBC and discovered that the targeted OCT showed an additional 15%−20% detection rate of tumors compared to the white light or fluorescent cystoscopy alone. The sensitivity and specificity of targeted OCT were significantly higher than those without the combination of OCT (100% vs 87.9% and 87.5% vs 62.5%, respectively). Moreover, Goh and colleagues revealed that OCT had the ability to discriminate the clinical stage of bladder tumor in a real-time manner [23]. The authors evaluated 32 patients who underwent cystoscopic biopsy or transurethral resection of the bladder tumor and showed that the use of OCT in addition to the standard cystoscopy correctly distinguished Ta, T1, and T2 tumors with a sensitivity of 90%, 75%, and 100%, and a specificity of 89%, 97%, and 90%, respectively.

However, there are still unresolved limitations of this novel imaging tool in terms of bladder cancer detection including the risk of false-positive readings of bladder inflammatory lesions, the inability to take accurate images on large tumors with broadened involvement, and the equipped limited probe size with limited endoscopic view for whole urinary bladder wall [4]. Again, additional clinical evidence are required before applying this technology into the real-world clinical practice (Figs. 10.8 and 10.9).

OTHER EMERGING IMAGING TECHNOLOGIES

There are other advanced imaging technologies in the developing stage to improve the accuracy in detecting bladder cancer. Confocal laser

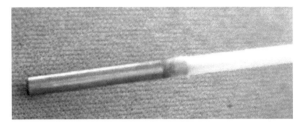

FIGURE 10.8 OCT probe inserted into the bladder via the working channel of the cystoscope sheath.

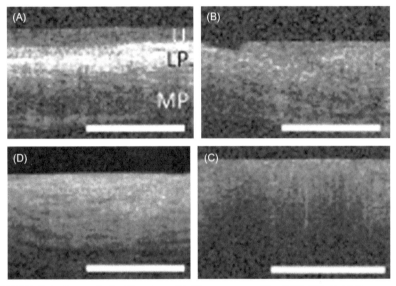

FIGURE 10.9 Layer of a healthy urinary bladder as generated by OCT. CIS: U + LP appear as single bright layer and MP is intact. T1: U + LP appear as single layer without clear demarcation with MP. T2: no evidence of horizontal structure. *CIS*, carcinoma in situ; *U*, urothelium; *LP*, lamina propria; *MP*, muscularis propria.

endomicroscopy (CLE) is the combined imaging tool with confocal microscopy and fiber optics with the highest resolution, up to 2−5 μm. [24]. CLE can obtain the microscopic, real-time, and histopathologic imaging data that provide optical biopsy in the suspicious lesions in vivo [25]. Two-photon laser microscopy is one of the fluorescence imaging techniques displaying the ability to detect autofluorescence of both cells as well as the extracellular matrix in the ultraviolet range and visualize the three-dimensional localization of target molecules in the living cells [26]. The ratio of distinct fluorescence of normal and malignant cells is used to differentiate them [27]. High-frequency endoluminal ultrasound shows a high resolution with significantly greater depth of penetration (up to 20 mm) improving the diagnostic accuracy for the larger and invasive tumors [28]. Specific molecular imaging agents conjugated with fluorophores, such as fluorescently labeled CD47 antibody, improve the visualization of tumorous lesions, and also reduce the false-positive readings by the inflammatory changes in the urinary bladder. Further studies are required to determine the suitability of these emerging technologies for accurately detecting bladder cancer [29].

CONCLUSIONS

In this chapter, several novel endoscopic imaging modalities for diagnosing and surveilling bladder cancer are reviewed. These include NBI, fluorescence cystoscopy, optical coherence, and other emerging technologies. Though the new imaging tools still do not replace the pathological confirmation of specimens where additional trials are desirable for their clinical use, they hold great potential to accurately detect cancer and estimate the oncological outcomes among patients with bladder cancer in the near future.

REFERENCES

[1] Siegel RL, Miller KD, Jemal A. Cancer statistics, 2016. CA Cancer J Clin 2016;66(1):7−30.

[2] Hall MC, Chang SS, Dalbagni G, Pruthi RS, Seigne JD, Skinner EC, et al. Guideline for the management of nonmuscle invasive bladder cancer (stages Ta, T1, and Tis): 2007 update. J Urol 2007;178(6):2314−30.

[3] Babjuk M, Bohle A, Burger M, Capoun O, Cohen D, Comperat EM, et al. EAU guidelines on non-muscle-invasive urothelial carcinoma of the bladder: update 2016. Eur Urol 2017;71(3):447−61.

[4] Hale NE, Deem S. Advances in cystoscopic surveillance of superficial bladder cancer: detection of the invisible tumor. Med Instrum 2013;1−5.

[5] Kolodziej A, Krajewski W, Matuszewski M, Tupikowski K. Review of current optical diagnostic techniques for non-muscle-invasive bladder cancer. Cent European J Urol 2016;69(2):150−6.

[6] Liu JJ, Droller MJ, Liao JC. New optical imaging technologies for bladder cancer: considerations and perspectives. J Urol 2012;188(2):361−8.

[7] Gono K. Narrow band imaging: technology basis and research and development history. Clin Endosc 2015;48(6):476−80.

[8] Naselli A, Puppo P. Narrow band imaging and bladder cancer: when and how. Urologia 2015;82(Suppl 2):S5−8.

[9] Naselli A, Hurle R, Puppo P. The role of narrow-band imaging in the management of non-muscle-invasive bladder cancer. Expert Rev Anticancer Ther 2012;12(12):1523−8.

[10] Bryan RT, Billingham LJ, Wallace DM. Narrow-band imaging flexible cystoscopy in the detection of recurrent urothelial cancer of the bladder. BJU Int 2008;101(6):702−5 discussion 5-6.

[11] Li K, Lin T, Fan X, Duan Y, Huang J. Diagnosis of narrow-band imaging in non-muscle-invasive bladder cancer: a systematic review and meta-analysis. Int J Urol 2013;20(6):602−9.

[12] Xiong Y, Li J, Ma S, Ge J, Zhou L, Li D, et al. A meta-analysis of narrow band imaging for the diagnosis and therapeutic outcome of non-muscle invasive bladder cancer. PloS One 2017;12(2):e0170819.

[13] Altobelli E, Zlatev DV, Liao JC. Role of narrow band imaging in management of urothelial carcinoma. Curr Urol Rep 2015;16(8):58.

[14] Shah JB, Kamat AM. Fluorescence cystoscopy for nonmuscle invasive bladder cancer: is the honeymoon over for the blue light special? Cancer 2011;117(5):882−3.

[15] Oude Elferink P, Witjes JA. Blue-light cystoscopy in the evaluation of non-muscle-invasive bladder cancer. Ther Adv Urol 2014;6(1):25−33.

[16] Burger M, Grossman HB, Droller M, Schmidbauer J, Hermann G, Dragoescu O, et al. Photodynamic diagnosis of non-muscle-invasive bladder cancer with hexaminolevulinate cystoscopy: a meta-analysis of detection and recurrence based on raw data. Eur Urol 2013;64(5):846−54.

[17] Chou R, Selph S, Buckley DI, Fu R, Griffin JC, Grusing S, et al. Comparative effectiveness of fluorescent versus white light cystoscopy for initial diagnosis or surveillance of bladder cancer on clinical outcomes: systematic review and meta-analysis. J Urol 2017;197(3 Pt 1):548−58.

[18] Cauberg EC, de Bruin DM, Faber DJ, van Leeuwen TG, de la Rosette JJ, de Reijke TM. A new generation of optical diagnostics for bladder cancer: technology, diagnostic accuracy, and future applications. Eur Urol 2009;56(2):287−96.

[19] Zysk AM, Nguyen FT, Oldenburg AL, Marks DL, Boppart SA. Optical coherence tomography: a review of clinical development from bench to bedside. J Biomed Opt 2007; 12(5):051403.

[20] Gupta M, Su LM. Current and evolving uses of optical coherence tomography in the genitourinary tract. Curr Urol Rep 2015;16(3):15.

[21] Kharchenko S, Adamowicz J, Wojtkowski M, Drewa T. Optical coherence tomography diagnostics for onco-urology. Review of clinical perspectives. Cent European J Urol 2013;66(2):136−41.

[22] Schmidbauer J, Remzi M, Klatte T, Waldert M, Mauermann J, Susani M, et al. Fluorescence cystoscopy with high-resolution optical coherence tomography imaging as an adjunct reduces false-positive findings in the diagnosis of urothelial carcinoma of the bladder. Eur Urol 2009;56(6):914−19.

[23] Goh AC, Tresser NJ, Shen SS, Lerner SP. Optical coherence tomography as an adjunct to white light cystoscopy for intravesical real-time imaging and staging of bladder cancer. Urology 2008;72(1):133−7.

[24] Neumann H, Kiesslich R, Wallace MB, Neurath MF. Confocal laser endomicroscopy: technical advances and clinical applications. Gastroenterology 2010;139(2):388−92 92 e1-2.

[25] Wu K, Liu JJ, Adams W, Sonn GA, Mach KE, Pan Y, et al. Dynamic real-time microscopy of the urinary tract using confocal laser endomicroscopy. Urology 2011;78 (1):225−31.

[26] Imanishi Y, Lodowski KH, Koutalos Y. Two-photon microscopy: shedding light on the chemistry of vision. Biochemistry 2007;46(34):9674−84.

[27] Perry SW, Burke RM, Brown EB. Two-photon and second harmonic microscopy in clinical and translational cancer research. Ann Biomed Eng 2012;40(2):277−91.

[28] Kondabolu S, Khan SA, Whyard J, Diblasio C, Ayyala M, Pentyala S. The role of endoluminal ultrasonography in urology: current perspectives. Int Braz J Urol 2004;30 (2):96−101.

[29] Pan Y, Volkmer JP, Mach KE, Rouse RV, Liu JJ, Sahoo D, et al. Endoscopic molecular imaging of human bladder cancer using a CD47 antibody. Sci Transl Med 2014;6(260) 260ra148.

Section III

Pathology and Staging

Chapter 11

Histological Classification of Bladder Tumors

Young A. Kim[1] and Kyung C. Moon[2]

[1]Seoul Metropolitan Government Boramae Hospital, Seoul, South Korea, [2]Seoul National University College of Medicine, Seoul, South Korea

Chapter Outline

UROTHELIAL NEOPLASMS

WHO Classification of Tumors of Urinary Tract

The fourth edition of "WHO classification of tumors of the urinary system and male genital organs" is published in 2016, which is summarized in Table 11.1 [1].

Noninvasive Urothelial Lesions

Urothelial Proliferation of Uncertain Malignant Potential

1. Definition and clinical features

    Urothelial proliferation of uncertain malignant potential is an urothelial lesion showing a thickening of the urothelium without cytologic atypia and no true papillary architecture. This lesion is frequently seen in patients with a history of papillary urothelial lesions.

2. Pathologic features

    Cystoscopically, this lesion can be seen as a focal elevated lesion or may show no gross abnormality.

    Microscopically, urothelial layer is markedly thickened and arranged in undulating folds, but well-formed papillae are not found (Fig. 11.1).

Bladder Cancer. DOI: http://dx.doi.org/10.1016/B978-0-12-809939-1.00011-4

TABLE 11.1 Summary of 2016 WHO Classification of Tumors of the Urinary Tract

Urothelial Tumors	Neuroendocrine Tumors
Infiltrating urothelial carcinoma	Small cell neuroendocrine carcinoma
Urothelial carcinoma in situ	Large cell neuroendocrine carcinoma
Noninvasive papillary urothelial carcinoma, low grade	Well-differentiated neuroendocrine tumor
Noninvasive papillary urothelial carcinoma, high grade	Paraganglioma
Papillary urothelial neoplasm of low malignant potential	*Melanocytic tumors*
Urothelial papilloma	Malignant melanoma
Inverted urothelial papilloma	Nevus
Urothelial proliferation of uncertain malignant potential	Melanosis
Urothelial dysplasia	*Mesenchymal tumors*
Urothelial dysplasia	Rhabdomyosarcoma
Squamous cell neoplasms	Leiomyosarcoma
Pure squamous cell carcinoma	Angiosarcoma
Verrucous carcinoma	Inflammatory myofibroblastic tumor
Squamous cell papilloma	Perivascular epithelioid cell tumor
Glandular neoplasms	Solitary fibrous tumor
Adenocarcinoma	Leiomyoma
Villous adenoma	Hemangioma
Urachal carcinoma	Granular cell tumor
Tumors of Müllerian type	Neurofibroma
Clear cell carcinoma	*Hematopoietic and lymphoid tumors*
Endometrioid carcinoma	*Miscellaneous tumors*

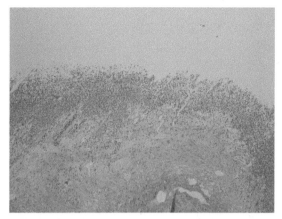

FIGURE 11.1 Urothelial proliferation of uncertain malignant potential. Microscopically, urothelial layer shows markedly increased thickness with undulating folds. Well-formed papillae are not identified. Cytologic atypia is absent or minimal.

Cytological atypia is absent or minimal. It can be found adjacent to the low-grade papillary neoplasms.

3. Prognosis

The 5-year risk of subsequently developing urothelial neoplasia is almost 40%, so this lesion is regarded as an early manifestation of low-grade papillary urothelial neoplasm [2−4].

Urothelial Dysplasia

1. Definition and clinical features

Urothelial dysplasia is a flat lesion with features of cytological and architectural atypia that fall short of the criteria for carcinoma in situ (CIS) [5]. De novo lesion is rare, so clinical symptoms are associated with accompanying papillary or invasive carcinoma.

2. Pathologic features

Grossly, urothelial dysplasia usually appears normal.

Microscopically, urothelial dysplasia shows mild loss of polarity, focal nuclear crowding and nuclear enlargement or irregularity but not the degree seen in urothelial CIS (Fig. 11.2).

3. Prognosis

Progression rate of urothelial dysplasia is reported to be 15%−19% [6,7].

Urothelial CIS

1. Definition and clinical features

Urothelial CIS is a flat noninvasive urothelial lesion composed of cytologically malignant cells. CIS is usually seen in association with high-grade

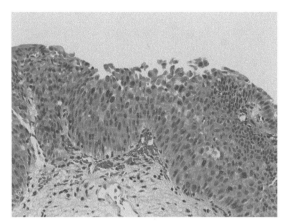

FIGURE 11.2   Urothelial dysplasia. Microscopically, urothelium revealed mild loss of polarity, focal nuclear crowding, and nuclear enlargement or irregularity. The degree of cytologic atypia is less than those in urothelial CIS.

papillary or invasive urothelial carcinoma. Pure form of CIS accounts only for 1%−3% of newly diagnosed cases of bladder cancer [8,9].

2. Pathologic features

   Grossly, CIS appears as an erythematous lesion. Microscopically, malignant tumor cells have large pleomorphic nuclei with one or multiple nucleoli, and there is architectural disorder with haphazardly arranged nuclei and nuclear crowding (Fig. 11.3A). Tumor cells of CIS are often discohesive, and in some cases only a few atypical cells are present clinging to the basement membrane (Fig. 11.3B). Sometimes, the tumor cells show pagetoid spread (Fig. 11.3C).

   Immunohistochemistry may be helpful in differentiating CIS from urothelial atypia. CK20 is positive in full thickness of CIS while being only positive in umbrella cells of normal urothelium (Fig. 11.3D). Diffuse expression of p53 is shown in most of the CIS cases [10,11].

3. Prognosis

   Up to 25% cases of CIS progress to invasive disease. Failure to intravesical therapy has been associated with disease progression and is an indication for early cystectomy [12,13].

Urothelial Papilloma

1. Definition and clinical features

   Urothelial papilloma is a papillary urothelial neoplasm lined by urothelium of normal appearance and thickness. Most cases occur in less than 50 years of age. The main symptom is microscopic or gross hematuria.

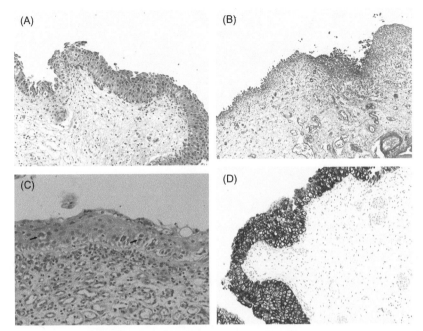

FIGURE 11.3   Urothelial CIS. (A) Microscopically, urothelium shows haphazardly arranged nuclei and nuclear crowding. The malignant tumor cells show large pleomorphic nuclei with one or multiple nucleoli. (B) Tumor cells of CIS often show clinging pattern with discohesive nature. (C) Sometimes, pagetoid spread pattern (*arrow*) was identified. (D) Immunohistochemical staining of CK20 shows positivity in full thickness of CIS.

2. Pathologic features

   Grossly, urothelial papilloma presents as a single small exophytic papillary lesion.

   Microscopically, urothelial papilloma has delicate fibrovascular cores and simple papillary structures with minimal epithelial confluence between papillae. Overly urothelium is not thickened and there is no cellular atypia (Fig. 11.4).

3. Prognosis

   Recurrence and progression are rare in de novo cases. The treatment of choice is complete transurethral resection [14,15].

Inverted Urothelial Papilloma

1. Definition and clinical features

   Inverted urothelial papilloma is an urothelial neoplasm with a complex, anastomosing inverted growth pattern and absent to minimal

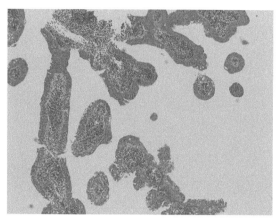

FIGURE 11.4 Urothelial papilloma. Microscopically, urothelial papilloma shows fibrovascular cores and simple papillary structures with no cellular atypia.

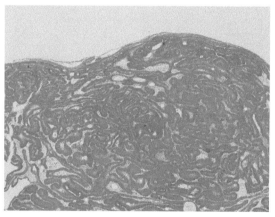

FIGURE 11.5 Inverted urothelial papilloma. Microscopically, inverted urothelial papilloma arises from surface epithelium and shows complex trabecular, inverted growth pattern with minimal cytologic atypia.

cytological atypia. Inverted urothelial papilloma constitutes less than 1% of all bladder neoplasm. Main presenting symptom is hematuria.

2. Pathologic features

Grossly, it presents as raised, polypoid lesion with a smooth overlying surface.

Microscopically, this lesion arises from surface epithelium with invagination into lamina propria. It showed complex trabecular, inverted growth pattern with minimal cytological atypia (Fig. 11.5) [16,17].

3. Prognosis

Inverted papilloma is treated with transurethral resection and the recurrence rate is very low (less than 2%) [18].

Papillary Urothelial Neoplasm of Low Malignant Potential

1. Definition and clinical features

    Papillary urothelial neoplasm of low malignant potential (PUNLMP) is a papillary urothelial tumor with minimal atypia and thickened urothelium. Main initial symptom is gross or microscopic hematuria. However, urine cytology is negative in most cases.

2. Pathologic features

    Grossly, it is a single or multiple exophytic papillary lesions of variable size.

    Microscopically, tumors are composed of delicate papillae lined by thickened urothelium but no other architectural abnormalities (Fig. 11.6A). Nuclei of the tumor cells are slightly enlarged and more crowded and show monotonous appearance (Fig. 11.6B). Mitoses are very rare and only limited to basal layer [5].

3. Prognosis

    PUNLMPs have a significantly lower rate of recurrence than papillary low-grade urothelial carcinoma and have a very low rate of stage progression [19−22].

Noninvasive Papillary Urothelial Carcinoma, Low Grade

1. Definition and clinical features

    Noninvasive papillary urothelial carcinoma, low-grade, is a papillary urothelial proliferation with some degree of disorder in architectural and cytological features at medium power magnification. However, invasion beyond the basement membrane is not observed (Ta). Most common symptom is painless intermittent hematuria.

2. Pathologic features

    Grossly, there are single or multiple exophytic lesions with variable sizes.

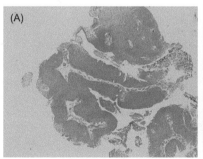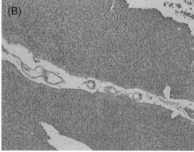

FIGURE 11.6 Papillary urothelial neoplasm of low malignant potential. (A) Microscopically, papillary urothelial neoplasm of low malignant potential shows delicate papillae lined by thickened urothelium with no other architectural abnormalities. (B) Tumor cells show crowded and slightly enlarged nuclei with monotonous appearance.

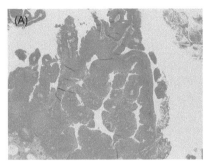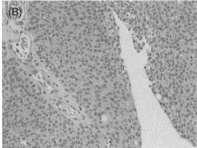

FIGURE 11.7 Noninvasive papillary urothelial carcinoma, low grade. (A) Microscopically, relatively ordered architectural and cytological features with branching delicate papillae are identified at low magnification. (B) At high magnification, the loss of polarity, nuclear pleomorphism, and irregularity are easily identified.

Microscopically, low-grade lesions have delicate papillae with extensive branching. At low magnification, they give the impression of relative order in architectural and cytological features (Fig. 11.7A). However, at medium power, the loss of polarity, nuclear irregularity, and pleomorphism are easily seen (Fig. 11.7B). Mitoses are usually found away from basement membrane [5,23].

3. Prognosis

The recurrence and stage progression rates are 50% and 10% for low-grade carcinoma, respectively [24].

Noninvasive Papillary Urothelial Carcinoma, High Grade

1. Definition and clinical features

Noninvasive papillary urothelial carcinoma, high-grade, is a papillary urothelial proliferation with marked architectural and cytological disorder at low power magnification. However, invasion beyond the basement membrane is not observed (Ta). Most common symptom is painless intermittent hematuria.

2. Pathologic features

Grossly, there are single or multiple exophytic lesions with variable sizes. High-grade lesions are more hyperemic and nontranslucent.

Microscopically, in high-grade lesions, papillae are frequently fused forming apparently solid masses. Nuclear size variation, irregularity, and pleomorphism are readily recognized at low to medium magnification (Fig. 11.8). Mitoses are frequent including abnormal ones and may be seen at any level of epithelium [5,25].

3. Prognosis

In high-grade carcinoma, the recurrence rate is 60%, and the rates of progression to lamina propria (T1) and invasion of muscularis propria are 25% and 5%, respectively [26].

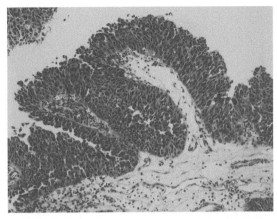

FIGURE 11.8 Noninvasive papillary urothelial carcinoma, high grade. Microscopically, tumor cells show marked nuclear size variation, irregularity, and pleomorphism. The papillae are frequently fused and formed solid masses.

Infiltrating Urothelial Carcinoma

1. Definition and clinical features

Infiltrating urothelial carcinoma is an urothelial carcinoma with the invasion beyond the basement membrane. It is the most common malignant neoplasm of the urinary tract. Bladder cancer is three to four times more common in men than in women, and median age at diagnosis is 65−70 years [27−29]. Most common symptom is painless gross hematuria, followed by urgency, nocturia, and dysuria.

2. Pathologic features

Grossly, most of infiltrating urothelial carcinomas is polypoid, sessile, or ulceroinfiltrative. Associated CIS is indicated by erythematous areas.

Invasive urothelial carcinoma is well known for its histologic diversity. Many of these are so distinct that they are now separated as specific variants, which are discussed in detail later in this chapter [30,31]. Invasive urothelial carcinoma presents wide variety of growth pattern, such as solid sheet, large and small nests, trabeculae, cords, and single cells (Fig. 11.9). The majority of invasive urothelial carcinomas are high-grade, which means prominent nuclear pleomorphism and high mitotic rates with abnormal mitotic figures. Desmoplastic stromal reaction is also prominent in most of the cases.

Immunohistochemically, uroplakin III and GATA3 are commonly used specific markers for urothelial carcinoma [11]. Urothelial carcinoma also expresses CK7, CK20, high-molecular weight cytokeratin, and p63.

3. Prognosis

Depth of invasion, especially muscularis propria invasion is the most important prognostic determinant in invasive urothelial carcinoma.

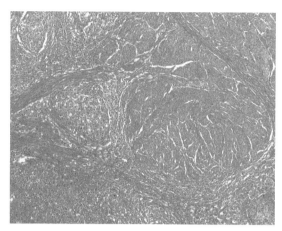

FIGURE 11.9 Infiltrating urothelial carcinoma. Microscopically, invasive urothelial carcinoma shows variable growth patterns including solid sheet, large and small nests, trabeculae, cords, and single cells.

Accompanying CIS increases the risk of progression to muscle-invasive tumor up to 50% [32]. High-grade tumors have poorer prognosis than low-grade tumors although most of invasive urothelial carcinomas are high grade [32].

Urothelial Carcinoma with Divergent Differentiation

Urothelial carcinomas occasionally can have areas with nonurothelial differentiation such as squamous, glandular, or trophoblastic differentiation.

Urothelial Carcinoma with Squamous Differentiation

1. Definition and clinical features

    Squamous differentiation of urothelial carcinoma is defined by the presence of squamous cell carcinoma area having intercellular bridge, keratin pearl, or keratinization with typical urothelial carcinoma. The incidence of squamous or glandular differentiation in urothelial carcinoma has been reported in about 7%−18% [33−35]. Squamous differentiation is more common than glandular differentiation of urothelial carcinoma.

2. Pathologic features

    Grossly, urothelial carcinomas with squamous differentiation frequently form muscle-invasive mass lesion (Fig. 11.10A).

    Microscopically, squamous differentiation is characterized by keratinization and intercellular bridge. These features are found in various proportions with typical urothelial carcinoma component (Fig. 11.10B).

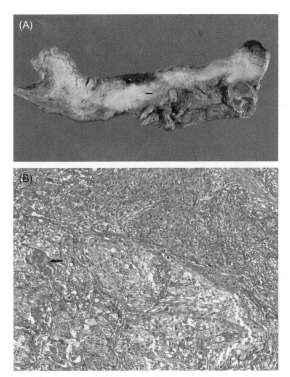

FIGURE 11.10 Urothelial carcinoma with squamous differentiation. (A) Gross photograph of urothelial carcinoma with squamous differentiation shows a muscle-invasive mass at the cut section. (B) Microscopically, both urothelial carcinoma component (upper right) and squamous cell carcinoma area (lower left) are found in this case with keratinization (*arrow*).

Sometimes, only urothelial CIS lesion can be found as urothelial carcinoma components.

3. Differential diagnosis

Pure squamous cell carcinoma is included in the differential diagnosis. They do not have the urothelial carcinoma components, and keratinizing squamous metaplasia of nonneoplastic urothelium is often found in pure squamous cell carcinomas.

4. Prognosis

Squamous or glandular differentiation is frequently found in high-stage urothelial carcinoma [34,35]. Prognostic significance of squamous or glandular differentiation of urothelial carcinoma is controversial [33,35]. Some studies showed that squamous or glandular differentiation of urothelial carcinoma is an independent predictor of survival, but other studies could not reveal the prognostic significance of squamous or glandular differentiation in survival analysis.

Urothelial Carcinoma with Glandular Differentiation

1. Definition and clinical features

   Glandular differentiation of urothelial carcinoma is defined by the presence of glandular components within the urothelial carcinoma. It is less common than squamous differentiation of urothelial carcinoma. Rarely squamous and glandular differentiation can be found in the same cases.

2. Pathologic features

   Grossly, urothelial carcinomas with glandular differentiation frequently form muscle-invasive mass lesion.

   Microscopically, areas of glandular differentiation are found with typical urothelial carcinoma component (Fig. 11.11). Glandular components frequently resemble the colonic adenocarcinoma. Less commonly, mucinous adenocarcinoma or signet ring cell carcinoma components can be found.

   Immunohistochemically, glandular components of urothelial carcinoma can occasionally express CDX2 and CK20 like colonic adenocarcinoma [36].

3. Differential diagnosis

   Pure adenocarcinoma or urachal carcinoma is included in the differential diagnosis. They do not have the urothelial carcinoma components.

4. Prognosis

   Urothelial carcinoma with squamous and/or glandular differentiation is frequently found in higher stage urothelial carcinoma [33,35].

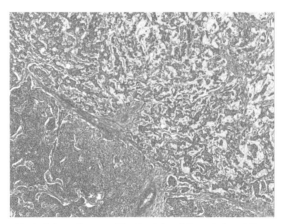

FIGURE 11.11 Urothelial carcinoma with glandular differentiation. Microscopically, typical urothelial carcinoma component (lower left) and component of carcinoma with glandular differentiation (upper right) are identified.

Urothelial Carcinoma with Trophoblastic Differentiation

1. Definition and clinical features

Trophoblastic differentiation of urothelial carcinoma is defined by the presence of syncytiotrophoblastic giant cells or choriocarcinoma components. Patients with urothelial carcinoma with trophoblastic differentiation show elevated serum β-human chorionic gonadotropin (β-hCG) level. In fact, serum β-hCG level is also frequently elevated in patients with high-grade urothelial carcinoma without trophoblastic differentiation and can be a prognostic factor for urothelial carcinoma [37].

2. Pathologic features

Microscopically, this tumor contains syncytiotrophoblastic giant cells or choriocarcinoma components with typical high-grade urothelial carcinoma (Fig. 11.12A). Syncytiotrophoblastic giant cells or choriocarcinoma components are rarely found in routine hematoxylin-eosin (HE) sections of urothelial carcinoma. However, high-grade urothelial carcinomas frequently show immunoreactivity for β-hCG without morphologic evidence of syncytiotrophoblastic giant cells or trophoblastic differentiation.

Immunohistochemistry for β-hCG shows positive staining (Fig. 11.12B).

Variants of Urothelial Carcinoma

Nested Variant

1. Definition and clinical features

Nested variant of urothelial carcinoma is defined by the invasive urothelial carcinoma composed of bland-appearing small urothelial nests resembling von Brunn nests.

It is very rare with an incidence of 0.3% of invasive urothelial carcinomas. The patient age ranged from 42 to 90 years, and this tumor is more common in men [38].

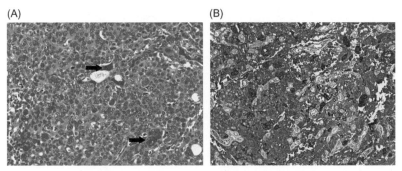

(A)   (B)

FIGURE 11.12   Urothelial carcinoma with trophoblastic differentiation. (A) Microscopically, multinucleated syncytiotrophoblastic giant cells (*arrows*) are seen. (B) β-HCG immunoreactivity is identified in this case with trophoblastic differentiation.

2. Pathologic features

Nested variant is composed of irregular, confluent small nests infiltrating the lamina propria and proper muscle layer (Fig. 11.13). This tumor can have area of conventional urothelial carcinoma. The tumor cells in infiltrating nests have minimal to mild atypia. Sometimes tubule or microcyst formation can be found. Large nested variant of urothelial carcinoma is another variation of nested variant consisting of large infiltrating nests with bland cytology (Fig. 11.14) [39].

Immunohistochemical features of nested variant are similar to those of conventional urothelial carcinomas showing positive staining for CK7, CK20, and p63 [40].

3. Differential diagnosis

Nested variant urothelial carcinomas can be confused with some benign conditions such as von Brunn nest or nephrogenic adenoma due to bland cytology of nested variant.

4. Prognosis

Nested variants of urothelial carcinoma show unfavorable prognosis similar to conventional high-grade infiltrating urothelial carcinomas [41]. This variant is also commonly associated with muscle invasion, extravesical extension, and metastasis [38].

Micropapillary Variant

1. Definition and clinical features

Micropapillary variant of urothelial carcinoma is defined by microscopic features consisting of micropapillary architecture on mucosal surface and infiltrating small and tight nests surrounded by lacuna-like space.

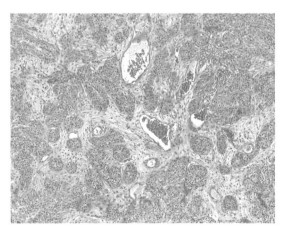

FIGURE 11.13 Urothelial carcinoma, nested variant. Microscopically, nested urothelial carcinoma shows infiltrating irregular, confluent small nests with minimal to mild cytologic atypia.

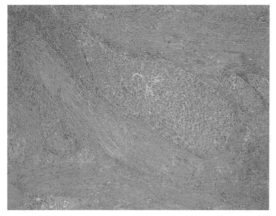

FIGURE 11.14   Urothelial carcinoma, large nested variant. Photomicrograph of a large nested variant of urothelial carcinoma with invasion of the muscularis propria.

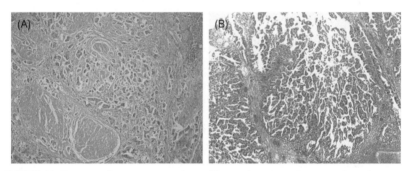

FIGURE 11.15   Urothelial carcinoma, micropapillary variant. (A) Microscopically, micropapillary variant of urothelial carcinoma shows small infiltrating urothelial nests without fibrovascular core and resembles lymphovascular invasion. (B) Noninvasive micropapillary components arising from the main papillary core are shown in the surface of urothelium.

The incidence of micropapillary variant has been reported about 1%−8% of urothelial carcinomas, and male to female ratio is 5:1 to 10:1 [42,43].

2. Pathologic features

Gross findings of micropapillary variant of urothelial carcinoma are not specific. It can be papillary, polypoid, ulcerated, or infiltrative mass [43,44].

Microscopically, micropapillary variant of urothelial carcinoma is composed of small infiltrating urothelial nests without fibrovascular core, and these nests are surrounded by empty space resembling lymphovascular invasion (Fig. 11.15A). Noninvasive micropapillary components can be present in the surface urothelium (Fig. 11.15B). True lymphovascular invasion is also common. The nuclei of tumor cells are typically high grade. This variant is commonly admixed with conventional high-grade urothelial carcinoma, other variants of urothelial carcinomas, and/or urothelial CIS [45,46]. The proportion of micropapillary components is variable.

Micropapillary components are frequently positive for CK7, CK20, and uroplakin III; but p63 expression of micropapillary variant is relatively lower than conventional urothelial carcinomas [40,47,48]. HER2 protein overexpression or *HER2* gene amplification is more frequently present in micropapillary variant of urothelial carcinoma than in conventional urothelial carcinoma [49].

3. Differential diagnosis

Micropapillary variant of urothelial carcinomas can be confused with metastatic ovarian serous carcinoma or metastatic micropapillary carcinoma of other organs such as breast.

4. Prognosis

Micropapillary variant is frequently muscle invasive at presentation and also frequently shows lymph node and distant metastasis [50]. Prognosis of this variant is generally poorer than conventional urothelial carcinoma [50,51].

Plasmacytoid Variant

1. Definition and clinical features

Plasmacytoid variant of urothelial carcinoma is a rare and aggressive variant containing plasma cell–like tumor cells.

This rare variant constitutes about 0.5% of urothelial carcinomas, and males are more commonly affected [52–54]. Main initial presenting symptom is hematuria.

2. Pathologic features

At microscopy, the tumor cells are small- to medium-sized single cells with eccentric hyperchromatic nuclei and amphophilic or eosinophilic cytoplasm resembling plasma cells (Fig. 11.16A). The proportion of plasmacytoid component ranged from 30% to 100%, and this variant can be admixed with conventional urothelial carcinoma or other variants such as micropapillary variant [54].

Plasmacytoid variants of urothelial carcinoma express CK7, CK20, and CD138 (Fig. 11.16B, C). And this variant frequently shows HER2 protein overexpression and *HER2* gene amplification (Fig. 11.16D) [54].

3. Differential diagnosis

Plasmacytoma should be considered in differential diagnosis. Immunostaining for cytokeratin can differentiate plasmacytoid variant urothelial carcinoma from plasmacytoma.

4. Prognosis

Plasmacytoid variant urothelial carcinoma frequently presents at a high stage and has a poor prognosis [55].

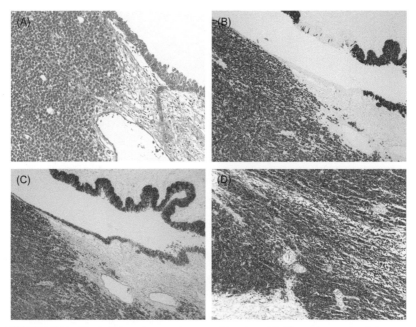

FIGURE 11.16   Urothelial carcinoma, plasmacytoid variant. (A) Photomicrograph of plasmacy-toid variant of urothelial carcinoma shows tumor cells with eccentric hyperchromatic nuclei and amphophilic or eosinophilic cytoplasm resembling plasma cells. The tumor cells revealed immu-noreactivity for CK7 (B), CD138 (C), and HER2 protein overexpression (D).

Sarcomatoid Carcinoma

1. Definition and clinical features

    Sarcomatoid carcinomas of urinary bladder have both malignant spin-dle cell or malignant mesenchymal tumor components and malignant epithelial tumor components.

    A main presenting symptom of sarcomatoid carcinoma is gross hematuria-like conventional urothelial carcinoma. Mean age of patients is 72 years, and males are more commonly affected [56].

2. Pathologic features

    Malignant epithelial tumor components can be urothelial carcinoma, squamous cell carcinoma, adenocarcinoma, or small-cell carcinoma [56]. Sarcomatoid components can show variable morphology including spin-dle cell sarcoma, pleomorphic sarcoma, or heterologous elements such as chondrosarcoma, osteosarcoma, rhabdomyosarcoma, or liposarcoma (Fig. 11.17A, B) [57].

    Sarcomatoid components frequently express both epithelial markers such as cytokeratin or epithelial membrane antigen and mesenchymal markers such as vimentin (Fig. 11.17C) [56].

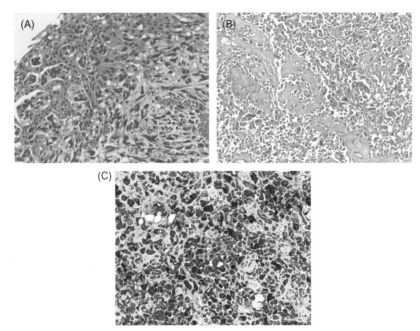

FIGURE 11.17 Sarcomatoid carcinoma. Microscopically, sarcomatoid carcinoma can have atypical spindle cells (lower right) (A) or heterologous elements such as osteosarcoma (B). (C) Immunoreactivity for CK was identified at osteosarcoma component of sarcomatoid carcinoma.

3. Differential diagnosis

Pure sarcomas of urinary bladder can be considered in differential diagnosis. Sarcomatoid carcinoma has malignant epithelial components and frequently expresses cytokeratin.

4. Prognosis

Sarcomatoid carcinomas of urinary bladder frequently present at high stage in initial diagnosis.

NONUROTHELIAL NEOPLASMS

Epithelial Tumors

Squamous Cell Carcinoma of Urinary Bladder

1. Definition and clinical features

Squamous cell carcinoma of urinary bladder is a malignant epithelial neoplasm consisting of pure squamous cell components.

Risk factors of squamous cell carcinoma of urinary bladder include chromic schistosomial infection, bladder stone, and long-term catheterization. Major presenting symptom is a hematuria and dysuria [58].

2. Pathologic features

Grossly, squamous cell carcinomas of urinary bladder show exophytic, ulcerated, or solid appearance [58]. Unaffected mucosa of urinary bladder frequently reveals whitish change representing squamous metaplasia (Fig. 11.18A).

Microscopically, squamous cell carcinoma of urinary bladder has identical features of squamous cell carcinomas of other sites such as keratin pearl, individual keratinization, or intercellular bridges (Fig. 11.18B). By definition, urothelial carcinoma components should not be included. Nonneoplastic mucosa adjacent to the tumor frequently reveals squamous metaplasia (Fig. 11.18C)

3. Differential diagnosis

Urothelial carcinoma with squamous differentiation should be included in differential diagnosis, and the presence of urothelial carcinoma components or urothelial CIS supports the diagnosis of urothelial carcinoma.

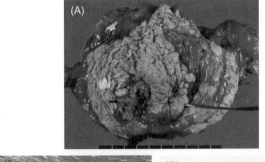

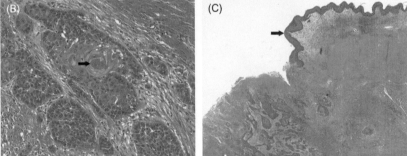

FIGURE 11.18   Squamous cell carcinoma. (A) Gross photograph of squamous cell carcinoma of urinary bladder shows exophytic and ulcerated mass (*arrow*). Whitish change representing squamous metaplasia was shown in unaffected mucosa of urinary bladder. (B) Keratin pearl formation (*arrow*) and individual keratinization were identified. (C) Squamous metaplasia (*arrow*) of nonneoplastic mucosa adjacent to the tumor is frequently seen (upper right).

4. Prognosis

Squamous cell carcinomas of urinary bladder are frequently of high stage at presentation and show poor prognosis [58,59].

Adenocarcinoma of Urinary Bladder

1. Definition and clinical features

Adenocarcinoma of urinary bladder consists purely of malignant glandular elements without association with urothelial carcinoma or squamous cell carcinoma.

Pure adenocarcinoma of urinary bladder is rare. Gross hematuria is the most frequent symptom.

2. Pathologic features

Adenocarcinoma of urinary bladder can show various histologic features including enteric type adenocarcinoma, NOS (not otherwise specified) type adenocarcinoma, mucinous adenocarcinoma, or signet ring cell carcinoma (Fig. 11.19A, B). The enteric type is similar to colonic adenocarcinoma. Mucinous type contains abundant mucin with some floating tumor cell clusters.

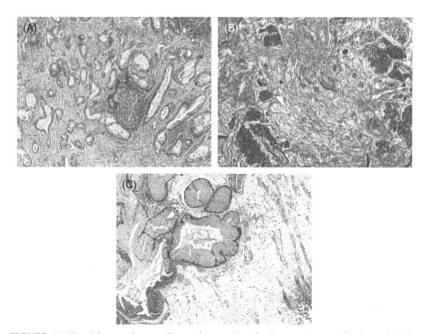

FIGURE 11.19 Adenocarcinoma. Photomicrographs of adenocarcinoma of urinary bladder showing histologic features of enteric type adenocarcinoma (A) and mucinous adenocarcinoma with signet ring cell components (B). (C) Intestinal type cystitis glandularis can be confused with adenocarcinoma of urinary bladder, but this lesion shows no cytologic atypia.

In immunohistochemical staining, adenocarcinoma of urinary bladder commonly expresses CK20 and may express CK7 and CDX2.

3. Differential diagnosis

The differential diagnostic considerations include secondary adenocarcinomas especially from colon. Microscopic features and immunohistochemical findings of colonic adenocarcinoma can be similar to those of adenocarcinoma of urinary bladder. Frequent nuclear beta-catenin positivity of colonic adenocarcinoma can be helpful in differential diagnosis. Intestinal type cystitis glandularis also can be confused with adenocarcinoma of urinary bladder, but this lesion resembles normal colonic mucosa without cytologic atypia (Fig. 11.19C).

4. Prognosis

Adenocarcinomas of urinary bladder also show poor prognosis due to its frequent presence at high stage and show poor prognosis.

Urachal Carcinoma

1. Definition and clinical features

Urachal carcinoma is defined by an invasive carcinoma arising from urachal remnant. Most of urachal carcinomas are adenocarcinoma, but urothelial or squamous carcinoma can arise.

It is less common than nonurachal primary adenocarcinoma of urinary bladder. Mean age of patients has been reported as 58 years, and this tumor is more common in men [60].

2. Pathologic features

Grossly, urachal carcinoma is mainly located to dome of urinary bladder. On cut sections, urachal carcinoma shows predominant invasion of the muscularis or deeper tissues (Fig. 11.20A).

Microscopically, urachal adenocarcinoma can have variable histologic pattern such as enteric type, NOS (not otherwise specified) type, mucinous type, signet ring cell type, and mixed type (Fig. 11.20B, C). Enteric type and NOS type are common histologic type of urachal adenocarcinoma [60]. Urachal remnants are frequently present. Diagnosis of urachal adenocarcinoma can be made from clinicopathologic considerations. Location of tumor, histologic findings, and clinical situations are important to exact diagnosis. Some diagnostic criteria of urachal adenocarcinoma have been proposed [60,61]. Gopalan et al. used the following diagnostic criteria [60]: (1) Location of the tumor in the dome/anterior wall, (2) epicenter of carcinoma in the bladder wall, (3) absence of widespread cystitis cystica/glandularis beyond the dome/anterior wall, and (4) absence of a known primary elsewhere.

In immunohistochemical staining, urachal adenocarcinomas frequently express CK7, CK20, and CDX2 (Fig. 11.20D)

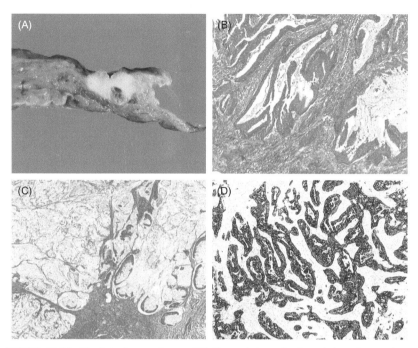

FIGURE 11.20 Urachal adenocarcinoma. (A) Gross photograph of urachal carcinoma shows invasion of the muscularis and deeper tissues at a cut section. Microscopically, urachal carcinoma can show histologic patterns of enteric type (B) and mucinous type (C). (D) Immunoreactivity for CK20 is frequently seen.

3. Differential diagnosis

Nonurachal primary adenocarcinoma of urinary bladder and involvement of colonic adenocarcinoma are main differential diagnostic considerations. The above-mentioned diagnostic criteria help the differential diagnosis.

Clear-Cell Adenocarcinoma

1. Definition and clinical features

Clear-cell adenocarcinoma is a distinct morphologic variant of adenocarcinoma of urinary bladder or urethra and resembles the clear-cell adenocarcinoma of female genital tract.

It is very rare. This tumor is more frequently developed in urethra than in urinary bladder and commonly occurs in female with hematuria or dysuria [62].

2. Pathologic features

Clear-cell adenocarcinoma of urinary bladder and urethra shows mixed growth pattern, solid, tubular, papillary, or cystic (Fig. 11.21A). Flat to cuboidal tumor cells have clear to eosinophilic cytoplasm

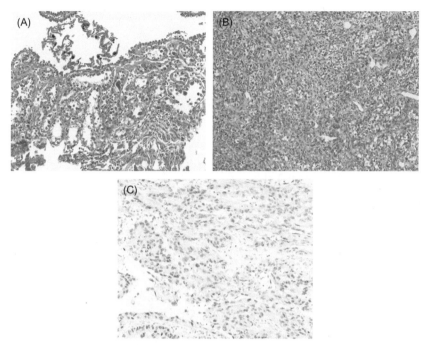

FIGURE 11.21 Clear-cell adenocarcinoma. Microscopically, clear-cell adenocarcinoma shows tubular or cystic (A) or solid growth pattern (B) and is composed of cuboidal tumor cells with clear to eosinophilic cytoplasm. (C) Nuclear expression of PAX8 is typically identified.

(Fig. 11.21B). Hobnail appearance can be present. Urethral clear-cell adenocarcinoma is frequently associated with urethral diverticulum [62].

In immunohistochemical staining, typically PAX2 and PAX8 are positive in nuclei (Fig. 11.21C). CK7 and AMACR are also frequently positive.

3. Differential diagnosis

Nephrogenic adenoma (nephrogenic metaplasia) can be confused with clear-cell adenocarcinoma. Nephrogenic adenoma also expresses PAX2 and PAX8 and can show similar histology to clear-cell adenocarcinoma. However, nephrogenic adenoma is usually in small size and does not show nuclear pleomorphism.

Neuroendocrine Tumors

Small-Cell Neuroendocrine Carcinoma

1. Definition and clinical features

Small-cell neuroendocrine carcinoma of urinary bladder is highly malignant neuroendocrine tumor histologically resembling pulmonary small-cell carcinoma.

It is an extremely rare tumor with the incidence of 0.35%−1.8% of all urinary bladder cancers [63].

2. Pathologic features

Grossly, this tumor can be present as polypoid mass with extensive infiltration.

Histological features of small-cell neuroendocrine carcinoma of urinary bladder are identical to those of small-cell carcinoma of lung or other sites (Fig. 11.22A). The tumor consists of sheets or nests of uniform small- to medium-sized tumor cells with scant cytoplasm, hyperchromatic nuclei, nuclear molding, and finely stippled chromatin. Mitotic figures are common. Small-cell neuroendocrine carcinoma can be admixed with other type carcinomas such as conventional urothelial carcinoma, squamous cell carcinoma, or adenocarcinoma of about 50% of cases (Fig. 11.22B).

Neuroendocrine markers, synaptophysin, chromogranin A, and CD56 are positive (Fig. 11.22C). TTF-1, a marker of pulmonary small-cell

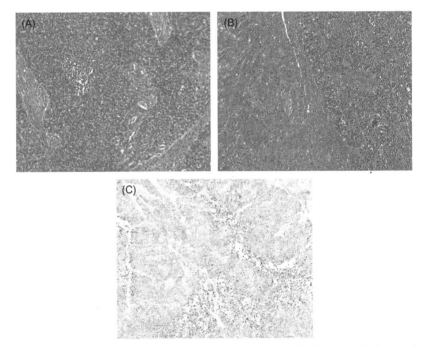

FIGURE 11.22 Small-cell neuroendocrine carcinoma. (A) Small-cell neuroendocrine carcinoma of urinary bladder is histologically identical to small-cell carcinoma of lung or other sites and consists of uniform small- to medium-sized tumor cells with scant cytoplasm, hyperchromatic nuclei, and finely stippled chromatin. (B) Conventional urothelial carcinoma component (left) and small-cell neuroendocrine carcinoma component (right) are found in this case. (C) Immunoreactivity for synaptophysin is observed.

carcinoma, is also positive in up to 40% of small-cell neuroendocrine carcinoma of urinary bladder [63].

3. Differential diagnosis

Poorly differentiated invasive urothelial carcinoma can be considered in differential diagnosis, and positive staining of neuroendocrine markers in small-cell neuroendocrine carcinoma is helpful in differential diagnosis.

4. Prognosis

Small-cell neuroendocrine carcinoma of urinary bladder is a highly aggressive tumor with poor prognosis especially in higher stage [64]. Neoadjuvant chemotherapy can induce the pathologic downstaging and correlates with higher survival rate [65].

Well-Differentiated Neuroendocrine Tumor

1. Definition and clinical features

Well-differentiated neuroendocrine tumor of urinary bladder is potentially malignant neoplasm showing neuroendocrine differentiation. This tumor was formerly called as carcinoid.

It is extremely rare and has been reported in approximately 30 cases in English literatures.

2. Pathologic features

Reported cases are small size. The tumors locate subepithelial area. Tumor cells are uniform cuboidal or columnar cells with inconspicuous nucleoli and finely stippled chromatin. Mitosis is infrequent, and necrosis is not present. The tumor cells are arranged in pseudoglandular, acinar, or cribriform structures (Fig. 11.23A) [66]. Neuroendocrine markers such as synaptophysin, chromogranin A, or CD56 are positive in this tumor (Fig. 11.23B).

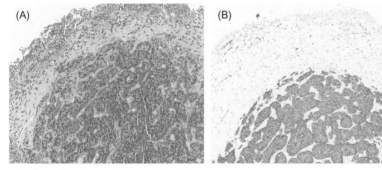

FIGURE 11.23 Well-differentiated neuroendocrine tumor (carcinoid). (A) Microscopically, well-differentiated neuroendocrine tumor of urinary bladder shows pseudoglandular or acinar structures. (B) Synaptophysin immunohistochemistry shows positive in this tumor.

Paraganglioma

1. Definition and clinical features

    Paraganglioma is a neuroendocrine neoplasm derived from paraganglia cells.

    Paraganglioma of urinary bladder accounts for less than 0.5% of neoplasms of urinary bladder. Presenting symptoms include hypertension, headache, hematuria, syncope/palpitation, and micturition attack [67].

2. Pathologic features

    Grossly, paragangliomas are well circumscribed and multinodular (Fig. 11.24A) and ranged from 1 to 9 cm [67,68].

    Microscopically, tumor cells are commonly arranged nested or zellballen pattern, but diffuse growth pattern is noted in about 20% of cases [68]. Tumor cells have round to polygonal shape with abundant amphophilic to eosinophilic cytoplasm (Fig. 11.24B). The nuclei are centrally located and have vesicular chromatin.

    Tumor cells of paraganglioma express neuroendocrine markers such as chromogranin A and synaptophysin, and are negative for cytokeratin

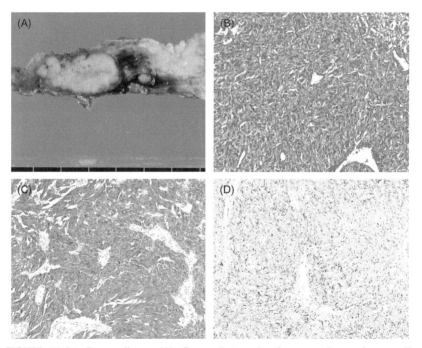

FIGURE 11.24 Paraganglioma. (A) Gross photograph of paraganglioma shows well-circumscribed multinodular mass. (B) Microscopically, paraganglioma consists of round to polygonal tumor cells with abundant amphophilic to eosinophilic cytoplasm. (C) Synaptophysin immunohistochemistry shows positive in tumor cells. (D) S100 protein is expressed in the sustentacular cells.

(Fig. 11.24C). S100 protein is expressed in the sustentacular cells, but sustentacular cells are not always present (Fig. 11.24D).

3. Differential diagnosis

Paraganglioma can be misdiagnosed as invasive urothelial carcinoma, especially in transurethral resection specimens [68].

4. Prognosis

Recurrence rate and metastasis have been reported in 14.2% and 9.4%, respectively. Localized tumors show good prognosis, but patients with locally advanced or metastatic disease have poor prognosis [67].

Mesenchymal Tumors

Leiomyoma

1. Definition and clinical features

Leiomyoma is a benign mesenchymal tumor showing smooth muscle differentiation. This tumor is rare but the most common benign mesenchymal tumor of urinary bladder.

2. Pathologic features

Grossly, leiomyoma of urinary bladder is relatively well-circumscribed whitish mass with whirling pattern in cut surface (Fig. 11.25A).

Microscopically, leiomyoma is composed of bland spindle cells with eosinophilic cytoplasm. The tumor cells are arranged in fascicular pattern (Fig. 11.25B). Mitotic figures are not present, and cytologic atypia is absent or minimal. There is no necrosis.

In immunohistochemistry, tumor cells are positive for smooth muscle actin and desmin (Fig. 11.25C).

Inflammatory Myofibroblastic Tumor

1. Definition and clinical features

Inflammatory myofibroblastic tumor is a neoplasm of fibroblastic and myofibroblastic spindle cells with inflammatory infiltrates. This tumor commonly occurs in children and young adults. Presenting symptoms are hematuria and irritative or obstructive urinary symptoms.

2. Pathologic features

Grossly, inflammatory myofibroblastic tumor frequently form protruding polypoid mass.

Microscopically, the tumor is composed of loosely arranged spindle cells admixed with inflammatory cells including plasma cells and eosinophils (Fig. 11.26A). Cellularity is variable, and edematous or myxoid stroma can be present.

In immunohistochemistry, the majority of cases express smooth muscle actin. ALK is also expressed in a subset of cases (Fig. 11.26B, C). *ALK* gene rearrangement can be also present in some cases.

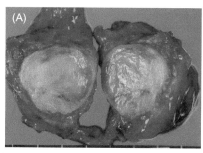

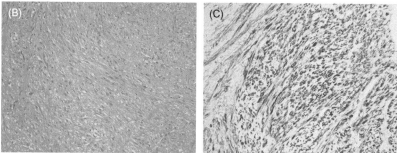

FIGURE 11.25   Leiomyoma. (A) Gross photograph of leiomyoma of urinary bladder shows relatively well-circumscribed whitish mass with whirling pattern at a cut section. (B) Microscopically, leiomyoma is composed of bland spindle cells with fascicular arrangement. (C) Immunoreactivity for smooth muscle actin is observed.

3. Differential diagnosis

Leiomyosarcoma, rhabdomyosarcoma, and sarcomatoid carcinoma can be considered in differential diagnosis.

4. Prognosis

Local recurrence rate has been reported as 10%–25%.

Rhabdomyosarcoma

1. Definition and clinical features

Rhabdomyosarcoma is a malignant mesenchymal tumor showing skeletal muscle differentiation.

It is the most common sarcoma of urinary bladder in children and very rare in adults. Presenting symptoms are hematuria, obstructive symptoms, or abdominal mass.

2. Pathologic features

Grossly, embryonal rhabdomyosarcoma of urinary bladder are typically present as polypoid mass (Fig. 11.27A).

Rhabdomyosarcoma can be divided into some variants such as embryonal, alveolar, spindle cell, or pleomorphic rhabdomyosarcomas. Embryonal rhabdomyosarcoma is the most common variant in urinary

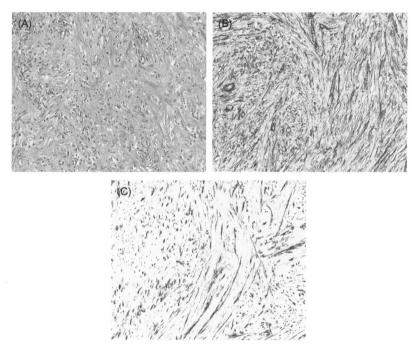

FIGURE 11.26 Inflammatory myofibroblastic tumor. (A) Microscopically, inflammatory myo-fibroblastic tumor is composed of loosely arranged spindle cells admixed with inflammatory cells including plasma cells and eosinophils. (B) Smooth muscle actin is expressed in tumor cells. (C) Immunoreactivity for ALK is observed in a subset of cases.

bladder. The tumor cells of embryonal rhabdomyosarcoma are round to spindle cells (Fig. 11.27B). Cross striations in cytoplasm is occasionally found. The underlying stroma can be myxoid.

In immunohistochemistry, rhabdomyosarcomas express desmin and myogenin (Fig. 11.27C, D).

3. Differential diagnosis

Inflammatory myofibroblastic tumor should be considered in differential diagnosis in children. Myogenin immunohistochemistry can help the differential diagnosis.

4. Prognosis

Rhabdomyosarcomas generally have poor prognosis. But chemotherapy improves the survival, especially in children [69].

Other Mesenchymal Tumors

Hemangioma (Fig. 11.28), leiomyosarcoma, granular cell tumor (Fig. 11.29), and neurofibroma can occur in urinary bladder.

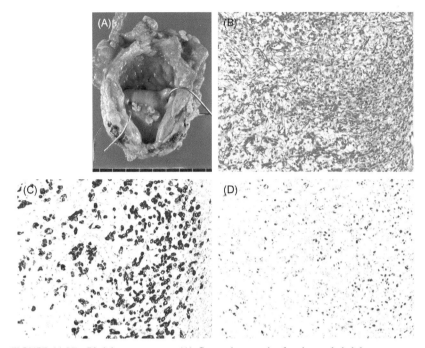

FIGURE 11.27 Rhabdomyosarcoma. (A) Gross photograph of embryonal rhabdomyosarcoma shows polypoid (botryoid) mass. (B) Microscopically, embryonal rhabdomyosarcoma consists of round to spindle cells with myxoid stroma. Immunoreactivity for desmin (C) and myogenin (D) is observed.

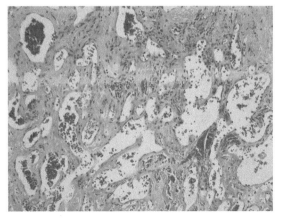

FIGURE 11.28 Hemangioma. Microscopically, hemangioma consists of blood vessels with cytologically bland endothelial cells.

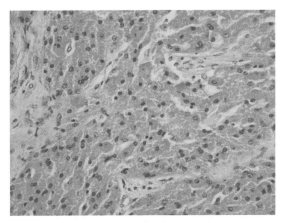

FIGURE 11.29   Granular cell tumor. Microscopically, granular cell tumor consists of round tumor cells with abundant granular eosinophilic cytoplasm.

REFERENCES

[1]   Moch H, Humphrey PA, Ulbright TM, Reuter V. WHO classification of tumours of the urinary system and male genital organs. Lyon, France: International Agency for Research on Cancer; 2016.

[2]   Readal N, Epstein JI. Papillary urothelial hyperplasia: relationship to urothelial neoplasms. Pathology 2010;42:360–3.

[3]   Chow NH, Cairns P, Eisenberger CF, et al. Papillary urothelial hyperplasia is a clonal precursor to papillary transitional cell bladder cancer. Int J Cancer 2000;89:514–18.

[4]   Taylor DC, Bhagavan BS, Larsen MP, Cox JA, Epstein JI. Papillary urothelial hyperplasia. A precursor to papillary neoplasms. Am J Surg Pathol 1996;20:1481–8.

[5]   Epstein JI, Amin MB, Reuter VR, Mostofi FK. The World Health Organization/ International Society of Urological Pathology consensus classification of urothelial (transitional cell) neoplasms of the urinary bladder. Bladder Consensus Conference Committee. Am J Surg Pathol 1998;22:1435–48.

[6]   Cheng L, Cheville JC, Neumann RM, Bostwick DG. Natural history of urothelial dysplasia of the bladder. Am J Surg Pathol 1999;23:443–7.

[7]   Cheng L, Cheville JC, Neumann RM, Bostwick DG. Flat intraepithelial lesions of the urinary bladder. Cancer 2000;88:625–31.

[8]   Kakizoe T, Matumoto K, Nishio Y, Ohtani M, Kishi K. Significance of carcinoma in situ and dysplasia in association with bladder cancer. J Urol 1985;133:395–8.

[9]   Zincke H, Utz DC. Review of Mayo Clinic experience with carcinoma in situ. Urology 1986;27:288.

[10]   McKenney JK, Desai S, Cohen C, Amin MB. Discriminatory immunohistochemical staining of urothelial carcinoma in situ and non-neoplastic urothelium: an analysis of cytokeratin 20, p53, and CD44 antigens. Am J Surg Pathol 2001;25:1074–8.

[11]   Amin MB, Trpkov K, Lopez- Beltran A, Grignon D. Best practices recommendations in the application of immunohistochemistry in the bladder lesions: report from the International Society of Urologic Pathology consensus conference. Am J Surg Pathol 2014;38:e20–34.

[12] Cheng L, Cheville JC, Neumann RM, et al. Survival of patients with carcinoma in situ of the urinary bladder. Cancer 1999;85:2469–74.

[13] Gofrit ON, Pode D, Pizov G, et al. The natural history of bladder carcinoma in situ after initial response to bacillus Calmette-Guerin immunotherapy. Urol Oncol 2009;27:258–62.

[14] McKenney JK, Amin MB, Young RH. Urothelial (transitional cell) papilloma of the urinary bladder: a clinicopathologic study of 26 cases. Mod Pathol 2003;16:623–9.

[15] Magi-Galluzzi C, Epstein JI. Urothelial papilloma of the bladder: a review of 34 de novo cases. Am J Surg Pathol 2004;28:1615–20.

[16] Kunze E, Schauer A, Schmitt M. Histology and histogenesis of two different types of inverted urothelial papillomas. Cancer 1983;51:348–58.

[17] Amin MB, Smith SC, Reuter VE, et al. Update for the practicing pathologist: The International Consultation on Urologic Disease—European association of urology consultation on bladder cancer. Mod Pathol 2015;28:612–30.

[18] Picozzi S, Casellato S, Bozzini G, et al. Inverted papilloma of the bladder: a review and an analysis of the recent literature of 365 patients. Urol Oncol 2013;31:1584–90.

[19] Holmang S, Hedelin H, Anderstrom C, Holmberg E, Busch C, Johansson SL. Recurrence and progression in low grade papillary urothelial tumors. J Urol 1999;162:702–7.

[20] Pich A, Chiusa L, Formiconi A, Galliano D, Bortolin P, Navone R. Biologic differences between noninvasive papillary urothelial neoplasms of low malignant potential and low-grade (grade 1) papillary carcinomas of the bladder. Am J Surg Pathol 2001;25:1528–33.

[21] Campbell PA, Conrad RJ, Campbell CM, Nicol DL, MacTaggart P. Papillary urothelial neoplasm of low malignant potential: reliability of diagnosis and outcome. BJU Int 2004;93:1228–31.

[22] Pan C-C, Chang Y-H, Chen K-K, Yu H-J, Sun C-H, Ho DMT. Prognostic significance of the 2004 WHO/ISUP classification for prediction of recurrence, progression, and cancer-specific mortality of non-muscle-invasive urothelial tumors of the urinary bladder: a clinicopathologic study of 1,515 cases. Am J Clin Pathol 2010;133:788–95.

[23] Amin MB, McKenney JK, Paner GP, et al. ICUD-EAU International consultation on bladder cancer 2012: pathology. Eur Urol 2013;63:16–35.

[24] Lopez- Beltran A, Montironi R. Non-invasive urothelial neoplasms: according to the most recent WHO classification. Eur Urol 2004;46:170–6.

[25] Nishiyama N, Kitamura H, Maeda T, et al. Clinicopathological analysis of patients with non-muscle-invasive bladder cancer: prognostic value and clinical reliability of the 2004 WHO classification system. Jpn J Clin Oncol 2013;43:1124–31.

[26] Gontero P, Gillo A, Fiorito C, et al. Prognostic factors of high-grade Ta bladder cancers according to the WHO 2004 classification: are these equivalent to high-risk non-muscle-invasive bladder cancer?. Urol Int 2014;92:136–42.

[27] Kirkali Z, Chan T, Manoharan M, et al. Bladder cancer: epidemiology, staging and grading, and diagnosis. Urology 2005;66:4–34.

[28] Chavan S, Bray F, Lortet-Tieulent J, Goodman M, Jemal A. International variations in bladder cancer incidence and mortality. Eur Urol 2014;66:59–73.

[29] Siegel R, Ma J, Zou Z, Jemal A. Cancer statistics, 2014. CA Cancer J Clin 2014;64:9–29.

[30] Lopez- Beltran A, Cheng L. Histologic variants of urothelial carcinoma: differential diagnosis and clinical implications. Hum Pathol 2006;37:1371–88.

[31] Amin MB. Histological variants of urothelial carcinoma: diagnostic, therapeutic and prognostic implications. Mod Pathol 2009;22(Suppl. 2):S96–118.

[32] Sylvester RJ, van der Meijden APM, Oosterlinck W, et al. Predicting recurrence and progression in individual patients with stage Ta T1 bladder cancer using EORTC risk tables:

a combined analysis of 2596 patients from seven EORTC trials. Eur Urol 2006;49 466-5-discussion 75-7.

[33] Lee YJ, Moon KC, Jeong CW, Kwak C, Kim HH, Ku JH. Impact of squamous and glandular differentiation on oncologic outcomes in upper and lower tract urothelial carcinoma. PLoS One 2014;9:e107027.

[34] Billis A, Schenka AA, Ramos CC, Carneiro LT, Araujo V. Squamous and/or glandular differentiation in urothelial carcinoma: prevalence and significance in transurethral resections of the bladder. Int Urol Nephrol 2001;33:631−3.

[35] Kim SP, Frank I, Cheville JC, et al. The impact of squamous and glandular differentiation on survival after radical cystectomy for urothelial carcinoma. J Urol 2012;188:405−9.

[36] Lopez-Beltran A, Jimenez RE, Montironi R, et al. Flat urothelial carcinoma in situ of the bladder with glandular differentiation. Hum Pathol 2011;42:1653−9.

[37] Douglas J, Sharp A, Chau C, et al. Serum total hCG beta level is an independent prognostic factor in transitional cell carcinoma of the urothelial tract. Br J Cancer 2014;110:1759−66.

[38] Venyo AK. Nested variant of urothelial carcinoma. Adv Urol 2014;2014:192720.

[39] Cox R, Epstein JI. Large nested variant of urothelial carcinoma: 23 cases mimicking von Brunn nests and inverted growth pattern of noninvasive papillary urothelial carcinoma. Am J Surg Pathol 2011;35:1337−42.

[40] Paner GP, Annaiah C, Gulmann C, et al. Immunohistochemical evaluation of novel and traditional markers associated with urothelial differentiation in a spectrum of variants of urothelial carcinoma of the urinary bladder. Hum Pathol 2014;45:1473−82.

[41] Linder BJ, Frank I, Cheville JC, et al. Outcomes following radical cystectomy for nested variant of urothelial carcinoma: a matched cohort analysis. J Urol 2013;189:1670−5.

[42] Humphrey PA. Micropapillary urothelial carcinoma of the urinary tract. J Urol 2011;186:1071−2.

[43] Kwon GY, Ro JY. Micropapillary variant of urothelial carcinoma. Adv Urol 2011;2011:217153.

[44] Alvarado-Cabrero I, Sierra-Santiesteban FI, Mantilla-Morales A, Hernandez-Hernandez DM. Micropapillary carcinoma of the urothelial tract. A clinicopathologic study of 38 cases. Ann Diagn Pathol 2005;9:1−5.

[45] Johansson SL, Borghede G, Holmang S. Micropapillary bladder carcinoma: a clinicopathological study of 20 cases. J Urol 1999;161:1798−802.

[46] Amin MB, Ro JY, el-Sharkawy T, et al. Micropapillary variant of transitional cell carcinoma of the urinary bladder. Histologic pattern resembling ovarian papillary serous carcinoma. Am J Surg Pathol 1994;18:1224−32.

[47] Li W, Liang Y, Deavers MT, et al. Uroplakin II is a more sensitive immunohistochemical marker than uroplakin III in urothelial carcinoma and its variants. Am J Clin Pathol 2014;142:864−71.

[48] Lotan TL, Ye H, Melamed J, Wu XR, Shih Ie M, Epstein JI. Immunohistochemical panel to identify the primary site of invasive micropapillary carcinoma. Am J Surg Pathol 2009;33:1037−41.

[49] Schneider SA, Sukov WR, Frank I, et al. Outcome of patients with micropapillary urothelial carcinoma following radical cystectomy: ERBB2 (HER2) amplification identifies patients with poor outcome. Mod Pathol 2014;27:758−64.

[50] Wang JK, Boorjian SA, Cheville JC, et al. Outcomes following radical cystectomy for micropapillary bladder cancer versus pure urothelial carcinoma: a matched cohort analysis. World J Urol 2012;30:801−6.

[51] Sung HH, Cho J, Kwon GY, et al. Clinical significance of micropapillary urothelial carcinoma of the upper urinary tract. J Clin Pathol 2014;67:49−54.

[52] Lopez-Beltran A, Requena MJ, Montironi R, Blanca A, Cheng L. Plasmacytoid urothelial carcinoma of the bladder. Hum Pathol 2009;40:1023–8.

[53] Ro JY, Shen SS, Lee HI, et al. Plasmacytoid transitional cell carcinoma of urinary bladder: a clinicopathologic study of 9 cases. Am J Surg Pathol 2008;32:752–7.

[54] Kim B, Kim G, Song B, Lee C, Park JH, Moon KC. HER2 protein overexpression and gene amplification in plasmacytoid urothelial carcinoma of the urinary bladder. Dis Markers 2016;2016:8463731.

[55] Dayyani F, Czerniak BA, Sircar K, et al. Plasmacytoid urothelial carcinoma, a chemosensitive cancer with poor prognosis, and peritoneal carcinomatosis. J Urol 2013;189: 1656–61.

[56] Torenbeek R, Blomjous CE, de Bruin PC, Newling DW, Meijer CJ. Sarcomatoid carcinoma of the urinary bladder. Clinicopathologic analysis of 18 cases with immunohistochemical and electron microscopic findings. Am J Surg Pathol 1994;18:241–9.

[57] Cheng L, Zhang S, Alexander R, et al. Sarcomatoid carcinoma of the urinary bladder: the final common pathway of urothelial carcinoma dedifferentiation. Am J Surg Pathol 2011;35:e34–46.

[58] Lagwinski N, Thomas A, Stephenson AJ, et al. Squamous cell carcinoma of the bladder: a clinicopathologic analysis of 45 cases. Am J Surg Pathol 2007;31:1777–87.

[59] Riadh BS, El Atat R, Sfaxi M, Derouiche A, Kourda N, Chebil M. Clinical presentation and outcome of bladder schistosoma-unrelated squamous cell carcinoma: report on 33 consecutive cases. Clin Genitourin Cancer 2007;5:409–12.

[60] Gopalan A, Sharp DS, Fine SW, et al. Urachal carcinoma: a clinicopathologic analysis of 24 cases with outcome correlation. Am J Surg Pathol 2009;33:659–68.

[61] Sheldon CA, Clayman RV, Gonzalez R, Williams RD, Fraley EE. Malignant urachal lesions. J Urol 1984;131:1–8.

[62] Oliva E, Young RH. Clear cell adenocarcinoma of the urethra: a clinicopathologic analysis of 19 cases. Mod Pathol 1996;9:513–20.

[63] Ismaili N. A rare bladder cancer—small cell carcinoma: review and update. Orphanet J Rare Dis 2011;6:75.

[64] Choong NW, Quevedo JF, Kaur JS. Small cell carcinoma of the urinary bladder. The Mayo Clinic experience. Cancer 2005;103:1172–8.

[65] Lynch SP, Shen Y, Kamat A, et al. Neoadjuvant chemotherapy in small cell urothelial cancer improves pathologic downstaging and long-term outcomes: results from a retrospective study at the MD Anderson Cancer Center. Eur Urol 2013;64:307–13.

[66] Chen YB, Epstein JI. Primary carcinoid tumors of the urinary bladder and prostatic urethra: a clinicopathologic study of 6 cases. Am J Surg Pathol 2011;35:442–6.

[67] Beilan JA, Lawton A, Hajdenberg J, Rosser CJ. Pheochromocytoma of the urinary bladder: a systematic review of the contemporary literature. BMC Urol 2013;13:22.

[68] Zhou M, Epstein JI, Young RH. Paraganglioma of the urinary bladder: a lesion that may be misdiagnosed as urothelial carcinoma in transurethral resection specimens. Am J Surg Pathol 2004;28:94–100.

[69] Leuschner I, Harms D, Mattke A, Koscielniak E, Treuner J. Rhabdomyosarcoma of the urinary bladder and vagina: a clinicopathologic study with emphasis on recurrent disease: a report from the Kiel Pediatric Tumor Registry and the German CWS Study. Am J Surg Pathol 2001;25:856–64.

Chapter 12

Tumor, Nodes, Metastases (TNM) Classification System for Bladder Cancer

Jeong Hwan Park and Kyung Chul Moon

Seoul National University College of Medicine, Seoul, South Korea

Chapter Outline

AJCC/TNM STAGING SYSTEM OF BLADDER CANCER

The most recent staging system is 2017 American Joint Committee on Cancer/tumor, nodes, metastases (AJCC/TNM) staging system (eighth edition). The 2017 staging system of urinary bladder cancer has several changes in comparison with 2010 system. (1) Perivesical lymph node metastasis is classified as N1. (2) Substaging of M1 is proposed. M1a represents a non-regional lymph node metastasis, and M1b represents non-lymph-node distant metastases. (3) Stage groups III and IV are subdivided into IIIA/IIIB and IVA/IVB. The definitions of TNM in 2017 staging system and stage groupings are shown in Tables 12.1 and 12.2 [1].

Primary Tumor (T)

T0 is used when primary tumor is not identified after an initial diagnosis in the biopsy or transurethral resection (TUR). Ta and Tis represent non-invasive papillary urothelial carcinoma and flat urothelial carcinoma in situ (CIS), respectively.

T1 is for invasion into the lamina propria (Fig 12.1A). Determination of stromal invasion of urothelial carcinoma can be problematic. Some histologic features can help this problem. Invasive tumors are much more commonly

TABLE 12.1 The Definitions of TNM in 2017 AJCC/TNM Staging System for Bladder Cancer

T—Primary Tumor

TX	Primary tumor cannot be assessed
T0	No evidence of primary tumor
Ta	Non-invasive papillary carcinoma
Tis	Urothelial carcinoma in situ: "flat tumor"
T1	Tumor invades lamina propria (subepithelial connective tissue)
T2	Tumor invades muscularis propria
T2a	Tumor invades superficial muscularis propria (inner half)
T2b	Tumor invades deep muscularis propria (outer half)
T3	Tumor invades perivesical soft tissue
T3a	Microscopically
T3b	Macroscopically (extravesical mass)
T4	Extravesical tumor directly invades any of the following: prostatic stroma, seminal vesicles, uterus, vagina, pelvic wall, abdominal wall
T4a	Extravesical tumor invades directly into prostatic stroma, seminal vesicles, uterus, vagina
T4b	Extravesical tumor directly invades pelvic wall, abdominal wall

N—Regional Lymph Nodes

NX	Lymph nodes cannot be assessed
N0	No lymph node metastasis
N1	Single regional lymph node metastasis in the true pelvis (perivesical, obturator, internal and external iliac, or sacral lymph node metastasis)
N2	Multiple regional lymph node metastasis in the true pelvis (perivesical, obturator, internal and external iliac, or sacral lymph node metastasis)
N3	Lymph node metastasis to the common iliac lymph nodes

M—Distant Metastasis

M0	No distant metastasis
M1	Distant metastasis
M1a	Distant metastasis limited to lymph nodes beyond the common iliac lymph node
M1b	Non-lymph-node distant metastases

TABLE 12.2 Stage Groups in 2017 AJCC/TNM Staging System for Bladder Cancer

Stage Group	T	N	M
Stage 0a	Ta	N0	M0
Stage 0is	Tis	N0	M0
Stage I	T1	N0	M0
Stage II	T2a	N0	M0
Stage II	T2b	N0	M0
Stage IIIA	T3a, T3b, T4a	N0	M0
Stage IIIA	T1–T4a	N1	M0
Stage IIIB	T1–T4a	N2, N3	M0
Stage IVA	T4b	N0	M0
Stage IVA	Any T	Any N	M1a
Stage IVB	Any T	Any N	M1b

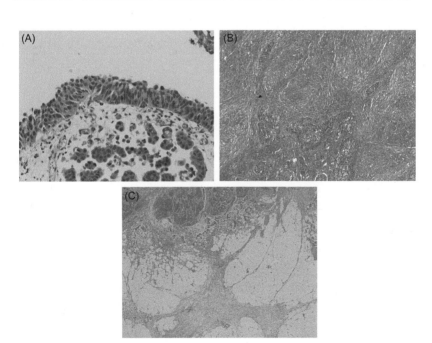

FIGURE 12.1   T categories of urothelial carcinoma of urinary bladder. (A) T1 invasive urothelial carcinoma with lamina propria invasion. (B) T2 invasive urothelial carcinoma with muscularis propria invasion. (C) T3 invasive urothelial carcinoma with perivesical fat invasion.

high-grade tumors. Single cell infiltration, absence of basement membrane, finger-like projections, stromal desmoplastic, or inflammatory reaction are helpful findings of stromal invasion of urothelial carcinoma. Papillary stalk invasion of an exophytic lesion is considered lamina propria invasion.

T2 is for invasion into the muscularis propria (Fig. 12.1B). T2 is subdivided based on invasion into superficial (inner half) (T2a) or deep muscularis propria (outer half) (T2b). Biopsy and TUR specimen may not contain muscularis propria and invasive carcinoma with no muscularis propria will need repeated procedure for determine depth of invasion. If invasion into whether the muscularis propria or muscularis mucosae is uncertain, this regard should be stated.

T3 represents invasion into the perivesical fat (Fig. 12.1C) and T3 is further divided according to microscopic perivesical fat invasion (T3a) or macroscopic invasion forming extravesical mass (T3b). As fat tissue can be found at all layers of urinary bladder wall, biopsy and TUR specimen cannot distinguish invasion into the perivesical fat.

T4 is used when primary tumor invades beyond urinary bladder. T4a is for invasion into prostatic stroma, seminal vesicles, uterus, or vagina. Subepithelial invasion of prostatic urethra does not constitute T4 staging. Prostatic stromal invasion of T4a category is defined as direct invasion of extravesical tumor into prostatic stroma. When prostatic stromal invasion originates from urothelial CIS extending into prostatic urethra, T2 category of urethral staging should be categorized. T4b is for invasion into the pelvic or abdominal wall.

Regional Lymph Nodes (N)

pNx is used when lymph nodes cannot be assessed. When no lymph nodes are examined, pNx should be assigned. pN0 means no lymph node metastasis. pN1 and pN2 represent single and multiple regional lymph nodes metastases in the true pelvis, respectively. Lymph nodes in true pelvis include perivesical, hypogastric, obturator, external iliac, or presacral lymph nodes. pN3 means metastases to the common iliac lymph nodes.

Distant Metastasis (M)

If distant metastasis is present, M category is designated as M1. M1a is defined as distant metastasis limited to lymph nodes beyond the common iliac lymph node, and M1b is defined as non-lymph-node distant metastases.

REFERENCE

[1] Amin MB, American Joint Committee on Cancer. AJCC cancer staging manual. 8th ed. Chicago, IL: Springer; 2017. p. 757−65.

Treatment for Nonmuscle Invasive Bladder Cancer (NMIBC)

Chapter 13

Risk Factors for Recurrence and Progression of Nonmuscle Invasive Bladder Cancer

Jae Young Park

Korea University Ansan Hospital, Ansan, South Korea

Chapter Outline

THE EORTC RISK TABLE AND THE CUETO SCORING MODEL

Several studies have attempted to evaluate risk factors for recurrence and progression in high-risk nonmuscle invasive bladder cancer (NMIBC) treated with bacillus Calmette-Guérin (BCG). To predict the probabilities of disease recurrence and progression, the European Organization for Research and Treatment of Cancer (EORTC) Genito-Urinary Cancers Group developed a scoring system and risk tables [1]. This prediction tool was built on data from 2596 patients diagnosed with Ta/T1 tumors who were randomized in seven previous EORTC Genito-Urinary Cancers Group trials. The scoring system was based on the six most relevant clinical and pathologic predictors of outcomes: number of tumors, tumor size, prior recurrence rate, T category, concomitant carcinoma in situ (CIS), and grade [2]. However, the data were limited by the low number of patients treated with BCG (7%) and immediate postoperative instillation of chemotherapy (<10%), and the fact

Bladder Cancer. DOI: http://dx.doi.org/10.1016/B978-0-12-809939-1.00013-8

that re-transurethral resection of the bladder tumor (TURBT) was not performed [3]. In order to overcome these flaws, the Club urológico español de tratamiento oncológico (CUETO) group developed a scoring model by analyzing 1062 patients with NMIBC from four randomized phase III trials treated only with BCG. Significant predictors for recurrence were female sex, age, history of recurrence, multiplicity, and presence of associated CIS. T1 stage and high grade were independent predictors of progression by multivariate Cox analysis [4]. With those 1062 patients a risk stratification model was developed to provide accurate estimates of recurrence (0−16) and progression (0−14) probability after BCG (Table 13.1) [5]. Patients were categorized into four groups by score: 0−4, 5−6, 7−9, 10−16 for recurrence and 0−4, 5−6, 7−9, 10−14 for progression.

Several studies to compare these two models have been performed very recently. An external validation of the EORTC tables in the 1062 patients of the CUETO group treated with BCG concluded that EORTC model more successfully stratified recurrence and progression in low and intermediate risks patients. However, the discriminative ability of the EORTC tables decreased for progression, and overestimated risks of recurrence and progression after BCG instillation [6]. Another external validation of 4689 patients with NMIBC in multicenter cohort showed that both models exhibited a poor discrimination for disease recurrence and progression (0.597 and 0.662, and 0.523 and 0.616, respectively, for the EORTC and CUETO models). The EORTC tables overestimated the risk of disease recurrence and progression in high-risk patients. The discrimination of the EORTC tables was even lower in the subgroup of patients treated with BCG (0.554 and 0.576 for disease recurrence and progression, respectively). Conversely, the discrimination of the CUETO model increased in BCG-treated patients (0.597 and 0.645 for disease recurrence and progression, respectively). However, both models overestimated the risk of disease progression in high-risk patients [7]. The longest follow-up of T1G3 patients treated with BCG in a single center revealed female sex or having CIS in the prostatic urethra as the only risk factors for time to recurrence, progression, and disease-related mortality [8]. They emphasize the importance of performing a biopsy of the prostatic urethra in patients with primary high-risk NMIBC as a first step to obtain the predictive information.

Some studies performed in Asia have also been published recently. A retrospective study of 363 Chinese patients with NMIBC concluded that the EORTC model showed more value in predicting recurrence and progression in these population than the CUETO risk tables, saying the concordance index using the EORTC and CUETO models was 0.711 and 0.663 for recurrence and 0.768 and 0.741 for progression, respectively [9]. Conversely, Japanese study concluded that CUETO model was a better predictor of tumor recurrence and progression in patients who underwent BCG immunotherapy [10]. CUETO model also showed more value in predicting recurrence and

TABLE 13.1 Factors by Weight to Calculate Recurrence and Progression Scores to Select Most Predictive Model (The CUETO Scoring Model) [5]

Factor	Recurrence Score	Progression Score
Gender:		
M	0	0
F	3	0
Age:		
Less than 60	0	0
60–70	1	0
Greater than 70	2	2
Recurrent tumor:		
No	0	0
Yes	4	2
No. of tumors:		
3 or less	0	0
Greater than 3	2	1
T category:		
Ta	0	0
T1	0	2
Associated Tis:		
No	0	0
Yes	2	1
Grade:		
G1	0	0
G2	1	2
G3	3	6
Total scores	0–16	0–14

progression in Korean patients [11]. In this study the concordance index of the EORTC and CUETO models was 0.759 and 0.836 for recurrence and 0.704 and 0.745 for progression, respectively, and the area under the receiver operating characteristics curve for the EORTC and CUETO models was 0.832 and 0.894 for recurrence and 0.722 and 0.724 for progression, respectively.

AGE

The EORTC model does not include age as a prognostic factor. The impact of age has been assessed in many studies. In a retrospective study of 2160 patients treated with primary TURBT, patients were divided into three subgroups depending on age, sex, stage, and grade [12]. Results showed that in young patients, compared with at least 50 years, bladder cancer occurs more frequently in men, and as low-grade and stage tumors. Age is also a patient characteristic widely associated with BCG response [13,14]. Despite some studies with larger cohorts have not shown the determining influence of age [8,15], the CUETO group showed that age was an independent predictive factor of progression [4]. Moreover, a phase II multicenter trial for BCG and IFN-α reported that aging appears to be related with a decreased response to intravesical immunotherapy [16].

SEX

Compared with men, women are more frequently diagnosed with tumors of a higher stage and tend to have a worse prognosis, supporting the hypothesis that gender independently influences bladder cancer development, progression, and mortality [17,18] In a study of 916 individuals presenting with T1 high-grade urothelial carcinoma, women were found to have a higher risk of disease recurrence (HR = 1.36, range: 1.07−1.72, $P = 0.012$), including those treated with BCG (HR = 1.72, range: 1.10−2.68, $P = 0.017$) than men [18]. Female gender has been found to be a negative prognostic factor for overall survival and cancer-specific survival (CSS) in patients with bladder cancer treated with TURBT and adjuvant radiotherapy or radiochemotherapy, independent of age at diagnosis, tumor stage and grade, concomitant CIS, lymphovascular invasion (LVI), tumor multifocality, and type of therapy [19]. Castelao et al. [20] suggested that women were at higher risk of bladder cancer associated with smoking. The risk in female smokers was statistically higher than in male smokers who smoke comparable number of cigarettes. Sex differences are also observed in stage adjusted survival. Among women the CSS rates are significantly worse, explained by the more frequent diagnosis of higher stage at presentation [21].

The role of gender in response to treatment in patients with NMIBC has not yet been clarified. Gender did not influence the response to intravesical BCG instillation in a series of 1021 patients with NMIBC (756 men and 265 women) [22]. On the other hand, in a series of 615 individuals who were newly diagnosed with urothelial carcinoma of the bladder, women had a fivefold higher risk of receiving intravesical treatments after TURBT than men, after adjusting for the effects of age, geographical area and tumor stage, grade, size, and multifocality ($P = 0.004$) [23]. The differential exposures to environmental factors such as tobacco and chemicals, and genetic, anatomic, hormonal, and societal factors could be additional causes of sex inequalities [17]. One study revealing the correlations of cytokine levels with the clinical outcomes after BCG therapy suggested that a good immunologic response to BCG was more frequent in men than in women [24]. Also the CUETO group found that female patients treated with BCG increased the risk of recurrence compared to male patients (HR = 1.71), and that male patients showed a significantly longer time to recurrence than female patients [4]. However, multivariate analyses did not show any significant relationship between sex and progression [4].

SIZE AND MULTIFOCALITY

Although size and multifocality are classical prognostic factors for recurrence and progression of NMIBC [25], its predictive value for the BCG response is controversial [13]. One study analyzing 132 patients with initial T1G3 revealed that only the presence of three risk factors such as multifocality, CIS, and size (3 cm or more) together seemed to predict an adverse oncological outcome in the bladder sparing approach for initial high-risk NMIBC [26]. In the CUETO group study, multifocality was found to be an independent factor of recurrence after BCG treatment but not predictive of progression [4].

HISTORY OF PREVIOUS RECURRENCES

The prognostic importance of a history of prior recurrences, or TURs, has not been categorically established. The CUETO group in a randomized study comparing standard 81 mg dose of BCG with 27 mg reported that prior bladder cancer resection was a significant factor affecting progression in multivariate analysis [15]. One study stratifying 191 NMIBC treated with BCG into primary versus nonprimary tumors revealed that nonprimary T1 NMIBC treated with BCG carried a significantly higher risk of progression to muscle invasive disease compared with primary tumors [27]. Recently, the CUETO group demonstrated increased the risk of progression in the patients with recurrent tumors treating BCG [4], whereas the other studies found a significant association only with recurrence [14,28].

STAGE AND GRADE

Several studies have analyzed the value of stage in BCG response. Herr et al. [29] in a multivariate analysis of 221 patients with NMIBC reported that BCG is less effective for tumor progression in T1 tumors than in Ta tumors. Recently, the CUETO group confirmed that T1 tumors were significantly correlated with progression in univariate and multivariate analysis compared with Ta stage [4].

Although grade did not correlate with recurrence or progression in either univariate or multivariate analysis in some reports [13], Millan-Rodriguez et al. [25] reported grade 3 as the main predictor of progression and mortality in a cohort of 1520 NMIBC. Moreover, in previous large studies comparing the efficacy of a threefold reduced dose (reduced dose, 27 mg) of intravesical BCG against the standard dose (81 mg) in patients with NMIBC, high grade was associated with shorter time to progression [15]. Also, Fernandez-Gomez et al. [4] reported grade as predictive of progression.

CONCOMITANT CIS AND CIS IN THE PROSTATIC URETHRA

Concomitant CIS is a known risk factor for both recurrence and progression and known as refractory to BCG [30,31], nevertheless long-term reports failed to confirm a relationship between CIS and the BCG response [32]. The CUETO group and Kakiashvili et al. [4,33] revealed that associated CIS was an independent factor for recurrence but not for progression. Conversely, the Southwest Oncology Group has demonstrated that CIS generally responds favorably to maintenance BCG immunotherapy [34]. The significance of involvement of the urothelium of the prostatic urethra, and/or prostate ducts in patients with bladder cancer, has been previously reported as a bad prognostic factor. Palou et al. [8] evaluated the incidence of CIS in the prostatic urethra of primary T1G3 NMIBC treated with BCG, which they routinely detected with cold-cup biopsy in a study with 146 patients. Results revealed that in 10.3% of cases, CIS was involved with prostatic urethra, and this factor was strongly related with recurrence and progression. They also suggested that prostatic urethra involvement should be done at the re-TUR if it has not been evaluated at the first TUR [8].

SUBSTAGING T1 BLADDER CANCER

Depth of lamina propria involvement allows the classification of high-risk NMIBC according to aggressiveness. Orsola et al. [35] revealed that those patients with deep lamina propria invasion (T1b/T1c) should be managed more aggressively, especially those with associated CIS. In a study analyzing 406 cases of T1 high grade from a series of 1515 NMIBC, substaging was performed using 0.5, 1.0, and 1.5 mm as thresholds to distinguish extensive from focal invasion [36]. The authors concluded that the substaging of T1 bladder cancer is feasible and can provide more precise prognostic information to identify a subset of patients with a more unfavorable prognosis. For the T1 substage, van Rhijn et al. [37] used a new system that discerns T1-microinvasive (T1m) and T1-extensive-invasive (T1e). They concluded that T1 substaging was possible in 100% of cases with this new system and very predictive of high-risk behavior.

LYMPHOVASCULAR INVASION

LVI is defined as the presence of carcinoma in an unequivocal endothelial lining or in the vascular wall [38]. Most articles stress the prognostic value of LVI, but there are still some doubts as to its use in clinical decision making owing to the poor diagnosis reproducibility [39]. This is why it would be necessary to reach a consensus on strict diagnostic criteria as soon as possible to be able to incorporate this prognostic factor in clinical practice [38]. In a study with 118 patients with newly diagnosed T1 high-risk NMIBC, and LVI confirmed in 33 patients (28.0%), the authors concluded that LVI in TUR specimens predicts disease progression and metastasis [40]. Other reports have demonstrated that LVI was associated with shorter survival in patients with stage I or II disease [41]. Moreover, Resnick et al. [42] confirmed LVI at TUR as useful prognostic information that should be incorporated into clinical decision making, particularly with regard to cystectomy for NMIBC.

EARLY RECURRENCE

The rate of residual and/or recurrent tumor at first cystoscopy has been reported to be as high as 57%, with a later progression rate of 34% [8]. In addition, it was reported that the 80% of the patients who did not presented complete response at 3 months showed progression [43]. Also previously, Herr et al. [29] found that bladder cancer recurrence within 1 year from intravesical BCG instillation was associated with progression. However, Brausi et al. [44] showed a marked difference in the recurrence rates at different centers in randomized EORTC trials, which could only be attributable to the quality of the TUR. In addition, it was reported that the recurrence and progression rates at first cystoscopy were only 8.2%−0.5% in patients that all presented muscle in the TUR specimen and treated with BCG, even without re-TUR [8].

MOLECULAR PREDICTIVE FACTORS

Despite many works have been done until now, no molecular marker has yet entered routine clinical practice. However, some of them have proved their predictive value in studies. The p53 protein serves as a "guardian of the genome" by inducing multiple mechanisms of cell cycle arrest after cellular insult [45]. p53 nuclear overexpression is an early event in BC that occurs in 48% of cases of bladder CIS [46]. Oh et al. [47] investigated the impact of p53 overexpression on tumor recurrence after BCG intravesical therapy in patients with NMIBC. They concluded that strong overexpression of p53 was predictive of recurrence in patients with NMIBC undergoing intravesical BCG treatment. In a series of 80 consecutive patients with pT1N0 NMIBC, expression of p53 was altered in 25% of patients and p53 was found to be independently associated with recurrence [hazard ratio (HR), 3.66; $P = 0.033$] [48]. pRb is known as a tumor suppressor gene involved in cell cycle control. Altered Rb expression can serve as a predictive marker of outcome in patients with high-risk NMIBC treated with BCG instillation [49]. p21 inhibits the activity of cyclin-dependent kinase and thus functions as a regulator of cell cycle progression [45]. One study performing immunohistochemical staining for p53 and p21 demonstrated that positive p21 expression was associated with bladder cancer recurrence and progression when adjusted for the effects of clinical stage and grade, and the combined p53/p21 expression status was independently associated with disease recurrence, progression, and CSS [50]. Ki 67 is an indicator of cell proliferation and a measure of cell growth. It is also an independent risk factor for progression in NMIBC and increased expression of Ki 67 is related to tumor grade, stage, recurrence, and progression of BC [45]. Besides the factors described earlier, the other molecular biomarkers are summarized in Table 13.2.

TABLE 13.2 Molecular Biomarkers in Bladder Cancer

Class	Marker	Prognostic Value
Cell cycle regulators	p21	Higher stage, recurrence, all-cause mortality
	p27	Higher grade, cancer-specific mortality
	Ki 67	Recurrence, progression
	Cyclin D	Low grade, low stage, recurrence
	Cyclin E	Low stage, recurrence, cancer-specific mortality
Apoptosis	Survivin	Recurrence, cancer-specific mortality, all-cause mortality
	Bcl2	Recurrence, cancer-specific mortality
	Caspase-3	Recurrence, cancer-specific mortality
Angiogenesis	Microvessel density	Recurrence, all-cause mortality
	VEGF	Microvessel density, high grade, recurrence
	FGFR3	Recurrence, cancer-specific mortality
Tumor suppressor genes	p53	Higher stage, recurrence, progression, cancer-specific and all-cause mortality
	pRb	Higher stage, recurrence, progression, cancer-specific and all-cause mortality

(Continued)

TABLE 13.2 (Continued)

Class	Marker	Prognostic Value
Proto-oncogenes and oncogenes	EGFR	Higher grade, progression, all-cause mortality
	Her-2 Neu	Recurrence, metastasis, cancer-specific mortality
	FGFR3	Low grade, low stage, recurrence and progression
Miscellaneous	GSTT1	Recurrence, progression, cancer-specific mortality
	NOS and PPAR	Progression, cancer-specific mortality
	HMOX1	Higher grade, recurrence and progression

Source: From Ather MH, Nazim SM. New and contemporary markers of prognosis in nonmuscle invasive urothelial cancer. Korean J Urol 2015;56:553−64. [45]

CONCLUSION

Many research revealed that age, sex, grade, size, multifocality, history of previous recurrences, stage, grade, CIS, T1 substaging, LVI, and early recurrence are the prognostic factors for recurrence, progression, and/or CSS in NMIBC. Moreover, the multifactorial prediction tools combining the risk factors described earlier such as the EORTC risk table and the CUETO scoring model were proved to be helpful to predict risk stratification in NMIBC. New molecular markers including p53, pRB, p21, Ki 67, and so on are increasingly studied and their predictive value in recurrence, progression, and mortality of BC proved continuously.

As the technologies develop fast and big data are available easily, even more interesting is the possibility of combining multimarker panels that could be used in routine clinical practice, as all these risk factors can be evaluated by history, pathology, immunohistochemistry, and molecular analysis. The risk factors described herein will be becoming widely available and cost-effective tools for reliable risk assessment in the near future, and it would provide precious information in counseling patients, in selecting them for appropriate treatments, and finally it would improve the prognosis in the patients with NMIBC.

REFERENCES

[1] Sylvester RJ, van der Meijden AP, Oosterlinck W, Witjes JA, Bouffioux C, Denis L, et al. Predicting recurrence and progression in individual patients with stage Ta T1 bladder cancer using EORTC risk tables: a combined analysis of 2596 patients from seven EORTC trials. Eur Urol 2006;49:466−77.

[2]   http://www.eortc.be/tools/bladdercalculator/ assessed 29 Aug 2016.

[3]   Kluth LA, Black PC, Bochner BH, Catto J, Lerner SP, Stenzl A, et al. Prognostic and prediction tools in bladder cancer: a comprehensive review of the literature. Eur Urol 2015;68:238−53.

[4]   Fernandez-Gomez J, Solsona E, Unda M, Martinez-Piñeiro L, Gonzalez M, Hernandez R, et al. Prognostic factors in patients with non−muscle-invasive bladder cancer treated with bacillus Calmette-Guérin: multivariate analysis of data from four randomized CUETO trials. Eur Urol 2008;53:992−1002.

[5]   Fernandez-Gomez J, Madero R, Solsona E, Unda M, Martinez-Piñeiro L, Gonzalez M, et al. Predicting nonmuscle invasive bladder cancer recurrence and progression in patients treated with bacillus Calmette-Guerin: the CUETO scoring model. J Urol 2009;182:2195−203.

[6]   Fernandez-Gomez J, Madero R, Solsona E, Unda M, Martinez-Piñeiro L, Ojea A, et al. The EORTC tables overestimate the risk of recurrence and progression in patients with non−muscle-invasive bladder cancer treated with bacillus Calmette-Guérin: external validation of the EORTC risk tables. Eur Urol 2011;60:423−30.

[7]   Xylinas E, Kent M, Kluth L, Pycha A, Comploj E, Svatek R, et al. Accuracy of the EORTC risk tables and of the CUETO scoring model to predict outcomes in non-muscle-invasive urothelial carcinoma of the bladder. Br J Cancer 2013;109:1460−6.

[8]   Palou J, Sylvester RJ, Faba OR, Parada R, Peña JA, Algaba F, et al. Female gender and carcinoma in situ in the prostatic urethra are prognostic factors for recurrence, progression, and disease-specific mortality in T1G3 bladder cancer patients treated with bacillus Calmette-Guérin. Eur Urol 2012;62:118−25.

[9]   Xu T, Zhu Z, Zhang X, Wang X, Zhong S, Zhang M, et al. Predicting recurrence and progression in Chinese patients with nonmuscle-invasive bladder cancer using EORTC and CUETO scoring models. Urology 2013;82:387−93.

[10] Kohjimoto Y, Kusumoto H, Nishizawa S, Kikkawa K, Kodama Y, Ko M, et al. External validation of European Organization for Research and Treatment of Cancer and Spanish Urological Club for Oncological Treatment scoring models to predict recurrence and progression in Japanese patients with non-muscle invasive bladder cancer treated with bacillus Calmette−Guérin. Int J Urol 2014;21:1201−7.

[11] Choi SY, Ryu JH, Chang IH, Kim T-H, Myung SC, Moon YT, et al. Predicting recurrence and progression of non-muscle-invasive bladder cancer in Korean patients: a comparison of the EORTC and CUETO models. Korean J Urol 2014;55:643−9.

[12] Poletajew S, Walędziak M, Fus Ł, Pomada P, Ciechańska J, Wasiutyński A. Urothelial bladder carcinoma in young patients is characterized by a relatively good prognosis. Ups J Med Sci 2012;117:47−51.

[13] Saint F, Salomon L, Quintela R, Cicco A, Hoznek A, Abbou CC, et al. Do prognostic parameters of remission versus relapse after bacillus Calmette−Guérin (BCG) immunotherapy exist?: analysis of a quarter century of literature. Eur Urol 2003;43:351−61.

[14] Takashi M, Wakai K, Hattori T, Furuhashi K, Ono Y, Ohshima S, et al. Multivariate evaluation of factors affecting recurrence, progression, and survival in patients with superficial bladder cancer treated with intravesical bacillus Calmette-Guerin (Tokyo 172 strain) therapy: significance of concomitant carcinoma in situ. Int Urol Nephrol 2002;33:41−7.

[15] Martinez-Pineiro J, Flores N, Isorna S, Solsona E, Sebastian J, Pertusa C, et al. Long-term follow-up of a randomized prospective trial comparing a standard 81 mg dose of intravesical bacille Calmette-Guerin with a reduced dose of 27 mg in superficial bladder cancer. BJU Int 2002;89:671−80.

[16] Joudi FN, Smith BJ, O'Donnell MA, Konety BR. The impact of age on the response of patients with superficial bladder cancer to intravesical immunotherapy. J Urol 2006;175:1634−40.

[17] Fajkovic H, Halpern JA, Cha EK, Bahadori A, Chromecki TF, Karakiewicz PI, et al. Impact of gender on bladder cancer incidence, staging, and prognosis. World J Urol 2011;29:457−63.

[18] Kluth LA, Fajkovic H, Xylinas E, Crivelli JJ, Passoni N, Rouprêt M, et al. Female gender is associated with higher risk of disease recurrence in patients with primary T1 high-grade urothelial carcinoma of the bladder. World J Urol 2013;31:1029−36.

[19] Keck B, Ott OJ, Häberle L, Kunath F, Weiss C, Rödel C, et al. Female sex is an independent risk factor for reduced overall survival in bladder cancer patients treated by transurethral resection and radio-or radiochemotherapy. World J Urol 2013;31:1023−8.

[20] Castelao JE, Yuan J-M, Skipper PL, Tannenbaum SR, Gago-Dominguez M, Crowder JS, et al. Gender-and smoking-related bladder cancer risk. J Natl Cancer Inst 2001;93:538−45.

[21] Mungan NA, Aben KK, Schoenberg MP, Visser O, Coebergh J-WW, Witjes JA, et al. Gender differences in stage-adjusted bladder cancer survival. Urology 2000;55:876−80.

[22] Boorjian SA, Zhu F, Herr HW. The effect of gender on response to bacillus Calmette-Guérin therapy for patients with non-muscle-invasive urothelial carcinoma of the bladder. BJU Int 2010;106:357−61.

[23] Puente D, Malats N, Cecchini L, Tardon A, García-Closas R, Serra C, et al. Gender-related differences in clinical and pathological characteristics and therapy of bladder cancer. Eur Urol 2003;43:53−62.

[24] Saint F, Patard JJ, Maille P, Soyeux P, Hoznek A, Salomon L, et al. Prognostic value of at helper 1 urinary cytokine response after intravesical bacillus Calmette-Guérin treatment for superficial bladder cancer. J Urol 2002;167:364−7.

[25] Millan-Rodriguez F, Chechile-Toniolo G, Salvador-Bayarri J, Palou J, Vicente-Rodiguez J. Multivariate analysis of the prognostic factors of primary superficial bladder cancer. J Urol 2000;163:73−8.

[26] Denzinger S, Otto W, Fritsche HM, Roessler W, Wieland WF, Hartmann A, et al. Bladder sparing approach for initial T1G3 bladder cancer: do multifocality, size of tumor or concomitant carcinoma in situ matter? A long-term analysis of 132 patients. Int J Urol 2007;14:995−9.

[27] Alkhateeb SS, Van Rhijn BW, Finelli A, van der Kwast T, Evans A, Hanna S, et al. Nonprimary pT1 nonmuscle invasive bladder cancer treated with bacillus Calmette-Guerin is associated with higher risk of progression compared to primary T1 tumors. J Urol 2010;184:81−6.

[28] Losa A, Hurle R, Lembo A. Low dose bacillus Calmette-Guerin for carcinoma in situ of the bladder: long-term results. J Urol 2000;163:68−72.

[29] Herr H, Badalament R, Amato D, Laudone V, Fair W, Whitmore Jr W. Superficial bladder cancer treated with bacillus Calmette-Guerin: a multivariate analysis of factors affecting tumor progression. J Urol 1989;141:22−9.

[30] Millan-Rodriguez F, Chechile-Toniolo G, Salvador-Bayarri J, Palou J, Algaba F, Vicente-Rodriguez J. Primary superficial bladder cancer risk groups according to progression, mortality and recurrence. J Urol 2000;164:680−4.

[31] Ovesen H, Horn T, Steven K. Long-term efficacy of intravesical bacillus Calmette-Guerin for carcinoma in situ: relationship of progression to histological response and p53 nuclear accumulation. J Urol 1997;157:1655−9.

[32] Pansadoro V, Emiliozzi P, de Paula F, Scarpone P, Pansadoro A, Sternberg CN. Long-term follow-up of G3T1 transitional cell carcinoma of the bladder treated with intravesical bacille Calmette-Guerin: 18-year experience. Urology 2002;59:227–31.

[33] Kakiashvili DM, van Rhijn BW, Trottier G, Jewett MA, Fleshner NE, Finelli A, et al. Long-term follow-up of T1 high-grade bladder cancer after intravesical bacille Calmette-Guérin treatment. BJU Int 2011;107:540–6.

[34] Lamm DL, Blumenstein BA, Crissman JD, Montie JE, Gottesman JE, Lowe BA, et al. Maintenance bacillus Calmette-Guerin immunotherapy for recurrent TA, T1 and carcinoma in situ transitional cell carcinoma of the bladder: a randomized Southwest Oncology Group Study. J Urol 2000;163:1124–9.

[35] Orsola A, Trias I, Raventos C, Espanol I, Cecchini L, Bucar S, et al. Initial high-grade T1 urothelial cell carcinoma: feasibility and prognostic significance of lamina propria invasion microstaging (T1a/b/c) in BCG-treated and BCG-non-treated patients. Eur Urol 2005;48:231–8.

[36] Chang W-C, Chang Y-H, Pan C-C. Prognostic significance in substaging of T1 urinary bladder urothelial carcinoma on transurethral resection. Am J Surg Pathol 2012;36:454–61.

[37] van Rhijn BW, van der Kwast TH, Alkhateeb SS, Fleshner NE, van Leenders GJ, Bostrom PJ, et al. A new and highly prognostic system to discern T1 bladder cancer substage. Eur Urol 2012;61:378–84.

[38] Algaba F. Lymphovascular invasion as a prognostic tool for advanced bladder cancer. Curr Opin Urol 2006;16:367–71.

[39] Faba OR, Palou J. Predictive factors for recurrence progression and cancer specific survival in high-risk bladder cancer. Curr Opin Urol 2012;22:415–20.

[40] Cho KS, Seo HK, Joung JY, Park WS, Ro JY, Han KS, et al. Lymphovascular invasion in transurethral resection specimens as predictor of progression and metastasis in patients with newly diagnosed T1 bladder urothelial cancer. J Urol 2009;182:2625–31.

[41] Streeper NM, Simons CM, Konety BR, Muirhead DM, Williams RD, O'Donnell MA, et al. The significance of lymphovascular invasion in transurethral resection of bladder tumour and cystectomy specimens on the survival of patients with urothelial bladder cancer. BJU Int 2009;103:475–9.

[42] Resnick MJ, Bergey M, Magerfleisch L, Tomaszewski JE, Malkowicz SB, Guzzo TJ. Longitudinal evaluation of the concordance and prognostic value of lymphovascular invasion in transurethral resection and radical cystectomy specimens. BJU Int 2011;107:46–52.

[43] Solsona E, Iborra I, Dumont R, Rubio-Briones J, Casanova J, Almenar S. The 3-month clinical response to intravesical therapy as a predictive factor for progression in patients with high risk superficial bladder cancer. J Urol 2000;164:685–9.

[44] Brausi M, Collette L, Kurth K, van der Meijden AP, Oosterlinck W, Witjes J, et al. Variability in the recurrence rate at first follow-up cystoscopy after TUR in stage Ta T1 transitional cell carcinoma of the bladder: a combined analysis of seven EORTC studies. Eur Urol 2002;41:523–31.

[45] Ather MH, Nazim SM. New and contemporary markers of prognosis in nonmuscle invasive urothelial cancer. Korean J Urol 2015;56:553–64.

[46] Sarkis A, Dalbagni G, Cordon-Cardo C, Melamed J, Zhang Z, Sheinfeld J, et al. Association of P53 nuclear overexpression and tumor progression in carcinoma in situ of the bladder. J Urol 1994;152:388–92.

[47] Oh JJ, Ji SH, Choi DK, Gong IH, Kim TH, Park DS. A six-week course of bacillus Calmette-Guérin prophylaxis is insufficient to prevent tumor recurrence in nonmuscle invasive bladder cancer with strong-positive expression of p53. Oncology 2011;79:440–6.

[48]   Shariat SF, Bolenz C, Godoy G, Fradet Y, Ashfaq R, Karakiewicz PI, et al. Predictive value of combined immunohistochemical markers in patients with pT1 urothelial carcinoma at radical cystectomy. J Urol 2009;182:78−84.

[49]   Cormio L, Tolve I, Annese P, Saracino A, Zamparese R, Sanguedolce F, et al. Altered p53 and pRb expression is predictive of response to BCG treatment in T1G3 bladder cancer. Anticancer Res 2009;29:4201−4.

[50]   Shariat SF, Kim J, Raptidis G, Ayala GE, Lerner SP. Association of p53 and p21 expression with clinical outcome in patients with carcinoma in situ of the urinary bladder. Urology 2003;61:1140−5.

Chapter 14

Treatment for TaT1 Tumors

Seung W. Lee
Hanyang University Guri Hospital, Guri, South Korea

Chapter Outline

Bladder cancer includes noninvasive papillary carcinoma (Ta) that has not invaded the bladder wall beyond the inner layer. This early stage of bladder cancer is most often treated with transurethral resection of bladder tumor (TURBT). This may be followed either by observation (close follow-up without further treatment) or by intravesical therapy to try to keep the cancer from coming back. Of the intravesical treatments, immunotherapy with Bacille Calmette-Guerin (BCG) seems to be better than chemotherapy at both keeping cancers from coming back and from getting worse. But it also tends to have more side effects. Ta stage bladder cancers rarely need to be treated with more extensive surgery. Cystectomy (removal of the bladder) is considered only when there are many superficial cancers or when a superficial cancer continues to grow (or seems to be spreading) despite treatment. Stage I bladder cancers have grown into the connective tissue layer of the bladder wall but have not reached the muscle layer. If no other treatment is given, many patients will later get a new bladder cancer, which will often be more advanced. This is more likely to happen if the first cancer is high grade. If not all of the cancer was removed, options include either intravesical BCG or cystectomy (removal of part or all of the bladder).

Bladder Cancer. DOI: http://dx.doi.org/10.1016/B978-0-12-809939-1.00014-X

TRANSURETHRAL RESECTION OF BLADDER TUMOR

Endoscopic Surgical Management

TURBT is the initial form of treatment for all bladder cancers. It allows a reasonably accurate estimate of tumor stage and grade and the need for additional treatment. Patients with single, low-grade, noninvasive tumors may be treated with TURBT alone; those with superficial disease but high-risk features should be treated with transurethral resection (TUR) followed by selective use of intravesical therapy. TURBT alone has rarely been used in the management of patients with invasive bladder cancer because of a high likelihood of recurrence and progression. Such an approach has been used infrequently for carefully selected patients with comorbid medical conditions and either no residual disease or minimal disease only at restaging TUR of bladder tumor. TURBT is under regional or general anesthesia is the initial treatment for visible lesions and is performed to (1) remove all visible tumors and (2) provide specimens for pathologic examination to accurately determine stage and grade. Bimanual examination of the bladder is often performed with the patient under anesthesia before preparation and draping unless the tumor is clearly small and noninvasive, and is repeated after resection. Fixation or persistence of a palpable mass after resection suggests locally advanced disease, although the additional value of this maneuver in the era of modern imaging appears limited and may even be misleading [1].

Patients scheduled for cystoscopy or anesthetic cystoscopy with TURBT must have sterile urine documented prior to instrumentation. Sterility is usually presumed on the basis of a microscopic urinalysis showing no bacteria or white blood cells (WBCs). A urine culture is ideal but not always feasible for surveillance cystoscopy. The risk of urinary tract infection with instrumentation is approximately 1%. Therefore a single dose of fluoroquinolone is recommended for patients undergoing cystoscopy and a dose of intravenous antibiotics (i.e., cefazolin and gentamicin) for patients in the operating room. Allergies may prompt the use of alternative antibiotic regimens. Some patients need additional antibiotics based on a history of valvular heart disease. The American Heart Association guidelines recommend prophylaxis in these patients to prevent endocarditis. Administer 2 gm of ampicillin intravenously or intramuscularly at least 30 minutes before the procedure (or 2 gm of amoxicillin orally at least 1 hour before the procedure) in moderate-risk patients. In patients allergic to penicillin, vancomycin at a dosage of 1 gm intravenously over 1–2 hours, completed at least 30 minutes before the procedure, may be substituted. High-risk patients also receive 120 mg of gentamicin parenterally 30 minutes before the procedure, and they receive a second dose of ampicillin or amoxicillin 6 hours later.

Resection is performed using a 12- or 30-degree lens placed through a resectoscope sheath because this deflection allows visualization of the loop placed at this location. Continuous irrigation with the bladder filled only enough to visualize its contents minimizes bladder wall movement and lessens thinning of the detrusor through overdistention, which should reduce the risk of perforation [2]. Resection is performed piecemeal, delaying transection of any stalk until most tumor has been resected, to maintain countertraction. Friable, low-grade tumors can often be removed without the use of electrical energy because the nonpowered cutting loop will break off many low-grade tumors. This minimizes the chance of bladder perforation and unnecessary cautery damage or loss of specimens. Higher grade, more solid tumors and the base of all tumors require the use of cutting current; cautery yields hemostasis once the entire tumor has been resected. Lifting the tumor edge away from detrusor lessens the chance of perforation [3].

After primary TURBT, adjuvant intravesical BCG instillation is commonly used to manage high-grade T1 nonmuscle-invasive bladder tumor (NMIBC) [4].

T1 of high cellular grade (HGT1), the subset of NMIBC with the highest risk of progression, may exhibit histopathological, clinical, and biological characteristics of invasive tumors. Even though classically 30% of these tumors have been considered to progress [5], updated data show a 21% progression rate [6]. Therefore, a notable proportion of HGT1 behave in a relatively indolent manner and up to one-third resolve ad interim after standard treatment [7,8]. This wide range of tumor biology highlights the need to risk stratify these patients.

Unfortunately, for high-risk NMIBC, both European Organisation for Research and Treatment of Cancer (EORTC) and Spanish Urological Club for Oncological Treatment (CUETO) scoring systems have poor discriminating ability and limited predictive value, tending to overestimate progression [6,9].

As a result, there is a need to reexamine management of HGT1 bladder cancer. Standard initial treatment is based on endoscopic TUR, and intravesical immunotherapy with BCG. A repeat transurethral resection (reTUR) is recommended by guidelines to rule out understaging, even though for an array of reasons, reTUR remains underutilized with no higher than 7.7% of HGT1 patients reportedly undergoing this second procedure even at tertiary care centers [10]. ReTUR may improve outcome but adds morbidity and is probably unnecessary in over 60% of cases, while 6.5%−30% might still progress [11,12]. Conversely, prolongation of conservative treatment and deferring radical cystectomy may allow progression and decrease cancer-specific survival (CSS) [12,13]. Deciding upon ideal timing for cystectomy is one of the most difficult clinical decisions in urology and an ongoing area of controversy. This major surgical procedure requires urinary diversion, is associated with substantial morbidity (50%−67% complication rate) and up to 9% mortality [14], and may represent overtreatment [7]. Therefore identifying those cases of HGT1 suitable for organ preservation and differentiating them from those that will most benefit from a timely cystectomy is a major challenge and key to improving outcomes.

However, whether preventive intravesical chemotherapy should be performed in selected cases of high-grade T1 remains a moot point [15]. T1 tumors, which represent approximately 25% of NMIBCs, are defined as lamina propria (LP) invasion without muscle invasion in the bladder wall [16]. The mitomycin was first described at the end of the 1980s [17]. It consists mostly of scattered, discontinuous smooth muscle fascicles adjacent to intermediate-sized blood vessels lying parallel to the mucosa in the LP. Invasion depth in the bladder wall, a crucial prognostic factor for bladder neoplasms, defines the current TNM classification [18].

After all visible tumor has been resected, an additional pass of the cutting loop or a cold-cup biopsy can be obtained to send to pathology separately to determine the presence of muscle invasion of the tumor base.

Resection of diverticular tumors presents significant risk of bladder wall perforation, and accurate staging is difficult to achieve in this circumstance because the underlying detrusor is absent. Invasion beyond the diverticular LP involves perivesical fat (stage T3a by definition). Low-grade diverticular tumors are best treated with a combination of resection and fulguration of the base. Conservative resection can be followed with subsequent repeat resection if the final pathologic interpretation is high grade. High-grade tumors require adequate sampling of the tumor base, often including perivesical fat, despite the near certainty of bladder perforation. An indwelling catheter usually allows healing within a few days. Partial or radical cystectomy should be strongly considered for high-grade diverticular lesions.

FLUORESCENCE-GUIDED RESECTION

The European Association of Urology (EAU) guidelines recommend fluorescence-guided resection, as it is more sensitive than white-light (WL) cystoscopy alone for detection of tumors, particularly carcinoma in situ (CIS) [19]. The Food and drug association (FDA) has approved blue-light (BL) cystoscopy with hexaminolevulinate (Cysview) as an adjunct to white-light cystoscopy in patients suspected or known to have nonmuscle-invasive papillary cancer of the bladder on the basis of a prior cystoscopy. This technique is not a replacement for random bladder biopsies or other procedures used in the detection of bladder cancer and is not for repetitive use.

BL cystoscopy with hexaminolevulinate detects more Ta/T1 bladder cancer lesions than does WL cystoscopy alone [20,21]. Patients with Ta or T1 tumors, at least one of the tumors was seen only with fluorescent cystoscopy in 16% of patients [22]. Improved detection leads to improved tumor resection, as every tumor detected is resected in the same TURBT [23].

Complications of TURBT and Bladder Biopsy

The major complications of uncontrolled hematuria and clinical bladder perforation occur in fewer than 5% of cases, although a majority of patients will exhibit contrast agent extravasation indicative of minor perforation if cystography is performed. The incidence of perforation can be reduced by attention to technical details, avoiding overdistention of the bladder, and using anesthetic paralysis during the resection of significant lateral wall lesions to lessen an obturator reflex response. The vast majority of perforations are extraperitoneal, but intraperitoneal rupture is possible when tumors are resected at the dome [24]. The risk of tumor seeding from perforation appears to be low [25]. Management of extraperitoneal perforation by prolonged urethral catheter drainage is usually possible. Intraperitoneal perforation is less likely to close spontaneously and usually requires open or laparoscopic surgical repair. Moreover, large, bulky tumors and those that appear to be muscle invasive are often best resected in a staged manner because it is believed that repeat resection can more safely remove residual tumor if indicated.

More recently, as bipolar technology has emerged and improved, its application has extended to TURBT, with a potential benefit of decreased risk of bladder perforation from obturator reflex and decreased risk of TUR syndrome. With bipolar technology, the active and return electrodes are very close together on the loop so that the current does not travel through the patient's body to an external pad, as is the case with monopolar cautery. This also allows for the use of nonconductive isotonic irrigation fluid, mitigating the aforementioned risks of TUR syndrome [26]. Wang and colleagues were the first to report on bipolar TURBT and compared the pathologic specimens from 11 patients who underwent bipolar TURBT with a matched historic cohort of 11 patients who underwent standard monopolar TURBT [27]. Yang and associates retrospectively compared clinical and pathologic results in 115 patients who underwent bipolar ($n = 64$) versus monopolar ($n = 51$) TURBT [28]. Postoperative change in hemoglobin (-0.58 ± 0.91 g/dL vs -0.95 ± 1.28 g/dL, $P = .038$) and mean duration of catheterization (2.20 ± 0.96 d vs 2.65 ± 1.45 d, $P = .026$) favored the bipolar TURBT group. No difference in the grade of thermal damage was noted between the two groups as well. Furthermore, reducing the power settings to 50-W cutting and 40-W coagulation may reduce the incidence of obturator nerve reflex and bladder perforation to close to zero while still maintaining diagnostic and therapeutic efficacy [29].

As long as resection of the ureteral orifice is performed with pure cutting current, scarring is minimal and obstruction unlikely. Traditionally, TURBT was performed using monopolar electrocautery to provide the necessary energy for resecting the tumor and cauterizing blood vessels.

Repeat Transurethral Resection of Bladder Tumor

Repeat TURBT is often indicated if high-grade tumor is identified. Repeat TURBT is usually appropriate in the evaluation of T1 tumors because a repeat TURBT can demonstrate worse prognostic findings in up to 25% of specimens [30].

Laser Therapy

Lasers are not optimal for the treatment of new bladder lesions as tissue samples are requisite to determine depth of invasion (stage) and tumor grade. Appropriate patients for this therapy have papillary, low-grade tumors and a history of low-grade, low-stage tumors. Laser coagulation allows minimally invasive ablation of tumors up to 2.5 cm in size. The most significant complication of laser therapy is forward scatter of laser energy to adjacent structures, resulting in perforation of a hollow, viscous organ such as overlying bowel.

Office-Based Endoscopic Management

Low-grade recurrences and small tumor (typically <0.5 cm, but up to 1 cm diameter) can be managed safely in the office setting with the use of diathermy or laser ablation [16]. Instillation of viscous or injectable 1%−2% lidocaine through a catheter and a dwelling time of 15−30 minutes yields satisfactory mucosal analgesia.

CONSERVATIVE MANAGEMENT

Certain patients with low risk and recurrent NIMBC may be managed conservatively with office fulguration of the lesions or even cystoscopic surveillance. Only those patients with a well-documented history of low-grade Ta tumors have been considered for such an approach, in that the surgical and anesthetic risks of multiple repeated TURBTs in these patients may exceed the low risk of disease progression. Certainly, larger experiences and confirmatory trials are indicated to validate and support a conservative approach.

Fluorescence Cystoscopy and Narrowband Imaging

Photodynamic diagnosis (PDD) has emerged as a viable adjunct to WL kcystoscopy to assist in the performance of a complete TURBT [31]. Lesions can be missed using WL cystoscopy, and PDD has been developed to assist in the detection of these lesions, reduce the rate of recurrence, and improve the completeness of resection. PDD exploits the photodynamic properties of several compounds, including hexaminolevulinate (HAL) (Hexvix, Cysview, Photocure; Oslo, Norway) and 5-aminolevulinic acid (5-ALA).

Approximately 1 hour prior to planned TURBT, 50 mL of reconstituted solution of HAL is instilled into the emptied bladder via an intravesical catheter. Following installation, protoporphyrin IX accumulates preferentially in neoplastic tissue, producing a clearly demarcated red fluorescence with illumination with blue-violet light (380–440 nm). Cysview (HAL hydrochloride) was approved by the US FDA in 2010 for use with the Karl Storz D-Light C PDD system with the BL setting as an adjunct to the WL setting in the detection of nonmuscle-invasive papillary cancer of the bladder in patients suspected or known to have lesions on the basis of a prior cystoscopy.

A recent metaanalysis reviewed the raw data from prospective studies on 1345 patients with known or suspected NIMBC on whom HAL and BL as an adjunct to WL cystoscopy [32]. The EAU guidelines on nonmuscle-invasive bladder cancer recommend PDD in patients who are suspected of harboring a high-grade tumor for guidance of TURBT. It is possible that BL HAL-assisted TURBT improves completeness and quality of resection and might obviate the need for perioperative intravesical instillation of chemotherapy or a second TURBT, but further study is needed in this area to test this hypothesis.

While 5-ALA is not currently approved for routine clinical use for the detection of bladder cancer in Europe or the United States, it has been extensively studied in numerous clinical trials. Furthermore, orally applied 5-ALA has been approved in Europe to enhance intraoperative detection of malignant glioma. The study evaluated the clinical value of PDD with intravesical ($n = 75$) and oral ($n = 135$) instillation of 5-ALA and PDD-guided TURBT for NIMBC in a multiinstitutional retrospective study in 210 patients [33]. Rates of recurrence were compared with historical control subjects who underwent TURBT with WL cystoscopy. 5-ALA-guided TURBT improved detection of CIS, as 72.1% of flat lesions (including dysplasia and CIS) could only be detected with BL 5-ALA-assisted TURBT. The route of administration of 5-ALA (oral vs intravesical) did not affect diagnostic accuracy or recurrence-free survival.

The management of nonmuscle-invasive bladder cancer is expensive, stemming from high recurrence rates necessitating repeat TURBT and frequent surveillance cystoscopies. As HAL and 5-ALA have been shown to help increase the detection and reduce the recurrence of nonmuscle-invasive bladder cancer, this technology may reduce the cost of bladder cancer management. The study assessed the cost effectiveness of BL HAL-assisted cystoscopy as an adjunct to WL cystoscopy versus WL cystoscopy alone at the time of initial TURBT and noted a cost savings of nearly $5000 in the PDD group in their model over a 5-year projected period [34,35].

NARROWBAND IMAGING

Narrowband imaging technology takes advantage of the hypervascular nature of bladder cancer to aid in differentiation of normal urothelium. WL is filtered into two bandwidths of 415 and 540 nm, which is preferentially absorbed by hemoglobin in hypervascular neoplastic tissues. A recent meta-analysis evaluated the diagnostic accuracy of NBI-assisted cystoscopy compared with WL cystoscopy for nonmuscle-invasive bladder cancer [36] NBI detected tumors in an additional 17% of patients and found an additional 24% of tumors compared with WL cystoscopy. No difference in the rate of false-positive tumor detection was noted between NBI and WL cystoscopy. NBI may be a useful adjunct for the detection and management of nonmuscle-invasive bladder cancer.

Perioperative Intravesical Therapy

Chemotherapy should be withheld in patients with extensive resection or when there is concern about perforation. BCG can never be safely administered immediately after TURBT because the risk of bacterial sepsis is high.

Mitomycin C appears to be the most effective adjuvant intravesical chemotherapeutic agent perioperatively, although epirubicinis used in Europe and direct comparative studies are lacking [37]. Consistent with its proposed mechanism of action to prevent tumor cell implantation, a single dose administered within 6 hours lessens recurrence rates, whereas a dose 24 hours later does not [38,39], and maintenance therapy does not reduce the risk further [40]. Although local irritative symptoms are the most common complications of postoperative instillation, serious sequelae and rare deaths have occurred, especially in patients with perforation during resection [41].

REFERENCES

[1] Ploeg M, Kiemeney LA, Smits GA, et al. Discrepancy between clinical staging through bimanual palpation and pathological staging after cystectomy. Urol Oncol 2012;30(3):247–51.

[2] Koch MO, Smith Jr. JA. Natural history and surgical management of superficial bladder cancer (stages Ta/T1/Tis). In: Vogelzang N, Miles BJ, editors. Comprehensive textbook of genitourinary oncology. Baltimore: Lippincott Williams & Wilkins; 1996. p. 405–15.

[3] Holzbeierlein JM, Smith Jr. JA. Surgical management of noninvasive bladder cancer (stages Ta/T1/CIS). Urol Clin North Am 2000;27:15–24, vii–viii.

[4] Babjuk M, Oosterlinck W, Sylvester R, et al. EAU guidelines on non-muscle-invasive urothelial carcinoma of the bladder, the 2011 update. Eur Urol 2011;59:997.

[5] Sylvester RJ, van der Meijden AP, Oosterlinck W, Witjes JA, Bouffioux C, Denis L, et al. Predicting recurrence and progression in individual patients with stage Ta T1 bladder cancer using EORTC risk tables: a combined analysis of 2596 patients from seven EORTC trials. Eur Urol 2006;49(3): 466–465, discussion 475–477.

[6] Van den Bosch S, Alfred Witjes J. Long-term cancer-specific survival in patients with high-risk, non-muscle-invasive bladder cancer and tumour progression: a systematic review. Eur Urol 2011;60(3):493–500.

[7] Pansadoro V, Emiliozzi P, de Paula F, Scarpone P, Pansadoro A, Sternberg CN. Long-term follow-up of G3T1 transitional cell carcinoma of the bladder treated with intravesical Bacille Calmette-Guérin: 18-year experience. Urology 2002;59(2):227−31.

[8] Jakse G, Algaba F, Malmström P, Oosterlinck W. A second-look TUR in T1 transitional cell carcinoma: why? Eur Urol 2004;45(5):539−46, discussion 546.

[9] Xylinas E, Kent M, Kluth L, Pycha A, Comploj E, Svatek RS, et al. Accuracy of the EORTC risk tables and of the CUETO scoring model to predict outcomes in non-muscle-invasive urothelial carcinoma of the bladder. Br J Cancer 2014;109(6):1460−6.

[10] Skolarus TA, Ye Z, Montgomery JS, Weizer AZ, Hafez KS, Lee CT, et al. Use of restaging bladder tumor resection for bladder cancer among medicare beneficiaries. Urology 2011;78(6):1345−9.

[11] Divrik RT, Sahin AF, Yildirim U, Altok M, Zorlu F. Impact of routine second transurethral resection on the long-term outcome of patients with newly diagnosed pT1 urothelial carcinoma with respect to recurrence, progression rate, and disease-specific survival: a prospective randomized clinical trial. Eur Urol 2010;58(2):185−90.

[12] Sfakianos JP, Kim PH, Hakimi AA, Herr HW. The effect of restaging transurethral resection on recurrence and progression rates in patients with nonmuscle invasive bladder cancer treated with intravesical bacillus Calmette-Guérin. J Urol 2014;191(2):341−5.

[13] Raj GV, Herr H, Serio AM, Donat SM, Bochner BH, Vickers AJ, et al. Treatment paradigm shift may improve survival of patients with high risk superficial bladder cancer. J Urol 2007;177(4):1283−6, discussion 1286.

[14] Aziz A, May M, Burger M, Palisaar RJ, Trinh QD, Fritsche HM, et al. PROMETRICS 2011 research group. Prediction of 90-day mortality after radical cystectomy for bladder cancer in a Prospective European Multicenter Cohort. Eur Urol 2013;66(1):156−63.

[15] Hautmann RE, Volkmer BG, Gust K. Quantification of the survival benefit of early versus deferred cystectomy in high-risk non-muscle invasive bladder cancer (T1 G3). World J Urol 2009;27:347.

[16] van Rhijn BW, Burger M, Lotan Y, et al. Recurrence and progression of disease in non-muscle-invasive bladder cancer: from epidemiology to treatment strategy. Eur Urol 2009;56:430.

[17] Dixon JS, Gosling JA. Histology and fine structure of the muscularis mucosae of the human urinary bladder. J Anat 1983;136:265.

[18] Bernardini S, Billerey C, Martin M, et al. The predictive value of muscularis mucosae invasion and p53 over expression on progression of stage T1 bladder carcinoma. J Urol 2001;165:42.

[19] Collado A, Chechile GE, Salvador J, et al. Early complications of endoscopic treatment for superficial bladder tumors. J Urol 2000;164:1529−32.

[20] Schmidbauer J, Witjes F, Schmeller N, Donat R, Susani M, Marberger M. Improved detection of urothelial carcinoma in situ with hexaminolevulinate fluorescence cystoscopy. J Urol 2004 Jan;171(1):135−8.

[21] Jichlinski P, Guillou L, Karlsen SJ, Malmström PU, Jocham D, Brennhovd B, et al. Hexyl aminolevulinate fluorescence cystoscopy: new diagnostic tool for photodiagnosis of superficial bladder cancer—a multicenter study. J Urol 2003 Jul;170(1):226−9.

[22] Stenzl A, Burger M, Fradet Y, Mynderse LA, Soloway MS, Witjes JA, et al. Hexaminolevulinate guided fluorescence cystoscopy reduces recurrence in patients with nonmuscle invasive bladder cancer. J Urol 2010 Nov;184(5):1907−13.

[23] Hermann GG, Mogensen K, Carlsson S, Marcussen N, Duun S. Fluorescence-guided transurethral resection of bladder tumours reduces bladder tumour recurrence due to less residual

tumour tissue in Ta/T1 patients: a randomized two-centre study. BJU Int 2011 Oct;108 (8 Pt 2):E297–303.

[24] Balbay MD, Cimentepe E, Unsal A, et al. The actual incidence of bladder perforation following transurethral bladder surgery. J Urol 2005;174:2260–2.

[25] Venkatramani V, Panda A, Manojkumar R, Kekre NS. Monopolar versus bipolar transurethral resection of bladder tumors: a single center, parallel arm, randomized, controlled trial. J Urol 2014 Jun;191(6):1703–7.

[26] Wang DS, Bird VG, Leonard VY, et al. Use of bipolar energy for transurethral resection of bladder tumors: pathologic considerations. J Endourol 2004 Aug;18(6):578–82.

[27] Yang SJ, Song PH, Kim HT. Comparison of deep biopsy tissue damage from transurethral resection of bladder tumors between bipolar and monopolar devices. Korean J Urol 2011 Jun;52(6):379–83.

[28] Gupta NP, Saini AK, Dogra PN, Seth A, Kumar R. Bipolar energy for transurethral resection of bladder tumours at low-power settings: initial experience. BJU Int 2011 Aug;108 (4):553–6.

[29] Schwaibold HE, Treiber U, Kuebler H, et al. Second transurethral resection detects histopathological changes worsening the prognosis in 25% of patients with T1 bladder cancer. J Urol 2000;163:153.

[30] Donat SM, North A, Dalbagni G, et al. Efficacy of office fulguration for recurrent low grade papillary bladder tumors less than 0.5 cm. J Urol 2004;171:636–9.

[31] Herr HW. Randomized trial of narrow-band versus white-light cystoscopy for restaging (second-look) transurethral resection of bladder tumors. Eur Urol 2015 Apr;67(4):605–8 [Medline].

[32] Burger M, Grossman HB, Droller M, et al. Photodynamic diagnosis of non-muscle-invasive bladder cancer with hexaminolevulinate cystoscopy: a meta-analysis of detection and recurrence based on raw data. Eur Urol 2013 Apr 8; [Medline].

[33] Inoue K, Fukuhara H, Shimamoto T, et al. Comparison between intravesical and oral administration of 5-aminolevulinic acid in the clinical benefit of photodynamic diagnosis for nonmuscle invasive bladder cancer. Cancer 2012 Feb 15;118(4):1062–74 [Medline].

[34] Garfield SS, Gavaghan MB, Armstrong SO, Jones JS. The cost-effectiveness of blue light cystoscopy in bladder cancer detection: United States projections based on clinical data showing 4.5 years of follow up after a single hexaminolevulinate hydrochloride instillation. Can J Urol 2013 Apr;20(2):6682–9 [Medline].

[35] Gendy R, Delprado W, Brenner P, Brooks A, Coombes G, et al. Repeat transurethral resection for non-muscle-invasive bladder cancer: a contemporary series. BJU Int 2015 Oct 21; [Medline].

[36] Li K, Lin T, Fan X, Duan Y, Huang J. Diagnosis of narrow-band imaging in non-muscle-invasive bladder cancer: a systematic review and meta-analysis. Int J Urol 2013 Jun;20 (6):602–9 [Medline].

[37] Witjes JA, Hendricksen K. Intravesical pharmacotherapy for non–muscleinvasive bladder cancer: a critical analysis of currently available drugs, treatment schedules, and long-term results. Eur Urol 2008;53(1):45–52.

[38] Isaka S, Okano T, Abe K, et al. Sequential instillation therapy with mitomycin C and Adriamycin for superficial bladder cancer. Cancer Chemother Pharmacol 1992;30:41.

[39] Sekine H, Fukui I, Yamada T. Intravesical mitomycin C and doxorubicin sequential therapy for carcinoma in situ of the bladder: a longer follow-up result. J Urol 1994;151:27–30.

[40] Tolley DA, Parmar MK, Grigor KM, et al. The effect of intravesical mitomycin C on recurrence of newly diagnosed superficial bladder cancer: a further report with 7 years of follow-up. J Urol 1996;155:1233.

[41] Oddens JR, van der Meijden AP, Sylvester R. One immediate postoperative instillation of chemotherapy in low risk Ta, T1 bladder cancer patients. Is it always safe? Eur Urol 2004;46:336−8.

Chapter 15

Treatment for Carcinoma In Situ

Jeong Hyun Kim

Kangwon National University School of Medicine, Chuncheon, South Korea

Chapter Outline

INTRODUCTION

Approximately 70%−80% of all patients with bladder cancer initially present with superficial diseases, and among these, approximately 70% present as stage Ta, 20% as T1, and 10% as carcinoma in situ (CIS) [1−2]. CIS is a high-grade carcinoma confined to the urothelium, with a flat nonpapillary configuration. Unlike a papillary tumor, CIS appears as reddened and velvety mucosa and is slightly elevated but sometimes not visible. Primary CIS (no previous or concurrent papillary tumors) can be distinguished from secondary CIS (with a history of papillary tumors) and concurrent CIS (in the presence of papillary tumors) [1]. Although confined to the urothelium in the same manner as stage Ta, CIS is regarded as a precursor lesion for the development of an invasive high-grade cancer [3]. Unlike low-grade Ta and T1 tumors, CIS is a highly malignant carcinoma that is at a high risk for progression to muscle-invasive disease and subsequently death, if left untreated [4]. Based on the untreated natural history of CIS, up to 83% of patients diagnosed with CIS experience progression to muscle-invasive disease and up to 39% have died of the disease [2].

CIS is diagnosed in most cases through a combination of cystoscopy, urine cytology, and multiple bladder biopsies [5]. Of these, the histology of bladder biopsies is a determinant to establish the diagnosis. It is difficult to detect and accurately assess flat lesions via cystoscopy. The mucosa may range from unremarkable to erythematous, edematous, or eroded, and lesions may be found

Bladder Cancer. DOI: http://dx.doi.org/10.1016/B978-0-12-809939-1.00015-1
213

both near an invasive tumor and at a distance from it [6]. Characteristic lesions are sometimes described as "red, velvety patches," although these findings are nonspecific. In CIS, a larger number cells float in the urine because the coherence and adherence of epithelial cells decreases. Therefore, CIS can always be detected via urine cytology with a sensitivity of approximately 60% and specificity of more than 90%, and a cold cup biopsy sometimes reveals a denudation in the specimens [7]. Within the limitations of random sampling and pathologic assessment, multiple bladder biopsies have a sensitivity of approximately 77% [8]. Photodynamic diagnosis (PDD) or fluorescence cystoscopy, which is performed using violet light after intravesical instillation of 5-aminolevulinic acid and hexaminolevulinic acid, reveals areas in the bladder that are suspicious for CIS but cannot be seen with white-light cystoscopy (WLC) (Fig. 15.1). Although the use of PDD increases the detection rates of CIS from 23–68% with WLC alone to 91–97% with WLC plus PDD [9–10], it has not yet been implemented on a regular basis in daily practice.

TREATMENT OF CIS

CIS is often multifocal and, unlike papillary tumors, cannot be treated by transurethral resection (TUR), with the result that CIS managed in this way

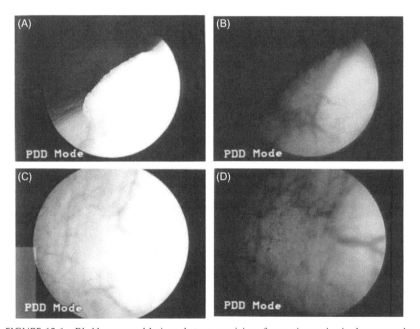

FIGURE 15.1 Bladder mucosal lesions that are suspicious for carcinoma in situ but cannot be seen with white-light cystoscopy (A, C) and can be detected by fluorescence cystoscopy (B, D), which is performed using violet light after intravesical instillation of 5-aminolevulinic acid and hexaminolevulinic acid.

frequently progresses to invasive cancer [1,11]. Until 1976, radical cystect-omy (RC) was considered the only definitive therapy for CIS [12]. However, in more recent decades, intravesical chemotherapy and immunotherapy are the most widely used initial conservative treatments. Cystectomy is generally reserved for patients in whom conservative treatment has failed, but it may sometimes be used as the initial treatment. If concurrent CIS is found in association with a muscle-invasive bladder cancer, the therapy for the patient is determined according to the invasive tumor. If concurrent CIS is found in association with a non-muscle-invasive bladder cancer (NMIBC; Ta or T1), TUR of all concomitant papillary tumors is mandatory for correct staging and grade determination. No consensus exists on whether conservative ther-apy (intravesical instillations) or aggressive therapy (cystectomy) should be employed, especially when there are concurrent high-grade papillary tumors.

INTRAVESICAL THERAPY

Intravesical bacillus Calmette–Guerin (BCG) is generally accepted as standard in the treatment of CIS [13]. The American Urological Association (AUA) and the European Association of Urology (EAU) guidelines also recommend intravesical BCG as the first-line therapy in CIS [14,15]. Several large-scale studies and meta-analyses have found the rate of complete response (CR) after BCG treatment to be quite high, averaging approximately 70% [16,17]. Administration is often performed in a 6- to 8-week course, composed of weekly 2 hour instillations of an approximately 80 mg suspension of BCG, fol-lowed by a second course for patients who do not achieve CR. Nevertheless, there are important limitations to drawing conclusions based on an overview of the CR rates from a number of different studies. There may be important differences between studies with respect to the definition of CIS, patient char-acteristics, and assessment of the response to treatment. Unfortunately, there is a relative paucity of randomized trials in patients with just CIS. Most trials also include patients with papillary tumors, and separate results are not always provided for the smaller subgroup of patients with CIS.

The long-term results of BCG therapy have been somewhat disappointing [11,18]. In a study by Talic et al., although the initial CR rate was 71%–72%, half of the patients developed a recurrence or progression within 2 years. Many of those with a recurrence developed an invasive carcinoma and ulti-mately had metastases [19]. Similarly, Chade et al. reported that the 5-year cumulative incidence of progression to cT1 or higher was 45% and progres-sion to cT2 or higher was 17% in a cohort of 155 patients with primary CIS managed with induction BCG only, while the CR rate at 6 months was 62% [20]. Therefore, maintenance treatment has been investigated as a possible solution. The efficacy of BCG maintenance specifically for CIS was deter-mined best in the Southwest Oncology Group (SWOG) 8507 trial comparing induction therapy only with induction plus maintenance in this randomized prospective study [21]. The CR rate at 3 months (after induction therapy) was 57% in the induction-only arm and 55% in the maintenance arm of the trial. The CR rate after 6 months increased to 68% in the induction-only arm and to 84% in the maintenance arm (after the first course of maintenance; $P = 0.004$). This trial demonstrated not only the benefits of maintenance BCG but also the potential delayed benefits of BCG in the treatment of CIS and the necessity of waiting for 6 months before assessing the response to treatment with a repeat bladder biopsy. Unfortunately, longer term outcomes for patients with CIS in SWOG 8507 were not reported separately, and there is a paucity of long-term data after maintenance therapy. However, these additional rounds of treatment carry the additional risks for side effects. Notably, in patients who have undergone BCG treatment, subsequent biopsy specimens may reveal changes similar to tuberculous cystitis, including acute and chronic inflammation, noncaseating granulomas, and reactive atypia with denudation and ulceration of the urothelium [22]. In some cases, these chronic inflammatory changes may hinder an evaluation for recurrent CIS.

The optimal duration of BCG maintenance is often debated because the 3-year period was arbitrarily determined, and prolonged therapy has a significant toxicity. A recent randomized controlled trial by the European Organization for Research and Treatment of Cancer (EORTC) compared the efficacy of one-third dose with full-dose BCG therapy in a 1- or 3-year course to optimize the efficacy of BCG while minimizing the toxicity [23]. In contrast to SWOG 8507 (16% completion rate for the full 3-year course), 35.2% of patients completed the 3-year course of full-dose BCG in the EORTC trial. There was no difference in the toxicity between a one-third dose and full dose, and interestingly, there was also no difference in the progression ($P = 0.85$) or survival rates ($P = 0.56$) in any of the treatment arms. However, the 3-year course of full-dose BCG was found to be more effective in high-risk patients than a 1-year course ($P = 0.0087$). This is important to note because CIS is classified as a high-risk disease. Therefore, 3-year maintenance therapy is recommended as the standard of care.

In addition to intravesical BCG, intravesical chemotherapy with drugs such as thiotepa, adriamycin, epirubicin, and mitomycin C (MMC) has been used in the treatment of CIS for more than 20 years. A review of 497 patients treated with intravesical chemotherapy revealed an overall CR rate of 48%, including 38% with thiotepa, 48% with doxorubicin, and 53% with MMC [1]. However, considerable variability was observed for the same drug from one study to the next. Several randomized trials have compared BCG to different chemotherapy regimens in patients with CIS [7], and the results indicate an overall CR rate of 68% for BCG and 49% for chemotherapy with overall disease-free rates of 51% and 27%, respectively (Tables 15.1 and 15.2). Thus, treatment with BCG showed an increase in both the CR rate and the overall percentage of patients remaining disease-free when compared to chemotherapy. Furthermore, Sylvester conducted a

TABLE 15.1 BCG vs Chemotherapy: CR Rate in Patients With CIS of the Urinary Bladder

Reference	BCG	Chemotherapy
BCG vs MMC		
Di Stasi	23/36	11/36
Vegt	26/38	8/12
Witjes	NA/24	NA/16
Lamm	17/31	16/35
Malmstrom	NA/41	NA/42
Total	66/105 (63%)	35/83 (42%)
BCG vs electro MMC		
Di Stasi	23/36 (64%)	21/36 (58%)
BCG vs Adriamycin		
Lamm	45/64	23/67
Martinez-Pineiro	NA/6	NA/6
Total	45/64 (70%)	23/67 (34%)
BCG vs Epirubicin		
De Reijke	55/84	47/84
Melekos	NA/4	NA/3
Total	55/84 (65%)	47/84 (56%)
BCG vs Thiotepa		
Martinez-Pineiro	NA/6	NA/5
BCG vs MMC +ADM		
Sekine	18/21 (86%)	17/21 (81%)
BCG +MMC vs MMC		
Witjes	NA/29	NA/36
Rintala	21/28	20/40
Total	21/28 (75%)	20/40 (50%)
Overall Total	205/302 (68%)	163/331 (49%)

NA, Data not available.
Source: From van der Meijden AP, Sylvester R, Oosterlinck W, Solsona E, Boehle A, Lobel B, et al. EAU guidelines on the diagnosis and treatment of urothelial carcinoma in situ. Eur Urol 2005;48:363.

TABLE 15.2 BCG vs Chemotherapy: Disease-Free Rate in Patients With CIS of the Urinary Bladder

Reference	BCG	Chemotherapy	Median Follow-up (years)
BCG vs MMC			
Di Stasi	17/36	9/36	3.6
Vegt	NA/38	NA/12	3.0
Witjes	11/22	7/16	7.2
Lamm	NA/31	NA/35	2.5
Malmstrom	23/41	14/42	5.3
Total	51/99 (52%)	30/94 (32%)	
BCG vs Electro MMC			
Di Stasi	17/36 (47%)	17/36 (47%)	3.6
BCG vs Adriamycin			
Lamm	26/64	8/67	5.4
Martinez-Pineiro	4/6	0/6	3.0
Total	30/70 (43%)	8/73 (11%)	
BCG vs Epirubicin			
De Reijke	37/84	16/84	5.6
Melekos	NA/4	NA/3	
Total	37/84 (44%)	16/84 (19%)	
BCG vs Thiotepa			
Martinez-Pineiro	4/6 (67%)	3/5 (60%)	3.0
BCG vs MMC +ADM			
Sekine	16/21 (76%)	6/21 (29%)	3.9
BCG +MMC vs MMC			
Witjes	NA/29	NA/36	
Rintala	20/28	17/40	2.8
Total	20/28 (71%)	17/40 (43%)	
Overall total	154/302 (51%)	97/353 (27%)	3.75

NA, Data not available.
Source: From van der Meijden AP, Sylvester R, Oosterlinck W, Solsona E, Boehle A, Lobel B, et al. EAU guidelines on the diagnosis and treatment of urothelial carcinoma in situ. Eur Urol 2005;48:363.

meta-analysis of randomized clinical trials and found that intravesical BCG significantly reduces the risk of disease progression in CIS by 35% relative to intravesical chemotherapy or a different form of immunotherapy [24]. Nevertheless, most studies in which BCG has been compared with intravesical chemotherapy do not delineate CIS from other stages of NMIBC [24]. In the EORTC Phase III trial, BCG was compared with epirubicin specifically in 168 patients with primary (23%), secondary (24%), and concurrent CIS (52%) [25]. Maintenance therapy was administered in both treatment arms. The overall CR rates for BCG and epirubicin were similar (65% vs 56%; $P = 0.21$), but the time to recurrence after CR was significantly longer in patients treated with BCG (median: 5.1 vs 1.4 year), and CIS recurrences were more frequently observed in patients treated with epirubicin (45% vs 16%). However, no differences were observed in this trial in the time to progression or duration of survival.

In randomized trials comparing BCG plus chemotherapy to BCG alone in CIS patients ($n = 304$) [26], no difference was found in the CR rate between the two treatment arms. However, based on a median follow-up of 56 months, there was a significantly longer disease-free interval in the BCG monotherapy arm: 80 of 145 (55%) patients were disease-free on BCG alone compared to 72 of 159 (45%) patients on a combination of BCG and MMC.

SECONDARY BLADDER-PRESERVING TREATMENT

While induction and maintenance intravesical BCG therapy may decrease the rate of progression or the need for RC in patients with CIS, approximately 50% of complete responders will not be disease-free and are therefore deemed to "fail" BCG [27]. BCG failure is described as the recurrence of a tumor after intravesical BCG therapy. However, this definition is complicated by the fact that failure comes in many forms with different implications regarding therapy options and prognosis. O'Donnell et al. stratified the definition into four categories: BCG intolerance, BCG resistance, BCG relapsing, and BCG refractory [28]. Of these, BCG refractory is defined as the absence of CR within 6 months after BCG induction. This also includes the progression of the disease within 3 months after the first cycle of BCG. Although these classifications can be helpful, it is ultimately up to the urologist to determine whether "BCG failure" has occurred. Before proceeding with additional therapy, it is important to consider the upper tracts and the prostatic urethra as possible sites of disease for all patients experiencing a recurrence of CIS after prior intravesical BCG therapy. Huguet et al. reported a 20% 5-year disease-specific survival in high-risk NMIBC for patients with prostatic urethral tumor involvement compared to 78% survival in patients without prostatic urethral involvement ($P < 0.0002$) [29].

Although RC is recommended in BCG-refractory CIS patients, second-line intravesical therapy can be considered in patients who are poor surgical candidates with a significant medical comorbidity or advanced age, or for those who have refused RC.

In some cases, interferon-α (INF-α) has been used in tandem with BCG, and this combination has shown a 50%–60% CR rate after BCG failure in several studies [30–32]. In a subsequent large Phase II trial on this combination therapy ($n = 1007$), 45% of BCG failure and 59% of BCG-naive patients remained disease-free at 24 months of median follow-up [33]. However, no clear advantage was observed over BCG monotherapy. Another Phase II trial determined that the factors affecting a significant recurrence after BCG and INF-α therapy in CIS were multifocality, large size (>5 cm), presence of T1, and two or more prior BCG failures [34]. Furthermore, a multicenter, prospective randomized study ($n = 670$) also found limited efficacy of this combination therapy with INF-α for CIS after two BCG failures [35]. Therefore, combination therapy with INF-α should not be used as the first-line therapy because it has not been shown to be effective.

Valrubicin is a derivative of the anthracycline doxorubicin, which has only been approved by the Food and Drug Administration (FDA) for the intravesical treatment of BCG-refractory CIS. In a Phase I-II trial [36], a dose of 200–900 mg valrubicin was instilled intravesically every week for 6 weeks, and minimal systemic absorption and toxicity were found. In a Phase III trial that included 90 patients with CIS despite multiple courses of intravesical therapies, 21% were disease-free at 9 months and only 8% were disease-free at 30 months, whereas 88% had a recurrence with 56% undergoing eventual cystectomy [37]. In a subsequent Phase II-III open-label study of 80 BCG refractory/intolerant patients, CR was 18% at 3 months and 4% at 2 years [38]. Thus, the benefit is marginal and does not warrant delaying RC in patients who can tolerate cystectomy, but it does offer an option in cases where RC is not possible.

Intravesical gemcitabine has demonstrated activity against BCG failure in high-risk NMIBC [39]. In a Phase II trial of 30 patients with NMIBC refractory to BCG therapy, 50% achieved a CR with a median follow-up of 19 months [40]. However, this was not durable because only two patients maintained CR at 23 and 29 months, respectively. In a subsequent SWOG Phase II trial for gemcitabine in recurrent NMIBC after two prior courses of BCG, CR was observed in 47% at 3 months, 28% at 1 year, and 21% at 2 years with maintenance therapy [41]. In this study, 20 of 47 patients had pure CIS. This is comparable to CR rates of 18%–21% in prior valrubicin studies [37,38], suggesting that gemcitabine may be a suitable alternative.

New device-assisted therapies have been developed to improve the delivery and efficacy of MMC, such as electromotive drug administration of MMC and intravesical hyperthermia with MMC instillation. Electromotive drug administration is based on the enhancement of intravesical chemotherapy transport by applying a current gradient between the drug and the bladder wall. Di Stasi et al. reported that in a prospective randomized study of 108 patients with

CIS, CR at 6 months was observed in 31% of passive MMC patients, 58% of electromotive MMC patients, and 64% of BCG patients [42]. Electromotive MMC administration appears to be most effective when alternated with BCG [43]. Meanwhile, Witjes et al. demonstrated that treatment with intravesical hyperthermia and MMC resulted in a CR rate of 92% in patients with CIS (17 BCG-naive and 34 BCG failures), and 50% had a durable response at 2 years [44].

However, all of these studies had small, heterogeneous treatment arms, and further studies are required in a CIS setting for both BCG-naive and BCG-refractory diseases to determine the optimal treatment schedule and the benefit for maintenance therapy.

RADICAL CYSTECTOMY

Patients who experience recurrence after intravesical BCG therapy have a poor prognosis, with a high risk of progression to muscle-invasive disease and death due to bladder cancer [45]. In one study, the 3-year bladder cancer–specific survival was 67% in patients initially presenting with muscle-invasive disease but was only 37% in patients whose disease progressed after intravesical treatment [46]. In general, the results are disappointing for conservative treatment after BCG failure, and therefore, RC is currently accepted as the standard treatment for most patients when intravesical treatment has failed [14,15]. Cookson et al. reported that 53% of BCG-treated patients experienced disease progression within 15 years, and 36% eventually underwent RC for progression or refractory/recurrent CIS [11]. However, the decision process to undergo RC is often difficult for patients and physicians, and this is especially true in terms of timing. Most studies show a negative selection bias against delayed RC because only patients progressing during or after conservative treatment receive radical treatment.

Currently, there is no clear consensus for further therapeutic management of patients with recurrent CIS of the urinary bladder. Furthermore, there is no reliable method to date to differentiate between those who will progress and those who will not [47]. Thus, doubt remains as to the best time point to abandon conservative treatment and to proceed to cystectomy. Herr et al. reported that patients with high-risk NMIBC (81% associated with CIS) who undergo RC less than 2 years after initial BCG treatment had a markedly higher 15-year disease-specific survival rate compared to those with RC after 2 years of follow-up (69% vs 26%, $P = 0.003$) [48]. In contrast, Cheng et al. reported that after controlling for age, patients who underwent early RC within 3 months after the initial diagnosis of CIS of the bladder have no survival benefit compared with those who did not ($P = 0.16$) [4]. Shariat et al. also noted that the time from TUR to RC is not associated with recurrence-free survival (RFS) and cancer-specific survival (CSS) in pathological CIS-only patients ($P \geq 0.103$) [49]. Furthermore, it is not clear whether delayed RC after failed BCG therapy results in differences in overall survival compared with immediate cystectomy in CIS of the bladder due to a lack of randomized clinical trials.

Another issue is that stage and grade disparity occurs frequently in patients treated with TUR after RC (Table 15.3), and this is one of the concerns [29,50]. Tilki et al. noted that approximately one-fourth of patients with clinical CIS refractory to intravesical therapy at the time of RC were up-staged to muscle-invasive disease (12% pT2, 5% pT3, and 6% pT4) [51], which is within the range reported in other series [29,52]. The Bladder Cancer Research Consortium found that 33% of patients treated with RC for clinical CIS had been up-staged to invasive disease ($\geq$pT1) at RC and that 27% had muscle-invasive bladder cancer [50]. However, pathological upgrading was found in 4% of patients and clinical overgrading was found in 10% of patients in another report, which is less frequent compared with stage disparity [53]. The same group specifically analyzed 99 patients with pathologic CIS only and found the preoperative staging to be clinical CIS only in 47%, cTa in 7%, cT1 in 23%, and cT2 in 23% (all with or without concomitant CIS) [49]. This stage disparity may be due to a sampling error with incomplete TUR, delay in the interval from TUR to RC, and a poor sensitivity of preoperative staging tools. Interestingly, in one series, these upstaging rates were more likely to be observed in patients who underwent RC after failing intravesical therapy than in those who underwent immediate RC (36.8 vs 14.3%, respectively) [52].

Although CIS theoretically has no access to the lymphatic channel or to blood vessels, lymphovascular invasion (LVI) and lymph node (LN) metastasis were sometimes found in patients who underwent RC for clinical CIS-only, possibly due to the aforementioned stage disparity (Table 15.3). Tilki et al. reported that 9% of patients had LVI and 5.8% of patients had metastasis to regional LNs in the final pathology after RC for clinical CIS-only, and these were associated with worse outcomes, with an increased risk of disease recurrence ($P = 0.043$ and 0.017, respectively) and cancer-specific mortality ($P = 0.001$ and 0.019, respectively) [51]. However, in two studies of patients with pathological CIS-only at RC, LN metastasis was less frequently found in 3%–4% of patients [49,54]. LN positivity is known to increase incrementally with advancing final pathological stage in the RC series for bladder cancer from the Bladder Cancer Research Consortium (0% for pTa, 2% for pTis, 4% for pT1, 14% for pT2, 35% for pT3, and 52% for pT4, respectively) [53]. Interestingly, there was no LN metastasis in the series that includes only patients with both clinical and pathological CIS [55]. To date, there is little evidence available to conclude the necessity of pelvic LN dissection during RC in patients with clinical CIS-only and the extent of LN dissection if necessary.

To date, most series have shown excellent disease-specific survival after RC in patients with clinical or pathological CIS-only (Table 15.3) [56]. Tilki

TABLE 15.3 Outcomes After Radical Cystectomy for CIS of the Urinary Bladder

	Study	Subjects, n	Follow-up, months	Clinical Stage	Pathologic Stage	Stage Disparity, n (%)	LNs (+), n (%)	LVI (+), n (%)	5-year RFS	5-year CSS	5-year OS
Clinical CIS	Tilki et al.	243	37.3	cTis	48% Tis 8% T0 8% Ta 13% T1 23% T2–T4	Same stage: 117 (48%) Downstaging: 39 (16%) Upstaging: 87 (36%)	14 (5.8%)	22 (9.1%)	74%	85%	NA
	Cheng et al.	138	132	cTis	NA		NA	NA	87%[a]	96%	75%
	Stein et al.	100	122	cTis	NA		NA	NA	85%	NA	78%
	Huang et al.	27	94	cTis	59.3% Tis 7.4% T0 11% T1 7.4% T2 14.8% T4a	Same stage: 16 (59.3%) Downstaging: 2 (7.4%) Upstaging: 9 (33.3%)	1 (3.7%)	NA	100%	NA	87%
	Amling et al.	23	60	cTis	34.8%Tis 34.8% T0 21.7% T1 8.7% T3	Same stage: 8 (34.8%) Downstaging: 8 (34.8%) Upstaging: 7 (30.4%)	0	NA	NA	100%	NA

(Continued)

TABLE 15.3 (Continued)

	Study	Subjects, n	Follow-up, months	Clinical Stage	Pathologic Stage	Stage Disparity, n (%)	LNs (+), n (%)	LVI (+), n (%)	5-year RFS	5-year CSS	5-year OS
Pathologic CIS	Shariat et al.	99	39.2	47% cTis 6% cTa 23% cT1 23% cT2	Tis	Same stage: 46 (47%) Downstaging: 46 (48%) Upstaging: 6 (6%)	3 (3%)	2 (2%)	83%	90.7%	NA
	Zehnder et al.	52	102	cTis	Tis		0	NA	94%		85%
	Hassan et al.	50	37.2	38% cTis 2% cTa 16% cT1 44% cT2	Tis	Same stage: 19 (38%) Downstaging: 30 (60%) Upstaging: 1 (2%)	2 (4%)	NA	88%[b]		NA

OS, overall survival; NA, not available.

[a]Progression-free survival.

[b]3-year RFS.

Modified from Casey RG, Catto JW, Cheng L, Cookson MS, Herr H, Shariat S, et al. Diagnosis and management of urothelial carcinoma in situ of the lower urinary tract: a systematic review. Eur Urol 2015;67:876—88.

et al. described a multicenter international cohort of 243 patients who underwent RC for primary CIS who had failed bladder-preserving therapy [51]. In their large series, overall 5-year RFS and CSS estimates were 74% and 85%, respectively. Shariat et al. reported excellent outcomes in patients with pathological CIS-only, with RFS estimates of 83.0% at 5 and 7 years after RC and disease-specific survival estimates of 90.7% at 5 years and 87.2% at 7 years after surgery [49]. Six patients (6%) died of bladder cancer. Similar results were reported in the University of Southern California RC series with 5- and 10-year RFS rates of 91% and 89%, respectively, for pathological CIS disease [57]. Remarkably, the series from Zehnder et al. that includes only patients with both clinical and pathologic CIS also demonstrated excellent outcomes with RFS rates of 94% at 5 years and 90% at 10 years after surgery [55].

Although limited data are available on the efficacy of RC for the treatment of patients with clinical CIS-only disease at the time of surgery, most series showed excellent disease-specific survival after RC for CIS-only. However, as many as 40%−50% of patients may have been overtreated [51]. Therefore, as with all high-risk NMIBC, a balance must be struck between overtreatment with RC and undertreatment with a subsequent disease progression when administering BCG [15,58,59], and there is yet an unmet need for more good-quality evidence.

CONCLUSIONS

CIS of the urinary bladder is a highly malignant disease that constitutes a major step in the progression to invasive cancer. Intravesical BCG remains the standard first-line therapy with the highest rate of CR as well as the highest long-term disease-free rate among intravesical treatment. Six weeks only of BCG provide suboptimal treatment, thus maintenance BCG treatment is required but the optimal maintenance schedule is not determined. Alternative intravesical therapy may be applicable in nonsurgical candidates and in patients who refuse cystectomy and new agents continue to be investigated. RC should be considered for BCG-refractory disease and currently shows adequate local disease control and excellent survival outcomes. There is a clear clinical unmet need for improved localized therapies, including novel intravesical agents, to enable more frequent bladder preservation without increasing the risk of progression.

REFERENCES

[1]   Lamm D, Herr H, Jakse G, Kuroda M, Mostofi FK, Okajima E, et al. Updated concepts and treatment of carcinoma in situ. Urol Oncol 1998;4:130−8.

[2]   van Rhijn BW, Burger M, Lotan Y, Solsona E, Stief CG, Sylvester RJ, et al. Recurrence and progression of disease in non-muscle-invasive bladder cancer: from epidemiology to treatment strategy. Eur Urol 2009;56:430−42.

[3]   Althausen AF, Prout Jr GR, Daly JJ. Non-invasive papillary carcinoma of the bladder associated with carcinoma in situ. J Urol 1976;116:575−80.

[4] Cheng L, Cheville JC, Neumann RM, Leibovich BC, Egan KS, Spotts BE, et al. Survival of patients with carcinoma in situ of the urinary bladder. Cancer 1999;85:2469—74.

[5] Kurth KH, Schellhammer PF, Okajima E, Akdas A, Jakse G, Herr HW, et al. Current methods of assessing and treating carcinoma in situ of the bladder with or without involvement of the prostatic urethra. Int J Urol 1995;2(Suppl 2):8—22.

[6] Cheng L, Lopez-Beltran A, MacLennan GT, Montironi R, Bostwick DG. Neoplasms of the urinary bladder. In: Bostwick DG, Cheng L, editors. Urologic surgical pathology. 2nd ed. Philadelphia: Elsevier/Mosby; 2008. p. 259—352.

[7] van der Meijden AP, Sylvester R, Oosterlinck W, Solsona E, Boehle A, Lobel B, et al. EAU guidelines on the diagnosis and treatment of urothelial carcinoma in situ. Eur Urol 2005;48:363—71.

[8] Murphy WM, Takezawa K, Maruniak NA. Interobserver discrepancy using the 1998World Health Organization/International Society of Urologic Pathology classification of urothelial neoplasms: practical choices for patient care. J Urol 2002;168:968—72.

[9] Kausch I, Sommerauer M, Montorsi F, Stenzl A, Jacqmin D, Jichlinski P, et al. Photodynamic diagnosis in non-muscle-invasive bladder cancer: a systematic review and cumulative analysis of prospective studies. Eur Urol 2010;57:595—606.

[10] Grossman HB, Stenzl A, Fradet Y, Mynderse LA, Kriegmair M, Witjes JA, et al. Long-term decrease in bladder cancer recurrence with hexaminolevulinate enabled fluorescence cystoscopy. J Urol 2012;188:58—62.

[11] Cookson MS, Herr HW, Zhang ZF, Soloway S, Sogani PC, Fair WR. The treated natural history of high risk superficial bladder cancer: 15-year outcome. J Urol 1997;158:62—7.

[12] Morales A, Eidinger D, Bruce AW. Intracavitary Bacillus Calmette-Guerin in the treatment of superficial bladder tumors. J Urol 1976;116:180—3.

[13] Kamat AM, Porten S. Myths and mysteries surrounding bacillus Calmette-Guérin therapy for bladder cancer. Eur Urol 2014;65:267—9.

[14] Hall MC, Chang SS, Dalbagni G, Pruthi RS, Seigne JD, Skinner EC, et al. Guideline for the management of nonmuscle invasive bladder cancer (stages Ta, T1, and Tis): 2007 update. J Urol 2007;178:2314—30.

[15] Babjuk M, Burger M, Zigeuner R, Shariat SF, van Rhijn BW, Compérat E, et al. EAU guidelines on non-muscle-invasive urothelial carcinoma of the bladder: update 2013. Eur Urol 2013;64:639—53.

[16] Lamm DL, Blumenstein BA, Crawford ED, Montie JE, Scardino P, Grossman HB, et al. A randomized trial of intravesical doxorubicin and immunotherapy with bacille Calmette-Guérin for transitional-cell carcinoma of the bladder. N Engl J Med 1991;325:1205—9.

[17] Lamm DL. BCG in perspective: advances in the treatment of superficial bladder cancer. Eur Urol 1995;27(Suppl 1):2—8.

[18] Takenaka A, Yamada Y, Miyake H, Hara I, Fujisawa M. Clinical outcomes of bacillus Calmette-Guérin instillation therapy for carcinoma in situ of urinary bladder. Int J Urol 2008;15:309—13.

[19] Talic RF, Hargreave TB, Bishop MC, Kirk D, Prescott S. Intravesical Evans bacille Calmette-Guérin for carcinoma in situ of the urinary bladder. Scottish Urological Oncology Group. Br J Urol 1994;73:645—8.

[20] Chade DC, Shariat SF, Godoy G, Savage CJ, Cronin AM, Bochner BH, et al. Clinical outcomes of primary bladder carcinoma in situ in a contemporary series. J Urol 2010;184:464—9.

[21] Lamm DL, Blumenstein BA, Crissman JD, Montie JE, Gottesman JE, Lowe BA, et al. Maintenance bacillus Calmette-Guerin immunotherapy for recurrent TA, T1 and

carcinoma in situ transitional cell carcinoma of the bladder: a randomized Southwest Oncology Group Study. J Urol 2000;163:1124—9.

[22]   Lopez-Beltran A, Luque RJ, Mazzucchelli R, Scarpelli M, Montironi R. Changes produced in the urothelium by traditional and newer therapeutic procedures for bladder cancer. J Clin Pathol 2002;55:641—7.

[23]   Oddens J, Brausi M, Sylvester R, Bono A, van de Beek C, van Andel G, et al. Final results of an EORTC-GU cancers group randomized study of maintenance bacillus Calmette-Guérin in intermediate- and high-risk Ta, T1 papillary carcinoma of the urinary bladder: one-third dose versus full dose and 1 year versus 3 years of maintenance. Eur Urol 2013;63:462—72.

[24]   Sylvester RJ, van der Meijden AP, Lamm DL. Intravesical bacillus Calmette-Guerin reduces the risk of progression in patients with superficial bladder cancer: a meta-analysis of the published results of randomized clinical trials. J Urol 2002;168:1964—70.

[25]   de Reijke TM, Kurth KH, Sylvester RJ, Hall RR, Brausi M, van de Beek K, et al. Bacillus Calmette-Guerin versus epirubicin for primary, secondary or concurrent carcinoma in situ of the bladder: results of a European Organization for the Research and Treatment of Cancer-Genito-Urinary Group Phase III Trial (30906). J Urol 2005;173:405—9.

[26]   Kaasinen E, Wijkström H, Malmström PU, Hellsten S, Duchek M, Mestad O, et al. Alternating mitomycin C and BCG instillations versus BCG alone in treatment of carcinoma in situ of the urinary bladder: a nordic study. Eur Urol 2003;43:637—45.

[27]   Sylvester RJ, van der Meijden AP, Witjes JA, Kurth K. Bacillus Calmette-Guerin versus chemotherapy for the intravesical treatment of patients with carcinoma in situ of the bladder: a meta-analysis of the published results of randomized clinical trials. J Urol 2005;174:86—91, discussion 91—2.

[28]   O'Donnell MA. Advances in the management of superficial bladder cancer. Semin Oncol 2007;34:85—97.

[29]   Huguet J, Crego M, Sabaté S, Salvador J, Palou J, Villavicencio H. Cystectomy in patients with high risk superficial bladder tumors who fail intravesical BCG therapy: pre-cystectomy prostate involvement as a prognostic factor. Eur Urol 2005;48:53—9, discussion 59.

[30]   Luciani LG, Neulander E, Murphy WM, Wajsman Z. Risk of continued intravesical therapy and delayed cystectomy in BCG-refractory superficial bladder cancer: an investigational approach. Urology 2001;58:376—9.

[31]   Lam JS, Benson MC, O'Donnell MA, Sawczuk A, Gavazzi A, Wechsler MH, et al. Bacillus Calmete-Guérin plus interferon-alpha2B intravesical therapy maintains an extended treatment plan for superficial bladder cancer with minimal toxicity. Urol Oncol 2003;21:354—60.

[32]   Punnen SP, Chin JL, Jewett MA. Management of bacillus Calmette-Guerin (BCG) refractory superficial bladder cancer: results with intravesical BCG and Interferon combination therapy. Can J Urol 2003;10:1790—5.

[33]   Joudi FN, Smith BJ, O'Donnell MA, National BCG-Interferon Phase 2 Investigator Group. Final results from a national multicenter phase II trial of combination bacillus Calmette-Guérin plus interferon alpha-2B for reducing recurrence of superficial bladder cancer. Urol Oncol 2006;24:344—8.

[34]   Rosevear HM, Lightfoot AJ, Birusingh KK, Maymí JL, Nepple KG, O'Donnell MA, et al. Factors affecting response to bacillus Calmette-Guérin plus interferon for urothelial carcinoma in situ. J Urol 2011;186:817—23.

[35]   Nepple KG, Lightfoot AJ, Rosevear HM, O'Donnell MA, Lamm DL, Bladder Cancer Genitourinary Oncology Study Group. Bacillus Calmette-Guérin with or without

interferon α-2b and megadose versus recommended daily allowance vitamins during induction and maintenance intravesical treatment of nonmuscle invasive bladder cancer. J Urol 2010;184:1915−19.

[36] Greenberg RE, Bahnson RR, Wood D, Childs SJ, Bellingham C, Edson M, et al. Initial report on intravesical administration of N-trifluoroacetyladriamycin-14-valerate (AD 32) to patients with refractory superficial transitional cell carcinoma of the urinary bladder. Urology 1997;49:471−5.

[37] Steinberg G, Bahnson R, Brosman S, Middleton R, Wajsman Z, Wehle M. Efficacy and safety of valrubicin for the treatment of Bacillus Calmette-Guerin refractory carcinoma in situ of the bladder. The Valrubicin Study Group. J Urol 2000;163:761−7.

[38] Dinney CP, Greenberg RE, Steinberg GD. Intravesical valrubicin in patients with bladder carcinoma in situ and contraindication to or failure after bacillus Calmette-Guérin. Urol Oncol 2013;31:1635−42.

[39] Di Lorenzo G, Perdonà S, Damiano R, Faiella A, Cantiello F, Pignata S, et al. Gemcitabine versus bacille Calmette-Guérin after initial bacille Calmette-Guérin failure in non-muscle-invasive bladder cancer: a multicenter prospective randomized trial. Cancer 2010;116:1893−900.

[40] Dalbagni G, Russo P, Bochner B, Ben-Porat L, Sheinfeld J, Sogani P, et al. Phase II trial of intravesical gemcitabine in bacille Calmette-Guérin-refractory transitional cell carcinoma of the bladder. J Clin Oncol 2006;24:2729−34.

[41] Skinner EC, Goldman B, Sakr WA, Petrylak DP, Lenz HJ, Lee CT, et al. SWOG S0353: Phase II trial of intravesical gemcitabine in patients with nonmuscle invasive bladder cancer and recurrence after 2 prior courses of intravesical bacillus Calmette-Guérin. J Urol 2013;190:1200−4.

[42] Di Stasi SM, Giannantoni A, Stephen RL, Capelli G, Navarra P, Massoud R, et al. Intravesical electromotive mitomycin C versus passive transport mitomycin C for high risk superficial bladder cancer: a prospective randomized study. J Urol 2003;170:777−82.

[43] Di Stasi SM, Giannantoni A, Giurioli A, Valenti M, Zampa G, Storti L, et al. Sequential BCG and electromotive mitomycin versus BCG alone for high-risk superficial bladder cancer: a randomised controlled trial. Lancet Oncol 2006;7:43−51.

[44] Alfred Witjes J, Hendricksen K, Gofrit O, Risi O, Nativ O. Intravesical hyperthermia and mitomycin-C for carcinoma in situ of the urinary bladder: experience of the European Synergo working party. World J Urol 2009;27:319−24.

[45] Stanisic TH, Donovan JM, Lebouton J, Graham AR. 5-year experience with intravesical therapy of carcinoma in situ: an inquiry into the risks of "conservative" management. J Urol 1987;138:1158−61.

[46] Schrier BP, Hollander MP, van Rhijn BW, Kiemeney LA, Witjes JA. Prognosis of muscle-invasive bladder cancer: difference between primary and progressive tumours and implications for therapy. Eur Urol 2004;45:292−6.

[47] Witjes JA. Bladder carcinoma in situ in 2003: state of the art. Eur Urol 2004;45:142−6.

[48] Herr HW, Sogani PC. Does early cystectomy improve the survival of patients with high risk superficial bladder tumors? J Urol 2001;166:1296−9.

[49] Shariat SF, Palapattu GS, Amiel GE, Karakiewicz PI, Rogers CG, Vazina A, et al. Characteristics and outcomes of patients with carcinoma in situ only at radical cystectomy. Urology 2006;68:538−42.

[50] Shariat SF, Palapattu GS, Karakiewicz PI, Rogers CG, Vazina A, Bastian PJ, et al. Discrepancy between clinical and pathologic stage: impact on prognosis after radical cystectomy. Eur Urol 2007;51:137−49.

[51] Tilki D, Reich O, Svatek RS, Karakiewicz PI, Kassouf W, Novara G, et al. Characteristics and outcomes of patients with clinical carcinoma in situ only treated with radical cystectomy: an international study of 243 patients. J Urol 2010;183:1757−63.

[52] Huang GJ, Kim PH, Skinner DG, Stein JP. Outcomes of patients with clinical CIS-only disease treated with radical cystectomy. World J Urol 2009;27:21−5.

[53] Shariat SF, Karakiewicz PI, Palapattu GS, Lotan Y, Rogers CG, Amiel GE, et al. Outcomes of radical cystectomy for transitional cell carcinoma of the bladder: a contemporary series from the Bladder Cancer Research Consortium. J Urol 2006;176(6 Pt 1): 2414−22, discussion 2422.

[54] Hassan JM, Cookson MS, Smith Jr JA, Johnson DL, Chang SS. Outcomes in patients with pathological carcinoma in situ only disease at radical cystectomy. J Urol 2004;172: 882−4.

[55] Zehnder P, Moltzahn F, Daneshmand S, Leahy M, Cai J, Miranda G, et al. Outcome in patients with exclusive carcinoma in situ (CIS) after radical cystectomy. BJU Int 2014;113: 65−9.

[56] Casey RG, Catto JW, Cheng L, Cookson MS, Herr H, Shariat S, et al. Diagnosis and management of urothelial carcinoma in situ of the lower urinary tract: a systematic review. Eur Urol 2015;67:876−88.

[57] Stein JP, Lieskovsky G, Cote R, Groshen S, Feng AC, Boyd S, et al. Radical cystectomy in the treatment of invasive bladder cancer: long-term results in 1,054 patients. J Clin Oncol 2001;19:666−75.

[58] Lockyer CR, Sedgwick JE, Gillatt DA. Beware the BCG failures: a review of one institution's results. Eur Urol 2002;42:542−6.

[59] Thomas F, Noon AP, Rubin N, Goepel JR, Catto JW. Comparative outcomes of primary, recurrent, and progressive high-risk non-muscle-invasive bladder cancer. Eur Urol 2013;63: 145−54.

Chapter 16

Treatment for T1G3 Tumor

Soodong Kim
Dong-A University Medical Center, Busan, South Korea

Chapter Outline

IMMEDIATE PROPHYLACTIC POSTTRANSURETHRAL RESECTION CHEMOTHERAPY INSTILLATION

Immediate single instillation (SI) therapy destroys circulating tumor cells after transurethral resection of bladder tumor (TURBT) and acts by an ablative effect on residual tumor cells at the resection site and on miniscule overlooked tumors. Four large meta-analyses showed that after TURBT, SI significantly reduces the recurrence rate compared with TURBT alone [1–4]. (Level 1a) In the most recent systematic review and individual patient data meta-analysis of 2278 eligible patients, immediate SI reduced the risk of recurrence, and only low-risk patients and intermediate-risk patients with a prior recurrence rate of less than or equal to one recurrence per year and a European Organization for Research and Treatment of Cancer (EORTC) recurrence score <5 benefitted from SI. It does not prolong either the time to progression or death from bladder cancer. The authors suggested that the instillation might be associated with an increase in the risk of death in high-risk patients, so it is not effective or recommended. Conversely, a sufficient number of delayed repeat chemotherapy instillations without SI can also reduce recurrence [5]. A meta-analysis showed a highly significant 44% reduction in the odds of recurrence (corresponding to an absolute difference

Bladder Cancer. DOI: http://dx.doi.org/10.1016/B978-0-12-809939-1.00016-3

of approximately 14%) at 1 year in favor of chemotherapy over TURBT alone, but no effect on tumor progression [6]. The duration and frequency of chemotherapy instillations remains controversial. Contraindications to its use include very deep resections, bladder perforation, and prior documented allergic reaction. Although several chemotherapeutic agents are used, the majority of centers use mitomycin C (MMC) (40 mg in 40 cm^3 of saline) as the prophylactic chemotherapeutic agent of choice [7].

SECONDARY TRANSURETHRAL RESECTION

For all cases of newly diagnosed high-grade T1, a secondary TUR 4−6 weeks after the primary TUR is strongly recommended. The advantages of a second TUR are threefold. First, a repeat resection of the previously resected site 2−6 weeks after the initial resection provides more accurate pathological staging information. This is particularly important because the probability of understaging high-grade T1 ranges from 20% to 70%, depending on the presence of muscularis propria in the sample, and persistent tumors in the second TUR specimens can be detected in 33%−55% of patients [8−11].

In addition to the diagnostic benefit, repeat TUR has the ability to detect and potentially clear residual tumor. Because at least 27% of patients harbor residual tumor (the highest reported rate is 62%), repeat resection might have a therapeutic benefit [9]. In some randomized controlled trials (RCTs), a second TUR decreased the recurrence rate compared to a single TUR, and patients in the repeat TUR group experienced a significantly improved 3-year recurrence-free survival (RFS) of 69% compared to 37% in the group without secondary TUR [12,13]. A third and recently appreciated advantage of repeat TUR is prognostication. Residual tumor in the second TUR specimen is associated with a poor prognosis. Of 92 patients with residual T1 cancer in the second TUR, 75 (82%) progressed to muscle invasion within 5 years compared to 49 of 260 (19%) who had no or non-T1 tumor detected on restaging TUR [14]. Based on these data, residual T1 tumor on repeat TUR was deemed a negative prognostic indicator and a potential indication for immediate cystectomy in high-grade T1 patients.

INTRAVESICAL BACILLUS CALMETTE−GUERIN THERAPY

Adjuvant intravesical bacillus Calmette−Guerin (BCG) immunotherapy is the treatment of choice for bladder preservation with high-grade T1 disease [15−17]. Standard induction therapy comprises 6 weekly instillations after a diagnosis of high-grade T1 disease following complete resection [7]. For preventing the recurrence of non-muscle-invasive bladder cancer (NMIBC), BCG after TURBT is superior to TURBT alone or chemotherapy after

TURBT in several meta-analyses [16−20]. Three recent RCTs of intermediate- and high-risk tumors compared BCG with epirubicin and interferon [21], MMC [22], or epirubicin alone [23] and confirmed the superiority of BCG for the prevention of tumor recurrence (Level 1a). Furthermore, two meta-analyses have demonstrated that BCG therapy prevents, or at least delays, the risk of tumor progression [15,17] (Level 1a).

BCG therapy might be associated with severe side effects with local or systemic symptoms. However, serious side effects occur in less than 5% of patients, and most cases can be treated effectively [24] (Level 1b). In addition, the maintenance schedule is not associated with an increased risk of side effects compared to an induction course [25]. The role of maintenance BCG therapy for high-grade T1 bladder cancer is supported by many lines of evidence [26]. The maintenance protocol consisted of three weekly BCG instillations at 3 and 6 months' post-TUR and semiannually thereafter for 3 years. Both the 5-year RFS (60% vs 41%, $P < 0.001$) and "worsening-free" survival (a proxy for progression-free survival [PFS] 76% vs 70%, $P = 0.04$) were improved with maintenance BCG [7].

IMMEDIATE OR EARLY CYSTECTOMY

Considering the high risk of recurrence, progression, and cancer death of high-grade T1 disease treated conservatively, radical cystectomy (RC) can be performed as an immediate procedure (directly after NMIBC diagnosis) or an early procedure (after BCG failure).

As a therapeutic option, RC has a number of advantages. First, RC provides the most definitive opportunity for cure. Table 16.1 lists the contemporary series in which T1 tumors were treated immediately or early with RC. The disease-specific survival (DSS) for these patients ranges between approximately 80% and 90%. Second, understaged lesions will also be appropriately treated. Although restaging TUR refines local cancer staging, thereby decreasing the risk of understaging T1 lesions, approximately 13% of patients will still be understaged even after re-TUR [35]. Third, RC enables lymphadenectomy. Because up to 18% of T1 patients have positive lymph nodes, cystectomy can be both diagnostic and therapeutic with regard to nodal metastases. Fourth, RC obviates the need for repeated intravesical therapies and simplifies follow-up. However, there are several concerns about overtreatment, deterioration of the quality of life, and perioperative or long-term complications [33,36].

Thus, the potential benefit of RC must be weighed against the risk, morbidity, and impact on quality of life. It is reasonable to propose immediate RC in patients with high-grade T1 bladder cancer who are at the highest risk of progression based on the several factors including residual tumor on

TABLE 16.1 Contemporary Outcomes of High-Grade T1 Bladder Cancer Managed With Immediate or Early RC

Study	Time Frame	n	Median Follow-up (months)	Prior BCG (%)	Upstaging (%)	LN Positive (%)	Recurrence[a] (%)	DSS[a] (%)	OS[a] (%)
Herr and Sogani[b] [27]	1979–84	35	NR	100	NR	NR	NR	92	NR
Dutta et al.[b] [28]	1995–99	78	NR	37	40	12	NR	78	64
Thalmann et al. [29]	1980–99	29	47	0	41	14	21	69	54
Masood et al. [30]	1992–2002	30	57	30	27	NR	NR	88	NR
Bianco et al. [31]	1990–2000	66	48	27	27	9	78	78	NR
Lambert et al. [32]	1990–2005	104	NR	44	40	NR	48	93	87
Gupta et al. [33]	1984–2003	167	34	44	50	18	29	82	69
Denzinger et al. [34]	1995–2005	54	61	0	26	NR	NR	78	NR

BCG=bacillus Calmette-Guerin; LN=lymph node; DSS=disease-specific survival; OS=overall survival; NR=not reported; BCa=bladder cancer.

[a]Rates reported are those reported at study completion and are not necessarily 5-year actuarial values.

[b]"High-risk" superficial bladder cancer (exact proportion T1G3 not specified for Herr and Sogani; 80% for Dutta et al.).

Source: From Kulkarni GS, Hakenberg OW, Gschwend JE, Thalmann G, Kassouf W, Kamat A, et al. An updated critical analysis of the treatment strategy for newly diagnosed high-grade T1 (previously T1G3) bladder cancer. Eur Urol 2010;57:60–70, with permission.

re-TUR, lymphovascular invasion (LVI), variant histologies, and prostate involvement.

As mentioned in section Secondary Transurethral Resection, because patients with residual T1 on re-TUR have a worse prognosis than those with no residual tumor in terms of recurrence and PFS, RC is recommended. In one study, one-fourth of patients with residual T1 on re-TUR had carcinoma invading the bladder muscle, and RC should be considered for these patients [37].

The presence of LVIon TUR pathology was an independent predictor of disease-related mortality [38−42]. In a recent study, patients with LVI in their TURBT specimens had a shorter DSS than those without LVI, with a 5-year survival of 33.6% vs 62.9%, respectively, and the authors suggested that patients with this feature should be preferentially treated with RC [39].

Variant histologies in TUR specimens are associated with a worse prognosis, and aggressive intervention is necessary. One study contended that patients with high-risk NMIBC and variant histology should be offered early cystectomy, especially if the tumors harbor pure squamous, adenocarcinoma, sarcomatoid, plasmacytoid, or micropapillary disease [43]. Several studies noted that prostatic urethra involvement is an important prognostic factor in high-grade T1 disease [17,44,45]. In addition, early RC is strongly recommended for patients with BCG refractory tumors. A delay in RC might lead to decreased DSS [46] (Level 3). Several lines of evidence bolster the rationale for cystectomy in high-grade T1. A retrospective review of 219 patients with NMIBC who underwent cystectomy suggested that the number of TURs and instances of tumor upstaging in cystectomy specimens correlated with an increased prevalence of lymph node metastasis [47]. A similar study reported that early cystectomy seems to prolong cancer-specific survival compared to deferred cystectomy in high-risk, high-grade T1 patients [34]. Fig. 16.1 illustrates a possible treatment algorithm for newly diagnosed high-grade T1 tumors based on the information. It supports a bladder preservation regimen for patients without identifiable risk factors while helping to identify those individuals at risk for progression in whom immediate or early cystectomy should be performed.

OTHER TREATMENT MODALITIES

A limited number of reports have assessed the role of radiation therapy (RT) with or without chemotherapy for the treatment of high-grade T1. However, when compared with BCG, the results of RT have not been as encouraging. The largest RCT comparing RT to conservative therapy (observation or intravesical BCG/MMC) for T1G3 transitional cell carcinoma concluded that RT cannot be recommended for routine use as a bladder preservation strategy [48].

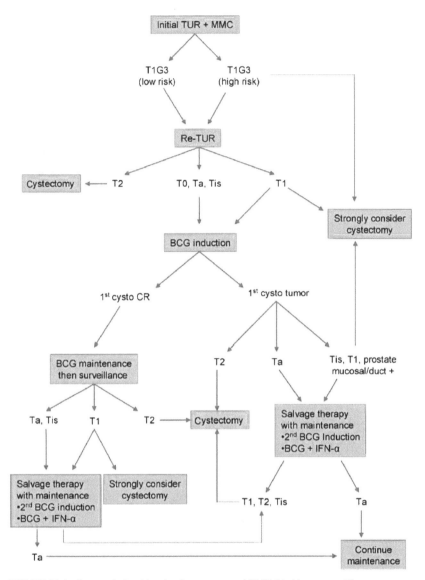

FIGURE 16.1 Proposed algorithm for the treatment of T1G3 bladder cancer. The management decisions are outlined in boxes. High-risk, high-grade T1 refers to tumors with associated risk factors for progression, whereas low-risk, high-grade T1 tumors lack any risk factors for progression. All pathology identified after the first cystoscopic assessment assumes adequate transurethral resection (i.e., reresection of T1 lesions). Although not explicitly stated, the treatment decisions for non-muscle-invasive recurrences are also influenced by the tumor grade (i.e., Ta, Grade 3 vs Ta, Grade 1) and require clinical judgment based on the specific circumstances of each case. *Source: From Kulkarni GS, Hakenberg OW, Gschwend JE, Thalmann G, Kassouf W, Kamat A, et al. An updated critical analysis of the treatment strategy for newly diagnosed high-grade T1 (previously T1G3) bladder cancer. Eur Urol 2010;57:60−70, with permission.*

REFERENCES

[1] Sylvester RJ, Oosterlinck W, Holmang S, Sydes MR, Birtle A, Gudjonsson S, et al. Systematic review and individual patient data meta-analysis of randomized trials comparing a single immediate instillation of chemotherapy after transurethral resection with transurethral resection alone in patients with stage pTa-pT1 urothelial carcinoma of the bladder: which patients benefit from the instillation? Eur Urol 2016;69:231—44.

[2] Sylvester RJ, Oosterlinck W, van der Meijden AP. A single immediate postoperative instillation of chemotherapy decreases the risk of recurrence in patients with stage Ta T1 bladder cancer: a meta-analysis of published results of randomized clinical trials. J Urol 2004;171: 2186—90, quiz 2435.

[3] Abern MR, Owusu RA, Anderson MR, Rampersaud EN, Inman BA. Perioperative intravesical chemotherapy in non-muscle-invasive bladder cancer: a systematic review and meta-analysis. J Natl Compr Canc Netw 2013;11:477—84.

[4] Perlis N, Zlotta AR, Beyene J, Finelli A, Fleshner NE, Kulkarni GS. Immediate post-transurethral resection of bladder tumor intravesical chemotherapy prevents non—muscle-invasive bladder cancer recurrences: an updated meta-analysis on 2548 patients and quality-of-evidence review. Eur Urol 2013;64:421—30.

[5] Sylvester RJ, Oosterlinck W, Witjes JA. The schedule and duration of intravesical chemotherapy in patients with non—muscle-inva- sive bladder cancer: a systematic review of the published results of randomized clinical trials. Eur Urol 2008;53:709—19.

[6] Huncharek M, McGarry R, Kupelnick B. Impact of intravesical chemotherapy on recurrence rate of recurrent superficial transitional cell carcinoma of the bladder: results of a meta-analysis. Anticancer Res 2001;21:765—9.

[7] Kulkarni GS, Hakenberg OW, Gschwend JE, Thalmann G, Kassouf W, Kamat A, et al. An updated critical analysis of the treatment strategy for newly diagnosed high-grade T1 (previously T1G3) bladder cancer. Eur Urol 2010;57:60—70.

[8] Herr HW. The value of a second transurethral resection in evaluating patients with bladder tumors. J Urol 1999;162:74—6.

[9] Ramírez-Backhaus M, Dominguez-Escrig J, Collado A, Rubio-Briones J, Solsona E. Restaging transurethral resection of bladder tumor for high-risk stage Ta and T1 bladder cancer. Curr Urol Rep 2012;13:109—14.

[10] Jahnson S, Wiklund F, Duchek M, Mestad O, Rintala E, Hellsten S, et al. Results of second-look resection after primary resection of T1 tumour of the urinary bladder. Scand J Urol Nephrol 2005;39:206—10.

[11] Vasdev N, Dominguez-Escrig J, Paez E, Johnson MI, Durkan GC, Thorpe AC. The impact of early re-resection in patients with pT1 high-grade non-muscle invasive bladder cancer. Ecancermedicalscience 2012;6:269.

[12] Kim W, Song C, Park S, Kim J, Park J, Kim SC, et al. Value of immediate second resection of the tumor bed to improve the effectiveness of transurethral resection of bladder tumor. J Endourol 2012;26:1059—64.

[13] Divrik T, Yildirim U, Eroglu AS, Zorlu F, Ozen H. Is a second transurethral resection necessary for newly diagnosed pT1 bladder cancer? J Urol 2006;175:1258—61.

[14] Herr HW, Donat SM, Dalbagni G. Can restaging transurethral resection of T1 bladder cancer select patients for immediate cystectomy? J Urol 2007;177:75—9.

[15] Sylvester RJ, van der Meijden AP, Lamm DL. Intravesical bacillus Calmette-Guerin reduces the risk of progression in patients with superficial bladder cancer: a meta-analysis of the published results of randomized clinical trials. J Urol 2002;168:1964—70.

[16] Shelley MD, Wilt TJ, Court J, Coles B, Kynaston H, Mason MD. Intravesical bacillus Calmette-Guérin is superior to mitomycin C in reducing tumour recurrence in high-risk superficial bladder cancer: a meta-analysis of randomized trials. BJU Int 2004;93:485–90.

[17] Böhle A, Bock PR. Intravesical bacille Calmette-Guérin versus mitomycin C in superficial bladder cancer: formal meta-analysis of comparative studies on tumor progression. Urology 2004;63:682–6.

[18] Malmström PU, Sylvester RJ, Crawford DE, Friedrich M, Krege S, Rintala E, et al. An individual patient data meta-analysis of the long-term outcome of randomised studies comparing intravesical mitomycin C versus bacillus Calmette-Guerin for non-muscle-invasive bladder cancer. Eur Urol 2009;56:247–56.

[19] Shelley MD, Kyanston H, Court J, Wilt TJ, Coles B, Burgon K, et al. A systematic review of intravesical bacillus Calmette-Guerin plus transurethral resection vs transurethral resection alone in Ta and T1 bladder cancer. BJU Int 2001;88:209–16.

[20] Han RF, Pan JG. Can intravesical bacillus Calmette-Guerin reduce recurrence in patients with superficial bladder cancer? A meta-analysis of randomized trials. Urology 2006;67:1216–23.

[21] Duchek M, Johansson R, Jahnson S, Mestad O, Hellström P, Hellsten S, et al. Bacillus Calmette-Guérin is superior to a combination of epirubicin and interferon-alpha2b in the intravesical treatment of patients with stage T1 urinary bladder cancer. A prospective, randomized, Nordic study. Eur Urol 2010;57:25–31.

[22] Järvinen R, Kaasinen E, Sankila A, Rintala E, FinnBladder Group. Long-term efficacy of maintenance bacillus Calmette-Guerin versus maintenance mitomycin C instillation therapy in frequently recurrent TaT1 tumours without carcinoma in situ: a subgroup analysis of the prospective, randomised FinnBladder I study with a 20-year follow-up. Eur Urol 2009;56:260–5.

[23] Sylvester RJ, Brausi MA, Kirkels WJ, Hoeltl W, Calais Da Silva F, Powell PH, et al. Long-term efficacy results of EORTC genito-urinary group randomized phase 3 study 30911 comparing intravesical instillations of epirubicin, bacillus Calmette-Guerin, and bacillus Calmette-Guerin plus isoniazid in patients with intermediate- and high-risk stage Ta T1 urothelial carcinoma of the bladder. Eur Urol 2010;57:766–73.

[24] Hinotsu S, Akaza H, Naito S, Ozono S, Sumiyoshi Y, Noguchi S, et al. Maintenance therapy with bacillus Calmette-Guérin Connaught strain clearly prolongs recurrence-free survival following transurethral resection of bladder tumour for non-muscle-invasive bladder cancer. BJU Int 2011;108:187–95.

[25] van der Meijden AP, Sylvester RJ, Oosterlinck W, Hoeltl W, Bono AV, EORTC Genito-Urinary Tract Cancer Group. Maintenance bacillus Calmette-Guerin for Ta T1 bladder tumors is not associated with increased toxicity: results from a European Organisation for Research and Treatment of Cancer Genito-Urinary Group Phase III Trial. Eur Urol 2003;44:429–34.

[26] Lamm DL, Blumenstein BA, Crissman JD, Montie JE, Gottesman JE, Lowe BA, et al. Maintenance bacillus Calmette-Guerin immunotherapy for recurrent TA, T1 and carcinoma in situ transitional cell carcinoma of the bladder: a randomized Southwest Oncology Group Study. J Urol 2000;163:1124–9.

[27] Herr HW, Sogani PC. Does early cystectomy improve the survival of patients with high risk superficial bladder tumors? J Urol 2001;166:1296–9.

[28] Dutta SC, Smith Jr JA, Shappell SB, Coffey CS, Chang SS, Cookson MS. Clinical under staging of high risk nonmuscle invasive urothelial carcinoma treated with radical cystectomy. J Urol 2001;166:490–3.

[29] Thalmann GN, Markwalder R, Shahin O, Burkhard FC, Hochreiter WW, Studer UE. Primary T1G3 bladder cancer: organ preserving approach or immediate cystectomy? J Urol 2004;172:70−5.

[30] Masood S, Sriprasad S, Palmer JH, Mufti GR. T1G3 bladder cancer—indications for early cystectomy. Int Urol Nephrol 2004;36:41−4.

[31] Bianco Jr FJ, Justa D, Grignon DJ, Sakr WA, Pontes JE, Wood Jr. DP. Management of clinical T1 bladder transitional cell carcinoma by radical cystectomy. Urol Oncol 2004;22:290−4.

[32] Lambert EH, Pierorazio PM, Olsson CA, Benson MC, McKiernan JM, Poon S. The increasing use of intravesical therapies for stage T1 bladder cancer coincides with decreasing survival after cystectomy. BJU Int 2007;100:33−6.

[33] Gupta A, Lotan Y, Bastian PJ, Palapattu GS, Karakiewicz PI, Raj GV, et al. Outcomes of patients with clinical T1 grade 3 urothelial cell bladder carcinoma treated with radical cystectomy. Urology 2008;71:302−7.

[34] Denzinger S, Fritsche HM, Otto W, Blana A, Wieland WF, Burger M. Early versus deferred cystectomy for initial high-risk pT1G3 urothelial carcinoma of the bladder: Do risk factors define feasibility of bladder-sparing approach? Eur Urol 2008;53:146−52.

[35] Dalbagni G, Herr HW, Reuter VE. Impact of a second transurethral resection on the staging of T1 bladder cancer. Urology 2002;60:822−4.

[36] Hautmann RE, Abol-Enein H, Davidsson T, Gudjonsson S, Hautmann SH, Holm HV, et al. ICUD-EAU International Consultation on Bladder Cancer 2012: urinary diversion. Eur Urol 2013;63:67−80.

[37] Sternberg IA, Keren Paz GE, Chen LY, Herr HW, Dalbagni G. Role of immediate radical cystectomy in the treatment of patients with residual T1 bladder cancer on restaging transurethral resection. BJU Int 2013;112:54−9.

[38] Quek ML, Stein JP, Nichols PW, Cai J, Miranda G, Groshen S, et al. Prognostic significance of lymphovascular invasion of bladder cancer treated with radical cystectomy. J Urol 2005;174:103−6.

[39] Streeper NM, Simons CM, Konety BR, Muirhead DM, Williams RD, O'Donnell MA, et al. The significance of lymphovascular invasion in transurethral resection of bladder tumour and cystectomy specimens on the survival of patients with urothelial bladder cancer. BJU Int 2009;103(4):475−9.

[40] Lotan Y, Gupta A, Shariat SF, Palapattu GS, Vazina A, Karakiewicz PI, et al. Lymphovascular invasion is independently associated with overall survival, cause-specific survival, and local and distant recurrence in patients with negative lymph nodes at radical cystectomy. J Clin Oncol 2005;23:6533−9.

[41] May M, Bastian PJ, Brookman-May S, Burger M, Bolenz C, Trojan L, et al. Pathological upstaging detected in radical cystectomy procedures is associated with a significantly worse tumour-specific survival rate for patients with clinical T1 urothelial carcinoma of the urinary bladder. Scand J Urol Nephrol 2011;45:251−7.

[42] Cho KS, Seo HK, Joung JY, Park WS, Ro JY, Han KS, et al. Lymphovascular invasion in transurethral resection specimens as predictor of progression and metastasis in patients with newly diagnosed T1 bladder urothelial cancer. J Urol 2009;182:2625−30.

[43] Porten SP, Willis D, Kamat AM. Variant histology: role in management and prognosis of nonmuscle invasive bladder cancer. Curr Opin Urol 2014;24:517−23.

[44] Badalato GM, Gaya JM, Hruby G, Patel T, Kates M, Sadeghi N, et al. Immediate radical cystectomy vs conservative management for high grade cT1 bladder cancer: Is there a survival difference? BJU Int 2012;110:1471−7.

[45] Babjuk M, Böhle A, Burger M, Capoun O, Cohen D, Comperat EM, et al. EAU Guidelines on non-muscle-invasive urothelial carcinoma of the bladder: update 2016. Eur Urol 2016 Jun 17; pii: S0302-2838(16)30249-4.

[46] Raj GV, Herr H, Serio AM, Donat SM, Bochner BH, Vickers AJ, et al. Treatment paradigm shift may improve survival of patients with high risk superficial bladder cancer. J Urol 2007;177:1283−6, discussion 1286.

[47] Wiesner C, Pfitzenmaier J, Faldum A, Gillitzer R, Melchior SW, Thuroff JW. Lymph node metastases in non-muscle invasive bladder cancer are correlated with the number of transurethral resections and tumour upstaging at radical cystectomy. BJU Int 2005;95:301−5.

[48] Harland SJ, Kynaston H, Grigor K, Wallace DM, Beacock C, Kockelbergh R, et al. A randomized trial of radical radiotherapy for the management of pT1G3 NXM0 transitional cell carcinoma of the bladder. J Urol 2007;178:807−13.

Chapter 17

Single, Immediate, Postoperative Intravesical Chemotherapy

Jae Heon Kim
Soonchunhyang University, Seoul, South Korea

Chapter Outline

INTRODUCTION

Bladder cancer (BCa) is the 11th most frequent cancer worldwide [1]. It is the eighth leading cause of cancer death among men in the United States [2]. In comparison to other types of cancer, BCa entails a high burden of medical expense owing to frequent recurrence and aggravation.

Transurethral resection of bladder tumor (TURBT) is the gold standard treatment option as the initial therapeutic and diagnostic approach for suspected BCa. TURBT provides effective therapeutic and prognostic benefits in non-muscle-invasive bladder cancer (NMIBC). However, TURBT alone is not an optimal treatment strategy for NMIBC because of the high recurrence rate of BCa. Although TURBT guarantees complete tumor resection in most cases of NMIBC, the recurrence rate of BCa is as high as 80%. To date, various strategies have been attempted to prevent the local recurrence of BCa following TURBT because treatment of recurrent BCa is related with high

Bladder Cancer. DOI: http://dx.doi.org/10.1016/B978-0-12-809939-1.00017-5
241

financial cost. Recurrent BCa is the most expensive solid tumor to treat, especially when it stems from NMIBC [3].

Although there is some discrepancy about the strength of this recommendation, both American Urological Association (AUA) and European Association of Urology (EAU) guidelines continue to recommend immediate postoperative intravesical chemotherapy (PIC) after TURBT [4,5]. Moreover, recent meta-analyses [6,7] provide firm evidence for the effectiveness of immediate PIC by demonstrating a reduced likelihood of recurrence of suspected NMIBC.

There are two current important issues regarding the use of PIC in suspected NMIBC. These issues are the underuse rate and disparities in usage among urologists. In this chapter, although weighed the current status of PIC practice pattern (rate of singe, immediate PIC, and etiologies of disparity pattern), efficacy, mechanism of action, and future tasks to overcome current limitative role of single, immediate PIC are introduced in here.

EFFICACY OF SINGLE, IMMEDIATE PIC

Immediate PIC following TURBT for all localized blood cancers is strongly recommended by the EAU guidelines published in 2011 and 2013 for low- and intermediate-risk BCa patients and as an option for high-risk BCa patients [8–10]. The AUA guidelines support the use of immediate PIC after TURBT because it may decrease the risk of recurrence of NMIBC [11]. The possible mechanism for early recurrence of NMIBC following TURBT is implantation of floating BCa cells into the healthy bladder epithelium, and immediate PIC exerts a protective effect against early implantation of cancer cells [12].

To reduce the recurrence rate after TURBT, single, immediate PIC is recommended after almost all instances of TURBT. Exceptions are rare and include suspected injury or perforation of the bladder [9,13–15]. Although there have been some controversy about the actual preventive effect on recurrence, all arguments are now in favor of performing PIC after TURBT for NMIBC [13,14,16]. PIC is known to have a critical role in delaying and preventing tumor recurrence after TURBT by destroying circulating and residual tumor cells at the location of TURBT [9,17].

Gudjonsson et al. [18] found in a prospective randomized multicenter study that immediate PIC after TURBT for NMIBC may reduce the likelihood of tumor recurrence. However, the positive benefits of immediate PIC were minimized in patients in the intermediate- or high-risk groups. Moreover, Bohle et al. [19] reported the results of a randomized, double-blind placebo-controlled study showing that immediate PIC using gemcitabine after TURBT was not superior to a placebo regarding postoperative recurrence-free interval. They concluded that improved TURBT techniques and the use of a continuous irrigation system have greater positive effects than immediate PIC in terms of recurrence-free survival [19]. Both studies assessed the clinical benefits of immediate PIC for high-risk groups as being minimal and identified cases where multiple instillation therapy would be indicated [4,18]. Similarly, Dobruch et al. [16] concluded, from the results of a meta-analysis, that immediate PIC ought not to be recommended routinely because the clinical benefits were small regarding recurrence rates in patients with multiple tumors. This created a severe controversy for urologists and also agencies that establish guidelines. Concerning this issue, Abern et al. [6], in their meta-regression analysis, found that individual tumor risk factors such as recurrence, multifocal pattern, high grade, and T1 stage have no effect on the clinical outcomes of immediate PIC in NMIBC.

Recently, Kang et al. [20] reported that a single, immediate administration of PIC using pirarubicin, mitomycin, or epirubicin is associated with prolonged recurrence-free survival following TURBT in NMIBC patients, although only pirarubicin also reduced disease progression by their analysis using indirect comparison.

Recently, Seo et al. [21] reported that there was no difference between patients who underwent immediate PIC and patients who did not. This finding may have resulted from a selection bias: those patients who undergo immediate PIC may be at particularly high risk for recurrence because there are marked disparities in performing immediate PIC in Korea. In their report, there was no difference in the rate of additional operations or adjuvant systemic chemotherapy among patients with PIC and patients without PIC in the first year following TURBT (15.4% vs 15.0%, $P = 0.604$). Moreover, during the observational period, there was no difference in the frequency of repeat operations or administration of adjuvant systemic chemotherapy in patients given PIC and patients not given PIC (31.0% vs 32.08%, $P = 0.061$). There was no difference in the rate of repeat operations or adjuvant systemic chemotherapy according to immediate PIC (13.9% vs 15.5%, $P = 0.107$).

Most recent meta-analysis about the efficacy of single, immediate PIC showed that it reduces the risk of recurrence in NMIBC. However, the reducing effect is only confined to low-risk group of NMIBC [22].

MECHANISMS OF ACTION OF CURRENT AVAILABLE CHEMOTHERAPEUTIC AGENTS AS SINGLE, IMMEDIATE PIC

Current available agents are described in Tables 17.1 and 17.2. Their classification of drug, mechanism of action, and benefits and side effects are described [23]. To date, clinical evidence of single, immediate PIC is not sound except in cases when using mitomycin C (MMC). Contraindications include deep resection, bladder perforation, and prior allergy to the agent [24].

TABLE 17.1 Chemotherapeutic Agents for Single, Immediate PIC and Their Mechanism of Action

Chemotherapeutic Agents	Types of Agents (Mechanism of Action)
MMC	Antibiotic (competence for transformation: inhibition of DNA synthesis)
Thiotepa	Alkylating agent, organophosphorus compound (intracavitary effusions secondary to diffuse or localized neoplastic diseases of various serosal cavities)
Doxorubicin	Anthracycline drug, topoisomerase inhibitors (inhibition of DNA synthesis)
Valrubicin	Semisynthetic analog of the anthracycline (inhibition of DNA synthesis)
Pirarubicin	Anthracycline drug, topoisomerase inhibitors (inhibition of DNA synthesis)
Epirubicin	Anthracycline drug, topoisomerase inhibitors (intercalating DNA strands)
Gemcitabine	Nucleoside (inhibiting processes required for DNA synthesis)

Treatment strategies for intravesical therapy of NMIBC have not changed significantly over the past three decades. Intravesical irrigation is usually done with MMC, epirubicin, and valrubicin. An upcoming agent is gemcitabine, but this is not yet considered standard.

MMC, an antitumor antibiotic agent is usually indicated at the dose of 40 mg during PIC [25]. The EUA guidelines recommend 20−40 mg as the standard dose of MMC. MMC has been shown its efficacy with response rates of 40%−50%, and to date, MMC is regarded as one of the standard chemotherapy agents in the treatment of NMIBC [26]. In two recent studies, MMC was compared with bacillus Calmette−Guerin (BCG) in terms of prevention effect for recurrence, which showed relatively lower effect [27,28].

However, recently, Arends et al. compared 24 months recurrence-free survival with chemohyperthermia versus BCG therapy, which revealed the favorable outcome by MMC in terms of safety and recurrence-free survival rate [29]. In view of the recent worldwide shortages of BCG, this study shed a light for PIC with MMC to replace the role of BCG treatment in intermediate- and high-risk papillary NMIBC patient.

Although the use rate is decreasing, thiotepa is also used as intravesical chemotherapy in NMIBC. Thiotepa includes three patterns of treatment: (1) prophylactic treatment to prevent seeding of tumor cells; (2) adjunctive treatment at the time of biopsy; (3) therapeutic option to prevent recurrence

TABLE 17.2 Benefits and Adverse Events of Single, Immediate PIC Using Chemotherapeutic Agents

Chemotherapeutic Agents	Benefits	Adverse Events
MMC	Low molecular weight (improved bladder wall penetration)	General adverse events (dysuria, hematuria, and storage symptoms), Allergic skin reaction, possible systemic absorption
Thiotepa	Low molecular weight (well bladder wall penetration)	Systemic absorption causing myelosuppression
Doxorubicin	High molecular weight (low systemic absorption)	General adverse events
Valrubicin	High molecular weight (low systemic absorption)	General adverse events
Pirarubicin	High molecular weight (low systemic absorption)	General adverse events
Epirubicin	High molecular weight (low systemic absorption)	General adverse events
Gemcitabine	Lipid solubility, high molecular weight (low systemic absorption)	General adverse events

Source: From Porten SP, Leapman MS, Greene KL. Intravesical chemotherapy in non-muscle-invasive bladder cancer. Indian J Urol 2015;31(4):297−303.

after TURBT [30]. Although many studies have shown the success rate as up to 55% of success rate with 30 mg of thiotepa, there exists systemic absorption causing myelosupression with thrombocytopenia and leucopenia [30].

The new promising agent, gemcitabine has well-known antitumor activity in the treatment of metastatic BCa [31], which triggered the possibility of its intravesical usage in NMIBC. Moreover, gemcitabine has pharmacologic superiority to other agents that it has high mucosal but low plasma absorption [32]. The optimal dosage with proven safety is up to 2000 mg in 50 mL saline [33,34].

Among the other chemotherapeutic agents, Kang et al. [20] reported that pirarubicin has reduced disease progression compared with other agents. Figs. 17.1 and 17.2 are showing the proven hazard ratio for recurrence-free

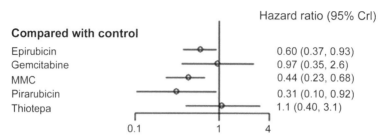

FIGURE 17.1 Pooled hazard ratio and 95% credible intervals (*CrIs*) for recurrence-free survival [20]. *Source: From Kang M, Jeong CW, Kwak C, Kim HH, Ku JH. Single, immediate postoperative instillation of chemotherapy in non-muscle invasive bladder cancer: a systematic review and network meta-analysis of randomized clinical trials using different drugs. Oncotarget 2016;7(29):45479−45488.*

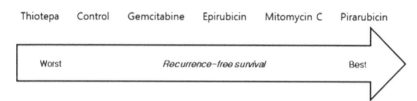

FIGURE 17.2 Ranking of treatments in terms of recurrence-free survival benefit. Each treatment was ranked using percentages from 2000 iterations [20]. *Source: From Kang M, Jeong CW, Kwak C, Kim HH, Ku JH. Single, immediate postoperative instillation of chemotherapy in non-muscle invasive bladder cancer: a systematic review and network meta-analysis of randomized clinical trials using different drugs. Oncotarget 2016;7(29):45479−45488.*

survival, which shows favorable benefit with MMC, epirubicin, and pirarubicin.

RATE OF SINGLE, IMMEDIATE PIC

Although current guidelines strongly recommend the use of immediate PIC after TURBT and meta-analyses support this recommendation, the actual performance rate of immediate PIC is low. It has recently been demonstrated that there is a marked low rate of immediate PIC after TURBT in NMIBC in both the United States and in European countries [35−38].

Although the AUA and EAU guidelines both support the use of immediate PIC and recent meta-analyses also support the use of immediate PIC, the performance rate of immediate PIC remains low. Although a recent report by Palou-Redorta et al. found a relatively high rate of immediate PIC in European countries, i.e., 43.3% [38], most studies have shown a much lower rate of immediate PIC following TURBT, just 0.32%−3.2%. Moreover, the pattern of usage shows marked disparities between urologists, hospitals, provinces, and countries [35−37]. Recently, Kowallick et al. [36] showed that immediate PIC remains greatly underutilized, at just 2.6%, according to the American College of Surgeons National Surgical Quality Improvement Program (ACS-NSQIP) database.

In the most recent report using Korea National Health Data [21], the rate of PIC use within 60 days from the index date was 11.0% (2457 cases). A total of 6.6% (1487) of cases were treated during initial hospital admission (immediate PIC), and a total of 0.2% (40) of cases were given PIC within 7 days in an outpatient department. A total of 3.6% (803) of cases were given PIC within 8−30 days from the index date, and a total of 0.6% (127) of cases received PIC within 31−60 days from the index date. Among the possible PIC regimens, MMC was the most popular regimen (2024 cases, 91.4%).

DISPARITY OF SINGLE, IMMEDIATE PIC

A recent nationwide cross-sectional study in the United States showed a large disparity in the use of immediate PIC after TURBT among urologists [39]. Causal factors of this large disparity include compliance on the part of healthcare providers and patients. Factors regarding compliance of healthcare providers include surgeons' decisions or preferences, the number of surgeons available, the amount of education surgeons receive, nursing care, and the preparedness of pharmacists [38,39].

Although Chamie et al. [35] reported that Asian patients had a higher compliance rate than did those of other races, no direct investigation into the underuse rate of PIC in Asia has been done, except in Korea. Seo et al. [21] attempted to measure the real rate of immediate PIC after TURBT for suspected NMIBC using the national health database system and to investigate the potential role of immediate PIC in preventing or reducing the need for additional treatment because of recurrence.

Recently, Cookson et al. [39] showed nationwide heterogeneity in clinical practice patterns of immediate PIC, and, moreover, they reported that the majority of urologists in the United States have no experience with immediate PIC. Only 2% of urologists use immediate PIC 100% of the time, whereas 17% of them perform the procedure only 50% of the time, and the majority of urologists (67%) never perform immediate PIC. Neither geographical region nor practice setting (academic training hospital or private local hospital) were associated with the pattern of immediate PIC use. This implies that individual disparities between urologists are at least to some extent responsible for the low rate of immediate PIC. In our data, among the top five hospitals where TURBT is most commonly performed, the use of immediate PIC showed marked variation (from 0% to 23.5%).

ETIOLOGY OF THE LOW USE RATE OF SINGLE, IMMEDIATE PIC AND ITS DISPARITY

Table 17.3 summarizes the possible etiologies for the low rate of use of single, immediate PIC and for the associated disparities. There have been several studies on the reasons for the underuse and variation in use of immediate PIC after TURBT [35,38,39]. There are many reasons for the low use of immediate PIC in real practice. Suggested reasons for the underuse of immediate PIC include increased financial expense associated with the need for extra postoperative nursing care after TURBT and difficulties in coordinating support for patients following PIC between the operating room, pharmacy, and recovery room [39].

However, there are more fundamental reasons for the low rate of immediate PIC. First of all, the EAU or AUA guidelines could be thought of as impractical and not applicable because immediate PIC has to be performed before pathologic confirmation of cancer type and even before confirmation of local staging. Many urologists are reluctant to use immediate PIC because they believe that the effectiveness of immediate PIC in intermediate- or high-risk tumors cannot be guaranteed [38]. Mischaracterization of tumor stage may result in the underestimation of the risk of recurrence of NMIBC. For instance, the final pathological stage is inconsistent with the cystoscopic clinical stage approximately 30% of time [14]. This ambiguity during surgery may influence the urologist's decision regarding immediate PIC.

Another explanation is that many urologists do not agree with the guidelines and do not perform the recommendations put forth by those guidelines. Given the results of univariate analysis, Chamie et al. [35] reported that there was no significant change in the percentage of subjects who complied with care after publication of clinical practice guidelines. This finding was also prominent in provider-level compliance. Recently, Burks et al. [40] reported important issues associated with the implementation of clinical guidelines. Simply disseminating published guidelines is not enough to form treatment

TABLE 17.3 Etiologies for the Low Rate of Use of Single, Immediate PIC and for its Disparities

Increased cost expense

Nonequipment of extra postoperative nursing care, operating room, pharmacy, and recovery room

Mischaracterization of tumor stage, which may result in the underestimation of recurrence risk for NMIBC

Inconsistence in degree of recommendation by AUA or EAU guidelines

Low evidence of immediate PIC in preventing recurrence or progression from RCTs strategies and reduce disparities; there must also be an understanding of the logistic and practical barriers involved in implementing the guidelines.

Moreover, although those two guidelines support immediate PIC to prevent recurrence of BCa after TURBT, the degree of the recommendation is inconsistent. The AUA guidelines consider immediate PIC only as an optional treatment, granting PIC much less importance as a treatment strategy as compared with the EAU guidelines. The AUA guidelines do not actually recommend immediate PIC for all low-risk groups of BCa patients, and they state that "the health outcomes of the interventions are not sufficiently well known to permit meaningful decisions, or preferences are unknown or equivocal." The AUA guidelines also mention the negative issues surrounding immediate PIC, including financial issues, the inability to confirm tumor pathology before administering PIC, and the side effects of PIC regimens [18,41]. This inconsistency in the guidelines contributes to the clinical disparity in performance of immediate PIC.

TECHNIQUE TO OVERCOME THE CURRENT LIMITATIVE EFFICACY OF PIC

Those techniques to optimize the passive diffuse of chemotherapeutic agents consist of optimization in delivery and contact time and consequent enhanced absorption and action of chemotherapeutic agents. Classically, those techniques include urine alkalization, dose escalation (40 mg of MMC), and voluntary dehydration with urinary volume [42,43]. However, recently, thermal manipulation and electromotive drug administration (EMDA) have been proposed. Hyperthermic treatment using MMC has been shown to the efficacy by enhancing the cytotoxic action against tumor cells [44]. Chemohyperthermic delivery of MMC could be introduced using indwelling bladder radiofrequency applicator in NMIBC patients. EMDA of MMC includes the delivery of an electric current through the bladder. Recently, Di Stasi et al. showed favorable clinical outcome using 20 mA EMDA of MMC therapy compared with passive MMC and BCG instillation in high-risk NMIBC [45].

FUTURE TASKS FOR OVERCOMING THE LOW RATE OF SINGLE, IMMEDIATE PIC

Although recent, updated systematic reviews or meta-analyses by Abern et al. [6] and Perlis et al. [7] support the use of immediate PIC after TURBT in terms of prolongation of recurrence-free survival and a reduction in early recurrence, there have been several studies that are critical of the effect of immediate PIC in suspected NMIBC [5,18,41]. Even the most recent network meta-analysis could not solve this issue [20]. The most important issue for the indication of immediate PIC is that a tumor lacks Level I positive evidence for multiple and recurrent tumors, high-grade tumors, and disease progression.

Negatives exist from an oncologic, clinical point of view, but also from an economic point of view. Rao et al. [41] reported that routine immediate PIC significantly lowered the overall cost of hospitalization because of a reduction in recurrence, but these benefits were diminished because of the use of outpatient immediate PIC.

To overcome the low rate of immediate PIC and the disparities in clinical practice, several tasks must be undertaken. The current need for clinical urologists to treat suspected NMIBC is clear. Encouraging the use of immediate PIC for suspected NMIBC and preparing well-designed randomized controlled trials (RCTs) are matters of urgency. To overcome preconceptions or misunderstandings among urologists about immediate PIC regarding its clinical benefits or side effects, education could be a key factor. One study revealed successful improvement in the rate of immediate PIC after a reasonable amount of education was provided [40]. Burks et al. [40] emphasized the importance of giving correct advice on enhancing the quality of care received by NMIBC patients. They suggested a multidimensional approach including clinician education, local logistical activities, and ensuring adequate pharmacy and staffing resources.

However, the most urgent need is for well-designed, high-qualified RCTs. Although several meta-analyses exist on this issue, a common pitfall of those studies is that they include low-quality RCTs. Although an initial meta-analysis on this issue performed by Sylvester et al. [15] clearly reported the importance of immediate PIC, those authors did not consider the low quality of the included studies. This initial meta-analysis greatly affected both the current AUA and EAU guidelines.

The fundamental reason for the need for qualified RCTs is that most meta-analyses that greatly impact current practice in treating NMIBC do not consider disease-free interval. Most studies have adopted recurrence rate as the main outcome. Before the meta-analysis that had time to recurrence (recurrence-free interval) as its end point, which was done by Perlis et al. [2], all meta-analyses were based on a decrease in recurrence rate. With more qualified RCTs, the more precise measure of disease-free interval can be investigated and then additional treatment after TURBT, including immediate PIC, can be judged objectively in terms of its real efficacy and positive effects. Moreover, clinicians have to be aware of the fact that recurrence risk was not guideline-based, but was instead assessed by the subjective decision of individual urologists.

Perils et al. [7] criticized the studies included in their recent meta-analysis using the important concepts of risk-of-bias and quality-of-evidence assessment. Contemporary methodology suggests a low quality of evidence for the examined outcomes. Thus, RCTs with careful randomization and blinding are still needed to clarify the real usefulness of immediate PIC in NMIBC cohorts.

CONCLUSION

To date, immediate PIC following TURBT is thought to have a beneficial effect on recurrence while causing minimal adverse events. However, due to a low quality of evidence, well-designed RCTs with proper blinding and placebos are warranted. Besides, a consensus is lacking among urologists about the real indications for PIC, the optimal chemotherapeutic agent, and the optimal timing of PIC. More concern has to be taken to improve the rate of use of immediate PIC after TURBT for suspected NMIBC. Moreover, high-quality RCTs are warranted in the near future.

REFERENCES

[1]   Song HN, Go SI, Lee WS, Kim Y, Choi HJ, Lee US, et al. Population-based regional cancer incidence in Korea: comparison between urban and rural areas. Cancer Res Treat 2016;48(2):789−97.

[2]   Patel SG, Cohen A, Weiner AB, Steinberg GD. Intravesical therapy for bladder cancer. Expert Opin Pharmacother 2015;16(6):889−901.

[3]   Chavan S, Bray F, Lortet-Tieulent J, Goodman M, Jemal A. International variations in bladder cancer incidence and mortality. Eur Urol 2014;66(1):59−73.

[4]   Babjuk M, Oosterlinck W, Sylvester R, Kaasinen E, Bohle A, Palou-Redorta J, et al. EAU guidelines on non-muscle-invasive urothelial carcinoma of the bladder, the 2011 update. Eur Urol 2011;59(6):997−1008.

[5]   Hall MC, Chang SS, Dalbagni G, Pruthi RS, Seigne JD, Skinner EC, et al. Guideline for the management of nonmuscle invasive bladder cancer (stages Ta, T1, and Tis): 2007 update. J Urol 2007;178(6):2314−30.

[6]   Abern MR, Owusu RA, Anderson MR, Rampersaud EN, Inman BA. Perioperative intravesical chemotherapy in non-muscle-invasive bladder cancer: a systematic review and meta-analysis. J Natl Compr Canc Netw 2013;11(4):477−84.

[7]   Perlis N, Zlotta AR, Beyene J, Finelli A, Fleshner NE, Kulkarni GS. Immediate post-transurethral resection of bladder tumor intravesical chemotherapy prevents non-muscle-invasive bladder cancer recurrences: an updated meta-analysis on 2548 patients and quality-of-evidence review. Eur Urol 2013;64(3):421−30.

[8]   Babjuk M, Burger M, Zigeuner R, Shariat SF, van Rhijn BW, Comperat E, et al. EAU guidelines on non-muscle-invasive urothelial carcinoma of the bladder: update 2013. Eur Urol 2013;64(4):639−53.

[9]   Babjuk M, Oosterlinck W, Sylvester R, Kaasinen E, Bohle A, Palou-Redorta J, et al. EAU guidelines on non-muscle-invasive urothelial carcinoma of the bladder. Eur Urol 2008;54 (2):303−14.

[10] Brausi M, Witjes JA, Lamm D, Persad R, Palou J, Colombel M, et al. A review of current guidelines and best practice recommendations for the management of nonmuscle invasive bladder cancer by the International Bladder Cancer Group. J Urol 2011;186(6):2158−67.

[11] Colonna M, Bossard N, Guizard AV, Remontet L, Grosclaude P, le reseau F. Descriptive epidemiology of thyroid cancer in France: incidence, mortality and survival. Ann Endocrinol (Paris) 2010;71(2):95−101.

[12] Heney NM, Ahmed S, Flanagan MJ, Frable W, Corder MP, Hafermann MD, et al. Superficial bladder cancer: progression and recurrence. J Urol 1983;130(6):1083−6.

[13] Lim D, Izawa JI, Middlebrook P, Chin JL. Bladder perforation after immediate postoperative intravesical instillation of mitomycin C. Can Urol Assoc J 2010;4(1):E1−3.

[14] Oosterlinck W, Sylvester R, Babjuk M, Kaasinen E, Bohle A, Palou-Redorta J, et al. Should all patients receive an immediate chemotherapeutic drug instillation after resection of papillary bladder tumors? Eur Urol 2011;59(3):374−6.

[15] Sylvester RJ, Oosterlinck W, van der Meijden AP. A single immediate postoperative instillation of chemotherapy decreases the risk of recurrence in patients with stage Ta T1 bladder cancer: a meta-analysis of published results of randomized clinical trials. J Urol 2004;171(6 Pt 1):2186−90, quiz 435.

[16] Dobruch J, Herr H. Should all patients receive single chemotherapeutic agent instillation after bladder tumour resection? BJU Int 2009;104(2):170−4.

[17] van Rhijn BW, van der Kwast TH, Alkhateeb SS, Fleshner NE, van Leenders GJ, Bostrom PJ, et al. A new and highly prognostic system to discern T1 bladder cancer substage. Eur Urol 2012;61(2):378−84.

[18] Gudjonsson S, Adell L, Merdasa F, Olsson R, Larsson B, Davidsson T, et al. Should all patients with non-muscle-invasive bladder cancer receive early intravesical chemotherapy after transurethral resection? The results of a prospective randomised multicentre study. Eur Urol 2009;55(4):773−80.

[19] Bohle A, Leyh H, Frei C, Kuhn M, Tschada R, Pottek T, et al. Single postoperative instillation of gemcitabine in patients with non-muscle-invasive transitional cell carcinoma of the bladder: a randomised, double-blind, placebo-controlled phase III multicentre study. Eur Urol 2009;56(3):495−503.

[20] Kang M, Jeong CW, Kwak C, Kim HH, Ku JH. Single, immediate postoperative instillation of chemotherapy in non-muscle invasive bladder cancer: a systematic review and network meta-analysis of randomized clinical trials using different drugs. Oncotarget 2016;7 (29):45479−88.

[21] Seo GH, Kim JH, Ku JH. Clinical practice pattern of immediate intravesical chemotherapy following transurethral resection of a bladder tumor in Korea: national health insurance database study. Sci Rep 2016;6:22716.

[22] Sylvester RJ, Oosterlinck W, Holmang S, Sydes MR, Birtle A, Gudjonsson S, et al. Systematic review and individual patient data meta-analysis of randomized trials comparing a single immediate instillation of chemotherapy after transurethral resection with transurethral resection alone in patients with stage pTa-pT1 urothelial carcinoma of the bladder: which patients benefit from the instillation? Eur Urol 2016;69(2):231−44.

[23] Porten SP, Leapman MS, Greene KL. Intravesical chemotherapy in non-muscle-invasive bladder cancer. Indian J Urol 2015;31(4):297−303.

[24] Kulkarni GS, Hakenberg OW, Gschwend JE, Thalmann G, Kassouf W, Kamat A, et al. An updated critical analysis of the treatment strategy for newly diagnosed high-grade T1 (previously T1G3) bladder cancer. Eur Urol 2010;57(1):60−70.

[25] Malmstrom PU. Intravesical therapy of superficial bladder cancer. Crit Rev Oncol Hematol 2003;47(2):109−26.

[26]   Witjes JA, Hendricksen K. Intravesical pharmacotherapy for non-muscle-invasive bladder cancer: a critical analysis of currently available drugs, treatment schedules, and long-term results. Eur Urol 2008;53(1):45−52.

[27]   Gardmark T, Jahnson S, Wahlquist R, Wijkstrom H, Malmstrom PU. Analysis of progression and survival after 10 years of a randomized prospective study comparing mitomycin-C and bacillus Calmette-Guerin in patients with high-risk bladder cancer. BJU Int 2007;99(4):817−20.

[28]   Ojea A, Nogueira JL, Solsona E, Flores N, Gomez JM, Molina JR, et al. A multicentre, randomised prospective trial comparing three intravesical adjuvant therapies for intermediate-risk superficial bladder cancer: low-dose bacillus Calmette-Guerin (27 mg) versus very low-dose bacillus Calmette-Guerin (13.5 mg) versus mitomycin C. Eur Urol 2007;52(5):1398−406.

[29]   Arends TJ, Nativ O, Maffezzini M, de Cobelli O, Canepa G, Verweij F, et al. Results of a randomised controlled trial comparing intravesical chemohyperthermia with mitomycin C versus bacillus Calmette-Guerin for adjuvant treatment of patients with intermediate- and high-risk non-muscle-invasive bladder cancer. Eur Urol 2016;69(6):1046−52.

[30]   Barlow LJ, Benson MC. Experience with newer intravesical chemotherapy for high-risk non-muscle-invasive bladder cancer. Curr Urol Rep 2013;14(2):65−70.

[31]   Stadler WM, Kuzel T, Roth B, Raghavan D, Dorr FA. Phase II study of single-agent gemcitabine in previously untreated patients with metastatic urothelial cancer. J Clin Oncol 1997;15(11):3394−8.

[32]   Cozzi PJ, Bajorin DF, Tong W, Nguyen H, Scott J, Heston WD, et al. Toxicology and pharmacokinetics of intravesical gemcitabine: a preclinical study in dogs. Clin Cancer Res 1999;5(9):2629−37.

[33]   Dalbagni G, Russo P, Sheinfeld J, Mazumdar M, Tong W, Rabbani F, et al. Phase I trial of intravesical gemcitabine in bacillus Calmette-Guerin-refractory transitional-cell carcinoma of the bladder. J Clin Oncol 2002;20(15):3193−8.

[34]   Laufer M, Ramalingam S, Schoenberg MP, Haisfield-Wolf ME, Zuhowski EG, Trueheart IN, et al. Intravesical gemcitabine therapy for superficial transitional cell carcinoma of the bladder: a phase I and pharmacokinetic study. J Clin Oncol 2003;21(4):697−703.

[35]   Chamie K, Saigal CS, Lai J, Hanley JM, Setodji CM, Konety BR, et al. Compliance with guidelines for patients with bladder cancer: variation in the delivery of care. Cancer 2011;117(23):5392−401.

[36]   Kowalik C, Gee JR, Sorcini A, Moinzadeh A, Canes D. Underutilization of immediate intravesical chemotherapy following TURBT: results from NSQIP. Can J Urol 2014;21 (3):7266−70.

[37]   Madeb R, Golijanin D, Noyes K, Fisher S, Stephenson JJ, Long SR, et al. Treatment of nonmuscle invading bladder cancer: do physicians in the United States practice evidence based medicine? The use and economic implications of intravesical chemotherapy after transurethral resection of bladder tumors. Cancer 2009;115(12):2660−70.

[38]   Palou-Redorta J, Roupret M, Gallagher JR, Heap K, Corbell C, Schwartz B. The use of immediate postoperative instillations of intravesical chemotherapy after TURBT of NMIBC among European countries. World J Urol 2014;32(2):525−30.

[39]   Cookson MS, Chang SS, Oefelein MG, Gallagher JR, Schwartz B, Heap K. National practice patterns for immediate postoperative instillation of chemotherapy in nonmuscle invasive bladder cancer. J Urol 2012;187(5):1571−6.

[40] Burks FN, Liu AB, Suh RS, Schuster TG, Bradford T, Moylan DA, et al. Understanding the use of immediate intravesical chemotherapy for patients with bladder cancer. J Urol 2012;188(6):2108–13.

[41] Rao PK, Stephen Jones J. Routine perioperative chemotherapy instillation with initial bladder tumor resection: a reconsideration of economic benefits. Cancer 2009;115 (5):997–1004.

[42] Wientjes MG, Badalament RA, Au JL. Use of pharmacologic data and computer simulations to design an efficacy trial of intravesical mitomycin C therapy for superficial bladder cancer. Cancer Chemother Pharmacol 1993;32(4):255–62.

[43] Wientjes MG, Dalton JT, Badalament RA, Dasani BM, Drago JR, Au JL. A method to study drug concentration-depth profiles in tissues: mitomycin C in dog bladder wall. Pharm Res 1991;8(2):168–73.

[44] van der Heijden AG, Verhaegh G, Jansen CF, Schalken JA, Witjes JA. Effect of hyperthermia on the cytotoxicity of 4 chemotherapeutic agents currently used for the treatment of transitional cell carcinoma of the bladder: an in vitro study. J Urol 2005;173 (4):1375–80.

[45] Di Stasi SM, Giannantoni A, Stephen RL, Capelli G, Navarra P, Massoud R, et al. Intravesical electromotive mitomycin C versus passive transport mitomycin C for high risk superficial bladder cancer: a prospective randomized study. J Urol 2003;170 (3):777–82.

Chapter 18

Second Transurethral Resection of Bladder Cancer

Won Jae Yang

Soonchunhyang University Hospital, Seoul, South Korea

Chapter Outline

Transurethral resection of the bladder (TURB) is the essential surgical proce-dure to diagnose, stage, and treat non-muscle-invasive-blood cancer (NMIBC) [1]. Although TUR is a frequently performed operation familiar to urologists, complete tumor removal is not always possible, whether as a result of excessive tumor volume, anatomic inaccessibility, or risk of perfo-ration [2]. However, even in in the absence of these circumstances, second (so-called, restaging, repeat, or re-) TUR to manage high-risk NMIBC is now widely accepted because it improves clinical staging, detects more tumors than initial TUR, and reduces the rate of recurrence and progression [3].

Accumulating evidence supports the importance of second TUR for NMIBC.

DETECTION OF RESIDUAL TUMOR

Second TUR can detect residual tumor. TUR aims to resect all visible tumors completely; however, the rate of residual tumor detected by a second TUR is considerably high. The risk is higher in multiple tumors and high-grade lesions and increases with the stage of the original tumor. In studies that sep-arately evaluated Ta and T1 tumors, disease persistence was detected for

Bladder Cancer. DOI: http://dx.doi.org/10.1016/B978-0-12-809939-1.00018-7

35%—65% of Ta tumors (Table 18.1) [4—9] and for 33%—80% of T1 tumors (Tables 18.2 and 18.3) [4,5,8,9,10—14].

Second TUR may not be helpful for low-grade papillary tumors. However, Ta high-grade tumors show a relevant rate of persistent tumor at second resection. Lazica et al. demonstrated that residual tumor was found in 41.4% of patients having Ta high-grade tumors in the first TUR [6]. Herr and Donat have summarized their data on routine second TUR including 701 patients with pT1 tumors and revealed residual disease in 78% of patients (pTa 23%, pT1 25%, and upstaging to muscularis propria 30%) (Table 18.3) [8].

REDUCTION OF STAGING ERRORS

Second TUR can reduce staging errors. Underestimation of the depth of tumor invasion is critical, particularly when muscle-invasive disease is missed. A second TUR could improve the quality of the procedure especially when the muscle is not sampled during the initial resection [15]. Herr and Donat reported 15% of patients with clinical stage T1 disease, and muscle in the specimen were upstaged to T2 versus 45% if no muscle was present (Table 18.3) [8]. Dutta et al. reported a 64% rate of understaging in T1 tumors if muscle was absent in the specimen versus only a 30% rate if muscle was present [16]. In fact, detrusor muscle in the first, apparently complete TUR specimen is a surrogate marker of resection quality and predicts risk of early recurrence [17]. Mariappan et al. reported that the presence of detrusor muscle in the specimen was associated to the recurrence rate at the first follow-up cystoscopy. The probability of a recurrence in the first follow-up cystoscopy was 2.9 times higher in the absence of muscle in the previous TUR [17].

TABLE 18.1 Results of Second TUR After Ta (No Available Data of Present Muscle in the First TUR)

Study	Patients, n	Residual Tumor, %	Upstaging, %
Schips et al. [4]	31	38.7	6.5
Ali et al. [5]	30	40	20
Lazica et al. [6]	87 (HG)	41.4	5.7
Vasdev et al. [7]	49	49	10
Herr and Donat [8]	396 (HG)	65	15
*Grimm et al. [9]	83	35	8

HG, high grade, *present detrusor muscle in the first TUR.

TABLE 18.2 Results of Second TUR After T1 (No Available Data of Present Muscle in the First TUR)

Study	Patients, n	Residual Tumor, %	Upstaging, %
Schips et al. [4]	76	32.9	7.9
Divrik et al. [10]	105	33.3	7.6
Zurkirchen et al. [11]	115	37	
Schwaibold et al. [12]	136	52	10
Herr and Donat [13]	247	55.9	
Ali et al. [5]	61	67.2	26.2

TABLE 18.3 Results of Second TUR after T1 (Data Available of Present Muscle in the First TUR)

Study	Muscle	Patients, n	Residual Tumor, %	Upstaging, %
Grimm et al. [9]	O	34	59	5.5
Herr and Donat [8]	O	421	75	15
	X	280	80	45
Brauers et al. [14]	X	42	65	24

Even in Ta disease, when muscle was not clearly stated to be present in the TUR specimens, upstaging has been reported in up to 15% [7,8], contrary to the 8% as reported by Grimm et al. when muscle was sampled (Table 18.1) [9].

IMPROVEMENT OF ONCOLOGIC OUTCOMES

Second TUR can improve outcomes of NMIBC. A 5-year observational study showed that 63% undergoing a second TUR had tumor-free bladders compared to 40% of patients after one TUR [9]. Progression to muscle invasion occurred in only two (3%) patients after second TUR [9].

Divrik et al. randomly assigned 210 patients with newly diagnosed T1 to second TUR or standard follow-up. Recurrence-free survival rates at 1, 2, and 3 years were 86.4%, 77.7%, and 68.7%, respectively, in the second TUR

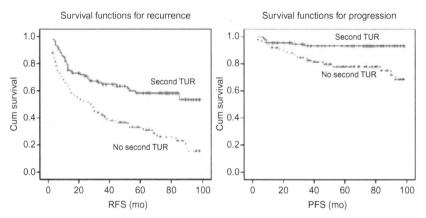

FIGURE 18.1 Recurrence-free (*RFS*) and progression-free survival (*PFS*) in pT1 bladder cancer patients after one versus second TUR [10].

group and 47.1%, 42.3%, and 37.0% in the TUR group, respectively. Second TUR was an independent predictor of recurrence in multivariable analysis in this series [10]. Fig. 18.1 shows longer recurrence-free (47 months) and progression-free (73 months) survival times after the second TUR rather than no second TUR (12 and 53 months, respectively). Overall survival in both groups was similar. However, only 2% of patients died of urothelial cancer after undergoing two TURs compared with 11% after one TUR [10].

STRENGTHENING THE RESPONSE TO BACILLUS CALMETTE–GUERIN THERAPY

A second TUR also appeared to improve the short-term response to bacillus Calmette–Guerin (BCG) if it was performed before instillation of BCG. Among the patients who underwent a single TUR before BCG therapy, 57% had residual or recurrent tumor at the first cystoscopy and 34% later had progression, compared with 29% patients who had residual or recurrent tumors and 7% who had progression after undergoing second TUR [18]. Fig. 18.2 shows that overall recurrence-free and progression-free survival was significantly better with BCG therapy after two versus one TUR [18].

SELECTION OF PATIENTS FOR EARLY CYSTECTOMY

Second TUR can help to select patients for cystectomy versus intravesical therapy. Fig. 18.3 shows progression-free survival of 710 patients with NMIBC who received BCG therapy after an initial (left) or restaged (right) TUR, stratified by stage and grade. After an initial TUR, all tumor categories appear to be appropriate candidates for intravesical treatments. However, the majority of patients with residual T1 disease on second TUR eventually

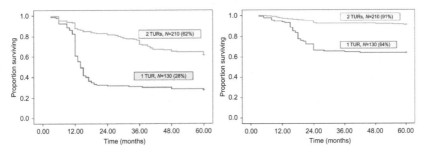

FIGURE 18.2   Recurrence-free (left) and progression-free (right) survival in 340 NMIBC patients treated with BCG after one versus two TURs [18].

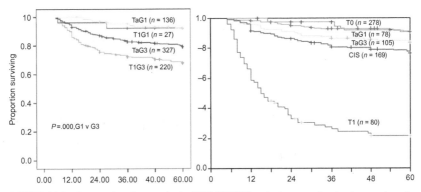

FIGURE 18.3   Progression-free survival of 710 NMIBC patients, according to stage and grade, after first (left) or second (right) TUR [19].

progressed (regardless of their original pathology), including many who responded initially to BCG therapy [19].

This has been confirmed in which patients having no tumor on repeat resection had fewer recurrences, longer times to tumor recurrence, and less progression than patients who underwent a single TUR [20]. Based on these findings, Herr et al. suggested that patients who have T1 NMIBC on a second TUR may be better served by immediate cystectomy rather than BCG therapy [21].

CANDIDATES OF SECOND TUR

Both American Urological Association (AUA) and European Association of Urology (EAU) guidelines recommend that a second or a restaging TUR should be performed when a high-grade or T1 tumor has been detected at initial TUR, as well as in all cases of incomplete resection or when muscle is not present for histological assessment [22,23]. There is no consensus on timing, but most authors recommend 1−6 weeks after initial resection [24]. Herr insisted that second TUR should include a thorough TUR of the primary tumor site, any overlooked tumors, and, all overt or suspected areas of carcinoma in situ because in the majority of cases, results are better when all tumors have been eradicated before subsequent intravesical treatments [21].

Surely, an additional surgery for the patient with a bladder tumor adds morbidity and may delay the implementation of adjuvant intravesical therapy. However, we should adhere to the recommendations of the AUA and EAU guidelines until larger prospective randomized trials clearly defining those cohorts of patients with NMIBC who really are going to benefit from routine second TUR [5].

REFERENCES

[1] Herr HW. The value of a second transurethral resection in evaluating patients with bladder tumors. J Urol 1999;162:74−6.

[2] Jones JS. Non-muscle-invasive bladder cancer (Ta, T1, and CIS). In: Wein AJ, Kavoussi LR, Partin AW, Peters CA, editors. Campbell-Walsh urology. 11th ed. Philadelphia: Elsevier; 2016. p. 2223−42.

[3] Bishr M, Lattouf JB, Latour M, Saad F. Tumour stage on re-staging transurethral resection predicts recurrence and progression-free survival of patients with high-risk non-muscle invasive bladder cancer. Can Urol Assoc J 2014;8:E306−310.

[4] Schips L, Augustin H, Zigeuner RE, Gallé G, Habermann H, Trummer H, et al. Is repeated transurethral resection justified in patients with newly diagnosed superficial bladder cancer? Urology 2002;59:220−3.

[5] Ali MH, Ismail IY, Eltobgy A, Gobeish A. Evaluation of second-look transurethral resection in restaging of patients with nonmuscleinvasive bladder cancer. J Endourol 2010;24:2047−50.

[6] Lazica DA, Roth S, Brandt AS, Böttcher S, Mathers MJ, Ubrig B. Second transurethral resection after Ta high-grade bladder tumor: a 4.5-year period at a single university center. Urol Int 2014;92:131−5.

[7] Vasdev N, McKiea C, Dominguez-Escrig J, et al. The role of early re-resection in pTaG3 transitional cell carcinoma of the urinary bladder. British. J Med Surg Urol 2011;4:158−65.

[8] Herr HW, Donat SM. Quality control in transurethral resection of bladder tumors. BJU Int 2008;102:1242−6.

[9] Grimm MO, Steinhoff C, Simon X, Spiegelhalder P, Ackermann R, Vogeli TA. Effect of routine repeat transurethral resection for superficial bladder cancer: a long-term observational study. J Urol 2003;170:433−7.

[10] Divrik RT, Sahin AF, Yildirim U, Altok M, Zorlu F. Impact of routine second TUR on the long-term outcome of patients with newly diagnosed pT1 urothelial carcinoma with respect to recurrence, progression rate, and disease-specific survival: a prospective randomized clinical trial. Eur Urol 2010;58:185−90.

[11] Zurkirchen MA, Sulser T, Gaspert A, Hauri D. Second transurethral resection of superficial transitional cell carcinoma of the bladder: a must even for experienced urologists. Urol Int 2004;72:99−102.

[12] Schwaibold HE, Sivalingam S, May F, Hartung R. The value of a second transurethral resection for T1 bladder cancer. BJU Int 2006;97:1199—201.

[13] Herr HW, Donat SM. A re-staging transurethral resection predicts early progression of superficial bladder cancer. BJU Int 2006;97:1194—8.

[14] Brauers A, Buettner R, Jakse G. Second resection and prognosis of primary high risk superficial bladder cancer: is cystectomy often too early? J Urol 2001;165:808—10.

[15] Ramirez-Backhaus M, Dominguez-Escrig J, Collado A, Rubio-Briones J, Solsona E. Restaging transurethral resection of bladder tumor for high-risk stage Ta and T1 bladder cancer. Curr Urol Rep 2012;13:109—14.

[16] Dutta SC, Smith Jr JA, Shappell SB, Coffey CS, Chang SS, Cookson MS. Clinical under staging of high risk nonmuscle invasive urothelial carcinoma treated with radical cystectomy. J Urol 2001;166:490—3.

[17] Mariappan P, Zachou A, Grigor KM, Edinburgh Uro-Oncology Group. Detrusor muscle in the first, apparently complete transurethral resection of bladder tumour specimen is a surrogate marker of resection quality, predicts risk of early recurrence, and is dependent on operator experience. Eur Urol 2010;57:843—9.

[18] Herr HW. Restaging transurethral resection of high risk superficial bladder cancer improves the initial response to BCG therapy. J Urol 2005;174:2134—7.

[19] Herr HW, Donat SM, Dalbagni G. Can restaging transurethral resection of T1 bladder cancer select patients for immediate cystectomy? J Urol 2007;177:75—9.

[20] Guevara A, Salomon L, Allory Y, Ploussard G, de la Taille A, Paul A, et al. The role of tumor-free status in repeat resection before intravesical BCG for high grade Ta,T1 and CIS bladder cancer. J Urol 2010;183:2161—4.

[21] Herr HW. Role of re-resection in non-muscle-invasive bladder cancer. Scientific World J 2011;11:283—8.

[22] Chang SS, Boorjian SA, Chou R, Clark PE, Daneshmand S, Konety BR, et al. Diagnosis and treatment of non-muscle invasive bladder cancer: AUA/SUO guideline. J Urol 2016; In Press.

[23] Babjuk M, Böhle A, Burger M, Capoun O, Cohen D, Compérat EM, et al. EAU guidelines on non-muscle-invasive urothelial carcinoma of the bladder: update 2016. Eur Urol 2016; In Press.

[24] Nieder AM, Brausi M, Lamm D, O'Donnell M, Tomita K, Woo H, et al. Management of stage T1 tumors of the bladder: International Consensus Panel. Urology 2005;66:108—25.

Chapter 19

Intravesical Chemotherapy

Sun Il Kim and Seol Ho Choo

Ajou University School of Medicine, Suwon, South Korea

Chapter Outline

INTRODUCTION

Intravesical chemotherapy for non-muscle-invasive bladder cancer (NMIBC) was first used in patients with multiple or large unresectable tumors in situ to supplement incomplete surgery with mixed response. Complete transurethral resection of bladder tumor (TURBT) has become the standard of care for NMIBC, and second resection is advocated to ensure that no residual tumor is left behind. Modern intravesical therapy is almost exclusively indicated as adjuvant therapy after complete TURBT of NMIBC or for primary treatment of carcinoma in situ (CIS). Bacillus Calmette—Guerin (BCG) is the most potent intravesical agent being the choice in NMIBC patients at intermediate and high risk of recurrence as it is the only agent proven to delay progression to muscle invasive cancer. Thus, intravesical chemotherapy beyond the immediate single instillation is best indicated in moderate risk patients for which its efficacy is at least comparable to BCG. Also,

Bladder Cancer. DOI: http://dx.doi.org/10.1016/B978-0-12-809939-1.00019-9

patients intolerant to the side effects of BCG are candidates for intravesical chemotherapy. Patients who have failed BCG but are unfit or refusing cystectomy constitute a subgroup of patients in which intravesical chemotherapy may be useful. As with BCG, intravesical chemotherapy beyond the immediate single instillation is used in induction (6−8 weeks) and maintenance (1−3 years) settings. Many chemotherapeutic agents are being used, but none is proven to be definitely superior to others in terms of efficacy and safety.

CHEMOTHERAPEUTIC AGENTS AND THEIR EFFICACY COMPARED TO CONTROL

Thiotepa

Thiotepa is the first FDA-approved chemotherapeutic agent against NMIBC. It is a low molecular weight (189 kd) nonspecific alkylating agent chemically related to nitrogen mustard. It can be absorbed through the bladder and cause myelosuppression resulting in thrombocytopenia and leukopenia. The toxicity seems to be dose-dependent as lower risk of leukopenia was observed when 30 mg was given compared to 60 mg [1]. Leukocyte and platelet count should be obtained before each treatment. Despite emergence of newer drugs with lesser toxicity, it is still being widely used in the United States and Europe due to its availability and a relatively low cost. Thiotepa is likely to be effective when given in a maintenance schedule only [2,3]. In an English multicenter trial, a single immediate post-TURBT instillation and additional monthly instillation for a total of five instillations both failed to reduce recurrence and progression [4].

Mitomycin C

Mitomycin C (MMC) is a moderately high molecular weight (334 kd) alkylating agent with low systemic absorption and little systemic toxicity. Dosage varies from 20 to 60 mg, the most common being 40 mg in 40 mL of saline. It is usually administered for 8 weeks followed by monthly instillation for a year as part of a maintenance protocol. Several randomized trials in which MMC were started within a few days after TURBT and maintained for at least 1 year where the majority of patients had low risk disease have reported significantly lower recurrence rate at 2−4 years compared to no treatment control (relative risk: 0.38−0.78) [5−8]. When MMC 40 mg was given within 24 hours of TURBT followed by four additional instillations without maintenance, the relative risk of recurrence was significantly reduced at 2 years (0.50) [9,10]. However, trials that gave eight weekly instillations of MMC 40 mg not including an immediate single instillation and without maintenance did not show significant reduction in recurrence [11,12]. In none of the presented trials did MMC reduce risk of cancer progression.

Doxorubicin

Doxorubicin is an anthracycline drug with a high molecular weight of 552 kd, thus is free of systemic side effect. It has mostly been studied in Europe. Dosage ranges from 10 to 100 mg. In randomized trials where doxorubicin 20−50 mg were given as eight induction therapy only or as maintenance therapy for at least 1 year, doxorubicin was associated with significantly reduced recurrence rate with relative risk ranging from 0.56 to 0.85 at 18 months to 3.4 years follow-up [5,11,13,14].

Epirubicin

Epirubicin is an anthracycline drug with the first clinical trial published in 1980. It is favored over doxorubicin because of better efficacy and fewer side effects [14]. Epirubicin 50 mg 8 weekly followed by monthly instillation for 1 year demonstrated efficacy equal to an immediate single instillation in reducing recurrence, and seems to be the optimal schedule in patients at low and intermediate risk [15]. In a cohort of mostly high-risk patients, 80 mg epirubicin was compared to 50 mg given in the same schedule of 8 weekly and monthly maintenance for 1 year. There was only marginal difference in recurrence rate between the two dosages (17.6% vs 25.0% vs 65.6%, control) with higher local side effects in the 80 mg arm [14]. An induction course of epirubicin 50 mg for 6 or 8 weeks followed by a less intensive maintenance schedule of single instillation at each follow-up visit for 2 years significantly delayed recurrence but without significantly reducing recurrence rate [16].

Gemcitabine

Gemcitabine is a nucleoside analog that became the first-line chemotherapeutic agent in combination with cisplatin in Stage 4 bladder cancer. Because of its efficacy against urothelial cancer, it was tried as an intravesical agent in various Phase 2 trials and demonstrated good efficacy and toxicity profile [17−19]. Results of some Phase 2 trials of intravesical gemcitabine in BCG failure patients are promising [20,21].

HEAD-TO-HEAD COMPARISON OF DIFFERENT CHEMOTHERAPEUTIC DRUGS

Different drugs have been compared to each other in many trials. Results are inconsistent largely depending on patient and tumor characteristics, drug dosages, and treatment schedules. Most studies reported nonsignificant difference in risk of recurrence and progression between drugs.

Thiotepa was the first to be challenged by MMC and doxorubicin. Randomized trials comparing thiotepa with MMC [22,23] and thiotepa with doxorubicin [24,25] failed to demonstrate superiority of MMC and doxorubicin over thiotepa in terms of recurrence.

Many trials have compared various doses of MMC and doxorubicin with similar efficacy in reducing recurrence [5,6,11,26], except for two studies that showed longer disease-free interval or recurrence-free survival in MMC [7,27].

Although epirubicin did not differ in recurrence-free survival compared to MMC [28], epirubicin was shown to be significantly better than doxorubicin in reducing recurrence [14]. However, two other trials did not show difference in recurrence-free survival [29] or number of recurrence and tumor free period [30].

In a Phase 3 multicenter study involving 109 recurrent cancer patients randomized to either MMC 40 mg 4 weekly followed by 10 monthly instillations or gemcitabine 2000 mg 6 weekly followed by 10 monthly instillations, gemcitabine showed significantly better recurrence-free survival compared to MMC, which was also true for Grade 3 cancers but not for lower grade cancers [31].

INDUCTION ONLY VS INDUCTION AND MAINTENANCE THERAPY

Whether maintenance intravesical therapy for long term is better than short-term therapy is still controversial.

In a study comparing 6 weekly instillations and long-term maintenance MMC 20 mg for 3 years following 6 weekly induction in intermediate and high-risk patients, recurrence-free survival was significantly better for long-term MMC arm [32].

Two studies with doxorubicin did not show benefit for maintenance therapy. In 220 low- and intermediate-risk patients randomized to doxorubicin 50 mg 13 times biweekly and 28 times for 6 months, no difference was found in recurrence rate [33]. In another trial with similar group of 146 patients randomized to doxorubicin 50 mg induction for 6 weeks and monthly instillations for 2 years following induction therapy, maintenance was not associated with reduced recurrence [34].

Several studies with epirubicin showed conflicting results. One study involving 138 patients showed no difference in recurrence-free survival at 3 years between 6 weekly epirubicin 40 mg induction therapy vs induction followed by 11 monthly instillation for 1 year [35]. A bigger study involving 395 intermediate risk patients randomized to immediate instillation of epirubicin 80 mg followed by 5 weekly instillations and to maintenance therapy of 16 installations over 1 year showed significantly better recurrence-free survival at 18 months but not lasting beyond [36]. Another trial randomized patients into two groups. One received nine installations of epirubicin 30 mg that was started within 24 hours of TURBT then continued at 2−3 days, 1 week, 2 weeks after TURBT, and once every 2 weeks for 10 weeks (9 total). The other group followed the same schedule but had 10 additional installations for 10 more months (19 total). The result showed a significantly better recurrence-free survival at 3 years for the second group (63.9% vs 85.2%) [37].

DIFFERENT DOSAGES AND SCHEDULES

Many investigators tried different dosages of drug delivered during different time schedule with limited conclusion on which therapy scheme is optimal. In a multicenter trial in which two different doses of thiotepa (30 and 60 mg) were given every 4 weeks for a maximum of 2 years, recurrence-free rate at 12 months was not significantly different [2]. Doxorubicin given at low or high concentration at short (4 weeks) or long term (2 years) did not show any difference in terms of number of recurrence [5,11]. In case of MMC, there was no significant difference in recurrence whether short term and more intensive schedule or longer term and less intensive schedule was used [26,38]. The results of two parallel prospective randomized studies by EORTC, one with 30 mg MMC and the other with 50 mg doxorubicin treatment designed to compare early (the day of resection) versus delayed (between 7 and 15 days after resection) installations and short-term (6 months) versus long-term (12 months) treatment indicated that in terms of recurrence rate and time to first recurrence, early and delayed treatment did not show any significant difference. Also, no significant difference was found between patients with and without maintenance therapy [39]. In a multicenter trial, equal doses of epirubicin 30 mg were given in two groups of patients, one group receiving 12 installations over 5 months and the other group 19 installations over 1 year. In this study, there was no significant difference in recurrence-free survival at 3 years [40]. In another multicenter trial, doubling total dose of epirubicin (12 weeks, 360 mg vs 6 weeks, 180 mg) significantly reduced recurrence [41]. In another multicenter trial comparing three different dosages of epirubicin (20 mg/40 mL, 30 mg/40 mL, and 40 mg/ml) given during different period of time with equal total dosage administered, more intense short-term epirubicin showed decreased recurrence compared to less intense and longer term installation [42]. In a multicenter study involving 731 patients that compared the efficacy of three different treatment schedule of epirubicin in which Group 1 received 4 weekly and 5 monthly installations (standard schedule), Group 2 received the same schedule as Group 1, but with an additional installation <48 hours after TURBT, and Group 3 received the same scheme as Group 1, but with additional instillations at 9 and 12 months (maintenance schedule); there was no difference in the 5-year recurrence-free period between the treatment groups [43]. In a small study that randomized 47 patients, single instillation of epirubicin 80 mg vs 40 mg every 6−8 weeks followed by monthly instillation for 10 months with total of 16−18 weeks did not show significant difference in recurrence-free survival at 1−5 years [28].

INTRAVESICAL CHEMOTHERAPY IN BCG UNRESPONSIVE PATIENTS

Although radical cystectomy is the treatment of choice in BCG refractory NMIBC patients, some patients who are medically unfit or simply refuse cystectomy will need alternative treatment options.

The efficacy of chemotherapy following BCG failure can find its rationale in a randomized controlled trial comparing MMC and BCG, where patients were allowed to crossover to the other arm in case of failure. In this study 19% of patients with second-line MMC achieved durable response compared to 39% with second-line BCG [44]. Usage of salvage intravesical gemcitabine has been studied in single-arm Phase 2 studies which showed moderate response in terms of prevention of recurrence [20,45]. Gemcitabine was also tried in BCG failure cases in randomized studies, showing significantly better recurrence-free survival in the gemcitabine arm compared to repeat BCG arm. However, progression-free survival did not differ between the two arms [21].

SEQUENTIAL USE OF INTRAVESICAL CHEMOTHERAPY AND BCG

Combination of chemotherapy and BCG was conceived to reduce side effects associated with BCG and enhance efficacy. Increased efficacy of chemotherapy and BCG combination was demonstrated in bladder cancer cell line treated with combination of the two resulting in potentiation of effect [46]. Chemical disruption of urothelium was shown to facilitate BCG attachment to fibronectin and enhance BCG-mediated antitumor activity [47]. However, randomized trial comparing sequential MMC and BCG versus BCG alone showed significantly worse recurrence-free survival in the sequential group. This result was partly explained by increased interval between BCG instillations and suboptimal number of BCG in the sequential group [48]. Similarly, EORTC Phase 2 trial comparing sequential MMC and BCG versus BCG alone in CIS patients did not show improvement of complete response in the sequential arm [49]. In another study comparing MMC and BCG and BCG alone, MMC was given 1 day before BCG instead of weekly alternating schedule to maximize BCG absorption. Although recurrence-free survival was significantly reduced in the sequential arm (hazard ratio of 0.57), higher

Grade 3 toxicity would limit its use to patients with high likelihood of recurrence [50].

Conversely, sequential therapy with MMC and BCG was compared with MMC alone. Two randomized trials comparing sequential combination of MMC and BCG with MMC alone in intermediate- and high-risk NMIBC patients did not show significant difference in terms of recurrence and progression. Also, the frequency of toxicity was not different between the two groups [51,52].

OPTIMIZING INTRAVESICAL CHEMOTHERAPY

Optimization of Drug Delivery

In an effort to enhance the suboptimal effect of standard adjuvant intravesical chemotherapy by enhancing drug delivery, several trials have been conducted that compared standard with optimized treatment method (decreasing urine volume, urine alkalinization, and high dose). Au et al. performed a multiinstitutional Phase III trial comparing standard and optimized treatment with 40 mg MMC, which showed a significantly longer median time to recurrence (29.1 months) and a greater recurrence-free fraction (41.0%) at 5 years in the optimized treatment arm compared to the standard arm (11.8 months and 24.6%) [53].

Thermochemotherapy

A novel method of drug administration, local microwave-induced hyperthermia was introduced to enhance drug delivery. Theoretical advantages combining thermal energy and chemotherapy include (1) increased cellular permeability leading to improved drug uptake and intracellular distribution in the malignant cells, (2) increased drug metabolism and reaction with DNA and inhibited DNA repair, and (3) lack in pathologic blood vessels nourishing the tumor of the ability to vasodilate in response to heat allowing the lesions to attain higher temperature compared with normal tissue [54,55]. Typically, the bladder wall is heated via the intravesical microwave applicator inserted through a transurethral catheter with real-time monitoring of temperature to be within 42.5−45.5°C range. In the initial randomized study in which tumors were pretreated at multiple sessions with MMC with or without hyperthermia, hyperthermia arm achieved significantly higher complete response rate (66% vs 22%) [55]. A systematic review on the role of combined intravesical chemotherapy and hyperthermia showed 59% reduction of recurrence compared to MMC alone and an improved bladder preservation rate (87.6%) [56]. The device was approved by the US FDA in 2008.

Electromotive Drug Administration

Electromotive drug administration (EMDA) uses an electric current to enhance transepithelial drug penetration. Experiment with human bladder tissue has shown that EMDA enhances transport of MMC across the urothelium, with EMDA achieving 4 to 6 times higher tissue concentration at all tissue depths compared to passive diffusion [57].

An electric current generated outside is conveyed into the bladder through an active electrode, which then flows across the bladder to a dispersive electrode applied to the skin. Typically, 15 mA electric current is maintained for 20 minutes during which time the drug is actively transported across the urothelium. A preliminary Phase 2 study comparing EMDA/MMC vs passive MMC demonstrated increased disease-free interval in EMDA/MMC group. The toxicity was tolerable [58].

In a study involving 108 patients, electromotive and passive administration of MMC 40 mg 6 weekly instillations with 10 additional monthly instillations were compared with BCG 81 mg given at the same schedule. At the median follow-up of 43 months, median time to recurrence was significantly longer in the electromotive group compared to passive MMC and BCG groups. In the pharmacokinetic study, peak plasma MMC was significantly higher following electromotive MMC than after MMC (43 vs 8 ng/mL), [59]. In another trial, 212 pT1 cancer patients were randomized into BCG 6 weekly and maintenance for 10 months vs BCG 2 weekly and EMDA/MMC 40 mg for 30 minutes once a week as one cycle for three cycles followed by 40 mg electromotive EMDA/MMC once a month for 2 months, followed by 81 mg BCG once a month as one cycle for three cycles. In this study, EMDA/MMC had higher disease-free interval, lower recurrence, lower progression, lower overall mortality, and lower disease-specific mortality. Side effects were comparable [60].

SIDE EFFECTS OF INTRAVESICAL THERAPY

Common side effects of intravesical chemotherapy include pollakisuria, dysuria, and hematuria. They are usually mild and self-limited. Systemic symptoms such as fever and nausea may also occur but are rare. Extravasation of chemotherapeutic agent can lead to severe inflammation and necrosis, and the consequences can be catastrophic leading to vesicoenteric, vesicovaginal, and vesicocutaneous fistula formation [61]. So, caution is required whenever intravesical chemotherapy is considered in patients suspected to have urinary extravasation. Thiotepa was shown to induce reduction in white blood cell or platelet count in 18% of patients. However, this decrease did not lead to any problem other than a delay in therapy [62]. In an experiment that measured plasma concentration following intravesical instillation of MMC in 31 patients after complete TUR, maximum plasma concentration never exceeded 31 ng/mL, which was less than 1% of the instilled dose. Also, instillation time (0.5 vs 1.0 hour) had no effect on plasma concentration. Only observed side effects were cystitis symptom, and there were no evidence of bone marrow suppression [63].

Comparison With BCG

Several studies compared occurrence of side effects between BCG and intra-vesical agents. Incidence of any local side effects were significantly higher in BCG vs MMC [64,65] and BCG vs epirubicin [66,67]. MMC [64,65,68] and epirubicin [66,67] showed lower incidence of systemic side effects or fever compared to BCG. As for gemcitabine, no difference in the incidence of local and systemic side effects was found compared to BCG [21,69,70]. Fever occurred more frequently with BCG compared to gemcitabine [21,70]. Inconsistency in the reported incidence of local and systemic side effects of BGC and doxorubicin between studies fails to put one drug in a superior position [24,71,72].

Chemical Cystitis

In a trial comparing maintenance regimen of thiotepa 60 or 30 mg vs no intra-vesical therapy, urinary tract symptoms were reported in 17% of patients with 60 mg arm, but none in 30 mg and no therapy arms [2]. In a trial comparing 6 weekly instillation of doxorubicin and MMC, main side effect was cystitis syndrome that appeared in 22% of doxorubicin and 8.9% of MMC [11]. When given in a maintenance setting, occurrence of cystitis syndrome was much higher with 48% in doxorubicin and 21% in MMC [26]. It is noteworthy that the incidence of side effects increases in relation to the number of instillations. In a study comparing epirubicin 40 mg maintained for 1 year with a total of 16−18 instillations vs MMC 40 mg with the same schedule, there was no sig-nificant difference in risk of urinary symptoms (13% vs 13%) [28]. Trial com-paring 1 year maintenance therapy of epirubicin 30 mg or 50 mg and doxorubicin 50 mg showed significantly higher local toxicity in doxorubicin than in the epirubicin group (36.7% vs 19.7%). Comparison of MMC 40 mg and gemcitabine 2000 mg both maintained for 1 year showed increased risk of chemical cystitis in the MMC than in the gemcitabine group (21.1% vs 5.5%) [31].

REFERENCES

[1] Watkins W, Kozak J, Flanagan M. Severe pancytopenia associated with the use of intrave-sical thio-TEPA. J Urol 1967;98(4):470−1.

[2] Koontz WJ, et al. The use of intravesical thio-tepa in the management of non-invasive car-cinoma of the bladder. J Urol 1981;125(3):307−12.

[3] Hirao Y, et al. A prospective randomized study of prophylaxis of tumor recurrence following transurethral resection of superficial bladder cancer—intravesical thio-TEPA versus oral UFT. Cancer Chemother Pharmacol 1992;30(Suppl):S26−30.

[4] The effect of intravesical thiotepa on tumour recurrence after endoscopic treatment of newly diagnosed superficial bladder cancer. A further report with long-term follow-up of a Medical Research Council randomized trial. Medical Research Council Working Party on Urological Cancer, Subgroup on Superficial Bladder Cancer. Br J Urol 1994;73 (6):632−8.

[5] Akaza H, et al. Comparative analysis of short-term and long-term prophylactic intravesical chemotherapy of superficial bladder cancer. Prospective, randomized, controlled studies of the Japanese Urological Cancer Research Group. Cancer Chemother Pharmacol 1987;20(Suppl):S91−6.

[6] Tsushima T, et al. Prophylactic intravesical instillation therapy with adriamycin and mitomycin C in patients with superficial bladder cancer. Cancer Chemother Pharmacol 1987;20(Suppl):S72−6.

[7] Gustafson H, et al. Prophylactic instillation therapy of superficial bladder cancer. A randomized study comparing mitomycin C and adriamycin with special reference to DNA ploidy. Scand J Urol Nephrol Suppl 1991;138:187−91.

[8] Krege S, et al. A randomized multicenter trial of adjuvant therapy in superficial bladder cancer: transurethral resection only versus transurethral resection plus mitomycin C versus transurethral resection plus bacillus Calmette-Guerin. Participating Clinics. J Urol 1996;156(3):962−6.

[9] Tolley DA, et al. *Effect of intravesical mitomycin C on recurrence of newly diagnosed superficial bladder cancer: interim report from the Medical Research Council Subgroup on Superficial Bladder Cancer (Urological Cancer Working Party).* Br Med J (Clin Res Ed) 1988;296(6639):1759−61.

[10] Tolley DA, et al. The effect of intravesical mitomycin C on recurrence of newly diagnosed superficial bladder cancer: a further report with 7 years of follow up. J Urol 1996;155(4):1233−8.

[11] Niijima T, Koiso K, Akaza H. Randomized clinical trial on chemoprophylaxis of recurrence in cases of superficial bladder cancer. Cancer Chemother Pharmacol 1983;11 (Suppl):S79−82.

[12] Kim H, Lee C. Intravesical mitomycin C instillation as a prophylactic treatment of superficial bladder tumor. J Urol 1989;141(6):1337−9.

[13] Kurth K, et al. Adjuvant chemotherapy for superficial transitional cell bladder carcinoma: long-term results of a European organization for research and treatment of cancer randomized trial comparing doxorubicin, ethoglucid and transurethral resection alone. J Urol 1997;158(2):378−84.

[14] Ali-El-Dein B, et al. Intravesical epirubicin versus doxorubicin for superficial bladder tumors (stages pTa and pT1): a randomized prospective study. J Urol 1997;158(1):68−74.

[15] Ali-El-Dein B, et al. Single-dose versus multiple instillations of epirubicin as prophylaxis for recurrence after transurethral resection of pTa and pT1 transitional-cell bladder tumours: a prospective, randomized controlled study. Br J Urol 1997;79(5):731−5.

[16] Melekos MD, et al. Intravesical instillations of 4-epi-doxorubicin (epirubicin) in the prophylactic treatment of superficial bladder cancer: results of a controlled prospective study. J Urol 1992;147(2):371−5.

[17]   Gontero P, et al. Phase II study to investigate the ablative efficacy of intravesical adminis-
       tration of gemcitabine in intermediate-risk superficial bladder cancer (SBC). Eur Urol
       2004;46(3):339−43.

[18]   Gårdmark T, et al. Randomized phase II marker lesion study evaluating effect of schedul-
       ing on response to intravesical gemcitabine in recurrent stage Ta urothelial cell carcinoma
       of the bladder. Urology 2005;66(3):527−30.

[19]   Bartoletti R, et al. Intravesical gemcitabine therapy for superficial transitional cell carci-
       noma: Results of a Phase II prospective multicenter study. Urology 2005;66(4):726−31.

[20]   Dalbagni G, et al. Phase II trial of intravesical gemcitabine in bacille Calmette-
       Guérin−refractory transitional cell carcinoma of the bladder. J Clin Oncol 2006;24
       (18):2729−34.

[21]   Di Lorenzo G, et al. Gemcitabine versus bacille Calmette-Guérin after initial bacille
       Calmette-Guérin failure in non-muscle-invasive bladder cancer. Cancer 2010;116
       (8):1893−900.

[22]   Zincke H, et al. Intravesical thiotepa and mitomycin C treatment immediately after trans-
       urethral resection and later for superficial (stages Ta and Tis) bladder cancer: a prospec-
       tive, randomized, stratified study with crossover design. J Urol 1985;134(6):1110−14.

[23]   Flanigan RC, et al. A trial of prophylactic thiotepa or mitomycin C intravesical therapy in
       patients with recurrent or multiple superficial bladder cancers. J Urol 1986;136(1):35−7.

[24]   Martinez-Pineiro JA, et al. Bacillus Calmette-Guerin versus doxorubicin versus thiotepa: a
       randomized prospective study in 202 patients with superficial bladder cancer. J Urol
       1990;143(3):502−6.

[25]   Bouffioux C, et al. Adjuvant chemotherapy of recurrent superficial transitional cell carci-
       noma: results of a European organization for research on treatment of cancer randomized
       trial comparing intravesical instillation of thiotepa, doxorubicin and cisplatin. The
       European Organization for Research on Treatment of Cancer Genitourinary Group. J Urol
       1992;148(2 Pt 1):297−301.

[26]   Huland H, et al. Comparison of different schedules of cytostatic intravesical instillations
       in patients with superficial bladder carcinoma: final evaluation of a prospective multicen-
       ter study with 419 patients. J Urol 1990;144(1):68−71 discussion 71−2.

[27]   Jauhiainen K, Alfthan O. Instillation of mitomycin C and doxorubicin in the prevention of
       recurrent superficial (Ta—T1) bladder cancer. Br J Urol 1987;60(1):54−9.

[28]   Liu B, et al. Randomized study of single instillation of epirubicin for superficial bladder
       carcinoma: long-term clinical outcomes. Cancer Invest 2006;24(2):160−3.

[29]   Eto H, et al. Comparison of the prophylactic usefulness of epirubicin and doxorubicin in
       the treatment of superficial bladder cancer by intravesical instillation: a multicenter ran-
       domized trial. Cancer Chemother Pharmacol 1994;35(1):S46−51.

[30]   Shuin T, et al. A phase II study of prophylactic intravesical chemotherapy with 4′-epirubi-
       cin in recurrent superficial bladder cancer: comparison of 4′-epirubicin and Adriamycin.
       Cancer Chemother Pharmacol 1994;35(1):S52−6.

[31]   Addeo R, et al. Randomized phase III trial on gemcitabine versus mytomicin in recurrent
       superficial bladder cancer: evaluation of efficacy and tolerance. J Clin Oncol 2010;28
       (4):543−8.

[32]   Friedrich MG, et al. Long-term intravesical adjuvant chemotherapy further reduces recur-
       rence rate compared with short-term intravesical chemotherapy and short-term therapy
       with bacillus Calmette-Guérin (BCG) in patients with non−muscle-invasive bladder carci-
       noma. Eur Urol 2007;52(4):1123−30.

[33] Rubben H, et al. Natural history and treatment of low and high risk superficial bladder tumors. J Urol 1988;139(2):283−5.

[34] Flamm J. Long-term versus short-term doxorubicin hydrochloride instillation after transurethral resection of superficial bladder cancer. Eur Urol 1990;17(2):119−24.

[35] Okamura K, et al. A randomized study of short-versus long-term intravesical epirubicin instillation for superficial bladder cancer. Nagoya University Urological Oncology Group. Eur Urol 1998;33(3):285−8 discussion 289.

[36] Serretta V, et al. A 1-year maintenance after early adjuvant intravesical chemotherapy has a limited efficacy in preventing recurrence of intermediate risk non-muscle-invasive bladder cancer. BJU Int 2010;106(2):212−17.

[37] Koga H, et al. A randomized controlled trial of short-term versus long-term prophylactic intravesical instillation chemotherapy for recurrence after transurethral resection of Ta/T1 transitional cell carcinoma of the bladder. J Urol 2004;171(1):153−7.

[38] Schwaibold H, et al. Long-term follow-up of cytostatic intravesical instillation in patients with superficial bladder carcinoma. Is short-term, intensive instillation better than maintenance therapy?. Eur Urol 1997;31(2):153−9.

[39] Bouffioux C, et al. Intravesical adjuvant chemotherapy for superficial transitional cell bladder carcinoma: results of 2 European organization for research and treatment of cancer randomized trials with mitomycin C and doxorubicin comparing early versus delayed instillations and short-term versus long-term treatment. J Urol 1995;153:934−41.

[40] Nomata K, et al. Intravesical adjuvant chemotherapy for superficial transitional cell bladder carcinoma: results of a randomized trial with epirubicin comparing short-term versus long-term maintenance treatment. Cancer Chemother Pharmacol 2002;50(4):266−70.

[41] Mitsumori K, et al. Early and large-dose intravesical instillation of epirubicin to prevent superficial bladder carcinoma recurrence after transurethral resection. BJU Int 2004;94(3):317−21.

[42] Kuroda M, et al. Effect of prophylactic treatment with intravesical epirubicin on recurrence of superficial bladder cancer—the 6th trial of the Japanese Urological Cancer Research Group (JUCRG): a randomized trial of intravesical epirubicin at dose of 20 mg/40 ml, 30 mg/40 ml, 40 mg/40 ml. Eur Urol 2004;45(5):600−5.

[43] Hendricksen K, et al. Comparison of three schedules of intravesical epirubicin in patients with non−muscle-invasive bladder cancer. Eur Urol 2008;53(5):984−91.

[44] Malmström PU, et al. 5-Year followup of a randomized prospective study comparing mitomycin C and bacillus Calmette-Guerin in patients with superficial bladder carcinoma. J Urol 1999;161(4):1124−7.

[45] Skinner EC, et al. SWOG S0353: phase II trial of intravesical gemcitabine in patients with nonmuscle invasive bladder cancer and recurrence after 2 prior courses of intravesical bacillus Calmette-Guérin. J Urol 2013;190(4):1200−4.

[46] Rajala P, et al. Cytostatic effect of different strains of Bacillus Calmette-Guérin on human bladder cancer cells in vitro alone and in combination with mitomycin C and Interferon-α. Urol Res 1992;20(3):215−17.

[47] Kavoussi LR, et al. Fibronectin-mediated Calmette-Guerin bacillus attachment to murine bladder mucosa. Requirement for the expression of an antitumor response. J Clin Invest 1990;85(1):62−7.

[48] Kaasinen E, et al. Alternating Mitomycin C and BCG instillations versus BCG alone in treatment of carcinoma in situ of the urinary bladder: a Nordic study. Eur Urol 2003;43(6):637−45.

[49] Oosterlinck W, et al. Sequential intravesical chemoimmunotherapy with mitomycin C and bacillus Calmette-Guérin and with bacillus Calmette-Guérin alone in patients with carcinoma in situ of the urinary bladder: results of an EORTC genito-urinary group randomized phase 2 trial (30993). Eur Urol 2011;59(3):438−46.

[50] Solsona E, et al. Sequential combination of mitomycin C plus bacillus Calmette-Guérin (BCG) is more effective but more toxic than BCG alone in patients with non−muscle-invasive bladder cancer in intermediate- and high-risk patients: final outcome of CUETO 93009, a randomized prospective trial. Eur Urol 2015;67(3):508−16.

[51] Witjes JA, et al. Results of a randomized phase III trial of sequential intravesical therapy with mitomycin C and bacillus Calmette-Guerin versus mitomycin C alone in patients with superficial bladder cancer. J Urol 1998;160(5):1668−71 discussion 1671−2.

[52] Rintala E, et al. Alternating mitomycin C and bacillus Calmette-Guerin instillation prophylaxis for recurrent papillary (stages Ta to T1) superficial bladder cancer. Finnbladder Group. J Urol 1996;156(1):56−9 discussion 59−60.

[53] Au JL, et al. Methods to improve efficacy of intravesical mitomycin C: results of a randomized phase III trial. J Natl Cancer Inst 2001;93(8):597−604.

[54] Herman TS, et al. Rationale for use of local hyperthermia with radiation therapy and selected anticancer drugs in locally advanced human malignancies. Int J Hyperthermia 1988;4(2):143−58.

[55] Colombo R, et al. Neoadjuvant combined microwave induced local hyperthermia and topical chemotherapy versus chemotherapy alone for superficial bladder cancer. J Urol 1996;155(4):1227−32.

[56] Lammers RJM, et al. The role of a combined regimen with intravesical chemotherapy and hyperthermia in the management of non-muscle-invasive bladder cancer: a systematic review. Eur Urol 2011;60(1):81−93.

[57] Di Stasi SM, et al. Electromotive versus passive diffusion of mitomycin C into human bladder wall: concentration-depth profiles studies. Cancer Res 1999;59(19):4912−18.

[58] Brausi M, et al. Intravesical electromotive administration of drugs for treatment of superficial bladder cancer: a comparative phase II study. Urology 1998;51(3):506−9.

[59] Di Stasi SM, et al. Intravesical electromotive mitomycin c versus passive transport mitomycin C for high risk superficial bladder cancer: a prospective randomized study. J Urol 2003;170(3):777−82.

[60] Di Stasi SM, et al. Sequential BCG and electromotive mitomycin versus BCG alone for high-risk superficial bladder cancer: a randomised controlled trial. Lancet Oncol 2006;7 (1):43−51.

[61] Dangle PP, Wang WP, Pohar KS. Vesicoenteric, vesicovaginal, vesicocutaneous fistula -an unusual complication with intravesical mitomycin. Can J Urol 2008;15(5):4269−72.

[62] Soloway MS, Ford KS. Thiotepa-induced myelosuppression: review of 670 bladder instillations. J Urol 1983;130(5):889−91.

[63] van Helsdingen PJ, et al. Mitomycin C resorption following repeated intravesical instillations using different instillation times. Urol Int 1988;43(1):42−6.

[64] Witjes WP, et al. Update on the Dutch cooperative trial: mitomycin versus bacillus Calmette-Guerin-Tice versus bacillus Calmette-Guerin RIVM in the treatment of patients with pTA-pT1 papillary carcinoma and carcinoma in situ of the urinary bladder. Dutch South East Cooperative Urological Group. Semin Urol Oncol 1996;14(1 Suppl 1):10−16.

[65] Ojea A, et al. A multicentre, randomised prospective trial comparing three intravesical adjuvant therapies for intermediate-risk superficial bladder cancer: low-dose bacillus

Calmette-Guerin (27 mg) versus very low-dose bacillus Calmette-Guerin (13.5 mg) versus mitomycin C. Eur Urol 2007;52(5):1398−406.

[66] de Reijke TM, et al. Bacillus Calmette-Guerin versus epirubicin for primary, secondary or concurrent carcinoma in situ of the bladder: results of a European Organization for the research and treatment of cancer—genito-urinary group phase III trial (30906). J Urol 2005;173(2):405−9.

[67] van der Meijden AP, et al. Intravesical instillation of epirubicin, bacillus Calmette-Guerin and bacillus Calmette-Guerin plus isoniazid for intermediate and high risk Ta, T1 papillary carcinoma of the bladder: a European Organization for Research and Treatment of Cancer genito-urinary group randomized phase III trial. J Urol 2001;166(2):476−81.

[68] DeBruyne FMJ, et al. Bacillus Calmette-Guérin versus mitomycin intravesical therapy in superficial bladder cancer. Urology 1992;40:11−15.

[69] Porena M, et al. Bacillus Calmette-Guérin versus gemcitabine for intravesical therapy in high-risk superficial bladder cancer: a randomised prospective study. Urol Int 2010;84 (1):23−7.

[70] Gontero P, et al. The impact of intravesical gemcitabine and 1/3 dose bacillus Calmette-Guérin instillation therapy on the quality of life in patients with nonmuscle invasive bladder cancer: results of a prospective, randomized, phase II trial. J Urol 2013;190 (3):857−62.

[71] Lamm DL, et al. A randomized trial of intravesical doxorubicin and immunotherapy with bacille Calmette−Guérin for transitional-cell carcinoma of the bladder. N Engl J Med 1991;325(17):1205−9.

[72] Hinotsu S, et al. Sustained prophylactic effect of intravesical bacille Calmette-Guérin for superficial bladder cancer: a smoothed hazard analysis in a randomized prospective study. Urology 2006;67(3):545−9.

Chapter 20

Immunotherapy: Bacille Calmette–Guérin

Chapter Outline

Bladder Cancer. DOI: http://dx.doi.org/10.1016/B978-0-12-809939-1.00020-5

Chapter 20.1

Indications for BCG

Sung Han Kim and Ho Kyung Seo

Research Institute and National Cancer Center, Goyang, South Korea

INTRODUCTION

The first report of Bacillus Calmette−Guérin (BCG) as an immunomodulator in cancer therapy was published in 1959 [1]. BCG is an attenuated mycobacterium developed as a vaccine for tuberculosis that has demonstrated antitumor activity in several different cancers, including urothelial carcinoma. The original regimen described by Morales included a percutaneous dose, which was discontinued after success with a similar intravesical regimen [2]. Efficacy of intravesical BCG instillation does not seem to be increased significantly when combined simultaneously with intradermal BCG vaccination.

In 1976, Morales et al. published a landmark paper on the favorable effects of intravesical BCG on outcomes in recurrent superficial bladder cancer in nine patients [2,3]. The first controlled trial showing similar results was published in 1980, and BCG received FDA approval for the treatment of superficial bladder cancer in 1990 [4]. In recent days, intravesical instillation of BCG, a live attenuated strain of *Mycobacterium bovis*, is the most effective adjuvant therapy after transurethral resection (TUR) of intermediate- or high-risk superficial bladder tumors, and is recommended as the first-line treatment for patients with carcinoma in situ (CIS) [5,6], for reducing the risk of short- and long-term recurrences [7]. Since then, several meta-analyses have shown that adjuvant intravesical treatment reduces recurrence of non-muscle invasive bladder cancer (NMIBC) [7,8]. The choice between adjuvant intravesical treatments, namely chemotherapy or BCG immunotherapy, depends on the need to reduced disease recurrence or progression. BCG immunotherapy is currently the most effective treatment for NMIBC and one of the most successful applications of immunotherapy to the treatment of cancer. NMIBC is a spectrum of fairly benign bladder tumors with a low recurrence rate and an extremely low rate of progression in patients classified as low risk and a high recurrence rate and progression in patients classified as high risk. Recurrences occur in the majority of high-risk patients, and a substantial percentage of these patients will experience progression to muscle-invasive bladder cancer (MIBC) during the course of their disease.

INDICATIONS OF INTRAVESICAL BCG

BCG can delay progression of high-risk bladder cancer, yet the long-term survival advantage is not fully defined. Intravesical BCG is indicated for treatment of high-grade Ta, T1, and/or CIS, and multifocal, large, low-grade Ta or recurrent low-grade Ta tumors.

Several guidelines, however, exist regarding the use of BCG in NMIBC, such as those by the American Urological Association (AUA) [9,10], the European Association of Urology (EAU) [11], the National Comprehensive Cancer Network (NCCN) [12,13], Canadian Urological Association (CUA) [14], and the International Consultation on Urological Diseases (ICUD) [15]. However, the guidelines are somewhat disparate, making implementation of the recommendations into routine practice difficult for the practicing urologist, although each of these guidelines are based on large-scale literature reviews on similar available data.

The AUA risk stratification by AUA/Society of Urologic Oncology (SUO) Guideline in 2016 [10] classified three risk categories as a low-, intermediate-, and high-risk NMIBC. They recommended the use of BCG instillation only in either intermediate- or high-risk NMIBC. In an intermediate-risk patient, a clinician should consider administration of a 6-week course of induction intravesical chemotherapy or immunotherapy (moderate recommendation; evidence strength: Grade B). In a high-risk patient with newly diagnosed CIS, high-grade T1, or high-risk Ta urothelial carcinoma, a clinician should administer a 6-week induction course of BCG (strong recommendation; evidence strength: Grade B). In an intermediate-risk patient who completely responds to an induction course of intravesical chemotherapy, a clinician may utilize maintenance therapy (conditional recommendation; evidence strength: Grade C). In an intermediate-risk patient who completely responds to induction BCG, a clinician should consider maintenance BCG for 1 year, as tolerated (moderate recommendation; evidence strength: Grade C). In a high-risk patient who completely responds to induction BCG, a clinician should continue maintenance BCG for 3 years, as tolerated (moderate recommendation; evidence strength: Grade B).

Using similar definitions, the First International Consultation on Bladder Tumors (FICBT) defines low risk as low-grade Ta stage, and the NCCN defines low risk as G1–2 Ta stage [16,17]. The NCCN guidelines [18] list the use of intravesical BCG as preferred therapy, citing Category 1 data for high-grade Ta, all T1, and any Tis tumors.

The EAU guidelines [4,5,19] for classifying risk are based on the previously published European Organization for Research and Treatment of Cancer (EORTC) risk tables [20]. The individual estimated risk of recurrence and progression can be calculated in individual patients with Stage Ta and T1 bladder cancer by using the risk score introduced by a simplified risk group classification or EORTC risk table. They allow the user to estimate the probability of recurrence and progression in patients with Stage Ta and T1 bladder cancer, based on six different factors such as number of tumors, tumor size, prior recurrence rate, T-stage category, concomitant CIS, and nuclear grade [5,20]. In the intermediate- and high-risk patients, the protective effect of long-term therapy with BCG is more pronounced compared to chemotherapy [21,22].

After careful review and analysis of the EAU [11,19], NCCN [23,24], and AUA [10] recommendations for the management of NMIBC, a committee of internationally renowned leaders in bladder cancer management, known as the International Bladder Cancer Group (IBCG) identified current key influencing guidelines and published English language literature related to the treatment and management of NMIBC, available as of March 2008 [25,26]. They developed a treatment algorithm to build on the existing framework provided by the EAU, FICBT, NCCN, and AUA guidelines, and to provide consensus on the definitions of low-, intermediate-, high-risk, and very high-risk NMIBC, as well as practical recommendations for the management of patients in each of these risk categories [25,26]. IBCG recommended BCG therapy after TUR for intermediate-risk disease, and intravesical chemotherapy or BCG induction, plus maintenance should be initiated following complete TUR and with a single immediate instillation of chemotherapy. For intermediate-risk disease, intravesical BCG induction plus maintenance or intravesical chemotherapy was recommended. Other recommendations are (1) for high-risk disease, intravesical BCG induction plus maintenance after complete TUR; (2) for recurrences in low-risk patients, they recommend treating as intermediate-risk; (3) for recurrences in intermediate-risk patients, they recommend to consider risk category, and if still an intermediate-risk disease, then repeat chemotherapy or BCG induction plus maintenance after TUR; (4) if high-risk disease is diagnosed, BCG induction plus maintenance or radical cystectomy is needed; and (5) for high-grade recurrences in high-risk patients, radical cystectomy is preferred, but TUR plus additional intravesical instillations is also recommended if the patient is not suitable for cystectomy (Tables 20.1.1−20.1.3).

Low-Risk NMIBC: A Small Volume, Low-Grade Ta

Consensus exists for small, solitary, superficial low-grade tumors (Ta), with all groups agreeing that BCG is not indicated in this setting given the very low risk of disease progression. Although BCG has been used in marker lesion studies, it may be considered as overtreatment in low-risk patients. Recognizing this, the EORTC studied the ablative effect of one-fourth dose of BCG in a small study with 44 low- and intermediate-risk patients [18]. Although the complete response rate was promising (27/44, 61%), 54% of patients had dysuria and 39% had macroscopic hematuria. The AUA

TABLE 20.1.1 Risk Classifications According to Different Guidelines

2016 AUA/SUO Risk Stratification for NMIBC [10]

Low Risk	Intermediate Risk	High Risk
Low-grade solitary Ta ≤ 3 cm	Recurrence within 1 year, LG Ta	High-grade T1
Papillary urothelial neoplasm of low malignant potential	Solitary low-grade Ta > 3 cm	Any recurrent, high-grade Ta
	Low-grade Ta, multifocal	High-grade Ta > 3 cm (or multifocal)
	High-grade Ta, ≤ 3 cm	Any CIS
Low grade	Low grade	Any BCG failure in high-grade patient
		Any variant histology
		Any lymphovascular invasion
		Any high-grade prostatic urethral involvement

2016 EAU Risk Group Stratification [4,5]

Low-risk tumor	Primary, solitary, Ta, low grade/G1, < 3 cm, no CIS
Intermediate-risk tumors	All tumors not defined in the two adjacent categories (between the low and high risk)
High-risk tumors	Any of the following: • T1 tumor • High-grade/G3 tumor • CIS • Multiple and recurrent and large (> 3 cm) Ta G1G2 tumors (all conditions must be present in this point)

(Continued)

TABLE 20.1.1 (Continued)

2016 IBCG Risk Classification [26]

Low-Risk NMIBC	Intermediate-Risk NMIBC	High-Risk NMIBC	Very−High-Risk NMIBC
Ta low-grade tumors	Multifocal or multirecurrent low-grade Ta	T1	High-grade T1 + any of the following factors:
	Multiple tumors	CIS	• Large tumors
	Tumor size ≥ 3 cm	Any high grade	• Micropapillary variant histology
	Early recurrence <1 y		• Bladder/prostatic urethra CIS
	Frequent recurrences > 1/y		• Lymphovascular invasion
			• Multiple tumors

Source: Copyright from Elsevier Publisher and Maurizio Brausi; Adapted from Brausi M, Witjes JA, Lamm D, Persad R, Palou J, Colombel M, et al. A review of current guidelines and best practice recommendations for the management of nonmuscle invasive bladder cancer by the International Bladder Cancer Group. J Urol 2011;186 (6):2158−67.

TABLE 20.1.2 Comparison of Risk Stratification Definitions Proposed by EAU, AUA, NCCN, CUA, and FICBT Guidelines

Guidelines	Low Risk	Intermediate Risk	High Risk
EAU [19]	• Primary, solitary, small Ta • Low grade with no CIS	Multifocal Grade 2 Ta or solitary Grade 2 T1 (EORTC recurrence score = 1–17 and progression score = 2–6)	T1 tumor, any HG, CIS, multiple and recurrent and large (>3 cm) Grade 1–2 Ta tumors (EORTC progression score = 7–23)
AUA [9]	Small volume low-grade Ta	Multifocal or large volume low-grade Ta	HG Ta, all T1, or CIS
NCCN [23,27]	Low-grade Ta	Not specifically defined	All T1 tumors
CUA [14]	Low-grade Ta	Multifocal or multirecurrent low-grade Ta	T1, CIS, or any HG
FIBCT [5,15]	Low-grade Ta	• Low-grade Ta with high risk of recurrence • Recurrent low-grade Ta tumors	• Multifocal G2T1 • G3Ta-T1 • CIS • HG Ta • All T1
CUA [14]	Low-grade Ta	Multifocal or multirecurrent low-grade Ta	• HG T1, CIS, any HG disease • Very high risk: T1HG with variant features; T1HG with lymphovascular invasion; multiple and/or large T1HG; T1HG with concomitant bladder/prostatic CIS; persistent T1HG on restaging TUR; early HG recurrence at 3 months; and invasive tumors involving bladder diverticula

HG, high grade.

Source: Copyright from Elsevier Publisher and Maurizio Brausi; Adapted from Brausi M, Witjes JA, Lamm D, Persad R, Palou J, Colombel M, et al. A review of current guidelines and best practice recommendations for the management of nonmuscle invasive bladder cancer by the International Bladder Cancer Group. J Urol 2011;186 (6):2158–67.

TABLE 20.1.3 Comparison of Guideline Recommendation for Low-, Intermediate-, and High-Risk Disease

Guideline	Low Risk	Intermediate Risk	High Risk
EAU [19]	One immediate instillation of intravesical chemotherapy after TURBT	• One immediate instillation of intravesical chemotherapy after TURBT • 1-year full-dose BCG treatment (induction plus weekly instillations for 3 weeks at 3, 6, and 12 months), or instillations of chemotherapy (the optimal schedule is not known) for a maximum of 1 year	• Intravesical full-dose BCG instillations for 1–3 years or cystectomy • Very high risk: radical cystectomy or full-dose BCG instillations for 1–3 years
AUA/SUO [10]	A single postoperative instillation of intravesical chemotherapy (e.g., MMC or epirubicin) within 24 hours of TURBT	Induction BCG, a clinician should consider maintenance BCG for 1 year	• Intravesical BCG induction and, a second course of BCG for 3 years • Cystectomy
NCCN [12]	• TURBT • Consider single-dose intravesical chemotherapy within 24 hours (not immunotherapy) and/or induction intravesical chemotherapy	• Intravesical therapy: BCG (preferred) or mitomycin after repeat TURBT • Observation after repeat TURBT	• Intravesical therapy BCG (Category 1) or cystectomy
IBCG [25]	• TURBT • Immediate, single, postoperative instillation of chemotherapy	Intravesical chemotherapy or BCG induction + maintenance after complete TURBT and single, immediate instillation of chemotherapy	• BCG induction + maintenance should be initiated after complete TURBT and a single, immediate instillation of chemotherapy. (Note: Efficacy of single, immediate instillation of chemotherapy has not been studied in high-risk disease)

FICBT	• TURBT
	• Single, immediate postoperative instillation of chemotherapy
		• TURBT
		• Single, immediate postoperative instillation of chemotherapy followed by
		  • Induction BCG + maintenance for 1 year
		  • Maintenance intravesical chemotherapy of 6–12 months
			• Repeat TURBT
			• BCG induction + maintenance for at least 1 year
			• Radical cystectomy

CUA [14]	• TURBT and immediate postoperative instillation of a chemotherapeutic agent	• TURBT and immediate postoperative instillation of a chemotherapeutic agent • Intravesical BCG or chemotherapy induction + maintenance for a year	• TURBT and immediate postoperative instillation of a chemotherapeutic agent • Repeat TUR • Full dose of induction BCG and 3-year maintenance (early radical cystectomy for very high-risk patients)

TURBT, transurethral resection of bladder tumor.

Source: Copyright from Elsevier Publisher and Maurizio Brausi; Adapted from Brausi M, Witjes JA, Lamm D, Persad R, Palou J, Colombel M, et al. A review of current guidelines and best practice recommendations for the management of nonmuscle invasive bladder cancer by the International Bladder Cancer Group. J Urol 2011;186 (6):2158–67.

guideline also did not recommend intravesical BCG but rather chemotherapy in a small volume, low-grade Ta tumor [9].

Intermediate-Risk NMIBC: A Multifocal or Large Low-Grade Ta, or Recurrent Low-Grade Ta

For multiple and/or large or recurrent low-grade tumors, BCG therapy with or without maintenance is considered optional by EAU and AUA guidelines, and the IBCG [9,11,25]. The AUA's meta-analysis suggests 24% and 31% reduction in recurrence rates for BCG induction and maintenance, respectively [9]. The AUA recommended BCG therapy only in multifocal or large low-grade Ta, or recurrent low-grade Ta tumors (the intermediate-risk category), as well as mitomycin C (MMC) therapy. The EAU recommendation is predominantly based on the recent meta-analysis by Sylvester and colleagues [21], which demonstrated a 32% relative risk reduction with the use of BCG maintenance compared to intravesical chemotherapy. The IBCG recommendation is based on a risk assessment model [28]. By contrast, the NCCN guidelines do not specifically address these intermediate-risk tumors [12].

High-Risk NMIBC: High-Grade Ta, All T1 or CIS

BCG has been shown to provide a better, complete response, and disease-free and progression-free survival when compared to chemotherapy in the treatment of patients with high-risk disease. In a meta-analysis by the Cochrane group, induction BCG was found to be markedly superior to MMC therapy in high-risk but not in low-risk patients. Additionally, the NCCN guidelines list the use of intravesical BCG as preferred therapy, citing Category 1 data for high-grade Ta, all T1, and any Tis tumors [2]. The AUA recommended high-grade Ta, all T1, and CIS tumors susceptible to BCG therapy [9,10,28], and the EAU additionally recommends BCG therapy in multiple and recurrent and large-sized (> 3 cm) Grade 1−2 Ta tumors [5,6].

Ta High-Grade NMIBC

Patients with high-grade Ta bladder tumors are at high risk for recurrence, and more importantly, progression. Because of these findings, both the AUA and the EUA recommend initial intravesical treatment with BCG [9,11,19,26]. These recommendations are based on data from multiple meta-analyses that have shown a decrease in recurrence and progression following treatment of NMIBC with BCG [8,29−33]. A meta-analysis of six trials comparing TUR with TUR plus BCG concluded that TUR with intravesical BCG provides a significantly better prophylaxis for tumor recurrence in Ta and T1 tumors than TUR of bladder tumor alone [32]. Han and Pan [31] reviewed 25 trials of patients treated with TUR or TUR and BCG for all NMIBC and found tumor recurrences in 49.7% and 40.5%, respectively.

Similar findings have been replicated by multiple other meta-analyses [30,32,33]. In 2002, Sylvester et al. [7] reviewed 24 trials involving TUR or TUR and BCG for information on tumor progression. Those treated with TUR alone progressed in 13.8% of all cases, whereas only 9.8% progressed when treated with TUR and BCG therapy [7]. Bohle and Bock [29] obtained similar findings for the preventive role of BCG on progression in their meta-analysis. Decrease in progression was only noted in studies with maintenance therapy [7,29].

T1 Tumors

The goal of intravesical BCG in T1 tumors is to decrease the high rates of recurrence and progression once the invasive component is removed by TUR. For high-risk T1 papillary tumors, the efficacy of BCG after TUR has been demonstrated in several series, with recurrence rates of 16%–40% and progression rates of 4.4%–40%, a substantial improvement compared to TUR alone [34–40].

Multiple studies have shown the efficacy of BCG in decreasing the risk of recurrence as well. In some retrospective studies with T1 bladder tumors (especially for high grade or Grade 3), BCG was found to be superior to TUR alone or other intravesical agents [41,42], whereas others could not show such an effect [43,44]. Hara et al. [41] reported that the risk of recurrence was higher for patients who did not receive BCG irrespective of age, tumor size, multiplicity, the presence of CIS, or lymphovascular invasion; only one of seven patients who progressed received BCG. Patard et al. [42] reported an improved recurrence-free survival and progression-free survival, as well as a lower rate of deferred cystectomies among patients treated with TUR and intravesical BCG versus TUR alone. A meta-analysis of six trials comparing TUR with TUR plus BCG concluded that TUR with intravesical BCG provides a significantly better prophylaxis for tumor recurrence in T1 tumors than TUR alone [27]. Another meta-analysis of 25 trials revealed a statistically significant difference in the odds of tumor recurrence between patients treated with BCG and those treated without BCG. Of 2342 patients undergoing BCG therapy, 949 (40.5%) had tumor recurrence compared to 1205 (49.7%) of 2425 patients treated without BCG [26].

In contrast, in a retrospective nonrandomized study, Shahin et al. [44] failed to show a benefit of intravesical BCG in the progression-free survival of patients with T1G3 disease. During a median follow-up of 5.3 years, tumors progressed in 33% of patients treated with BCG and in 36% treated with TUR alone; deferred cystectomy was performed in 29% of patients who received BCG versus 31% treated with resection alone. In a recent report, among 288 patients placed on surveillance, the 5-year probability of freedom from recurrence was 45% for those receiving and 54% for those not receiving early BCG, but on a multivariable analysis, early BCG use was not significantly associated with recurrence [45].

The effect of intravesical BCG on progression is less evident in T1 lesions. The cumulative incidence of progression to MIBC was 12% and 10%, respectively, for those receiving and not receiving early BCG, whereas the cumulative incidence of deferred cystectomy before progression was 14% for those receiving and 15% for those not receiving early BCG after a median follow-up for survivors of 4.3 years. In a separate meta-analysis involving 4863 patients in 24 trials, 9.8% of the patients on BCG progressed versus 13.8% in the control group, which represents a 27% reduction in the odds of progression [7]. However, only patients receiving maintenance BCG benefited. The AUA guidelines [9,10] recommend an induction course of BCG for patients with T1 tumors, followed by maintenance therapy; radical cystectomy is considered as an option, particularly in patients who are at an increased risk of progression. The EAU guidelines [11,19] recommend an immediate instillation of chemotherapy followed by intravesical BCG with maintenance for at least 1 year. There has been a plethora of nonrandomized studies dealing with the role of BCG in the management of cT1 bladder cancer showing progression ranging from 10% to 54% [34,36,39,40,42,46−57].

Carcinoma In Situ

Before the adoption of BCG intravesical therapy, CIS reportedly progressed at an average rate of 7% per year [58]. The initial tumor-free response rate is as high as 84% [13,24,27,59−61]. Approximately 50% of patients experience a durable response for a median period of 4 years. Over a 10-year period, approximately 30% of patients remain free from tumor progression or recurrence; therefore, close follow-up is mandatory. The majority of these occur within the first 5 years [62]. Herr and coworkers [63] reported progression in 19% of initial responders at 5 years but found the rate to be 95% in nonresponders, and these findings have been confirmed by other investigators [64,65].

One controlled study provides important clinical information in the management of CIS. The SWOG study of 6-week induction followed by 3-week maintenance BCG vs standard 6-week induction without maintenance included 269 randomized patients with CIS. An increase in complete response (58% at 3 months to 68% at 6 months) was seen in the induction-only arm, suggesting that although residual CIS is a poor prognostic feature, it may take up to 6 months for the full complete response to occur. With three additional weekly BCG maintenance instillations beginning at 3 months, 64% of those with residual CIS at 3 months had resolution at 6 months, yielding an overall complete response rate of 84% [27]. With continued 3-week maintenance BCG after 3 months, >70% of patients with an initial complete response remained tumor-free for >5 years, which is a remarkable achievement considering that many series historically reported progression in 54% of patients with CIS within that same time frame [66].

CIS of the bladder is commonly associated with papillary tumors. In the presence of papillary tumors, all visible tumors should be resected prior to intravesical treatment. Following resection, patients should receive one immediate dose of chemotherapy. If CIS is present in the setting of muscle-invasive disease, therapy is determined by the invasive tumor. If CIS is present together with NMIBC, patients should undergo induction and mainte-nance therapy for a minimum of 1 year with BCG per recommendations of the AUA and EAU [9,11,67]. The AUA guidelines panel supported BCG as the preferred initial treatment option for CIS [9].

Tumor multiplicity and associated CIS increased the risk of progression. Substaging lesions on the basis of the presence or absence of muscularis muco-sae invasion in a series of 49 patients did not improve prediction of recurrence (69% vs 65%) or progression (22% vs 29%) after BCG therapy [68].

When BCG is compared directly to chemotherapy, BCG was similar or superior to other chemotherapy regimens after a review of 12 randomized trials comparing BCG to different chemotherapy regimens, including mito-mycin, electromotive mitomycin, adriamycin, epirubicin, thiotepa, mitomy-cin in conjunction with adriamycin, and BCG in conjunction with mitomycin [7,67]. Among the 845 patients with CIS, a total of 633 patients achieved complete response to therapy, in which the average complete response was 68% in patients treated with BCG and of 49% in those treated with different chemotherapeutic regimens [67]. The average disease-free rate in the BCG and other chemotherapeutic regimens groups of patients was 51% and 27%, respectively, over a median follow-up of 3.75 years. The complete response rate of chemotherapeutic agents such as thiotepa, doxorubicin, and mitomy-cin in CIS patients was 38%, 48%, and 53%, respectively [69], whereas the average complete response was 86.5 [70]. Another Phase II trial looking at the effects of BCG on CIS showed 83% complete response rate [71].

Although reports of the impact of BCG on tumor recurrence are compel-ling, and increasing complete response and disease-free survival rates were shown, the greater need is the potential for impact on progression. BCG has been shown to decrease the risk of progression in all patients with CIS when compared to either chemotherapy or different immunotherapies (12% pro-gression rate when treated with BCG compared to 16% for other treatments) [7]. In 403 patients with CIS, BCG reduced the risk of progression by 35% compared to intravesical chemotherapy. In a randomized trial of 86 patients with high-risk superficial disease, Herr and colleagues demonstrated a greater delay in interval progression for BCG patients versus TUR controls [28]. In addition, the cystectomy rate was significantly decreased for CIS patients treated with BCG (11% vs 55% for controls), as was the time to cystectomy. However, only 27% of patients were alive with an intact func-tioning bladder after a follow-up over 10–15 years, so this apparent advantage is temporary in many cases [29]. Available data suggest that BCG can delay progression of high-risk CIS bladder cancer, yet the long-term survival advantage is not fully defined.

Residual Tumor

Intravesical BCG can effectively treat residual papillary lesions, but it should not be used as a substitute for surgical resection. Investigators have demonstrated a nearly 60% response by residual tumor with intravesical BCG alone [59,64,72]. Carcinoma of the mucosa or the superficial ducts of the prostate can be adequately treated by BCG with a 50% tumor-free rate. A limited TUR or fulguration can be effective in decreasing tumor burden and facilitating exposure of the prostate surface to BCG administration [72,73].

CONTRAINDICATIONS TO BCG THERAPY

During the intravesical instillation in the event of a traumatic catheterization, the treatment should be delayed for several days to 1 week, depending on the extent of injury. Active urinary tract infection is often considered an indication to delay treatment until it has been managed, but recent publications question the need to avoid BCG in the presence of asymptomatic bacteriuria [74].

In general, BCG use in significantly immunosuppressed or immunocompromised patients should be avoided, owing to the infectious risk of BCG. However, other patients with mild immune impairment (e.g., due to steroid use for chronic obstructive pulmonary disease), well controlled HIV, or mature transplants, as well as healthy elderly patients can be treated successfully with minimal adverse effects and good efficacy [75]. In addition, medications such as statins or antiplatelet agents are not contraindications for BCG therapy. Although these drugs have a potentially negative effect on the immune response to BCG treatment, neither had an effect on the clinical efficacy of BCG therapy in multiple clinical studies [76–81]. Further absolute contraindications are suggested for patients, immediately after TUR (within previous 2 weeks), on the basis of the risk of intravasation and septic death, and patients with personal history of BCG sepsis, gross hematuria (intravasation risk), traumatic catheterization (intravasation risk), and total incontinence (patient will not retain agent).

Other relative contraindications are prosthetic valves or orthopedic hardware. However, a large Phase II study with BCG combination therapy reported no infectious complications in the absence of prophylactic antibiotics, suggesting this population represents a low-risk setting [82]. This recommendation is in concordance with the American Heart Association's guideline against antibiotic prophylaxis for genitourinary procedures such as urethral catheterization utilized in BCG administration [83]. Additional relative contraindications are as follows: advanced age, urinary tract infection

TABLE 20.1.4 Contraindications to BCG Administration

Absolute Contraindications

Immunosuppressed and immunocompromised patients*

Immediately after TUR (within previous 2 weeks) on the basis of the risk of intravasation and septic death

Personal history of BCG sepsis

Gross hematuria (intravasation risk)

Traumatic catheterization (intravasation risk)

Total incontinence (patient will not retain agent)

Relative Contraindications

Urinary tract infection (intravasation risk)

Liver disease (precludes treatment with isoniazid if sepsis occurs)

Personal history of tuberculosis (risk theorized but unknown)

Poor overall performance status

Advanced age

Source: Adapted from Jones JS. Non-muscle invasive bladder cancer (Ta, T1, and CIS). In: Wein AJ, editor. Campbell-Walsh Urology. 11th ed. China: Elsevier; 2016. p. 2212–5.

(intravasation risk), liver disease (precludes treatment with isoniazid if sepsis occurs), personal history of tuberculosis (risk theorized but unknown), and poor overall performance status [74,82,83].

Further potential contraindications such as urethral stenosis and active tuberculosis are also suggested in some series of studies; however, ureteral reflux and administration of anti–tumor necrosis factor medications (theoretically predispose to BCG sepsis) are still debatable as contraindications for BCG instillation because of insufficient data [83] (Table 20.1.4).

REFERENCES

[1] Old LJ, Clarke DA, Benacerraf B. Effect of bacillus Calmette-Guerin infection on transplanted tumours in the mouse. Nature 1959;184(Suppl 5):291–2.

[2] Morales A, Eidinger D, Bruce AW. Intracavitary bacillus Calmette-Guerin in the treatment of superficial bladder tumors. J Urol 1976;116(2):180–3.

[3] Oddens J, Brausi M, Sylvester R, et al. Final results of an EORTC-GU cancers group randomized study of maintenance bacillus Calmette-Guérin in intermediate- and high-risk Ta, T1 papillary carcinoma of the urinary bladder: one-third dose versus full dose and 1 year versus 3 years of maintenance. Eur Urol 2013;63(3):462–72.

[4] Lamm DL, Thor DE, Harris SC, Reyna JA, Stogdill VD, Radwin HM. Bacillus Calmette-Guerin immunotherapy of superficial bladder cancer. J Urol 1980;124 (1):38–40.

[5] Brausi M, Witjes JA, Lamm D, Persad R, Palou J, Colombel M, et al. A review of current guidelines and best practice recommendations for the management of nonmuscle invasive bladder cancer by the International Bladder Cancer Group. J Urol 2011;186(6):2158−67.

[6] Ojea A, Nogueira JL, Solsona E, Flores N, Gomez JM, Molina JR, et al. A multicentre, randomised prospective trial comparing three intravesical adjuvant therapies for intermediate-risk superficial bladder cancer: low-dose bacillus Calmette-Guerin (27 mg) versus very low-dose bacillus Calmette-Guerin (13.5 mg) versus mitomycin C. Eur Urol 2007;52(5):1398−406.

[7] Sylvester RJ, van der MA, Lamm DL. Intravesical bacillus Calmette-Guerin reduces the risk of progression in patients with superficial bladder cancer: a meta-analysis of the published results of randomized clinical trials. J Urol 2002;168(5):1964−70.

[8] Gontero P, Bohle A, Malmstrom PU, O'Donnell MA, Oderda M, Sylvester R, et al. The role of bacillus Calmette-Guerin in the treatment of non-muscle-invasive bladder cancer. Eur Urol 2010;57(3):410−29.

[9] Hall MC, Chang SS, Dalbagni G, Pruthi RS, Seigne JD, Skinner EC, et al. Guideline for the management of nonmuscle invasive bladder cancer (stages Ta, T1, and Tis): 2007 update. J Urol 2007;178(6):2314−30.

[10] Chang SS, Boorjian SA, Chou R, Clark PE, Daneshmand S, Konety BR, et al. Diagnosis and treatment of non-muscle invasive bladder cancer: AUA/SUO guideline. J Urol 2016.

[11] Babjuk M, Burger M, Zigeuner R, Shariat SF, van Rhijn BW, Comperat E, et al. EAU guidelines on non-muscle-invasive urothelial carcinoma of the bladder: update 2013. Eur Urol 2013;64(4):639−53.

[12] Clark PE, Agarwal N, Biagioli MC, Eisenberger MA, Greenberg RE, Herr HW, et al. Bladder cancer. J Natl Compr Canc Netw 2013;11(4):446−75.

[13] Lamm DL, Riggs DL, Bugaj M, et al. Prophylaxis in bladder cancer: a meta-analysis. J Urol 2000;163:151−5.

[14] Kassouf W, Traboulsi SL, Kulkarni GS, Breau RH, Zlotta A, Fairey A, et al. CUA guidelines on the management of non-muscle invasive bladder cancer. Can Urol Assoc J 2015;9(9−10):E690−704.

[15] Burger M, Oosterlinck W, Konety B, Chang S, Gudjonsson S, Pruthi R, et al. ICUD-EAU International Consultation on Bladder Cancer 2012: non-muscle-invasive urothelial carcinoma of the bladder. Eur Urol 2013;63(1):36−44.

[16] National Comprehensive Cancer Network. NCCN Clinical Practice Guidelines in Oncology. 2017. https://www.nccn.org/professionals/physician_gls/pdf/bladder.pdf.

[17] Nieder AM, Brausi M, Lamm D, O'Donnell M, Tomita K, Woo H, et al. Management of stage T1 tumors of the bladder: International Consensus Panel. Urology 2005;66(6 Suppl 1):108−25.

[18] Mack D, Holtl W, Bassi P, Brausi M, Ferrari P, de Balincourt C, et al. The ablative effect of quarter dose bacillus Calmette-Guerin on a papillary marker lesion of the bladder. J Urol 2001;165(2):401−3.

[19] Babjuk M, Bohle A, Burger M, Capoun O, Cohen D, Comperat EM, et al. EAU guidelines on non-muscle-invasive urothelial carcinoma of the bladder: update 2016. Eur Urol 2016.

[20] Sylvester RJ, van der Meijden AP, Oosterlinck W, Witjes JA, Bouffioux C, Denis L, et al. Predicting recurrence and progression in individual patients with stage Ta T1 bladder cancer using EORTC risk tables: a combined analysis of 2596 patients from seven EORTC trials. Eur Urol 2006;49(3):466−75.

[21] Sylvester RJ, Brausi MA, Kirkels WJ, Hoeltl W, Calais Da Silva F, Powell PH, et al. Long-term efficacy results of EORTC genito-urinary group randomized phase 3 study

30911 comparing intravesical instillations of epirubicin, bacillus Calmette-Guerin, and bacillus Calmette-Guerin plus isoniazid in patients with intermediate- and high-risk stage Ta T1 urothelial carcinoma of the bladder. Eur Urol 2010;57(5):766−73.

[22] Malmstrom PU, Sylvester RJ, Crawford DE, Friedrich M, Krege S, Rintala E, et al. An individual patient data meta-analysis of the long-term outcome of randomised studies comparing intravesical mitomycin C versus bacillus Calmette-Guerin for non-muscle-invasive bladder cancer. Eur Urol 2009;56(2):247−56.

[23] National Comprehensive Cancer Network. NCCN Clinical Practice Guidelines in Oncology: Bladder Cancer. 2014.

[24] Lamm DL, Dehaven JI, Riggs DR. Keyhole limpet hemocyanin immunotherapy of bladder cancer: laboratory and clinical studies. Eur Urol 2000;37(Suppl 3):41−4.

[25] Lamm Dea. Clinical practice recommendations for the management of non−muscle invasive bladder cancer. Eur Urol 2008;(Suppl. 7):651−66.

[26] Kassouf W, Traboulsi SL, Schmitz-Drager B, Palou J, Witjes JA, van Rhijn BW, et al. Follow-up in non-muscle-invasive bladder cancer—International Bladder Cancer Network recommendations. Urol Oncol 2016;34(10):460−8.

[27] Lamm DL, Blumenstein BA, Crissman JD, Montie JE, Gottesman JE, Lowe BA, et al. Maintenance bacillus Calmette-Guerin immunotherapy for recurrent TA, T1 and carcinoma in situ transitional cell carcinoma of the bladder: a randomized Southwest Oncology Group Study. J Urol 2000;163(4):1124−9.

[28] Kamat AM, Witjes JA, Brausi M, Soloway M, Lamm D, Persad R, et al. Defining and treating the spectrum of intermediate risk nonmuscle invasive bladder cancer. J Urol 2014;192(2):305−15.

[29] Bohle A, Bock PR. Intravesical bacille Calmette-Guerin versus mitomycin C in superficial bladder cancer: formal meta-analysis of comparative studies on tumor progression. Urology 2004;63(4):682−6.

[30] Bohle A, Jocham D, Bock PR. Intravesical bacillus Calmette-Guerin versus mitomycin C for superficial bladder cancer: a formal meta-analysis of comparative studies on recurrence and toxicity. J Urol 2003;169(1):90−5.

[31] Han RF, Pan JG. Can intravesical bacillus Calmette-Guerin reduce recurrence in patients with superficial bladder cancer? A meta-analysis of randomized trials. Urology 2006;67 (6):1216−23.

[32] Shelley MD, Kynaston H, Court J, Wilt TJ, Coles B, Burgon K, et al. A systematic review of intravesical bacillus Calmette-Guerin plus transurethral resection vs transurethral resection alone in Ta and T1 bladder cancer. BJU Int 2001;88(3):209−16.

[33] Shelley MD, Wilt TJ, Court J, Coles B, Kynaston H, Mason MD. Intravesical bacillus Calmette-Guerin is superior to mitomycin C in reducing tumour recurrence in high-risk superficial bladder cancer: a meta-analysis of randomized trials. BJU Int 2004;93 (4):485−90.

[34] Cookson MS, Sarosdy MF. Management of stage T1 superficial bladder cancer with intravesical bacillus Calmette-Guerin therapy. J Urol 1992;148(3):797−801.

[35] Gohji K, Nomi M, Okamoto M, Takenaka A, Hara I, Okada H, et al. Conservative therapy for stage T1b, grade 3 transitional cell carcinoma of the bladder. Urology 1999;53 (2):308−13.

[36] Herr HW. Tumour progression and survival in patients with T1G3 bladder tumours: 15-year outcome. Br J Urol 1997;80(5):762−5.

[37] Hurle R, Losa A, Manzetti A, Lembo A. Intravesical bacille Calmette-Guerin in Stage T1 grade 3 bladder cancer therapy: a 7-year follow-up. Urology 1999;54(2):258−63.

[38] Hurle R, Losa A, Manzetti A, Lembo A. Upper urinary tract tumors developing after treatment of superficial bladder cancer: 7-year follow-up of 591 consecutive patients. Urology 1999;53(6):1144–8.

[39] Jimenez-Cruz JF, Vera-Donoso CD, Leiva O, Pamplona M, Rioja-Sanz LA, Martinez-Lasierra M, et al. Intravesical immunoprophylaxis in recurrent superficial bladder cancer (Stage T1): multicenter trial comparing bacille Calmette-Guerin and interferon-alpha. Urology 1997;50(4):529–35.

[40] Pansadoro V, Emiliozzi P, Defidio L, Donadio D, Florio A, Maurelli S, et al. Bacillus Calmette-Guerin in the treatment of stage T1 grade 3 transitional cell carcinoma of the bladder: long-term results. J Urol 1995;154(6):2054–8.

[41] Hara I, Miyake H, Takechi Y, Eto H, Gotoh A, Fujisawa M, et al. Clinical outcome of conservative therapy for stage T1, grade 3 transitional cell carcinoma of the bladder. Int J Urol 2003;10(1):19–24.

[42] Patard J, Moudouni S, Saint F, Rioux-Leclercq N, Manunta A, Guy L, et al. Tumor progression and survival in patients with T1G3 bladder tumors: multicentric retrospective study comparing 94 patients treated during 17 years. Urology 2001;58(4):551–6.

[43] Dalbagni G, Vora K, Kaag M, Cronin A, Bochner B, Donat SM, et al. Clinical outcome in a contemporary series of restaged patients with clinical T1 bladder cancer. Eur Urol 2009;56(6):903–10.

[44] Shahin O, Thalmann GN, Rentsch C, Mazzucchelli L, Studer UE. A retrospective analysis of 153 patients treated with or without intravesical bacillus Calmette-Guerin for primary stage T1 grade 3 bladder cancer: recurrence, progression and survival. J Urol 2003;169 (1):96–100.

[45] Dalbagni G, Kaag M, Cronin A, Vora K, Bochner B, Donat SM, et al. Variability of treatment selection among surgeons for patients with cT1 urothelial carcinoma. BJU Int 2010;106(10):1502–7.

[46] Baniel J, Grauss D, Engelstein D, Sella A. Intravesical bacillus Calmette-Guerin treatment for Stage T1 grade 3 transitional cell carcinoma of the bladder. Urology 1998;52 (5):785–9.

[47] Boccon-Gibod L, Leleu C, Herve JM, Belas M, Steg A. Bladder tumors invading the lamina propria (stage A/T1): influence of endovesical bacillus Calmette-Guerin therapy on recurrence and progression. Eur Urol 1989;16(6):401–4.

[48] Brake M, Loertzer H, Horsch R, Keller H. Long-term results of intravesical bacillus Calmette-Guerin therapy for stage T1 superficial bladder cancer. Urology 2000;55 (5):673–8.

[49] Brake M, Loertzer H, Horsch R, Keller H. Recurrence and progression of stage T1, grade 3 transitional cell carcinoma of the bladder following intravesical immunotherapy with bacillus Calmette-Guerin. J Urol 2000;163(6):1697–701.

[50] Dalbagni G, Herr HW. Current use and questions concerning intravesical bladder cancer group for superficial bladder cancer. Urol Clin North Am 2000;27(1):137–46.

[51] Eure GR, Cundiff MR, Schellhammer PF. Bacillus Calmette-Guerin therapy for high risk stage T1 superficial bladder cancer. J Urol 1992;147(2):376–9.

[52] Gunlusoy B, Degirmenci T, Arslan M, Nergiz N, Minareci S, Ayder AR. Recurrence and progression of T1G3 transitional cell carcinoma of the bladder treated with intravesical bacillus Calmette-Guerin. Urol Int 2005;75(2):107–13.

[53] Herr HW, Laudone VP, Badalament RA, Oettgen HF, Sogani PC, Freedman BD, et al. Bacillus Calmette-Guerin therapy alters the progression of superficial bladder cancer. J Clin Oncol 1988;6(9):1450–5.

[54] Hurle R, Losa A, Ranieri A, Graziotti P, Lembo A. Low dose Pasteur bacillus Calmette-Guerin regimen in stage T1, grade 3 bladder cancer therapy. J Urol 1996;156(5):1602–5.

[55] Kulkarni JN, Gupta R. Recurrence and progression in stage T1G3 bladder tumour with intravesical bacille Calmette-Guerin (Danish 1331 strain). BJU Int 2002;90(6):554–7.

[56] Pansadoro V, Emiliozzi P, depaula F, Scarpone P, Pizzo M, Federico G, et al. High grade superficial (G3t1) transitional cell carcinoma of the bladder treated with intravesical Bacillus Calmette-Guerin (BCG). J Exp Clin Cancer Res 2003;22(4 Suppl):223–7.

[57] Semper M JR, Solsona E, Fernandez J, Dorrego JM, et al. Treatment of carcinoma in situ of the bladder associated or not associated to non-muscle invasive transitional carcinoma using two different BCG doses: the standard or one third dose. A five year follow-up. Eur Urol Supp 2010;9:91.

[58] Zincke H, Utz DC, Farrow GM. Review of Mayo clinic experience with carcinoma in situ. Urology 1985;26(4 Suppl):39–46.

[59] Brosman SA. Experience with bacillus Calmette-Guerin in patients with superficial bladder carcinoma. J Urol 1982;128(1):27–30.

[60] De Jager R, Guinan P, Lamm D, Khanna O, Brosman S, De Kernion J, et al. Long-term complete remission in bladder carcinoma in situ with intravesical TICE bacillus Calmette Guerin. Overview analysis of six phase II clinical trials. Urology 1991;38(6):507–13.

[61] Hudson MA, Herr HW. Carcinoma in situ of the bladder. J Urol 1995;153(3 Pt 1):564–72.

[62] Herr HW, Wartinger DD, Fair WR, Oettgen HF. Bacillus Calmette-Guerin therapy for superficial bladder cancer: a 10-year follow-up. J Urol 1992;147(4):1020–3.

[63] Herr HW, Badalament RA, Amato DA, Laudone VP, Fair WR, Whitmore Jr. WF. Superficial bladder cancer treated with bacillus Calmette-Guerin: a multivariate analysis of factors affecting tumor progression. J Urol 1989;141(1):22–9.

[64] Coplen DE, Marcus MD, Myers JA, Ratliff TL, Catalona WJ. Long-term follow up of patients treated with 1 or 2, 6-week courses of intravesical bacillus Calmette-Guerin: analysis of possible predictors of response free of tumor. J Urol 1990;144(3):652–7.

[65] Harland SJ, Charig CR, Highman W, Parkinson MC, Riddle PR. Outcome in carcinoma in situ of bladder treated with intravesical bacille Calmette-Guerin. Br J Urol 1992;70 (3):271–5.

[66] Lamm DL. Carcinoma in situ. Urol Clin North Am 1992;19(3):499–508.

[67] van der Meijden AP, Sylvester R, Oosterlinck W, Solsona E, Boehle A, Lobel B, et al. EAU guidelines on the diagnosis and treatment of urothelial carcinoma in situ. Eur Urol 2005;48(3):363–71.

[68] Kondylis FI, Demirci S, Ladaga L, Kolm P, Schellhammer PF. Outcomes after intravesical bacillus Calmette-Guerin are not affected by substaging of high grade T1 transitional cell carcinoma. J Urol 2000;163(4):1120–3.

[69] Lamm D, Herr H, Jakse G, Kuroda M, Mostofi FK, Okajima E, et al. Updated concepts and treatment of carcinoma in situ. Urol Oncol 1998;4(4–5):130–8.

[70] Takenaka A, Yamada Y, Miyake H, Hara I, Fujisawa M. Clinical outcomes of bacillus Calmette-Guerin instillation therapy for carcinoma in situ of urinary bladder. Int J Urol 2008;15(4):309–13.

[71] Jakse G, Hall R, Bono A, Holtl W, Carpentier P, Spaander JP, et al. Intravesical BCG in patients with carcinoma in situ of the urinary bladder: long-term results of EORTC GU Group phase II protocol 30861. Eur Urol 2001;40(2):144–50.

[72] Schellhammer PF, Ladaga LE, Moriarty RP. Intravesical bacillus Calmette-Guerin for the treatment of superficial transitional cell carcinoma of the prostatic urethra in association with carcinoma of the bladder. J Urol 1995;153(1):53–6.

[73] Bretton PR, Herr HW, Kimmel M, Whitmore Jr. WF, Laudone V, Oettgen HF, et al. The response of patients with superficial bladder cancer to a second course of intravesical bacillus Calmette-Guerin. J Urol 1990;143(4):710−12. Discussion 23.

[74] Herr HW. Intravesical bacillus Calmette-Guerin outcomes in patients with bladder cancer and asymptomatic bacteriuria. J Urol 2012;187(2):435−7.

[75] Gaughan EM, Dezube BJ, Bower M, Aboulafia DM, Bohac G, Cooley TP, et al. HIV-associated bladder cancer: a case series evaluating difficulties in diagnosis and management. BMC Urol 2009;9:10.

[76] Berglund RK, Savage CJ, Vora KC, Kurta JM, Cronin AM. An analysis of the effect of statin use on the efficacy of bacillus Calmette-Guerin treatment for transitional cell carcinoma of the bladder. J Urol 2008;180(4):1297−300. discussion 300.

[77] Crivelli JJ, Xylinas E, Kluth LA, da Silva RD, Chrystal J, Novara G, et al. Effect of statin use on outcomes of non-muscle-invasive bladder cancer. BJU Int 2013;112(2):E4−12.

[78] Gee JR, Jarrard DF, Bruskewitz RC, Moon TD, Hedican SP, Leverson GE, et al. Reduced bladder cancer recurrence rate with cardioprotective aspirin after intravesical bacille Calmette-Guerin. BJU Int 2009;103(6):736−9.

[79] Hoffmann P, Roumeguere T, Schulman C, van Velthoven R. Use of statins and outcome of BCG treatment for bladder cancer. N Engl J Med 2006;355(25):2705−7.

[80] Joudi FN, Smith BJ, O'Donnell MA, Konety BR. The impact of age on the response of patients with superficial bladder cancer to intravesical immunotherapy. J Urol 2006;175 (5):1634−9.

[81] Kamat AM, Wu X. Statins and the effect of BCG on bladder cancer. N Engl J Med 2007;356(12):1276. author reply -7.

[82] Ehlers S. Why does tumor necrosis factor targeted therapy reactivate tuberculosis? J Rheumatol Suppl 2005;74:35−9.

[83] Jones JS. Non-muscle invasive bladder cancer (Ta, T1, and CIS). In: Wein AJ, editor. Campbell-Walsh Urology. 11th ed. China: Elsevier; 2016. p. 2212−5.

Chapter 20.2

Optimal BCG Schedule

Sung Han Kim and Ho Kyung Seo
Research Institute and National Cancer Center, Goyang, South Korea

INTRODUCTION

The improvement of survival outcomes of patients who undergo bacille Calmette−Guerin (BCG) immunotherapy that is observed in randomized control trials (RCTs) is confirmed in real-world practice research pattern. A review of data from about 24,000 patients with bladder cancer from the Surveillance, Epidemiology, and End Results (SEER)−Medicare database suggests that the use of BCG significantly reduces mortality (hazard ratio,

0.87), and deaths due to bladder cancer are reduced by 23% in patients with high-grade tumors [1]. Available data suggest that BCG can also delay the progression of high-risk bladder cancer, yet the long-term survival advantage is not fully defined. In contrast, no chemotherapy trial has achieved a significant reduction in progression [2]. Nevertheless, two meta-analyses have concluded that BCG reduces the risk of progression. Progression during a median follow-up period of 2.5 years was reduced by 27% (9.8% for BCG vs 13.8% for non-BCG) in one study [3] and by 23% (7.7% for BCG vs 9.4% for mitomycin C; MMC) during a median follow-up period of 26 months in another study [4]. In both studies, the superior results of BCG were seen only in trials using BCG maintenance therapy. While most agree on a 6-week induction cycle, a 6-week induction course alone is insufficient to obtain an optimal response in many patients, and maintenance therapy is a requisite. The American Urological Association (AUA) and The European Association of Urology (EAU) guidelines panel concluded that BCG appeared likely to reduce progression [5,6].

INDUCTION BCG REGIMEN: A 6-WEEK SCHEDULE

The original BCG protocol was initially conceived by a Canadian urologist, Morales, in 1972 [7]. He obtained the BCG strain manufactured at the Institut Armand-Frappier Research Centre. Morales suggested that to establish a delayed hypersensitivity reaction, a minimum of 3 weeks of treatment was necessary and would be gauged by an intradermal BCG injection. Additionally, he had determined that adverse effects resolved within 1 week, prompting him to adopt a weekly schedule. The Armand-Frappier BCG vaccine was packaged as 120 mg each and dispensed in six separate vials, therefore establishing a 6-week bladder instillation protocol. Systemic immune responses were higher after percutaneous vaccination than after intravesical administration alone. Therefore, the 6-week course of intravesical and percutaneous BCG suggested by Morales· was very effective [8]. The study revealed that 6-week intravesical plus percutaneous administrations resulted in a 12-fold reduction in bladder tumor recurrence. However, other RCTs failed to demonstrate the improved efficacy of percutaneous BCG in treating bladder cancer, and Morales wrote in the reply to an editorial comment to his landmark article that his regimen was arbitrary and might be modified in the future as additional data become available.

The success of the treatment proposed by Morales prompted the National Cancer Institute to request proposals for controlled human clinical trials using Morales' technique, and contracts were awarded to Lamm at the University of Texas in San Antonio and Pinsky at Memorial Sloan-Kettering Cancer Center (MSKCC) in New York. The initial BCG RCT, published in 1980, showed statistically significant reduction in tumor recurrence in 54 evaluable patients [9] and showed an advantage that increased with duration of follow-up time [10].

Similar results were reported in much higher risk patients in the MSKCC study [11]. Subsequent follow-up of these patients suggested that the benefit of a single 6-week course of intravesical plus percutaneous BCG provided long-term protection from tumor recurrence and even reduced disease progression. However, the 15-year follow-up of the MSKCC series showed the limitations of BCG protection without initiation of maintenance therapy. In Herr's [12] series, which was in agreement with the initial findings of a 10-year conferred protection in the MSKCC series [11], a significant reduction in tumor recurrence, disease progression, and mortality persisted for 10 years but was no longer significant at 15 years. While 6-week induction of BCG reduced recurrence, progression, and mortality at 10 years, this effect was not observed after 15 years, and patients remained at high risk for progression and development of disease in the prostatic urethra (24%) and upper urinary tracts (25%). The mortality rate was 32% in patients with disease progression into the upper urinary tracts and 44% in those with prostatic urothelial involvement [12]. Therefore, a 6-week induction course alone is insufficient to obtain an optimal response in many patients, and maintenance therapy is a requisite [13−16]. In additional animal studies, no benefit of BCG maintenance was seen at 9 months but a highly significant benefit was observed at 15 months [17].

Bohle and others reported, years later, that 6 weeks were ideal for maximum response to BCG although maintenance dosing enhanced response even further [4,18]. While most agree on a 6-week induction cycle, various maintenance schedules (if any at all) have also been implemented without a unifying consensus [19]. However, recent studies have failed to demonstrate that alternative schedules provide significant benefits. Early modifications, such as the omission of percutaneous vaccination and quarterly or monthly maintenance, although accepted, only marginally improve convenience or efficacy.

SECOND 6-WEEK INDUCTION SCHEDULE

The average additional response to a second induction course is 25% in those patients treated for prophylaxis and 30% in patients with carcinoma in situ (CIS) [3,4,20−23]. However, additional courses of BCG to treat refractory patients after a second 6-week course are accompanied by a significant risk of tumor progression in 20%−50% of patients [24]. Catalona and colleagues [25] reported roughly a 7% actual risk of progression in CIS with every additional course of BCG therapy. Response to BCG at 6 months can be used as a predictor of prognosis, with the number of patients developing progressive disease being significantly higher among nonresponders [26].

MAINTENANCE BCG REGIMEN

It has been proven that induction BCG is highly effective in reducing disease recurrence, but the role of maintenance BCG and its ability to reduce disease progression and mortality has been a matter of debate. Lamm [10] initially reported a fourfold reduction in the rate of tumor recurrence in patients treated with quarterly single BCG instillations. A controlled evaluation of this regimen in 1987 in 42 patients failed to show a significant reduction in tumor recurrence [27]. In the same year, Badalament et al. [28] reported an RCT involving 93 patients, which compared 6-week induction with monthly maintenance BCG, and found no significant benefit for maintenance therapy. These limitations of these studies are as follows: a relatively short follow-up period and lack of power; nevertheless, they had a major impact on clinical practice. Palou et al. [16] found that 6-week maintenance BCG every 6 months for 2 years was not significantly effective than induction alone in a study of 126 patients with CIS who were followed for an average of 79 months. Kamat and Porten stated in their article that RCTs of quarterly, monthly, and repeated 6-week BCG instillations, which aimed at maintaining the immune response, also failed to show a significant improvement of efficacy [29]. However, many urologists have adopted an initial 6-week BCG induction course followed by a repeat 6-week cycle at the time of tumor recurrence despite the absence of RCTs supporting this approach. Currently, all these results have led some experts to question the value of maintenance BCG, the optimal schedule, and to abandon its use [19].

Despite these "negative" studies, maintenance therapy may be the most important advancement in BCG treatment of bladder cancer since the introduction of Morales's original 6-week induction regimen. While other presumably inferior maintenance schedules have not achieved statistical significance in RCTs, a meta-analysis showed that induction plus maintenance BCG is superior to induction BCG alone and may be required as the most important benefit of BCG for the reduction of tumor progression [3]. A meta-analysis of 2000 patients with Ta, T1, and/or CIS disease found that patients receiving maintenance BCG had a statistically decreased rate of recurrence compared to those receiving induction therapy alone [30]. Based on another meta-analysis, maintenance BCG schedule was found to be essential in preventing disease progression [31].

SWOG TRIAL OF 3-WEEK MAINTENANCE SCHEDULE

By contrast to the prior failed maintenance therapy, the potential benefit of 3-week BCG maintenance, designed by the SWOG, taking into account the immunological principles, is different from the other BCG regimes, and it should not be considered in the same category as the other maintenance BCG regimens [13]. A controlled trial of 384 patients using an immunologically sound maintenance schedule, received a 6-week induction course followed by 3-week instillations at 3 and 6 months, and every 6 months thereafter for 3 years after routine cystoscopy at 3, 6, 12, 18, 24, 30, and 36 months. The estimated median recurrence-free survival was 76.8 months in the maintenance arm and 35.7 months in the control arm ($P = 0.0001$). The average recurrence-free survival was 111.5 months in the control arm and was not able to be estimated in the maintenance arm ($P = 0.04$). Overall, the 5-year survival rate was 78% in the control arm and 83% in the maintenance arm. No toxicities above Grade 3 were observed, yet only 16% of patients tolerated the full-dose schedule regimen (compliance in modern studies is higher than that in the original studies). Two-thirds of the patients who stopped receiving BCG because of side effects did so in the first 6 months, suggesting that the side effects do not increase appreciably with additional time on therapy. An interpretation that the intended full course of maintenance therapy cannot be accomplished in most patients because of side effects is misleading. Owing to the fact that the treatment group recovered better despite most patients having failed to complete the full course of therapy, the maximum benefit may have been achieved earlier. In summary, 3-week maintenance BCG markedly reduced long-term recurrence and worsening disease defined as stage progression or the requirement for cystectomy, radiation therapy, or systemic chemotherapy [13].

Shorter maintenance schedules and reduced dosages may accomplish the same results with less toxicity [13]. For high-grade T1 lesions or CIS, maintenance therapy has been proven to be effective in multiple studies [16]. The determination of whether the optimal treatment schedule should be as described in the SWOG study, monthly, or on some other schedule remains undefined, and optimal duration of a monthly maintenance schedule, if chosen, is unknown [13–15,32].

COMPARISON OF 3-WEEK BCG MAINTENANCE THERAPY TO SURGERY, CHEMOTHERAPY, OR OTHER IMMUNOTHERAPY

In the meta-analysis by Bohle et al. [4], all six comparison studies using maintenance BCG schedules found BCG to be clearly superior to MMC, whereas only one study reported statistical significance in groups not using maintenance BCG. However, the most convincing data are in the meta-analysis published by Sylvester et al. [3], with analysis of 24 studies comprising 4863 patients. BCG was compared with surgery, chemotherapy, or other immunotherapy with endpoints of disease progression and cancer-specific mortality being investigated. Disease progression was significantly reduced by 37% ($P < 0.001$); however, this benefit was only seen in patients receiving maintenance BCG. Bladder cancer mortality was reduced by 19%, but statistical significance was not achieved ($P = 0.20$) due to the short median follow-up of only 2.5 months. Malmström et al. [34] analyzed nine

RCTs comparing the long-term efficacy of intravesical MMC to BCG (induction alone and with maintenance) with time to first recurrence as the primary endpoint. BCG maintenance was found to confer a 32% reduction in the risk of recurrence compared to MMC, producing a statistically significant 4% difference against trials without BCG maintenance ($P < 0.001$). It was determined that for prophylaxis against recurrence, BCG maintenance was required to achieve the demonstrable superiority to MMC. Subsequent randomized clinical trials have shown that the 3-week, 3-year maintenance schedule used by the SWOG has achieved success that dwarfs that of other intravesical treatments [13]. In a European study of 957 patients with intermediate-to-high-risk bladder cancer without CIS, the 3-week maintenance schedule was compared to intravesical epirubicin chemotherapy using the same schedule. The 3-week maintenance BCG regimen significantly decreased recurrence ($P < 0.001$), metastasis ($P < 0.046$), and improved overall and disease-specific survival ($P < 0.023$) [1]. In a subsequent study assessing 3 years of BCG maintenance against 1 year maintenance therapy while maintaining a 3-week instillation schedule, full dose 3-week maintenance for 3 years significantly reduced recurrence compared to one-third dose of BCG maintenance for 1 year [35]. A subsequent reevaluation of the published data concluded that 3 years of maintenance therapy was supported by the literature but that patients with intermediate-risk disease may be equally managed with 1 year of maintenance [36].

THREE-WEEK MAINTENANCE SCHEDULE IN HIGH-GRADE TUMORS (INCLUDING CIS)

The recommendations for the use of BCG in high-grade tumors are relatively consistent across guidelines; variations mainly exist in the recommended duration of therapy. The AUA, EUA, and International Bladder Cancer Group (IBCG) advise BCG induction with 1–3 years of maintenance for all high-grade tumors [5,6,37]. The International Consultation on Urological Diseases (ICUD) guidelines for Ta high-grade tumors do not include maintenance BCG, remarking a lack of conclusive evidence about the effect of maintenance BCG on disease progression in these tumors. In addition, the efficacy of maintenance therapy in treating T1 disease has been a matter of debate [38]. CIS is the only condition for which maintenance is advised by ICUD, and the guideline also includes reinduction of BCG instillations if no response is detected at first evaluation [38]. The NCCN recommends BCG as the standard treatment for CIS only but includes BCG as the favorable choice of treatment for high-grade Ta and T1 tumors and suggests that maintenance should be considered [39].

In the population with CIS, complete response at 6 months in patients randomized to receive the initial 6-week BCG treatment only (induction arm) was 69% in comparison to 84% ($P < 0.01$) in patients randomized to receive the additional 3-week maintenance treatment (maintenance arm) [13]. In the maintenance arm, complete response increased from 55% at 3 months to 84% at 6 months (64% complete response in patients with treatment failure at 3 months). Even without additional BCG, 26% of patients with residual disease at 3 months in the induction arm went on to have complete response by 6 months, illustrating that 6 months is a preferred time to evaluate response.

Significant improvement in the treatment of CIS was confirmed by other RCTs with 3-week maintenance BCG, but no other treatment has Level 1 evidence of superiority to induction BCG. The most commonly used treatment, repeated 6-week instillations have been found to be ineffective in one RCT [40]. Five RCTs compared non-3-week maintenance schedules to BCG induction only [28]. None of these alternative maintenance schedules showed a statistically significant reduction in recurrence (range, 4%−22%; average, 7%). By contrast, two studies that compared 3-week maintenance to induction treatment alone showed a statistically significant 28% reduction in tumor recurrence [13,41]. Moreover, only the 3-week BCG maintenance schedule reduced disease progression and metastasis, as well as overall and cancer-specific mortality in RCTs [1,13].

Two other trials compared the 3-week maintenance BCG regimen with alternative agents [1,42]. EORTC 30911 compared the 3-week maintenance BCG with 3-week maintenance epirubicin chemotherapy with/without interferon-2 beta. BCG significantly reduced recurrence by 15%, metastasis by 45% ($P = 0.046$), and both overall ($P = 0.023$) and cancer-specific mortality ($P = 0.026$) [1]. No other intravesical treatment, BCG induction only, or non-3-week maintenance BCG schedule has achieved such success. Additionally, in the Duchek et al.'s randomized prospective study, at 24 months there was a significant difference in favor of BCG-treated patients regarding recurrence, although there was no difference in progression [42]. This effect was more pronounced in patients with concomitant CIS.

REFERENCES

[1] Sylvester RJ, Brausi MA, Kirkels WJ, Hoeltl W, Calais Da Silva F, Powell PH, et al. Long-term efficacy results of EORTC genito-urinary group randomized phase 3 study 30911 comparing intravesical instillations of epirubicin, bacillus Calmette-Guerin, and bacillus Calmette-Guerin plus isoniazid in patients with intermediate- and high-risk stage Ta T1 urothelial carcinoma of the bladder. Eur Urol 2010;57(5):766−73.

[2] Grossman HB, O'Donnell MA, Cookson MS, Greenberg RE, Keane TE. Bacillus calmette-guerin failures and beyond: contemporary management of non-muscle-invasive bladder cancer. Rev Urol 2008;10(4):281−9.

[3] Sylvester RJ, van der MA, Lamm DL. Intravesical bacillus Calmette-Guerin reduces the risk of progression in patients with superficial bladder cancer: a meta-analysis of the published results of randomized clinical trials. J Urol 2002;168(5):1964−70.

[4] Bohle A, Bock PR. Intravesical bacille Calmette-Guerin versus mitomycin C in superficial bladder cancer: formal meta-analysis of comparative studies on tumor progression. Urology 2004;63(4):682−6. discussion 6−7.

[5]   Hall MC, Chang SS, Dalbagni G, Pruthi RS, Seigne JD, Skinner EC, et al. Guideline for the management of nonmuscle invasive bladder cancer (stages Ta, T1, and Tis): 2007 update. J Urol 2007;178(6):2314–30.

[6]   Babjuk M, Burger M, Zigeuner R, Shariat SF, van Rhijn BW, Comperat E, et al. EAU guidelines on non-muscle-invasive urothelial carcinoma of the bladder: update 2013. Eur Urol 2013;64(4):639–53.

[7]   Herr HW, Morales A. History of bacillus Calmette-Guerin and bladder cancer: an immunotherapy success story. J Urol 2008;179(1):53–6.

[8]   Morales A, Eidinger D, Bruce AW. Intracavitary Bacillus Calmette-Guerin in the treatment of superficial bladder tumors. J Urol 1976;116(2):180–3.

[9]   Lamm DL, Thor DE, Harris SC, Reyna JA, Stogdill VD, Radwin HM. Bacillus Calmette-Guerin immunotherapy of superficial bladder cancer. J Urol 1980;124(1):38–40.

[10] Lamm DL. Bacillus Calmette-Guerin immunotherapy. J Urol 1987;138(2):391–2.

[11] Pinsky CM, Camacho FJ, Kerr D, Geller NL, Klein FA, Herr HA, et al. Intravesical administration of bacillus Calmette-Guerin in patients with recurrent superficial carcinoma of the urinary bladder: report of a prospective, randomized trial. Cancer Treat Rep 1985;69(1):47–53.

[12] Herr HW. Extravesical tumor relapse in patients with superficial bladder tumors. J Clin Oncol 1998;16(3):1099–102.

[13] Lamm DL, Blumenstein BA, Crissman JD, Montie JE, Gottesman JE, Lowe BA, et al. Maintenance bacillus Calmette-Guerin immunotherapy for recurrent TA, T1 and carcinoma in situ transitional cell carcinoma of the bladder: a randomized Southwest Oncology Group Study. J Urol 2000;163(4):1124–9.

[14] Lamm DL, Dehaven JI, Riggs DR. Keyhole limpet hemocyanin immunotherapy of bladder cancer: laboratory and clinical studies. Eur Urol 2000;37(Suppl 3):41–4.

[15] Lamm DL, Riggs DL, Bugaj M, et al. Prophylaxis in bladder cancer: a metaanalysis. J Urol 2000;163:151–5.

[16] Palou J, Laguna P, Millan-Rodriguez F, Hall RR, Salvador-Bayarri J, Vicente-Rodriguez J. Control group and maintenance treatment with bacillus Calmette-Guerin for carcinoma in situ and/or high grade bladder tumors. J Urol 2001;165(5):1488–91.

[17] Reichert DF, Lamm DL. Long term protection in bladder cancer following intralesional immunotherapy. J Urol 1984;132(3):570–3.

[18] Bohle A, Brandau S. Immune mechanisms in bacillus Calmette-Guerin immunotherapy for superficial bladder cancer. J Urol 2003;170(3):964–9.

[19] Herr HW, Dalbagni G, Donat SM. Bacillus Calmette-Guerin without maintenance therapy for high-risk non-muscle-invasive bladder cancer. Eur Urol 2011;60(1):32–6.

[20] Bretton PR, Herr HW, Kimmel M, Whitmore Jr. WF, Laudone V, Oettgen HF, et al. The response of patients with superficial bladder cancer to a second course of intravesical bacillus Calmette-Guerin. J Urol 1990;143(4):710–12. discussion 2–3.

[21] Coplen DE, Marcus MD, Myers JA, Ratliff TL, Catalona WJ. Long-term followup of patients treated with 1 or 2, 6-week courses of intravesical bacillus Calmette-Guerin: analysis of possible predictors of response free of tumor. J Urol 1990;144(3):652–7.

[22] Haaff EO, Catalona WJ, Ratliff TL. Detection of interleukin 2 in the urine of patients with superficial bladder tumors after treatment with intravesical BCG. J Urol 1986;136 (4):970–4.

[23] Kavoussi LR, Torrence RJ, Gillen DP, Hudson MA, Haaff EO, Dresner SM, et al. Results of 6 weekly intravesical bacillus Calmette-Guerin instillations on the treatment of superficial bladder tumors. J Urol 1988;139(5):935–40.

[24] Nadler RB, Catalona WJ, Hudson MA, Ratliff TL. Durability of the tumor-free response for intravesical bacillus Calmette-Guerin therapy. J Urol 1994;152(2 Pt 1):367–73.

[25] Catalona WJ, Hudson MA, Gillen DP, Andriole GL, Ratliff TL. Risks and benefits of repeated courses of intravesical bacillus Calmette-Guerin therapy for superficial bladder cancer. J Urol 1987;137(2):220–4.

[26] Orsola A, Palou J, Xavier B, Algaba F, Salvador J, Vicente J. Primary bladder carcinoma in situ: assessment of early BCG response as a prognostic factor. Eur Urol 1998;33 (5):457–63.

[27] Hudson MA, Ratliff TL, Gillen DP, Haaff EO, Dresner SM, Catalona WJ. Single course versus maintenance bacillus Calmette-Guerin therapy for superficial bladder tumors: a prospective, randomized trial. J Urol 1987;138(2):295–8.

[28] Badalament RA, Herr HW, Wong GY, Gnecco C, Pinsky CM, Whitmore Jr. WF, et al. A prospective randomized trial of maintenance versus nonmaintenance intravesical bacillus Calmette-Guerin therapy of superficial bladder cancer. J Clin Oncol 1987;5(3):441–9.

[29] Kamat AM, Porten S. Myths and mysteries surrounding bacillus Calmette-Guerin therapy for bladder cancer. Eur Urol 2014;65(2):267–9.

[30] Han RF, Pan JG. Can intravesical bacillus Calmette-Guerin reduce recurrence in patients with superficial bladder cancer? A meta-analysis of randomized trials. Urology 2006;67 (6):1216–23.

[31] van Rhijn BW, Burger M, Lotan Y, Solsona E, Stief CG, Sylvester RJ, et al. Recurrence and progression of disease in non-muscle-invasive bladder cancer: from epidemiology to treatment strategy. Eur Urol 2009;56(3):430–42.

[32] O'Donnell MA. Practical applications of intravesical chemotherapy and immunotherapy in high-risk patients with superficial bladder cancer. Urol Clin North Am 2005;32 (2):121–31.

[33] Borden Jr. LS, Clark PE, Hall MC. Bladder cancer. Curr Opin Oncol 2003;15(3):227–33.

[34] Malmstrom PU, Sylvester RJ, Crawford DE, Friedrich M, Krege S, Rintala E, et al. An individual patient data meta-analysis of the long-term outcome of randomised studies comparing intravesical mitomycin C versus bacillus Calmette-Guerin for non-muscle-invasive bladder cancer. Eur Urol 2009;56(2):247–56.

[35] Oddens J, Brausi M, Sylvester R, et al. Final results of an EORTC-GU cancers group randomized study of maintenance bacillus Calmette-Guérin in intermediate- and high-risk Ta, T1 papillary carcinoma of the urinary bladder: one-third dose versus full dose and 1 year versus 3 years of maintenance. Eur Urol 2013;63(3):462–72.

[36] Ehdaie B, Sylvester R, Herr HW. Maintenance bacillus Calmette-Guerin treatment of non-muscle-invasive bladder cancer: a critical evaluation of the evidence. Eur Urol 2013;64 (4):579–85.

[37] Lamm D. Clinical practice recommendations for the management of non–muscle invasive bladder cancer. Eur Urol 2008;(Suppl. 7):651–66.

[38] Burger M, Oosterlinck W, Konety B, Chang S, Gudjonsson S, Pruthi R, et al. ICUD-EAU International Consultation on Bladder Cancer 2012: non-muscle-invasive urothelial carcinoma of the bladder. Eur Urol 2013;63(1):36–44.

[39] Clark PE, Agarwal N, Biagioli MC, Eisenberger MA, Greenberg RE, Herr HW, et al. Bladder cancer. J Natl Comp Cancer Netw 2013;11(4):446–75.

[40] Gandhi NM, Morales A, Lamm DL. Bacillus Calmette-Guerin immunotherapy for genitourinary cancer. BJU Int 2013;112(3):288–97.

[41] Hinotsu S, Akaza H, Naito S, Ozono S, Sumiyoshi Y, Noguchi S, et al. Maintenance therapy with bacillus Calmette-Guerin Connaught strain clearly prolongs recurrence-free

survival following transurethral resection of bladder tumour for non-muscle-invasive bladder cancer. BJU Int 2011;108(2):187–95.

[42]   Duchek M, Johansson R, Jahnson S, Mestad O, Hellstrom P, Hellsten S, et al. Bacillus Calmette-Guerin is superior to a combination of epirubicin and interferon-alpha2b in the intravesical treatment of patients with stage T1 urinary bladder cancer. A prospective, randomized, Nordic study. Eur Urol 2010;57(1):25–31.

Chapter 20.3

Optimal Dose of BCG

Sung Han Kim and Ho Kyung Seo
Research Institute and National Cancer Center, Goyang, South Korea

COMPARISON OF THE EFFECTIVENESS AMONG FULL DOSE (81 MG) VS INTERMEDIATE LOW (27 MG) VS VERY LOW DOSE (13.5 MG)

Astram et al. [1] performed a meta-analysis of six clinical trials including Oden et al. [2], Martinez et al. [3], Semper et al. [4], Unda et al. [5], March et al. [6], and Ojea et al. [7] involving 2719 intermediate–high-risk non-muscle-invasive bladder cancer (NMIBC) patients to evaluate the effective dose and adverse effects of bacille Calmette–Guerin (BCG) doses in maintenance therapy. Full-dose (81 mg) BCG has superior outcomes in reducing recurrences compared to low-dose (27 mg) (Relative risks (RR), 0.86; 95% confidence interval [CI], 0.77–0.96; $I^2 = 0\%$ and $P = 0.008$) and very low-dose BCG (13.5 mg) (RR, 0.66; 95% CI, 0.49–0.89; $I^2 = 8.8\%$ and $P = 0.006$). About 20.1% of patients with low-dose BCG experience recurrence compared to 30% with very low dose [1]. Furthermore, there are no significant differences between each dose regarding local side effects, as proven in a meta-analysis of 1816 patients in two clinical trials ($P = 0.137$). However, full-dose BCG regimen has higher systemic side effects (25%) compared to low-dose (28.5%), and very low-dose BCG (15.5%; $P = 0.001$). The recurrence rate in full-dose (81 mg), low-dose (27 mg), and very low-dose BCG (13.5 mg) are 33.3%, 34.7%, and 30%, respectively. Low-dose BCG (27 mg) is superior to full-dose BCG when considering systemic side effects.

A randomized prospective trial comparing adjuvant therapy for intermediate-risk superficial bladder cancer between one-third dose (27 mg) and full-dose (81 mg) BCG and mitomycin C (MMC; 30 mg) suggests that the disease-free interval is significantly longer after treatment with 27 mg of

BCG, and the number of recurrence is lower in this group than in the 30-mg MMC group. This study suggests that the minimum effective dose of BCG is one-third (27 mg) of the standard dose (81 mg). One-sixth (13.5 mg) of the standard dose is not indicated as adjuvant treatment for superficial bladder cancer of intermediate risk, because it has the same efficacy as MMC at 30 mg but is more toxic. In fact, the toxicity level after administering one-sixth of the standard dose (13.5 mg) is similar to that observed after administering one-third (27 mg) of the standard dose [7].

March et al. [6] compared 30-mg MMC with 27-mg and 13.5-mg BCG as adjuvant therapy in medium- and low-risk superficial bladder cancer. The recurrence rate was lower in the 27-mg BCG group, and the time-to-recurrence was higher in this group. No significant differences between the other groups and no significant differences in adverse effects between the two BCG treatment groups were found.

EFFECTIVE DOSE REDUCTIONS TO MINIMIZE SIDE EFFECTS WITH OTHER IMMUNOSTIMULATING AGENTS

Several researchers have evaluated the potential for BCG dose reductions [8−11]. A decrease in toxicity with no statistical difference in efficacy has been noted in small series [12−14], although multifocal and high-grade tumors may respond better to full dosage. Some studies have shown an upregulation of the Th1 response with a lower dose of BCG.

Interferons (IFNs) are glycoproteins produced in response to antigenic stimuli. These agents have antitumor activities, including inhibition of nucleotide synthesis, upregulation of tumor antigens, antiangiogenic properties, and stimulation of cytokine release with enhanced T- and B-cell activation, as well as enhanced natural killer cell activity [15]. IFN-α has been the most extensively studied among the several subtypes. It is most active in doses of at least 100 million units, although optimal dose and administration schedule have yet to be determined [16,17].

IFN-α as a solitary agent is more expensive and less effective than BCG or intravesical chemotherapy in eradicating residual disease, preventing recurrence of papillary disease and treating carcinoma in situ (CIS) (20%−43% complete response). As a prophylactic agent, IFN-α alone demonstrated recurrence rates that were inferior to those of BCG alone (60%−16%) [18,19]. However, IFN-α has also been studied in a combination treatment regimen with either chemotherapy or BCG [20,21].

Several trials that investigated the combination of BCG and IFN-α have suggested the potential superiority of the combination, or the possibility of decreasing the dose of BCG, which may reduce side effects. Initial pioneering work by O'Donnell and colleagues [22] reported a 63% disease-free rate at 12 months and 53% at 24 months with the use of combination therapy. In a larger trial of 1000 patients, 231 patients with CIS were evaluated. In those patients who had CIS and were BCG-naive, the BCG and IFN-α combination treatment resulted in 59% disease-free status at 24 months [23]. Of the nonresponders to combination BCG and IFN-α, the majority of patients who experienced treatment failure with recurrence did so within 4 months of initial treatment [24].

Interleukin-2 (IL-2) is another immunostimulating agent similar to IFN-α that is used in combination with BCG. IL-2 is highly expressed after BCG stimulation and is a key component of the Th1 immune response. Preclinical data suggest a potential benefit and little toxicity [25]. Multiple studies have documented the potential use of intravesical IL-2 alone, with BCG, or with BCG and IFN-α [26]. Preclinical data identifying the efficacy of liposome-mediated intravesical IL-2 with biologic response modifiers have elucidated long-term T-cell memory against muscle-invasive blood cancer and NMIBC [27,28].

EFFICACY OF INTRAVESICAL BCG INSTILLATION IN BCG-INOCULATED AREA

Studies in Europe, where BCG inoculation for tuberculosis is more common than in North America, suggest that the dose may be safely reduced by half [3]. The difference in response to doing so in immunologically naive North Americans has not been understood, but Morales and colleagues [11] found a significant decrease in response rates (67% vs 37%), especially for patients with CIS and papillary bladder tumors.

REFERENCES

[1] Astram A, Khadijah A, Yuri P, Zulfan A, Mochtar CA, Danarto R, et al. Effective dose and adverse effects of maintenance Bacillus Calmette-Guerin in intermediate and high risk non-muscle invasive bladder cancer: a meta-analysis of randomized clinical trial. Acta Med Indones 2014;46(4):298–307.

[2] Oddens J, Brausi M, Sylvester R, Bono A, van de Beek C, van Andel G, et al. Final results of an EORTC-GU cancers group randomized study of maintenance bacillus Calmette-Guerin in intermediate- and high-risk Ta, T1 papillary carcinoma of the urinary bladder: one-third dose versus full dose and 1 year versus 3 years of maintenance. Eur Urol 2013;63 (3):462–72.

[3] Martinez-Pineiro JA, Flores N, Isorna S, Solsona E, Sebastian JL, Pertusa C, et al. Long-term follow-up of a randomized prospective trial comparing a standard 81 mg dose of intravesical bacille Calmette-Guerin with a reduced dose of 27 mg in superficial bladder cancer. BJU Int 2002;89(7):671–80.

[4] Semper M Jr, Solsona E, Fernandez J, Dorrego JM, et al. Treatment of carcinoma in situ of the bladder associated or not associated to non-muscle Invasive transitional carcinoma using two different BCG doses: the standard or one third dose. A five year follow-up. Eur Urol Supp 2010;9:91.

[5] Unda M, Solsona E, Gomez JM, Martines- Pineiro JA, Ojea A, CUETO group. Long-term follow up of the effectiveness of standard dose BCG (81 mg. Connaught strain) comparing with a three fold reduce dose (27 mg.) in high risk non muscle invasive bladder cancer. Eur Urol Supp 2009;8:284.

[6] Nogueira M, Solsona E, Unda M, Ojea A, et al. A multicenter and randomized prospective study comparing three intravesical therapies, two with Bacillus Calmette-Guérin immunotherapy and one with mitomycin-C chemotherapy in medium and low risk superficial bladder tumours. Eur Urol Supp 2002;1:101.

[7] Ojea A, Nogueira JL, Solsona E, Flores N, Gomez JM, Molina JR, et al. A multicentre, randomised prospective trial comparing three intravesical adjuvant therapies for intermediate-risk superficial bladder cancer: low-dose bacillus Calmette-Guerin (27 mg) versus very low-dose bacillus Calmette-Guerin (13.5 mg) versus mitomycin C. Eur Urol 2007;52(5):1398–406.

[8] Martinez-Pineiro JA, Solsona E, Flores N, Isorna S. Improving the safety of BCG immunotherapy by dose reduction. Cooperative Group CUETO. Eur Urol 1995;27(Suppl 1):13–18.

[9] Melekos MD, Chionis H, Pantazakos A, Fokaefs E, Paranychianakis G, Dauaher H. Intravesical bacillus Calmette-Guerin immunoprophylaxis of superficial bladder cancer: results of a controlled prospective trial with modified treatment schedule. J Urol 1993;149 (4):744–8.

[10] Pagano F, Bassi P, Piazza N, Abatangelo G, Drago Ferrante GL, Milani C. Improving the efficacy of BCG immunotherapy by dose reduction. Eur Urol 1995;27(Suppl 1):19–22.

[11] Morales A, Nickel JC, Wilson JW. Dose-response of bacillus Calmette-Guerin in the treatment of superficial bladder cancer. J Urol 1992;147(5):1256–8.

[12] Hurle R, Losa A, Ranieri A, Graziotti P, Lembo A. Low dose Pasteur bacillus Calmette-Guerin regimen in stage T1, grade 3 bladder cancer therapy. J Urol 1996;156(5):1602–5.

[13] Mack D, Frick J. Five-year results of a phase II study with low-dose bacille Calmette-Guerin therapy in high-risk superficial bladder cancer. Urology 1995;45(6):958–61.

[14] Pagano F, Bassi P, Milani C, Meneghini A, Maruzzi D, Garbeglio A. A low dose bacillus Calmette-Guerin regimen in superficial bladder cancer therapy: is it effective?. J Urol 1991;146(1):32–5.

[15] Naitoh J, Franklin J, O'Donnell MA, et al. Interferon alpha for the treatment of superficial bladder cancer. In: Baskin L, Hayward B, editors. Advances in bladder research. New York: Plenum; 1999.

[16] Belldegrun AS, Franklin JR, O'Donnell MA, Gomella LG, Klein E, Neri R, et al. Superficial bladder cancer: the role of interferon-alpha. J Urol 1998;159(6):1793–801.

[17] Torti FM, Shortliffe LD, Williams RD, Pitts WC, Kempson RL, Ross JC, et al. Alpha-interferon in superficial bladder cancer: a Northern California Oncology Group Study. J Clin Oncol 1988;6(3):476–83.

[18] Glashan RW. A randomized controlled study of intravesical alpha-2b-interferon in carcinoma in situ of the bladder. J Urol 1990;144(3):658–61.

[19] Kalble T, Beer M, Mendoza E, Ikinger U, Link M, Reichert HE, et al. [BCG vs interferon A for prevention of recurrence of superficial bladder cancer. A prospective randomized study] [in German]. Urologe A 1994;33(2):133–7.

[20] Bercovich E, Deriu M, Manferrari F, Irianni G. [BCG vs. BCG plus recombinant alpha-interferon 2b in superficial tumors of the bladder] [in Italian]. Arch Ital Urol Androl 1995;67(4):257–60.

[21] Stricker P, Pryor K, Nicholson T, Goldstein D, Golovsky D, Ferguson R, et al. Bacillus Calmette-Guerin plus intravesical interferon alpha-2b in patients with superficial bladder cancer. Urology 1996;48(6):957–61. discussion 61–2.

[22] O'Donnell MA, Luo Y, Chen X, Szilvasi A, Hunter SE, Clinton SK. Role of IL-12 in the induction and potentiation of IFN-gamma in response to bacillus Calmette-Guerin. J Immunol 1999;163(8):4246—52.

[23] Joudi FN, Smith BJ, O'Donnell MA, Konety BR. The impact of age on the response of patients with superficial bladder cancer to intravesical immunotherapy. J Urol 2006;175 (5):1634—9. discussion 9—40.

[24] Grossman HB, O'Donnell MA, Cookson MS, Greenberg RE, Keane TE. Bacillus Calmette-Guerin failures and beyond: contemporary management of non-muscle-invasive bladder cancer. Rev Urol 2008;10(4):281—9.

[25] Horinaga M, Harsch KM, Fukuyama R, Heston W, Larchian W. Intravesical interleukin-12 gene therapy in an orthotopic bladder cancer model. Urology 2005;66(2):461—6.

[26] Shapiro A GO, Pode D. The treatment of superficial bladder tumors with IL-2 and BCG. J Urol 2007;177—244.

[27] Horiguchi Y, Larchian WA, Kaplinsky R, Fair WR, Heston WD. Intravesical liposome-mediated interleukin-2 gene therapy in orthotopic murine bladder cancer model. Gene Ther 2000;7(10):844—51.

[28] Larchian WA, Horiguchi Y, Nair SK, Fair WR, Heston WD, Gilboa E. Effectiveness of combined interleukin 2 and B7.1 vaccination strategy is dependent on the sequence and order: a liposome-mediated gene therapy treatment for bladder cancer. Clin Cancer Res 2000;6(7):2913—20.

Chapter 20.4

BCG Toxicity

Sung Han Kim and Ho Kyung Seo
Research Institute and National Cancer Center, Goyang, South Korea

INTRODUCTION

Intravesical Bacillus Calmette—Guerin (BCG) instillation has many thera-peutic advantages. In a previous study, it was emphasized that approximately more than 95% of patients receiving intravesical BCG instillation tolerated BCG without significant morbidity. However, as with most cancer treat-ments, serious and potentially fatal toxicities can occur in a minority of patients [1].

Various local and systemic side effects occur following BCG instillation. The fastidious growth nature of BCG in culture and a doubling time of 24—48 hours contribute to the difficulty in its diagnostic isolation in many cases, despite a high clinical suspicion of BCG infection. In a number of case reports, acid-fast bacilli have not been demonstrated and organisms have not grown [2,3].

Most of the symptoms associated with intravesical BCG instillation are due to immune stimulation and cytokine production, which are required to effectively eradicate cancer cells. The mechanism by which BCG leads to the development of infectious complications is not fully understood. One explanation is that its mechanism of action as an immunotherapeutic agent is mediated by a helper T-cell cytokine profile known as the "Th1 response." [4] Considerable debate exists on whether infectious complications due to BCG represent a hypersensitivity reaction or ongoing active infection. The hypersensitivity hypothesis gained early attention based on the presence of granulomas and the absence of recoverable organisms.

In general, the adverse symptoms associated with BCG can begin after the second or third instillation and last for 1−2 days [5]. These symptoms may be associated with a more favorable antitumor response to BCG.

The possible side effects of local symptoms include bacterial or chemical cystitis, dysuria, urinary frequency, hematuria, granulomatous prostatitis, epididymitis, urethral obstruction, and contracted bladder. The most common local side effect was drug-induced cystitis, manifested as irritative voiding symptoms with negative urine culture, and hematuria that resolves in 48 hours without the need to stop BCG instillation [6−8]. Severe side effects associated with BCG result from intravenous absorption of the organism, most commonly from traumatic catheterization. While BCG sometimes is administered in cases showing the presence of hematuria, blood arising from a difficulty in placing the catheter is an absolute contraindication to BCG instillation. Systemic side effects include fever ($>39°C$), influenza-like symptoms, including general malaise and chills, BCG-induced lung infection, liver toxicity, and sepsis.

As previously mentioned, some rare serious systemic reactions of BCG, such as systemic granulomatous disease with high fever that can progress into multiple organ failure, can be caused by active infection, which results in immune responses. The onset of symptoms can occur months or even years after last instillation. This phenomenon may be due to the presence of BCG for a long time in body. Drug-related life-threatening side effects such as septic BCG could be caused by systemic BCG absorption [6]. Skin rash, arthralgia, and arthritis were classified as possible allergic reactions.

COMPLICATION CLASSIFICATIONS

The complications of BCG have been categorized by the intensity and duration of side effects [9]. One of the common classifications of BCG complications was suggested by the Cleveland Clinic, with an approach for the management of toxicity according to the severity of BCG complications (Table 20.4.1).

According to Cleveland Clinic Approach, BCG complications can be classified into Grades 1, 2, and 3 (Table 20.4.1).

TABLE 20.4.1 Management of BCG Toxicity (Cleveland Clinic Approach)

Grade 1: Mild to Moderate Symptoms <48 Hours

Mild or moderate irritative voiding symptoms, mild hematuria, fever <38.5°C

Assessment

Possible urine culture to rule out bacterial urinary tract infection

Symptom Management

Anticholinergics, topical antispasmodics (phenazopyridine), analgesics, non-steroidal antiinflammatory drugs

Asymptomatic prostatic granulomas that occur after BCG therapy can occasionally mimic prostate cancer clinically and/or radiographically. There is no evidence to support treatment in this setting [10].

Grade 2: Severe Symptoms and/or >48 Hours

Severe irritative voiding symptoms, hematuria, or symptoms lasting >48 hours

All maneuvers for Grade 1, along with the following:

Assessment

Urine culture, chest radiograph, liver function tests

Management

Consult immediately with physician experienced in management of mycobacterial infections and complications

Consider dose reduction to one-half to one-third of dose when instillations resume

Treat culture results as appropriate

Antimicrobial Agents

Administer isoniazid and rifampin, 300 mg/day and 600 mg/day, orally until symptom resolution

Do not use monotherapy

Observe for rifampin drug–drug interactions (e.g., warfarin)

Grade 3: Serious Complications (Hemodynamic Changes, Persistent High-Grade Fever)

Allergic Reactions (Joint Pain, Rash)

Perform all maneuvers described for Grades 1 and 2, plus the following: Isoniazid, 300 mg/day, and rifampin, 600 mg/day, for 3–6 months depending on response

Solid Organ Involvement (Epididymis, Liver, Lung, Kidney, Bone, Joint, and Prostate)

Isoniazid, 300 mg/day; rifampin, 600 mg/day; ethambutol, 15 mg/kg/day single daily dose for 3–6 months

Cycloserine often causes severe psychiatric symptoms and is to be strongly discouraged

(Continued)

TABLE 20.4.1 (Continued)

BCG is almost uniformly resistant to pyrazinamide, so this drug has no role

Consider prednisone, 40 mg/day, when response is inadequate or for septic shock (never given without effective antibacterial therapy)

Source: Adapted from Jones JS. Non-muscle invasive bladder cancer (Ta, T1, and CIS). In: Wein AJ, editor. Campbell-Walsh Urology. 11th ed. China: Elsevier; 2016. p. 2212−5.

PREVENTIVE MEASURES FOR SIDE EFFECTS

The occurrence of adverse effects is one of the main reasons why urologists try to avoid the use of BCG, particularly if it is not a high-risk disease. For such patients chemotherapeutic agents are often prescribed. Therefore, it is important to decrease BCG toxicity while maintaining its efficacy. BCG efficacy and toxicity are dose-dependent, and the problem lies in finding a very low BCG dose (13.5 mg) that is effective and has low toxicity. A reduction in side effects can be achieved in several ways. One of the best ways is reducing the BCG dose. Logarithmic dose reduction of BCG in patients with increasing side effects will typically prevent escalation of toxicity. Another way to decrease the side effects is lengthening of the instillation interval without loss of efficacy and the administration of an antituberculous drug.

Several investigators have evaluated the potential for BCG dose reduction [11−14]. In general, a decrease in toxicity with no statistical difference in efficacy has been noted in small series [15−17], although multifocal and high-grade tumors may respond better to full dosage (81 mg) [18]. Some studies have shown an upregulation of Th1 response at a lower dose of BCG. Two approaches to BCG immunotherapy were examined at the Padova University by specific Phase II and III trials designed to evaluate the possibility of reducing BCG-related side effects without compromising therapeutic efficacy [19]. The approaches include reducing the dose of BCG per instillation "low-dose" regimen and delaying the interval of the instillations "slow-rate" regimen. Lengthening of interval was also effective in decreasing the side effects without loss of efficacy.

A meta-analysis of four multiple RCTs involving 2360 intermediate- and high-risk patients with non-muscle-invasive bladder cancer was performed by Astram et al.; the effective dose and adverse effects of maintenance BCG were evaluated [20]. The incidence of local side effects after full-dose (81 mg), low-dose (27 mg), and very low-dose (13.5 mg) BCG instillation was 59.3 (537/905), 60.0 (708/1179), and 63.7% (176/276), respectively. Systemic side effects occurred in 25.4 (230/905), 28.5 (337/1179), and 15.5% (43/276), respectively. In a meta-analysis of local side effects in 1816 patients, no significant difference was observed ($P = 0.137$); however, lower dose was better in reducing systemic side effects ($P = 0.0001$). Among 544 patients given low-dose and very low-dose BCG, no significant difference was observed ($P = 0.400$) and ($P = 0.600$).

A recent RCT study by Brausi et al. showed comparative results for side effects between low-dose (27 mg) and full-dose (81 mg) intravesical BCG therapy [21]. It was concluded that no significant difference in toxicity according to dose (27 mg vs. 81 mg) or duration of treatment was observed. The comparison of a standard full dose (81 mg) with a reduced dose (27 mg) in superficial bladder cancer showed that the proportion of patients without toxicity, neither local nor systemic, was significantly higher in the reduced dose group than in the group administered standard dose. The differences in severe systemic toxicity were not significant, with 4.4% patients in the reduced dose group and 3.6% in the standard dose group. Neither life-threatening episodes nor sepsis was reported for either group. Granulomatous epididymitis and simultaneous polyneuropathy have been reported in patients administered a reduced dose but is unclear whether these side effects were caused by BCG.

Another way to reduce side effects is administration of anti-tuberculous drugs such as isoniazid (INH) [22,23] and antibiotic ofloxacin. Patients with continuing symptoms from earlier BCG administrations are best treated with antibiotics rather than forging ahead with more BCG. Antibiotic therapy may have a beneficial effect in treating or preventing systemic side effects of BCG therapy. However, it may also inhibit the effectiveness of BCG therapy if given routinely for urinary tract prophylaxis during the course of BCG therapy [24,25]. Quinolones in particular may affect the viability of BCG and should be avoided if possible during the course of BCG treatments [25]. While the use of fluoroquinolone prophylaxis has been shown to decrease the incidence of moderate-to-severe BCG-related adverse side effects [26], there were no differences in local or systemic adverse reactions after prophylactic administration of INH (300 mg) [27].

Another way to prevent or decrease the side effects of BCG or to treat patients with BCG failure or BCG-hypersensitive patients is to use other immunostimulating agents in combination with BCG at a reduced dose. Interferon alpha (IFN-α) has been studied in a combination treatment regimen with either chemotherapy or BCG [28,29]. Several trials investigated the combination of BCG and IFN-α and suggested the potential superiority of the combination or the possibility of decreasing the dose of BCG, which may subsequently reduce the side effects. Initial pioneering work by O'Donnell et al. [30] reported a 63% disease-free rate at 12 months and 53% at 24 months with the use of combination therapy. In a larger trial of 1000 patients, 231 patients with CIS were evaluated. In patients who had CIS and were BCG-naive, BCG and IFN-α combination treatment resulted in 59% disease-free status at 24 months [31]. Of the nonresponders to combination

BCG and IFN-α treatment, the majority of patients who experienced treatment failure with recurrence did so within 4 months of initial treatment [32].

Overall, intravesical treatment with IFN-α was well tolerated. The most common complications of IFN-α include flu-like symptoms, which are associated with cytokine release. Tori et al. reported 15 of 55 (27%) patients with such symptoms; these symptoms were self-limiting and did not require treatment modification. No cases of hematuria, irritative voiding symptoms, or perineal pain were reported in this series [33,34]. Malmstrom et al. reported adverse event rates of 37% and 48% with 50 and 80 million units of IFN-α, respectively. The most commonly reported adverse events were fever and urinary frequency, both occurring at a rate of 11% [34]. Long-term complications from IFN-α treatment include fatigue, weight loss, and anemia [35].

TREATMENTS FOR SIDE EFFECTS

Hematuria is usually self-limited but requires temporary discontinuation of the drug pending resolution. If symptoms persist, cystoscopy can be helpful in determining the etiology. Local symptoms are often managed successfully with expected strategies in conjunction with delayed treatment or dose reduction; however, other interventions such as oral pyridium, anticholinergics, quinolones, acetaminophen, steroids, or non-steroidal anti-inflammatory diseases may be required for the management of persistent toxicity. Urine cultures should always be obtained to rule out bacterial infection. Patients with evident symptoms of BCG infection such as epididymitis, hepatitis, or symptomatic prostatitis are treated with isoniazid plus rifampin 600 mg daily. In a European Organization for Research and Treatment of Cancer (EORTC) trial, intravesical epirubicin, BCG, and BCG plus isoniazid were compared in 957 patients. The results showed that isoniazid did not seem to reduce the side effects of BCG [5].

Tuncer et al. demonstrated the presence of BCG in the blood of patients receiving intravesical BCG. All patients with positive results had systemic symptoms [36]. Lamm et al. reported high fever (> 103°F) as the most common systemic complication, and it was observed in 2.9% of the patients [37]. To avoid sepsis, its systemic manifestations are usually managed by withholding BCG therapy until the symptoms resolve. BCG therapy may be discontinued when the severity of symptoms outweighs the benefit of treatment. Patients without fever may be treated conservatively [35]. To minimize toxicity, treatment should be avoided after recent transurethral resection, traumatic catheterization, or in the setting of an active urinary tract infection [35].

Another troubling complication of BCG therapy is granulomatous prostatitis, occurring in 1%–40% of patients after BCG therapy [35,38]. Granulomatous epididymo-orchitis, granulomatous hepatitis and pneumonitis, BCG sepsis, ureteral obstruction, and contracted bladder are other major sequelae of BCG therapy and are seen less frequently (<1% of patients) [35].

The most dangerous complication of BCG is systemic sepsis or hypersensitivity reaction or both, characterized by chills, fever, hypotension, confusion, and progressive multiple organ failure. However, the incidence of these adverse events is very low (0.4%) [7]. Patients with BCG sepsis require steroids in addition to gram-negative and antitubercular antibiotic therapy to reduce severe hypersensitivity, which can otherwise prove fatal. As the risk for bacterial sepsis and possibly death are high, BCG should never be used as an immediate postoperative intravesical instillation. Treatment should be initiated based on symptoms because cultures take time to return. BCG sepsis treatment includes isoniazid, rifampin, and prednisone, which should be administered for 6 months. Ethambutol may be added if symptoms persist; however, an infectious disease consultation is advised in complex cases [39]. To permit the continued use of BCG therapy in patients with mild-to-moderate BCG intolerance, dose reduction has been used in induction and maintenance therapy. Pagano et al. demonstrated similar efficacy for low-dose (75 mg) and full-dose (150 mg) Pasteur strain BCG in 120 patients. Complication rates improved with the low-dose regimen [17]. Similarly, Martinez-Pinero demonstrated similar efficacy with low-dose (27 mg) BCG and full dose (81 mg) in a comparison of 500 patients with superficial bladder cancer [11]. A lower rate of local and systemic complications was observed in patients randomized to the lower dose.

Serious late complications are also possible for intravesical BCG treatments [40–42]. Wolf et al. [42] reported a case of an 80-year-old patient presented with a BCG-infected, ruptured aortic aneurysm and aortic graft, 2 years after intravesical therapy.

SUMMARY

Intravesical BCG has higher efficacy and side effects than intravesical chemotherapy.

- BCG should be used cautiously for patients with low-risk disease owing to concern about side effects.
- Management of infectious complications of BCG is shown in Table 20.4.1.
- BCG is the only agent shown to delay or reduce high-grade tumor progression.
- The optimum dose and treatment schedule for BCG are undetermined; however, results are better with maintenance therapy, if tolerated.
- BCG is contraindicated in the setting of a disrupted urothelium because of the risk of intravasation and septic death.
- IFN-α has not been shown to have benefit compared to BCG for primary treatment. However, it appears to work well in combination with low-dose BCG, especially for salvage.

REFERENCES

[1] Brausi M OJ, Sylvester R et al. Bacillus Calmette-Guerin: one third dose versus full dose and one year versus three years of maintenance. Final results of EORTC GU Cancers Group randomized trial 30962 in non muscle invasive bladder cancer. AUA. 2012: http://www.aua2012; 2012 [cited 2012 November].

[2] Sylvester RJ, van der MA, Lamm DL. Intravesical bacillus Calmette-Guerin reduces the risk of progression in patients with superficial bladder cancer: a meta-analysis of the published results of randomized clinical trials. J Urol 2002;168(5):1964−70.

[3] Saint F, Kurth N, Maille P, Vordos D, Hoznek A, Soyeux P, et al. Urinary IL-2 assay for monitoring intravesical bacillus Calmette-Guerin response of superficial bladder cancer during induction course and maintenance therapy. Int J Cancer 2003;107 (3):434−40.

[4] Shintani Y, Sawada Y, Inagaki T, Kohjimoto Y, Uekado Y, Shinka T. Intravesical instillation therapy with bacillus Calmette-Guerin for superficial bladder cancer: study of the mechanism of bacillus Calmette-Guerin immunotherapy. Int J Urol 2007;14 (2):140−6.

[5] Mitropoulos DN. Novel insights into the mechanism of action of intravesical immunomodulators. In Vivo 2005;19(3):611−21.

[6] Case records of the Massachusetts General Hospital. Weekly clinicopathological exercises. Case 29-1998. A 57-year-old man with fever and jaundice after intravesical instillation of bacille Calmette-Guerin for bladder cancer. N Engl J Med 1998;339(12):831−7.

[7] Elkabani M, Greene JN, Vincent AL, VanHook S, Sandin RL. Disseminated Mycobacterium bovis after intravesicular bacillus Calmette-Guerin treatments for bladder cancer. Cancer Control 2000;7(5):476−81.

[8] Lamm DL. Efficacy and safety of bacille Calmette-Guerin immunotherapy in superficial bladder cancer. Clin Infect Dis 2000;31(Suppl 3):S86−90.

[9] Jones JS. Non-muscle invasive bladder cancer (Ta, T1, and CIS). In: Wein AJ, editor. Campbell-Walsh Urology. 11th ed. China: Elsevier; 2016. p. 2212−5.

[10] Suzuki T, Takeuchi M, Naiki T, Kawai N, Kohri K, Hara M, et al. MRI findings of granulomatous prostatitis developing after intravesical Bacillus Calmette-Guerin therapy. Clin Radiol 2013;68(6):595−9.

[11] Martinez-Pineiro JA, Solsona E, Flores N, Isorna S. Improving the safety of BCG immunotherapy by dose reduction. Cooperative Group CUETO. Eur Urol 1995;27(Suppl 1):13−18.

[12] Melekos MD, Chionis H, Pantazakos A, Fokaefs E, Paranychianakis G, Dauaher H. Intravesical bacillus Calmette-Guerin immunoprophylaxis of superficial bladder cancer: results of a controlled prospective trial with modified treatment schedule. J Urol 1993;149 (4):744−8.

[13] Pagano F, Bassi P, Piazza N, Abatangelo G, Drago Ferrante GL, Milani C. Improving the efficacy of BCG immunotherapy by dose reduction. Eur Urol 1995;27(Suppl 1):19−22.

[14] Morales A, Nickel JC, Wilson JW. Dose-response of bacillus Calmette-Guerin in the treatment of superficial bladder cancer. J Urol 1992;147(5):1256−8.

[15] Hurle R, Losa A, Ranieri A, Graziotti P, Lembo A. Low dose Pasteur bacillus Calmette-Guerin regimen in stage T1, grade 3 bladder cancer therapy. J Urol 1996;156 (5):1602−5.

[16] Mack D, Frick J. Five-year results of a phase II study with low-dose bacille Calmette-Guerin therapy in high-risk superficial bladder cancer. Urology 1995;45(6):958−61.

[17] Pagano F, Bassi P, Milani C, Meneghini A, Maruzzi D, Garbeglio A. A low dose bacillus Calmette-Guerin regimen in superficial bladder cancer therapy: is it effective?. J Urol 1991;146(1):32−5.

[18] Martinez-Pineiro JA, Flores N, Isorna S, Solsona E, Sebastian JL, Pertusa C, et al. Long-term follow-up of a randomized prospective trial comparing a standard 81 mg dose of intravesical bacille Calmette-Guerin with a reduced dose of 27 mg in superficial bladder cancer. BJU Int 2002;89(7):671−80.

[19] Bassi P, Spinadin R, Carando R, Balta G, Pagano F. Modified induction course: a solution to side-effects? Eur Urol 2000;37(Suppl 1):31−2.

[20] Astram A, Khadijah A, Yuri P, Zulfan A, Mochtar CA, Danarto R, et al. Effective dose and adverse effects of maintenance bacillus Calmette-Guerin in intermediate and high risk non-muscle invasive bladder cancer: a meta-analysis of randomized clinical trial. Acta Med Indones 2014;46(4):298−307.

[21] Brausi M, Oddens J, Sylvester R, Bono A, van de Beek C, van Andel G, et al. Side effects of bacillus Calmette-Guerin (BCG) in the treatment of intermediate- and high-risk Ta, T1 papillary carcinoma of the bladder: results of the EORTC genito-urinary cancers group randomised phase 3 study comparing one-third dose with full dose and 1 year with 3 years of maintenance BCG. Eur Urol 2014;65(1):69−76.

[22] Sylvester RJ, Brausi MA, Kirkels WJ, Hoeltl W, Calais Da Silva F, Powell PH, et al. Long-term efficacy results of EORTC genito-urinary group randomized phase 3 study 30911 comparing intravesical instillations of epirubicin, bacillus Calmette-Guerin, and bacillus Calmette-Guerin plus isoniazid in patients with intermediate- and high-risk stage Ta T1 urothelial carcinoma of the bladder. Eur Urol 2010;57 (5):766−73.

[23] van der Meijden AP, Brausi M, Zambon V, Kirkels W, de Balincourt C, Sylvester R. Intravesical instillation of epirubicin, bacillus Calmette-Guerin and bacillus Calmette-Guerin plus isoniazid for intermediate and high risk Ta, T1 papillary carcinoma of the bladder: a European Organization for Research and Treatment of Cancer genito-urinary group randomized phase III trial. J Urol 2001;166(2):476−81.

[24] Durek C, Brandau S, Ulmer AJ, Flad HD, Jocham D, Bohle A. Bacillus-Calmette-Guerin (BCG) and 3D tumors: an in vitro model for the study of adhesion and invasion. J Urol 1999;162(2):600−5.

[25] Durek C, Rusch-Gerdes S, Jocham D, Bohle A. Interference of modern antibacterials with bacillus Calmette-Guerin viability. J Urol 1999;162(6):1959−62.

[26] Colombel M, Saint F, Chopin D, Malavaud B, Nicolas L, Rischmann P. The effect of ofloxacin on bacillus Calmette−Guerin induced toxicity in patients with superficial blad-der cancer: results of a randomized, prospective, double-blind, placebo controlled, multi-center study. J Urol 2006;176(3):935−9.

[27] Vegt PD, van der Meijden AP, Sylvester R, Brausi M, Holtl W, de Balincourt C. Does isoniazid reduce side effects of intravesical bacillus Calmette-Guerin therapy in superficial bladder cancer? Interim results of European Organization for Research and Treatment of Cancer Protocol 30911. J Urol 1997;157(4):1246−9.

[28] Bercovich E, Deriu M, Manferrari F, Irianni G. [BCG vs. BCG plus recombinant alpha-interferon 2b in superficial tumors of the bladder] [in Italian]. Arch Ital Urol Androl 1995;67(4):257−60.

[29] Stricker P, Pryor K, Nicholson T, Goldstein D, Golovsky D, Ferguson R, et al. Bacillus Calmette-Guerin plus intravesical interferon alpha-2b in patients with superficial bladder cancer. Urology 1996;48(6):957−61. discussion 61−2.

[30] O'Donnell MA, Luo Y, Chen X, Szilvasi A, Hunter SE, Clinton SK. Role of IL-12 in the induction and potentiation of IFN-gamma in response to bacillus Calmette-Guerin. J Immunol 1999;163(8):4246−52.

[31] Joudi FN, Smith BJ, O'Donnell MA, Konety BR. The impact of age on the response of patients with superficial bladder cancer to intravesical immunotherapy. J Urol 2006;175 (5):1634−9. discussion 9−40.

[32] Grossman HB, O'Donnell MA, Cookson MS, Greenberg RE, Keane TE. Bacillus Calmette-Guerin failures and beyond: contemporary management of non-muscle-invasive bladder cancer. Rev Urol 2008;10(4):281−9.

[33] Torti FM, Shortliffe LD, Williams RD, Pitts WC, Kempson RL, Ross JC, et al. Alpha-interferon in superficial bladder cancer: a Northern California Oncology Group Study. J Clin Oncol 1988;6(3):476−83.

[34] Malmstrom PU. A randomized comparative dose-ranging study of interferon-alpha and mitomycin-C as an internal control in primary or recurrent superficial transitional cell carcinoma of the bladder. BJU Int 2002;89(7):681−6.

[35] Koya MP, Simon MA, Soloway MS. Complications of intravesical therapy for urothelial cancer of the bladder. J Urol 2006;175(6):2004−10.

[36] Tuncer S, Tekin MI, Ozen H, Bilen C, Unal S, Remzi D. Detection of bacillus Calmette-Guerin in the blood by the polymerase chain reaction method of treated bladder cancer patients. J Urol 1997;158(6):2109−12.

[37] Lamm DL. Complications of bacillus Calmette-Guerin immunotherapy. Urol Clin North Am 1992;19(3):565−72.

[38] Mukamel E, Konichezky M, Engelstein D, Cytron S, Abramovici A, Servadio C. Clinical and pathological findings in prostates following intravesical bacillus Calmette-Guerin instillations. J Urol 1990;144(6):1399−400.

[39] Pagano F, Bassi P, Galetti TP, Meneghini A, Milani C, Artibani W, et al. Results of contemporary radical cystectomy for invasive bladder cancer: a clinicopathological study with an emphasis on the inadequacy of the tumor, nodes and metastases classification. J Urol 1991;145(1):45−50.

[40] Alvarez-Mugica M, Gomez JM, Vazquez VB, Monzon AJ, Rodriguez JM, Robles LR. Pancreatic and psoas abscesses as a late complication of intravesical administration of bacillus Calmette-Guerin for bladder cancer: a case report and review of the literature. J Med Case Reports 2009;3:7323.

[41] Mangiarotti B, Trinchieri A, Marconato R, Pisani E. Skin abscess after intravesical instillation of bacillus Calmette-Guerin for prophylactic treatment of transitional cell carcinoma. J Urol 2002;168(3):1094−5.

[42] Wolf YG, Wolf DG, Higginbottom PA, Dilley RB. Infection of a ruptured aortic aneurysm and an aortic graft with bacille Calmette-Guerin after intravesical administration for bladder cancer. J Vasc Surg 1995;22(1):80−4.

FURTHER READING

Babjuk M, Burger M, Zigeuner R, Shariat SF, van Rhijn BW, Comperat E, et al. EAU guidelines on non-muscle-invasive urothelial carcinoma of the bladder: update 2013. Eur Urol 2013;64 (4):639−53.

Babjuk M, Bohle A, Burger M, Capoun O, Cohen D, Comperat EM, et al. EAU guidelines on non-muscle-invasive urothelial carcinoma of the bladder: update 2016. Eur Urol 2016.

Badalament RA, Herr HW, Wong GY, Gnecco C, Pinsky CM, Whitmore Jr. WF, et al. A prospective randomized trial of maintenance versus nonmaintenance intravesical bacillus Calmette-Guerin therapy of superficial bladder cancer. J Clin Oncol 1987;5 (3):441—9.

Baniel J, Grauss D, Engelstein D, Sella A. Intravesical bacillus Calmette-Guerin treatment for stage T1 grade 3 transitional cell carcinoma of the bladder. Urology 1998;52(5):785—9.

Belldegrun AS, Franklin JR, O'Donnell MA, Gomella LG, Klein E, Neri R, et al. Superficial bladder cancer: the role of interferon-alpha. J Urol 1998;159(6):1793—801.

Berglund RK, Savage CJ, Vora KC, Kurta JM, Cronin AM. An analysis of the effect of statin use on the efficacy of bacillus Calmette-Guerin treatment for transitional cell carcinoma of the bladder. J Urol 2008;180(4):1297—300. discussion 300.

Boccon-Gibod L, Leleu C, Herve JM, Belas M, Steg A. Bladder tumors invading the lamina propria (stage A/T1): influence of endovesical bacillus Calmette-Guerin therapy on recurrence and progression. Eur Urol 1989;16(6):401—4.

Bohle A, Bock PR. Intravesical bacille Calmette-Guerin versus mitomycin C in superficial bladder cancer: formal meta-analysis of comparative studies on tumor progression. Urology 2004;63(4):682—6. discussion 6—7.

Bohle A, Brandau S. Immune mechanisms in bacillus Calmette-Guerin immunotherapy for superficial bladder cancer. J Urol 2003;170(3):964—9.

Bohle A, Jocham D, Bock PR. Intravesical bacillus Calmette-Guerin versus mitomycin C for superficial bladder cancer: a formal meta-analysis of comparative studies on recurrence and toxicity. J Urol 2003;169(1):90—5.

Borden Jr. LS, Clark PE, Hall MC. Bladder cancer. Curr Opin Oncol 2003;15(3):227—33.

Brake M, Loertzer H, Horsch R, Keller H. Long-term results of intravesical bacillus Calmette-Guerin therapy for stage T1 superficial bladder cancer. Urology 2000;55(5):673—8.

Brake M, Loertzer H, Horsch R, Keller H. Recurrence and progression of stage T1, grade 3 transitional cell carcinoma of the bladder following intravesical immunotherapy with bacillus Calmette-Guerin. J Urol 2000;163(6):1697—701.

Brausi M, Witjes JA, Lamm D, Persad R, Palou J, Colombel M, et al. A review of current guidelines and best practice recommendations for the management of nonmuscle invasive bladder cancer by the International Bladder Cancer Group. J Urol 2011;186(6):2158—67.

Bretton PR, Herr HW, Kimmel M, Whitmore Jr. WF, Laudone V, Oettgen HF, et al. The response of patients with superficial bladder cancer to a second course of intravesical bacillus Calmette-Guerin. J Urol 1990;143(4):710—12. discussion 2—3.

Brosman SA. Experience with bacillus Calmette-Guerin in patients with superficial bladder carcinoma. J Urol 1982;128(1):27—30.

Burger M, Oosterlinck W, Konety B, Chang S, Gudjonsson S, Pruthi R, et al. ICUD-EAU International Consultation on Bladder Cancer 2012: non-muscle-invasive urothelial carcinoma of the bladder. Eur Urol 2013;63(1):36—44.

Catalona WJ, Hudson MA, Gillen DP, Andriole GL, Ratliff TL. Risks and benefits of repeated courses of intravesical bacillus Calmette-Guerin therapy for superficial bladder cancer. J Urol 1987;137(2):220—4.

Chang SS, Boorjian SA, Chou R, Clark PE, Daneshmand S, Konety BR, et al. Diagnosis and treatment of non-muscle invasive bladder cancer: AUA/SUO guideline. J Urol 2016.

Clark PE, Agarwal N, Biagioli MC, Eisenberger MA, Greenberg RE, Herr HW, et al. Bladder cancer. J Natl Comp Cancer Netw 2013;11(4):446—75.

Cookson MS, Sarosdy MF. Management of stage T1 superficial bladder cancer with intravesical bacillus Calmette-Guerin therapy. J Urol 1992;148(3):797—801.

Coplen DE, Marcus MD, Myers JA, Ratliff TL, Catalona WJ. Long-term followup of patients treated with 1 or 2, 6-week courses of intravesical bacillus Calmette-Guerin: analysis of possible predictors of response free of tumor. J Urol 1990;144(3):652–7.

Crivelli JJ, Xylinas E, Kluth LA, da Silva RD, Chrystal J, Novara G, et al. Effect of statin use on outcomes of non-muscle-invasive bladder cancer. BJU Int 2013;112(2):E4–12.

Dalbagni G, Herr HW. Current use and questions concerning intravesical bladder cancer group for superficial bladder cancer. Urol Clin North Am 2000;27(1):137–46.

Dalbagni G, Vora K, Kaag M, Cronin A, Bochner B, Donat SM, et al. Clinical outcome in a contemporary series of restaged patients with clinical T1 bladder cancer. Eur Urol 2009;56 (6):903–10.

Dalbagni G, Kaag M, Cronin A, Vora K, Bochner B, Donat SM, et al. Variability of treatment selection among surgeons for patients with cT1 urothelial carcinoma. BJU Int 2010;106 (10):1502–7.

De Jager R, Guinan P, Lamm D, Khanna O, Brosman S, De Kernion J, et al. Long-term complete remission in bladder carcinoma in situ with intravesical TICE bacillus Calmette Guerin. Overview analysis of six phase II clinical trials. Urology 1991;38(6):507–13.

Duchek M, Johansson R, Jahnson S, Mestad O, Hellstrom P, Hellsten S, et al. Bacillus Calmette-Guerin is superior to a combination of epirubicin and interferon-alpha2b in the intravesical treatment of patients with stage T1 urinary bladder cancer. A prospective, randomized, Nordic study. Eur Urol 2010;57(1):25–31.

Ehdaie B, Sylvester R, Herr HW. Maintenance bacillus Calmette-Guerin treatment of non-muscle-invasive bladder cancer: a critical evaluation of the evidence. Eur Urol 2013;64 (4):579–85.

Ehlers S. Why does tumor necrosis factor targeted therapy reactivate tuberculosis? J Rheumatol Suppl 2005;74:35–9.

Eure GR, Cundiff MR, Schellhammer PF. Bacillus Calmette-Guerin therapy for high risk stage T1 superficial bladder cancer. J Urol 1992;147(2):376–9.

Gandhi NM, Morales A, Lamm DL. Bacillus Calmette-Guerin immunotherapy for genitourinary cancer. BJU Int 2013;112(3):288–97.

Gaughan EM, Dezube BJ, Bower M, Aboulafia DM, Bohac G, Cooley TP, et al. HIV-associated bladder cancer: a case series evaluating difficulties in diagnosis and management. BMC Urol 2009;9:10.

Gee JR, Jarrard DF, Bruskewitz RC, Moon TD, Hedican SP, Leverson GE, et al. Reduced bladder cancer recurrence rate with cardioprotective aspirin after intravesical bacille Calmette-Guerin. BJU Int 2009;103(6):736–9.

Glashan RW. A randomized controlled study of intravesical alpha-2b-interferon in carcinoma in situ of the bladder. J Urol 1990;144(3):658–61.

Gohji K, Nomi M, Okamoto M, Takenaka A, Hara I, Okada H, et al. Conservative therapy for stage T1b, grade 3 transitional cell carcinoma of the bladder. Urology 1999;53(2):308–13.

Gontero P, Bohle A, Malmstrom PU, O'Donnell MA, Oderda M, Sylvester R, et al. The role of bacillus Calmette-Guerin in the treatment of non-muscle-invasive bladder cancer. Eur Urol 2010;57(3):410–29.

Gunlusoy B, Degirmenci T, Arslan M, Nergiz N, Minareci S, Ayder AR. Recurrence and progression of T1G3 transitional cell carcinoma of the bladder treated with intravesical bacillus Calmette-Guerin. Urol Int 2005;75(2):107–13.

Haaff EO, Catalona WJ, Ratliff TL. Detection of interleukin 2 in the urine of patients with superficial bladder tumors after treatment with intravesical BCG. J Urol 1986;136 (4):970–4.

Hall MC, Chang SS, Dalbagni G, Pruthi RS, Seigne JD, Skinner EC, et al. Guideline for the management of nonmuscle invasive bladder cancer (stages Ta, T1, and Tis): 2007 update. J Urol 2007;178(6):2314–30.

Han RF, Pan JG. Can intravesical bacillus Calmette-Guerin reduce recurrence in patients with superficial bladder cancer? A meta-analysis of randomized trials. Urology 2006;67 (6):1216–23.

Hara I, Miyake H, Takechi Y, Eto H, Gotoh A, Fujisawa M, et al. Clinical outcome of conservative therapy for stage T1, grade 3 transitional cell carcinoma of the bladder. Int J Urol 2003;10(1):19–24.

Harland SJ, Charig CR, Highman W, Parkinson MC, Riddle PR. Outcome in carcinoma in situ of bladder treated with intravesical bacille Calmette-Guerin. Br J Urol 1992;70 (3):271–5.

Herr HW. Tumour progression and survival in patients with T1G3 bladder tumours: 15-year outcome. Br J Urol 1997;80(5):762–5.

Herr HW. Extravesical tumor relapse in patients with superficial bladder tumors. J Clin Oncol 1998;16(3):1099–102.

Herr HW. Intravesical bacillus Calmette-Guerin outcomes in patients with bladder cancer and asymptomatic bacteriuria. J Urol 2012;187(2):435–7.

Herr HW, Morales A. History of bacillus Calmette-Guerin and bladder cancer: an immunotherapy success story. J Urol 2008;179(1):53–6.

Herr HW, Laudone VP, Badalament RA, Oettgen HF, Sogani PC, Freedman BD, et al. Bacillus Calmette-Guerin therapy alters the progression of superficial bladder cancer. J Clin Oncol 1988;6(9):1450–5.

Herr HW, Badalament RA, Amato DA, Laudone VP, Fair WR, Whitmore Jr. WF. Superficial bladder cancer treated with bacillus Calmette-Guerin: a multivariate analysis of factors affecting tumor progression. J Urol 1989;141(1):22–9.

Herr HW, Wartinger DD, Fair WR, Oettgen HF. Bacillus Calmette-Guerin therapy for superficial bladder cancer: a 10-year followup. J Urol 1992;147(4):1020–3.

Herr HW, Dalbagni G, Donat SM. Bacillus Calmette-Guerin without maintenance therapy for high-risk non-muscle-invasive bladder cancer. Eur Urol 2011;60(1):32–6.

Hinotsu S, Akaza H, Naito S, Ozono S, Sumiyoshi Y, Noguchi S, et al. Maintenance therapy with bacillus Calmette-Guerin Connaught strain clearly prolongs recurrence-free survival following transurethral resection of bladder tumour for non-muscle-invasive bladder cancer. BJU Int 2011;108(2):187–95.

Hoffmann P, Roumeguere T, Schulman C, van Velthoven R. Use of statins and outcome of BCG treatment for bladder cancer. N Engl J Med 2006;355(25):2705–7.

Horiguchi Y, Larchian WA, Kaplinsky R, Fair WR, Heston WD. Intravesical liposome-mediated interleukin-2 gene therapy in orthotopic murine bladder cancer model. Gene Ther 2000;7 (10):844–51.

Horinaga M, Harsch KM, Fukuyama R, Heston W, Larchian W. Intravesical interleukin-12 gene therapy in an orthotopic bladder cancer model. Urology 2005;66(2):461–6.

Hudson MA, Herr HW. Carcinoma in situ of the bladder. J Urol 1995;153(3 Pt 1):564–72.

Hudson MA, Ratliff TL, Gillen DP, Haaff EO, Dresner SM, Catalona WJ. Single course versus maintenance bacillus Calmette-Guerin therapy for superficial bladder tumors: a prospective, randomized trial. J Urol 1987;138(2):295–8.

Hurle R, Losa A, Manzetti A, Lembo A. Intravesical bacille Calmette-Guerin in Stage T1 grade 3 bladder cancer therapy: a 7-year follow-up. Urology 1999;54(2):258–63.

Hurle R, Losa A, Manzetti A, Lembo A. Upper urinary tract tumors developing after treatment of superficial bladder cancer: 7-year follow-up of 591 consecutive patients. Urology 1999;53(6):1144–8.

Jakse G, Hall R, Bono A, Holtl W, Carpentier P, Spaander JP, et al. Intravesical BCG in patients with carcinoma in situ of the urinary bladder: long-term results of EORTC GU Group phase II protocol 30861. Eur Urol 2001;40(2):144–50.

Jimenez-Cruz JF, Vera-Donoso CD, Leiva O, Pamplona M, Rioja-Sanz LA, Martinez-Lasierra M, et al. Intravesical immunoprophylaxis in recurrent superficial bladder cancer (Stage T1): multicenter trial comparing bacille Calmette-Guerin and interferon-alpha. Urology 1997;50 (4):529–35.

Kalble T, Beer M, Mendoza E, Ikinger U, Link M, Reichert HE, et al. [BCG vs interferon A for prevention of recurrence of superficial bladder cancer. A prospective randomized study] [in German]. Urologe A 1994;33(2):133–7.

Kamat AM, Porten S. Myths and mysteries surrounding bacillus Calmette-Guerin therapy for bladder cancer. Eur Urol 2014;65(2):267–9.

Kamat AM, Wu X. Statins and the effect of BCG on bladder cancer. N Engl J Med. 2007;356 (12):1276. author reply -7.

Kamat AM, Witjes JA, Brausi M, Soloway M, Lamm D, Persad R, et al. Defining and treating the spectrum of intermediate risk nonmuscle invasive bladder cancer. J Urol 2014;192 (2):305–15.

Kassouf W, Traboulsi SL, Kulkarni GS, Breau RH, Zlotta A, Fairey A, et al. CUA guidelines on the management of non-muscle invasive bladder cancer. Can Urol Assoc J 2015;9(9–10): E690–704.

Kassouf W, Traboulsi SL, Schmitz-Drager B, Palou J, Witjes JA, van Rhijn BW, et al. Follow-up in non-muscle-invasive bladder cancer—International Bladder Cancer Network recommendations. Urol Oncol 2016.

Kavoussi LR, Torrence RJ, Gillen DP, Hudson MA, Haaff EO, Dresner SM, et al. Results of 6 weekly intravesical bacillus Calmette-Guerin instillations on the treatment of superficial bladder tumors. J Urol 1988;139(5):935–40.

Kondylis FI, Demirci S, Ladaga L, Kolm P, Schellhammer PF. Outcomes after intravesical bacillus Calmette-Guerin are not affected by substaging of high grade T1 transitional cell carcinoma. J Urol 2000;163(4):1120–3.

Kulkarni JN, Gupta R. Recurrence and progression in stage T1G3 bladder tumour with intravesical bacille Calmette-Guerin (Danish 1331 strain). BJU Int 2002;90(6):554–7.

Lamm Dea. Clinical practice recommendations for the management of non–muscle invasive bladder cancer. Eur Urol 2008;(Suppl. 7):651–66.

Lamm D, Herr H, Jakse G, Kuroda M, Mostofi FK, Okajima E, et al. Updated concepts and treatment of carcinoma in situ. Urol Oncol 1998;4(4–5):130–8.

Lamm DL. Bacillus Calmette-Guerin immunotherapy. J Urol 1987;138(2):391–2.

Lamm DL. Carcinoma in situ. Urol Clin North Am 1992;19(3):499–508.

Lamm DL, Thor DE, Harris SC, Reyna JA, Stogdill VD, Radwin HM. Bacillus Calmette-Guerin immunotherapy of superficial bladder cancer. J Urol 1980;124(1):38–40.

Lamm DL, Riggs DL, Bugaj M, et al. Prophylaxis in bladder cancer: a metaanalysis. J Urol 2000;163:151–5.

Lamm DL, Blumenstein BA, Crissman JD, Montie JE, Gottesman JE, Lowe BA, et al. Maintenance bacillus Calmette-Guerin immunotherapy for recurrent TA, T1 and carcinoma in situ transitional cell carcinoma of the bladder: a randomized Southwest Oncology Group Study. J Urol 2000;163(4):1124–9.

Lamm DL, Dehaven JI, Riggs DR. Keyhole limpet hemocyanin immunotherapy of bladder cancer: laboratory and clinical studies. Eur Urol 2000;37(Suppl 3):41−4.

Larchian WA, Horiguchi Y, Nair SK, Fair WR, Heston WD, Gilboa E. Effectiveness of combined interleukin 2 and B7.1 vaccination strategy is dependent on the sequence and order: a liposome-mediated gene therapy treatment for bladder cancer. Clin Cancer Res 2000;6 (7):2913−20.

Mack D, Holtl W, Bassi P, Brausi M, Ferrari P, de Balincourt C, et al. The ablative effect of quarter dose bacillus Calmette-Guerin on a papillary marker lesion of the bladder. J Urol 2001;165(2):401−3.

Malmstrom PU, Sylvester RJ, Crawford DE, Friedrich M, Krege S, Rintala E, et al. An individual patient data meta-analysis of the long-term outcome of randomised studies comparing intravesical mitomycin C versus bacillus Calmette-Guerin for non-muscle-invasive bladder cancer. Eur Urol 2009;56(2):247−56.

March N SE, Unda M, Ojea A, et al. A multicenter and randomized prospective study comparing three intravesical therapies, two with Bacillus Calmette-Guérin immunotherapy and one with mitomycin-C chemotherapy in medium and low risk superficial bladder tumours. Eur Urol Supp 2002;1:101.

Morales A, Eidinger D, Bruce AW. Intracavitary Bacillus Calmette-Guerin in the treatment of superficial bladder tumors. J Urol 1976;116(2):180−3.

Nadler RB, Catalona WJ, Hudson MA, Ratliff TL. Durability of the tumor-free response for intravesical bacillus Calmette-Guerin therapy. J Urol 1994;152(2 Pt 1):367−73.

Naitoh J FJ, O'Donnell MA, et al. Interferon alpha for the treatment of superficial bladder cancer. In: Baskin L, Hayward B, editors. Advances in bladder research. New York: Plenum; 1999.

National Comprehensive Cancer Network. NCCN Clinical Practice Guidelines in Oncology. 2017. https://www.nccn.org/professionals/physician_gls/pdf/bladder.pdf.

Network NCC. Clinical practice guidelines in oncology. NCCN; 2007.

Nieder AM, Brausi M, Lamm D, O'Donnell M, Tomita K, Woo H, et al. Management of stage T1 tumors of the bladder: International Consensus Panel. Urology 2005;66(6 Suppl 1):108−25.

Oddens J, Brausi M, Sylvester R, Bono A, van de Beek C, van Andel G, et al. Final results of an EORTC-GU cancers group randomized study of maintenance bacillus Calmette-Guerin in intermediate- and high-risk Ta, T1 papillary carcinoma of the urinary bladder: one-third dose versus full dose and 1 year versus 3 years of maintenance. Eur Urol 2013;63 (3):462−72.

O'Donnell MA. Practical applications of intravesical chemotherapy and immunotherapy in high-risk patients with superficial bladder cancer. Urol Clin North Am 2005;32(2):121−31.

Ojea A, Nogueira JL, Solsona E, Flores N, Gomez JM, Molina JR, et al. A multicentre, randomised prospective trial comparing three intravesical adjuvant therapies for intermediate-risk superficial bladder cancer: low-dose bacillus Calmette-Guerin (27 mg) versus very low-dose bacillus Calmette-Guerin (13.5 mg) versus mitomycin C. Eur Urol 2007;52 (5):1398−406.

Old LJ, Clarke DA, Benacerraf B. Effect of Bacillus Calmette-Guerin infection on transplanted tumours in the mouse. Nature 1959;184(Suppl 5):291−2.

Orsola A, Palou J, Xavier B, Algaba F, Salvador J, Vicente J. Primary bladder carcinoma in situ: assessment of early BCG response as a prognostic factor. Eur Urol 1998;33 (5):457−63.

Palou J, Laguna P, Millan-Rodriguez F, Hall RR, Salvador-Bayarri J, Vicente-Rodriguez J. Control group and maintenance treatment with bacillus Calmette-Guerin for carcinoma in situ and/or high grade bladder tumors. J Urol 2001;165(5):1488−91.

Pansadoro V, Emiliozzi P, Defidio L, Donadio D, Florio A, Maurelli S, et al. Bacillus Calmette-Guerin in the treatment of stage T1 grade 3 transitional cell carcinoma of the bladder: long-term results. J Urol 1995;154(6):2054−8.

Pansadoro V, Emiliozzi P, depaula F, Scarpone P, Pizzo M, Federico G, et al. High grade superficial (G3t1) transitional cell carcinoma of the bladder treated with intravesical Bacillus Calmette-Guerin (BCG). J Exp Clin Cancer Res 2003;22(4 Suppl):223−7.

Patard J, Moudouni S, Saint F, Rioux-Leclercq N, Manunta A, Guy L, et al. Tumor progression and survival in patients with T1G3 bladder tumors: multicentric retrospective study comparing 94 patients treated during 17 years. Urology 2001;58(4):551−6.

Pinsky CM, Camacho FJ, Kerr D, Geller NL, Klein FA, Herr HA, et al. Intravesical administration of bacillus Calmette-Guerin in patients with recurrent superficial carcinoma of the urinary bladder: report of a prospective, randomized trial. Cancer Treat Rep 1985;69 (1):47−53.

Reichert DF, Lamm DL. Long term protection in bladder cancer following intralesional immunotherapy. J Urol 1984;132(3):570−3.

Schellhammer PF, Ladaga LE, Moriarty RP. Intravesical bacillus Calmette-Guerin for the treatment of superficial transitional cell carcinoma of the prostatic urethra in association with carcinoma of the bladder. J Urol 1995;153(1):53−6.

Semper M JR, Solsona E, Fernandez J, Dorrego JM, et al. Treatment of carcinoma in situ of the bladder associated or not associated to non-muscle Invasive transitional carcinoma using two different BCG doses: the standard or one third dose. A five year follow-up. Eur Urol Supp 2010;9:91.

Shahin O, Thalmann GN, Rentsch C, Mazzucchelli L, Studer UE. A retrospective analysis of 153 patients treated with or without intravesical bacillus Calmette-Guerin for primary stage T1 grade 3 bladder cancer: recurrence, progression and survival. J Urol 2003;169 (1):96−100.

Shapiro A GO, Pode D. The treatment of superficial bladder tumors with IL-2 and BCG. J Urol 2007;177−244.

Shelley MD, Kynaston H, Court J, Wilt TJ, Coles B, Burgon K, et al. A systematic review of intravesical bacillus Calmette-Guerin plus transurethral resection vs transurethral resection alone in Ta and T1 bladder cancer. BJU Int 2001;88(3):209−16.

Shelley MD, Wilt TJ, Court J, Coles B, Kynaston H, Mason MD. Intravesical bacillus Calmette-Guerin is superior to mitomycin C in reducing tumour recurrence in high-risk superficial bladder cancer: a meta-analysis of randomized trials. BJU Int 2004;93(4):485−90.

Sylvester RJ, van der Meijden AP, Oosterlinck W, Witjes JA, Bouffioux C, Denis L, et al. Predicting recurrence and progression in individual patients with stage Ta T1 bladder cancer using EORTC risk tables: a combined analysis of 2596 patients from seven EORTC trials. Eur Urol 2006;49(3). 466-5; discussion 75−7.

Takenaka A, Yamada Y, Miyake H, Hara I, Fujisawa M. Clinical outcomes of bacillus Calmette-Guerin instillation therapy for carcinoma in situ of urinary bladder. Int J Urol 2008;15(4):309−13.

Unda M, Solsona E, Gomez JM, Martines- Pineiro JA, Ojea A, CUETO Group. Long-term follow up of the effectiveness of standard dose BCG (81 mg Connaught strain) comparing with a three fold reduce dose (27 mg) in high risk non muscle invasive bladder cancer. Eur Urol Supp 2009;8:284.

van der Meijden AP, Sylvester R, Oosterlinck W, Solsona E, Boehle A, Lobel B, et al. EAU guidelines on the diagnosis and treatment of urothelial carcinoma in situ. Eur Urol 2005;48 (3):363–71.

van Rhijn BW, Burger M, Lotan Y, Solsona E, Stief CG, Sylvester RJ, et al. Recurrence and progression of disease in non-muscle-invasive bladder cancer: from epidemiology to treatment strategy. Eur Urol 2009;56(3):430–42.

Zincke H, Utz DC, Farrow GM. Review of Mayo Clinic experience with carcinoma in situ. Urology 1985;26(4 Suppl):39–46.

Chapter 21

Treatment of Failure of Intravesical Therapy

Sunghyun Paick
Konkuk University Medical Center, Seoul, South Korea

Chapter Outline

Although intravesical Bacillus Calmette—Guerin (BCG) is currently the recommended first-line treatment for high-risk, non-muscle-invasive bladder cancer (NMIBC), it can be complicated by recurrence and progression. Traditionally, recurrent or persistent disease after an initial 6-week course of BCG has been referred to as BCG failure, although this is a heterogeneous term that encompasses a number of different clinical scenarios. BCG failure has been divided into four subcategories by the International Bladder Cancer Group [1]:

BCG refractory: Failure to achieve a disease-free status at 6 months after initial BCG therapy if on maintenance/failure to achieve a disease-free status at 3 months after initial BCG therapy if re-treated.

BCG resistant: Recurrence or persistence of disease at 3 months after induction cycle.

BCG relapsing: Recurrence of disease after achieving a disease-free status by 6 months.

BCG intolerant: Less than adequate course of therapy terminated due to a serious adverse event.

A patient who has failed BCG therapy only has two options. One is to proceed with an immediate radical cystectomy (RC) and the other is to undergo alternative procedures to preserve the bladder. Immediate RC is the standard of care after failure of intravesical therapy, including BCG. There is much evidence that an immediate RC in this setting offers the most accurate

Bladder Cancer. DOI: http://dx.doi.org/10.1016/B978-0-12-809939-1.00021-7

pathological staging and improves disease-specific survival. However, many patients are unfit or unwilling to undergo an RC. In that case, alternative procedures such as concurrent radiochemotherapy and photodynamic therapy (PDT) to preserve the bladder are available, but both are considered oncologically inferior and RC remains the standard of care.

IMMEDIATE RC

Most clinicians and guidelines agree that patients in whom BCG fails should be offered an RC as the gold standard oncologic treatment because they are at significant risk for disease progression, which entails a drastically worse prognosis [2−5].

Several factors support an immediate RC in patients with the highest risk of NMIBC:

1. High rates of clinical−pathological stage discrepancy in NMIBC.

   A total of 27%−51% of patients with T1 bladder tumors were upstaged to muscle-invasive tumors during an RC [6−8]. Residual tumors found on repeated transurethral resection of bladder tumor (TURBT) in these patients are associated with an 82% probability of developing muscle invasion [9]. In a series of 3207 patients who underwent an RC, 243 had only carcinoma in situ (CIS) before surgery, but 36% of patients were upstaged to invasive cancer (pT1−T4) and 22.6% of patients were upstaged to muscle-invasive disease after an RC [10]. The following are the factors associated with high risk of tumor progression to muscle invasion: high grade and deep invasion into the lamina propria, diffuse CIS, tumors in the diverticula, substantial involvement of the distal ureters or prostatic urethra, refractory to initial therapy, or too large or anatomically inaccessible to complete endoscopic remove [11−16].

   Each occurrence of T1 tumors is also associated with a 5%−10% chance of metastasis [17].

   These data offer compelling evidence of the potential to underestimate disease status and recommend an immediate RC in patients with high-risk NMIBC.
2. Patients initially presenting with NMIBC who progress to muscle invasion have a worse prognosis than patients initially presenting with muscle-invasive disease [3,5,18]. The 3-year bladder cancer-specific survival after an RC due to muscle-invasive bladder cancer was 67% in the primary group and 37% in the progressive group [5].
3. A delay in an RC might lead to decreased disease-specific survival. Survival rates (10-year cancer-specific survival) for patients with initial T1 high-grade tumors who opted for an early versus a deferred RC were significantly different, at 78% vs 51% [19]. A study by Herr et al. demonstrated similar results. The survival rate of patients who underwent an

early RC for NMIBC (less than 2 years after initial BCG therapy) was 92%, while that of patients in the delayed group was only 56% [17].

A delay in RC of even 12 weeks is associated with poorer survival. Some of these procedures do not seem to be "early" enough [20]. Therefore, if RC is indicated, it should be performed as soon as possible.

However, an RC with urinary diversion has considerable morbidity, including gastrointestinal, genitourinary, infectious, and wound-related complications totaling over 60% of RC patients within 90 days of surgery, even in high-volume centers of excellence and regardless of open versus robotic approaches [21,22]. Mortality after RC may increase substantially in older patients, but patients with bladder tumors are usually old. Due to these reasons, in the United States, only 42% of patients between 75 and 79 years old and 29% of patients between 80 and 84 years old underwent an RC [23]. Thus, the risks of RC and urinary diversion must be weighed and carefully balanced against the risks of disease progression and a potential loss of the opportunity for cure in high-risk patients.

RADIOCHEMOTHERAPY

NMIBC is superficially located inside the body at the lumen. Thus, an external beam radiation therapy with or without systemic chemotherapy is not an appropriate treatment method. However, maximal debulking by TURBT, radiation, and chemotherapy have been the strategies for the treatment of patients with muscle-invasive bladder cancer who are unsuitable for major surgery or refuse RC. In addition, this method can be an alternative treatment to an RC for an NMIBC too. There is much evidence that the addition of chemotherapy to radical radiotherapy improves outcomes in patients, at least in the setting of muscle-invasive disease [24,25]. Therefore, if it is possible, radiochemotherapy is recommended instead of radiation monotherapy.

A study by Wo et al. reported findings of 17 patients who underwent radiochemotherapy after maximal TURBT following T2 recurrence after BCG failure for NMIBC [26]. During a 7-year follow-up, only 1 patient required a cystectomy, 10 patients (59%) were free of any bladder tumor recurrence, and disease-specific survival was 70%. Weiss et al. followed-up 141 patients with high-risk T1 disease who were treated with radiochemotherapy (in 80% patients) or radiation only (in 20% patients) after maximal TURBT [27]. Tumor progression at 5 and 10 years was 19% and 30%, respectively. Disease-specific survival rates were 82% and 73% at 5 and 10 years, respectively. More than 80% of survivors preserved their bladder. Unfortunately, prior BCG use for the cohort was not described. These interesting results cannot specifically answer the question of the role of radiochemotherapy in the treatment of NMIBC after BCG failure. Currently, the North American multicenter, cooperative Radiation Therapy Oncology

TABLE 21.1 Previous Clinical Studies of Radiochemotherapy for NMIBC

Study	Treatment	No. Patients	Status of Patients	Results	Comments
Weiss et al. (2006) [27]	TURBT and radiochemotherapy (in 80% patients) or radiation only (in 20%)	141	High-risk T1 bladder cancer	88% CR at restaging TURBT 19% progression at 5 years 73% DSS at 10 years 51% OS at 10 years	Over 80% of survivors could retain their native bladder Around 70% were "delighted" or "pleased" with their urinary function
Wo et al. (2009) [26]	TURBT and radiochemotherapy	17	T2 recurrence after failure of BCG therapy for T1 bladder cancer	70% DSS at 7 years 59% OS at 7 years	At 7 years, 54% of patients were alive with intact bladders and free of invasive recurrence

CR, complete response; DSS, disease-specific survival; OS, overall survival.

Group (RTOG) protocol RTOG 0926 is evaluating the role of radiochemotherapy (61.2 Gy with concurrent cisplatin or 5-fluorouracil plus mitomycin C) after maximum TURBT for patients with high-risk T1 bladder cancer following BCG failure, for whom the next therapy would have been RC [28]. This trial will hopefully clarify the role of trimodal therapy in treating patients with high-risk NMIBC and previous BCG failure (Table 21.1).

PHOTODYNAMIC THERAPY

PDT works on the principle of exciting photosensitized bladder tumor cells with a specific wavelength of intravesical light, leading to their destruction.

PDT for bladder cancer initially used hematoporphyrin derivatives administered intravenously followed by focal intravesical light treatments of papillary tumors or whole-bladder treatments for CIS [29,30]. Although these therapies were modestly effective at treating lesions, there were notable side effects. Almost all patients had cutaneous photosensitivity requiring them to avoid sunlight for 4–6 weeks and an appreciable rate of bladder capacity loss. In these studies, usability of PDT for BCG failure could not be estimated because patients with BCG failure were in the minority.

TABLE 21.2 Previous Clinical Studies of PDT for Bladder Tumor

Study	Agent	Administration Method	No. Patients	Response, % Early	Response, % Late	Adverse Effects	Comments
Nseyo et al. (1987) [30]	Photofrin II	Intravenous	23	83.3	30.4	Irritating LUTS, bladder shrinkage	Small number of BCG failure patients
Uchibayashi et al. (1995) [35]	Hematoporphyrin derivative	Intravenous	34	73.5 (3 months)	22 (24 months)	Skin photosensitivity, transient bladder capacity decrease	Unclear on what prior therapies are
Waidelich et al. (2001) [31]	5-ALA	Intravenous	11		46 (18 months)	Transient frequency, urgency	
Berger et al. (2003) [32]	5-ALA	Intravesical	31		52 (24 months)	Dysuria due to urinary tract infection, hematuria	No dose-limiting toxicity
Bader et al. (2003) [33]	HAL	Intravesical	17	52.9 (6 months)	11.8 (21 months)	Irritative bladder symptoms, infection, gross hematuria	No dose-limiting toxicity
Lee et al. (2013) [34]	Radachlorin	Intravenous	34	90.9 (12 months)	64.4 (24 months)	LUTS, infection, hematuria	Prospective trial, safe with no dose-limiting toxicity

LUTS, lower urinary tract symptoms; HAL, hexaminolevulinate.

The 5-aminolevulinic acid (5-ALA, a protoporphyrin IX precursor preferentially absorbed by malignant cells) is another photosensitizing agent that can be used for PDT. A study by Waidelich et al. performed PDT by an oral administration of 5-ALA in 24 patients with rapidly recurring, multifocal, BCG refractory, superficial pTa-pT1, transitional cell carcinoma of the bladder, and CIS [31]. Seven of 24 (29%) patients were recurrence-free, 4 (17%) progressed, and 3 (13%) underwent an RC. Noted side effects included nausea, hypotension, tachycardia, and some skin sensitivity. Immediately after the oral administration of 5-ALA, hypotension and tachycardia occurred in 19 and 10 patients, respectively, with previously known severe cardiovascular disease.

To prevent cutaneous photosensitivity or other systemic reactions, intravesically administered photosensitizing agents have also been used. A study by Berger et al. reported findings of a cohort of patients with recurrent BC treated with intravesical 5-ALA [32]. Side effects were tolerable, there were no phototoxic skin reactions, and only 13% had persistent dysuria or lower urinary tract symptoms. However, in a small group with BCG failure (10 patients) and after a mean follow-up of 23.7 months, 6 patients had a recurrence. Use of a similar agent, hexaminolevulinate has also been reported, although the outcomes have been modest, with only 11% disease-free patients at 21 months in a diverse cohort of patients with bladder cancer [33].

Radachlorin, a third photosensitizer, has also been investigated in a prospective trial of 34 patients with high-risk NMIBC and BCG failure [34]. This trial demonstrated that intravenous infusion of radachlorin was also safe without significant adverse events, and all patients were tumor-free at 3 months, with 91%, 64.4%, and 60.1% remaining disease-free at 12, 24, and 30 months, respectively.

These studies are small and underpowered to assess efficacy. Thus, PDT is not a realistic option for patients with BCG failure and is only available in highly specialized centers (Table 21.2).

REFERENCES

[1] Nieder AM, Brausi M, Lamm D, O'Donnell M, Tomita K, Woo H, et al. Management of stage T1 tumors of the bladder: International Consensus Panel. Urology 2005;66:108−25.

[2] Brausi M, Witjes JA, Lamm D, Persad R, Palou J, Colombel M, et al. A review of current guidelines and best practice recommendations for the management of nonmuscle invasive bladder cancer by the International Bladder Cancer Group. J Urol 2011;186:2158−67.

[3] van den Bosch S, Alfred Witjes JA. Long-term cancer-specific survival in patients with high-risk, non-muscle-invasive bladder cancer and tumour progression: a systematic review. Eur Urol 2011;60:493−500.

[4] Catalona WJ, Hudson MA, Gillen DP, Andriole GL, Ratliff TL. Risks and benefits of repeated courses of intravesical bacillus Calmette-Guerin therapy for superficial bladder cancer. J Urol 1987;137:220−4.

[5] Schrier BP, Hollander MP, van Rhijn BW, Kiemeney LA, Witjes JA. Prognosis of muscle-invasive bladder cancer: difference between primary and progressive tumours and implications for therapy. Eur Urol 2004;45:292−6.

[6] Fritsche HM, Burger M, Svatek RS, Jeldres C, Karakiewicz PI, Novara G, et al. Characteristics and outcomes of patients with clinical T1 grade 3 urothelial carcinoma treated with radical cystectomy: results from an international cohort. Eur Urol 2010;57:300−9.

[7] Turker P, Bostrom PJ, Wroclawski ML, van Rhijn B, Kortekangas H, Kuk C, et al. Upstaging of urothelial cancer at the time of radical cystectomy: factors associated with upstaging and its effect on outcome. BJU Int 2012;110:804−11.

[8] Shariat SF, Palapattu GS, Karakiewicz PI, Rogers CG, Vazina A, Bastian PJ, et al. Discrepancy between clinical and pathologic stage: impact on prognosis after radical cystectomy. Eur Urol 2007;51:137−49.

[9] Herr HW. High-risk superficial bladder cancer: transurethral resection alone in selected patients with T1 tumor. Semin Urol Oncol 1997;15:142−6.

[10] Tilki D, Reich O, Svatek RS, Karakiewicz PI, Kassouf W, Novara G, et al. Characteristics and outcomes of patients with clinical carcinoma in situ only treated with radical cystectomy: an international study of 243 patients. J Urol 2010;183:1757−63.

[11] Palou J, Sylvester RJ, Faba OR, Parada R, Pena JA, Algaba F, et al. Female gender and carcinoma in situ in the prostatic urethra are prognostic factors for recurrence, progression, and disease -specific mortality in T1G3 bladder cancer patients treated with bacillus Calmette -Guerin. Eur Urol 2012;62:118−25.

[12] Sylvester RJ, van der Meijden AP, Oosterlinck W, Witjes JA, Bouffioux C, Denis L, et al. Predicting recurrence and progression in individual patients with stage Ta T1 bladder cancer using EORTC risk tables: a combined analysis of 2596 patients from seven EORTC trials. Eur Urol 2006;49:466-5.

[13] Fernandez-Gomez J, Madero R, Solsona E, Unda M, Martinez-Pineiro L, Gonzalez M, et al. Predicting nonmuscle invasive bladder cancer recurrence and progression in patients treated with bacillus Calmette-Guerin: the CUETO scoring model. J Urol 2009;182:2195−203.

[14] Kamat AM, Gee JR, Dinney CP, Grossman HB, Swanson DA, Millikan RE, et al. The case for early cystectomy in the treatment of non -muscle invasive micropapillary bladder carcinoma. J Urol 2006;175:881−5.

[15] Parmar MK, Freedman LS, Hargreave TB, Tolley DA. Prognostic factors for recurrence and follow up policies in the treatment of superficial bladder cancer: report from the British Medical Research Council Subgroup on Superficial Bladder Cancer (Urological Cancer Working Party). J Urol 1989;143:284−8.

[16] Kurth KH, Denis L, Bouffioux C, Sylvester R, Debruyne FM, Pavone-Macaluso M, et al. Factors affecting recurrence and progression in superficial bladder tumours. Eur J Cancer 1995;31A:1840−6.

[17] Herr HW, Sogani PC. Does early cystectomy improve the survival of patients with high risk superficial bladder tumors? J Urol 2001;166:1296−9.

[18] Breau RH, Karnes RJ, Farmer SA, Thapa P, Cagiannos I, Morash C, et al. Progression to detrusor muscle invasion during urothelial carcinoma surveillance is associated with poor prognosis. BJU Int 2014;113:900−6.

[19] Denzinger S, Fritsche HM, Otto W, Blana A, Wieland WF, Burger M. Early versus deferred cystectomy for initial high-risk pT1G3 urothelial carcinoma of the bladder: do risk factors define feasibility of bladder-sparing approach? Eur Urol 2008;53:146−52.

[20] Sanchez-Ortiz RF, Huang WC, Mick R, Van Arsdalen KN, Wein AJ, Malkowicz SB. An interval longer than 12 weeks between the diagnosis of muscle invasion and cystectomy is associated with worse outcome in bladder carcinoma. J Urol 2003;169:110−15.

[21] Shabsigh A, Korets R, Vora KC, Brooks CM, Cronin AM, Savage C, et al. Defining early morbidity of radical cystectomy for patients with bladder cancer using a standardized reporting methodology. Eur Urol 2009;55:164−74.

[22] Bochner BH, Dalbagni G, Sjoberg DD, Silberstein J, Keren Paz GE, Donat SM, et al. Comparing open radical cystectomy and robot-assisted laparoscopic radical cystectomy: a randomized clinical trial. Eur Urol 2015;67:1042−50.

[23] Hall MC, Chang SS, Dalbagni G, Pruthi RS, Seigne JD, Skinner EC, et al. Guideline for the management of nonmuscle invasive bladder cancer (stages Ta, T1, and Tis): 2007 update. J Urol 2007;178:2314−30.

[24] James ND, Hussain SA, Hall E, Jenkins P, Tremlett J, Rawlings C, et al. Radiotherapy with or without chemotherapy in muscle-invasive bladder cancer. N Engl J Med 2012;366:1477−88.

[25] Coppin CM, Gospodarowicz MK, James K, Tannock IF, Zee B, Carson J, et al. Improved local control of invasive bladder cancer by concurrent cisplatin and preoperative or definitive radiation. The National Cancer Institute of Canada Clinical Trials Group. J Clin Oncol 1996;14:2901−7.

[26] Wo JY, Shipley WU, Dahl DM, Coen JJ, Heney NM, Kaufman DS, et al. The results of concurrent chemo-radiotherapy for recurrence after treatment with bacillus Calmette-Guerin for non-muscle-invasive bladder cancer: is immediate cystectomy always necessary? BJU Int 2009;104:179−83.

[27] Weiss C, Wolze C, Engehausen DG, Ott OJ, Krause FS, Schrott KM, et al. Radiochemotherapy after transurethral resection for high-risk T1 bladder cancer: an alternative to intravesical therapy or early cystectomy? J Clin Oncol 2006;24:2318−24.

[28] Kamat AM, Flaig TW, Grossman HB, Konety B, Lamm D, O'Donnell MA, et al. Expert consensus document: consensus statement on best practice management regarding the use of intravesical immunotherapy with BCG for bladder cancer. Nat Rev Urol 2015;12:225−35.

[29] Prout Jr GR, Lin CW, Benson Jr R, Nseyo UO, Daly JJ, Griffin PP, et al. Photodynamic therapy with hematoporphyrin derivative in the treatment of superficial transitional-cell carcinoma of the bladder. N Engl J Med 1987;317:1251−5.

[30] Nseyo UO, Dougherty TJ, Sullivan L. Photodynamic therapy in the management of resistant lower urinary tract carcinoma. Cancer 1987;60:3113−19.

[31] Waidelich R, Stepp H, Baumgartner R, Weninger E, Hofstetter A, Kriegmair M. Clinical experience with 5-aminolevulinic acid and photodynamic therapy for refractory superficial bladder cancer. J Urol 2001;165:1904−7.

[32] Berger AP, Steiner H, Stenzl A, Akkad T, Bartsch G, Holtl L. Photodynamic therapy with intravesical instillation of 5-aminolevulinic acid for patients with recurrent superficial bladder cancer: a single-center study. Urology 2003;61:338−41.

[33] Bader MJ, Stepp H, Beyer W, Pongratz T, Sroka R, Kriegmair M, et al. Photodynamic therapy of bladder cancer? − a phase I study using hexaminolevulinate (HAL). Urol Oncol 2013;31:1178−83.

[34] Lee JY, Diaz RR, Cho KS, Lim MS, Chung JS, Kim WT, et al. Efficacy and safety of photodynamic therapy for recurrent, high grade nonmuscle invasive bladder cancer refractory or intolerant to Bacille Calmette-Guerin immunotherapy. J Urol 2013;190:1192−9.

[35] Uchibayashi T, Koshida K, Kunimi K, Hisazumi H. Whole bladder wall photodynamic therapy for refractory carcinoma in situ of the bladder. Br J Cancer 1995;71:625−8.

Treatment for Muscle-Invasive Bladder Cancer (MIBC)

Chapter 22

Neoadjuvant Chemotherapy for Muscle-Invasive Bladder Cancer

Ho Kyung Seo[1], Whi-An Kwon[2] and Sung Han Kim[1]

[1]*Research Institute and National Cancer Center, Goyang, South Korea,* [2]*Wonkwang University Sanbon Hospital, Gunpo, South Korea*

Chapter Outline

INTRODUCTION

Bladder cancer is diagnosed in approximately 74,000 patients in the United States and approximately 450,000 new cases are diagnosed worldwide each year. Bladder cancer is the fourth most common cancer in men and the 11th most common cancer in women, with approximately 165,000 related deaths worldwide [1,2]. In Korea, the Korean National Cancer Registry reported that bladder cancer was the 12th most common type of cancer during 2013, with an estimated 3762 newly diagnosed patients [3]. Approximately 20% of all newly diagnosed bladder cancer cases involve muscle-invasive bladder cancer (MIBC), and 20% of non-muscle-invasive bladder cancers (NMIBCs) eventually progress to muscle-invasive disease [4,5]. Radical cystectomy and bilateral pelvic lymphadenectomy are the standard treatment for MIBC. However, nearly half of all patients who undergo only radical cystectomy will progress to metastatic disease within 2 years, which eventually results in death [6−8].

Bladder Cancer. DOI: http://dx.doi.org/10.1016/B978-0-12-809939-1.00022-9

Neoadjuvant chemotherapy (NAC) is an effective treatment for controlling various types of solid tumors, such as breast and colon cancers [9–13]. Multiple randomized controlled studies have been performed to define the effectiveness of cisplatin-based NAC before cystectomy for bladder cancer. Unfortunately, many of these studies were limited by inadequate statistical power and the absence of a standardized surgical approach, and were unable to clearly demonstrate a survival advantage for NAC. Grossman et al. [14] performed a prospective study of patients with MIBC in 2003 and found that cisplatin-based NAC provided an improved survival rate, and a 2005 meta-analysis of 11 prospective studies confirmed the benefits of NAC [15]. The National Comprehensive Cancer Network and the European Association of Urology guidelines have subsequently recommended NAC as a standard treatment for MIBC [16,17].

BASIS OF NAC FOR BLADDER CANCER

The goal of NAC is to remove micrometastases, reduce recurrence, and increase survival. In theory, micrometastases respond better to chemotherapy, compared to treatment for macrometastases that are accompanied by radiographically detected distant metastasis [18]. Compared to adjuvant chemotherapy (AC), NAC provides several advantages. First, patients tolerate NAC treatment better, as it is administered before surgery compromises their physical status, and postoperative complications can result in delayed chemotherapy administration. Second, it is easier to evaluate the tumor's response to NAC because the NAC is administered before the tumor is resected. Third, NAC can potentially downstage bulky and locally advanced tumors, which increases the likelihood of achieving the negative surgical margins that predict local recurrence after cystectomy. Finally, micrometastases can be effectively treated at an early stage. Nevertheless, NAC is associated with several disadvantages, such as delaying definitive local therapy for patients who do not respond the chemotherapy. These patients can experience disease progression, the development of chemotherapy-associated complications (e.g., infection that can preclude surgery), and the possibility of overtreatment [19–21].

RESPONSE OF BLADDER CANCER TO NAC

In metastatic breast and colon cancers, chemotherapy provides response rates of 35%–60% [22–25] and 17%–36% [26], respectively. Bladder cancer is also sensitive to chemotherapy, and treatment for metastatic bladder cancer using methotrexate, vinblastine, doxorubicin, and cisplatin (MVAC chemotherapy) provides a response rate of 50%–70% and complete remission in 12%–40% of cases [27–30]. Thus, it is possible that NAC using MVAC may be useful for treating bladder cancer. Many studies have explored the role of NAC in MIBC although most studies were underpowered to detect a significant difference in the survival rate and the surgical techniques were an important confounding factor.

The European Organization for Research and Treatment of Cancer (EORTC) and the Medical Research Council (MRC) performed the largest Phase III trial of NAC for bladder cancer (BA06 30894) [31]. That study investigated the effectiveness of cisplatin, methotrexate, and vinblastine (CMV)—based NAC in patients with MIBC (T2—T4a, N0/X, and M0) who were treated using cystectomy and/or radiotherapy (RT). Between 1989 and 1995, the study recruited 976 patients and performed a median follow-up of 8.0 years (cystectomy alone: $n = 212$, chemotherapy followed by cystectomy: $n = 216$, RT alone: $n = 210$, chemotherapy followed by RT: $n = 193$, RT + cystectomy: $n = 33$, chemotherapy followed by RT + cystectomy: $n = 33$, missing data: $n = 79$). The results revealed that CMV provided a 16% reduction in the risk of death (hazard ratio [HR]: 0.84, 95% confidence interval [CI]: 0.72—0.99; $P = 0.037$), a 23% reduction in the risk of metastases or death (HR: 0.77, 95% CI: 0.66—0.90; $P = 0.001$), a 13% reduction in the risk of local disease or death (HR: 0.87, 95% CI: 0.75—1.01; $P = 0.067$), an 18% reduction in the risk of disease or death (HR: 0.82, 95% CI: 0.70—0.95; $P = 0.008$), and a 4% reduction in the risk of locoregional relapse (HR: 0.96, 95% CI: 0.80—1.15; $P = 0.632$). In the subgroup analyses, the authors evaluated 403 patients who had received RT (RT alone: $n = 210$, chemotherapy followed by RT: $n = 193$) and 428 patients who had undergone cystectomy (cystectomy alone: $n = 212$, chemotherapy followed by cystectomy: $n = 216$). CMV treatment provided 20% and 26% reductions in the risk of death for the RT and cystectomy groups, respectively (RT, HR: 0.80, 95% CI: 0.63—1.02; $P = 0.07$; cystectomy, HR: 0.74, 95% CI: 0.57—0.96; $P = 0.022$). In terms of locoregional disease-free survival, there was some evidence that CMV provided a greater benefit before cystectomy (HR: 0.74, 95% CI: 0.58—0.95; $P = 0.019$), compared to before RT (HR: 0.91, 95% CI: 0.73—1.14; $P = 0.417$). However, the study was limited by the fact that the CMV regimen was not considered a standard of care for MIBC and has never been compared to MVAC. In addition, approximately 40% of the patients in the chemotherapy and local therapy arms received RT and not radical cystectomy.

The Southwestern Oncology Group (SWOG) 8710 study evaluated 317 patients with MIBC (cT2—T4aN0) and compared patients who underwent radical cystectomy alone or three cycles of MVAC NAC before radical cystectomy [14]. The authors found that patients who underwent only radical cystectomy had a 33% higher risk of mortality, compared to patients who received NAC (HR: 1.33, 95% CI: 1.00—1.76). The median survival was 46 months (95% CI: 25—60 months) among patients in the cystectomy group and 77 months (95% CI: 55—104 months) among patients in the combination therapy group. At 5 years, 57% of the patients in the combination therapy group were alive, compared to 43% in the cystectomy group ($P = 0.06$). Approximately 38% of the patients in the chemotherapy arm achieved pT0 status at the time of the cystectomy, compared to 15% in the control arm ($P < 0.001$). In addition, subgroup analyses revealed that MVAC NAC improved the survival rates among patients with $\geq$ T3 stage, positive lymph nodes, positive surgical margins, and resection of >10 lymph nodes. These studies (BA06 30894 and SWOG 8710) are summarized in Table 22.1.

A meta-analysis of 10 prospective randomized studies analyzed 2688 patients who had received NAC and found that this treatment provided a significant increase in overall survival (45%−50%, HR: 0.87, 95% CI: 0.78−0.98, $P = 0.016$), a 5% absolute benefit at 5 years, and a 13% reduction in the risk of death [36]. These results provided Level 1 evidence to support the use of NAC for clinically localized MIBC [14,37,38]. The Advanced Bladder Cancer meta-analysis also evaluated updated data from 3005 patients in 11 randomized NAC trials [15]. The meta-analysis revealed that a significant survival benefit was associated with platinum-based combination chemotherapy (HR: 0.86, 95% CI: 0.77−0.95; $P = 0.003$), which provided a 5% absolute improvement in survival at 5 years. There was also a significant disease-free survival benefit associated with the platinum-based combination chemotherapy (HR: 0.78, 95% CI: 0.71−0.86; $P < 0.0001$). Those results are similar to the results from the EORTC and MRC trial, which was the largest trial in the analysis. Based on the randomized trial results and the subsequent meta-analyses, it appears that cisplatin-based NAC is associated with an overall survival advantage of 5%−6% and a pathologic Complete Remission (pCR) rate of 30%−40%. The results from meta-analyses of Phase III trials for NAC are summarized in Table 22.2.

The current National Comprehensive Cancer Network guidelines list dose-dense MVAC or gemcitabine and cisplatin (GC) as optimal choices for NAC in patients with cT2−T4aN0M0 urothelial cancer [40]. The European Association of Urology guidelines currently recommend NAC using cisplatin-based combination therapy for T2−T4acN0M0 bladder cancer (http://uroweb.org/guideline/bladder-cancer-muscle-invasive-and-metastatic/). The American Society of Clinical Oncology has recently endorsed the European Association of Urology guidelines [41].

SURROGATE MARKERS FOR THE EFFICACY OF NAC

Downstaging of bladder cancer is a surrogate marker for evaluating the efficacy of NAC [42]. Many studies have reported that pCR is associated with improved disease-free survival and overall survival [14,42,43]. The SWOG 8710 study also revealed that compared to surgery alone, MVAC NAC provided a significantly higher pCR rate (38% vs 15%, $P < 0.001$), a better 5-year survival rate (57% vs 42%), and a better overall survival (median: 77 months vs 46 months, $P = 0.06$). Furthermore, 85% of the patients who

TABLE 22.1 Randomized Clinical Trials of NAC in MIBC

Study	Number of Patients	Randomization	Results
BA06 30894 [31]	976 (cT2–T4aN0M0)	Three cycles of CMV + cystectomy and/or RT vs cystectomy and/or RT alone	23% reduction in the risk of metastases or death (HR, 0.77; 95% CI, 0.66–0.90; $P = .001$) after CMV. Risk reduction in overall survival by 16% with CMV (HR: 0.84; 95% CI, 0.72–0.99; $P = 0.037$)
SWOG 8710 [14]	317 (cT2–T4aN0M0)	Three cycles of MVAC + cystectomy vs cystectomy alone	Improvement in pathologic complete response rate (38% vs 15%; $P < 0.001$). Overall survival improvement with MVAC (77 vs 46 months; $P = 0.06$)
WMURG/ ABCSG group [32]	255 (cT2–T4M0)	Cisplatin-based chemotherapy + RT vs RT alone	No difference in survival. The control groups faring marginally better than the chemotherapy groups (OR: 1.13)
Martinez group [33]	122 (cT2–4aNx-2M0)	Three cycles of cisplatin-based chemotherapy + cystectomy vs cystectomy alone	No difference in survival. However, the survival of the responders was significantly better than that of nonresponders ($P = 0.0142$), with specific death rate of 26.3% and 62.5%, respectively.
Sengeløv group [34]	153 (cT2–T4bNX-3M0)	Three cycles of cisplatin-based chemotherapy + cystectomy and/or RT vs cystectomy and/or RT alone	No difference in survival. The actuarial 5-year OS rate for all 153 patients was 29% and 29% for both treatment groups
Sherif group [35]	620 (cT1G3, T2–T4aNXM0)	Two cycles of cisplatin-based chemotherapy + preoperative RT and cystectomy vs preoperative RT and cystectomy	Risk reduction in overall survival by 20% with NAC (HR: 0.80; 95% CI, 0.64–0.99; $P = 0.049$)

WMURG, West Midlands Urological Research Group; ABCSG, Australian Bladder Cancer Study Group; CMV, Cisplatin+methotrexate+vinblastine; OR, odds ratio; OS, overall survival.

TABLE 22.2 Meta-Analyses of NAC Phase III Trials for MIBC

Study	Journal	Type of Treatment	Number of Trials	No. of Patients	Therapy	OS (HR)	DFS (HR)
Advanced bladder cancer meta-analysis collaboration, 2003 [36]	Lancet	Neoadjuvant	10	2688	Cisplatin-based	0.87 (0.78–0.98), $P = 0.016$ A 5% absolute survival benefit at 5 years	Insufficient data for analysis
Winquist et al., 2004 [39]	The Journal of Urology	Neoadjuvant	11	2605	Cisplatin-based	0.90 (0.82–0.99), $P = 0.002$	Insufficient data for analysis
Advanced bladder cancer meta-analysis collaboration, 2005 [15]	European Urology	Neoadjuvant	11	3005	Cisplatin-based	0.86 (0.77–0.95), $P = 0.003$ 5% absolute survival benefit at 5 years	0.78 (0.71–0.86), $P < 0.0001$

OS, overall survival; DFS, disease-free survival.

achieved pCR survived for >5 years, and this outcome was closely associated with long-term survival [14]. The recent Nordic Cystectomy Trials (I and II) also found that there was a close association between downstaging after NAC and improved survival, as the survival rate increased by 31.3% in patients who achieved pCR and by 17.9% in patients with downstaged NMIBC [44]. Thus, these results indicated that downstaging after NAC was a strong surrogate marker that could detect patients who were resistant to anticancer chemotherapy [44]. Moreover, the pCR rate after NAC ranges from 7% to 43% [37], and the 5-year survival rate for patients who achieve pCR is 85%–95% [14,45,46]. The pathological response (PaR) rates from recent studies are summarized in Table 22.3.

ANTICANCER AGENTS AND DURATIONS FOR NAC

Although many studies have found that NAC provides increased survival among patients with MIBC, there is no consensus regarding the agents or durations that are most appropriate for treatment. The current evidence indicates that cisplatin-based combination regimens are the recommended treatment, and the common regimens include three-cycle treatments using CMV (based on the EORTC/MRC study) or MVAC (based on the SWOG 8710 study) [14,27,47]. Furthermore, dose-dense MVAC or accelerated MVAC with prophylactic granulocyte-colony stimulating factor can increase the concentration and strength of MVAC. This regimen has been extensively studied among patients with locally advanced or metastatic bladder cancer, who receive 3–4 cycles of MVAC with granulocyte-colony stimulating factor treatment every 2 weeks. Although this regimen did not increase the survival rate, it does increase progression-free survival and exhibits relatively low toxicity [48,49]. Its efficacy has been observed in two single-group studies [50,51], although no prospective randomized trials have confirmed the efficacy of NAC using dose-dense MVAC. The first study evaluated 39 patients with MIBC (cN1: 43%) who received a dose-dense MVAC regimen (every 14 days for 4 cycles) which provided a PaR of 49% (19/39) and a pCR rate of 26% (10/39). The average follow-up period was 24 months, and the 1-year disease-free survival rate was higher among patients who achieved PaR, compared with patients who did not (89% vs 67%, HR: 2.6, 95% CI: 0.80–8.1) [50]. The second study evaluated 40 patients with MIBC (cN1: 7%) who received three cycles of an accelerated MVAC regimen, which provided pCR in 15 patients (38%) and downstaging to non-muscle-invasive disease in six patients (14%) [51]. Nevertheless, these studies were limited by their small sample sizes, possible sampling bias, and nonrandomized designs.

Combination therapy using GC provides similar efficacy and lower toxicity, compared to MVAC chemotherapy, in patients with metastatic bladder cancer. However, MVAC therapy provided a slightly better HR of 0.78 (95% CI: 0.40–1.54; $P = 0.48$) [52]. No prospective randomized trials have

TABLE 22.3 Summary of Comparative Studies Assessing Complete Pathologic Response and Partial Pathologic Response After Different NAC Regimens

Study	Year	Study Design	No. Patients Treated With Chemotherapy vs Cystectomy Only	Patient Characteristics	pCR (%)	5-Year Survival Rate (%)
Martinez group [33]	1995	Three cycles of cisplatin-based chemotherapy + cystectomy vs cystectomy alone	62 vs 60	cT2–4aNx-2M0	19.6 vs 3.4	NA
Sengeløv group [34]	2002	Three cycles of cisplatin-based chemotherapy + cystectomy and/or RT vs cystectomy and/or RT alone	79 vs 74	cT2–T4bNX-3M0	NA	29 vs 29
SWOG 8710 [14]	2003	MVAC vs cystectomy only	153 vs 154	cT2–4aN0M0	38 vs 15	57 vs 42
Sherif group [35]	2004	Two cycles of cisplatin-based chemotherapy + preoperative RT and cystectomy vs preoperative RT and cystectomy	306 vs 314	cT1G3, T2–T4aNXM0	NA	56 vs 48
Nordic Cystectomy Trials [44]	2011	Cisplatin-based NAC vs cystectomy only	225 vs 224	T2–T4aNXM0	22.7 vs 12.5	88.2 vs 57.1
BA06 30894 [31]	2011	Three cycles of CMV + cystectomy and/or RT vs cystectomy and/or RT alone	491 vs 485	cT2–T4aN0M0	NA	56 vs 50

NA, not available.

evaluated GC combination therapy for NAC, although an international retrospective study of 19 North American and European centers evaluated 935 patients with bladder cancer who received NAC (T2−T4a, cN0) [30]. In that study, GC was used for 64% of the cases, MVAC was used for 20% of the cases, and other therapies were used for 15% of the cases. There was no significant difference in the pCR rates of the GC and MVAC groups (23.9% vs 24.5%, $P = 0.2$) although these rates were lower than the rate for MVAC in the INT-0800 study. This discrepancy is likely related to differences in the patient populations, although selection bias, use of support and salvage therapies, and differences in staging and diagnosis may also have affected those findings. Nevertheless, the North American and European study revealed that GC therapy is a useful alternative to MVAC therapy for NAC among elderly patients or patients with comorbidities, who might not be able to receive MVAC.

NAC FOR PATIENTS WITH RENAL INSUFFICIENCY

The efficacy of NAC has been proven in patients with normal renal function, clinical stage $\geq$ T2, and negative lymph nodes, which is typically based on a standard dose of cisplatin [42]. However, renal insufficiency can cause poor performance status and may contraindicate platinum-based chemotherapy [12]. Furthermore, renal insufficiency frequently occurs in patients with a bladder tumor that is near one or both ureters, and previous studies of NAC have found that approximately 30%−50% of all patients were not eligible for standard chemotherapy because of renal insufficiency [53,54]. Carboplatin is a reasonable alternative to cisplatin for patients with metastatic bladder cancer and renal insufficiency [55] although carboplatin is less effective than cisplatin [56−59]. Therefore, careful consideration is warranted when carboplatin is being considered in place of cisplatin for NAC, as there are no concrete data regarding NAC in patients who cannot receive cisplatin.

SELECTING SURGERY BASED ON THE RESPONSE TO NAC

Radical cystectomy must be performed after completing NAC for bladder cancer, regardless of the clinical response. This is because only radical cystectomy and bilateral pelvis lymphadenectomy can accurately evaluate the efficacy of chemotherapy, even if the tumor exhibits good response to NAC. In the SWOG S0219 trial, 77 patients with bladder cancer (T2−T4a) received three cycles of chemotherapy using paclitaxel, carboplatin, and gemcitabine; the cases were subsequently restaged and the risk of residual cancer was evaluated among patients who achieved a complete clinical response [52]. In that study, 34 patients achieved a complete clinical response (46%), and 10 of the 34 patients had undergone immediate radical cystectomy. Among these 10 patients, 6 patients (60%) had a continuous tumor in the bladder tissue, which indicates that radical cystectomy should be performed regardless of the tumor's response to NAC.

NAC AND AC

No prospective randomized trial has directly compared NAC and AC. Although the initial studies of AC found promising results, they were ultimately terminated because of limited patient enrollment [60−63]. Nevertheless, AC is extensively used throughout the world although there is no high-level evidence to support this approach. One single-center retrospective study evaluated 146 patients who received systemic perioperative chemotherapy for cT2−T4aN0−N2M0 bladder cancer (73 patients received NAC, 73 patients received AC). That study did not identify significant differences in disease-specific survival ($P = 0.46$) or overall survival ($P = 0.76$) between the NAC and AC groups, although patients who received GC NAC exhibited better disease-specific survival, compared to patients who received GC AC (HR: 10.6, 95% CI: 1.01−112.2; $P = 0.049$) [64]. Therefore, based on these findings, NAC is currently the preferred treatment regimen [65]. The results from meta-analyses of Phase III trials for NAC are summarized in Table 22.3, and the ongoing studies are summarized in Table 22.4

TRENDS IN THE CLINICAL APPLICATION OF NAC

Cisplatin-based NAC provides a better survival benefit, compared to locoregional treatment. Despite the evidence supporting NAC, it continues to be underused in the clinical setting, and <20% of patients who are undergoing radical cystectomy receive NAC [66−68]. An analysis of 7161 patients with Stage III bladder cancer in the National Bladder Cancer Database revealed that 1.2% of the patients had received NAC [69]. Furthermore, only 12% of patients with bladder cancer (T2−T4aN0M0) receive NAC in North American academic referral centers [70]. A Korean study evaluated 1324 patients who underwent radical cystectomy and found that only 7.3% and 18.1% of these patients received NAC or AC, respectively [71]. Between 2003 and 2005, 4.6% of Korean patients with MIBC and no lymph node involvement received NAC before radical cystectomy although this proportion increased to 8.4% during 2010−13. Thus, the clinical use of NAC in Korea has significantly increased ($P < 0.005$) although the absolute frequency of NAC among these patients remains at <10% [71].

SUMMARY

The standard treatment for MIBC includes radical cystectomy and bilateral pelvis lymphadenectomy although approximately 50% of these cases progress to metastatic disease within 2 years, which eventually leads to death.

TABLE 22.4 Ongoing Trials of Neoadjuvant Therapy in MIBC

Institution	Regimen	Eligibility	Primary Endpoint	Study Phase	Estimated Enrollment	Estimated Completion Date	Trial ID
University Hospitals Bristol NHS Foundation Trust	Cisplatin and Cabazitaxel	cT2–4a/N0	<pT2	2	30	May 2017	NCT01616875
Memorial Sloan Kettering Cancer Center	Dose-dense GC	cT2–4a/N0	<pT2	2	46	April 2017	NCT01589094
University Hospital, Rouen	HD-MVAC vs. GC	cT2–4a/N0	PFS at 3 years	3	500	August 2021	NCT01812369
Sun Yat-sen University	Intra-arterial GC chemotherapy	pT3–4, N1–3, M0	Cancer PFS rate	3	212	December 2021	NCT01627197

HD, high dose; PFS, progressive free survival rate; NHS, National Health Service (United Kingdom).

Cisplatin-based NAC should be considered before radical cystectomy in all patients with MIBC (cT2−T4aN0M0) and preserved renal function.

In the neoadjuvant setting, cisplatin-based regimens, including MVAC and CMV, have shown overall survival benefits. The widely used regimen of GC has produced similar clinical outcomes and may be an appropriate alternative in cases who cannot receive MVAC (e.g., because of comorbidities or advanced age). NAC with dose-dense MVAC showed safety and promising pathological complete response rates (26%−38%).

REFERENCES

[1] Stewart B, Wild C. World Cancer Report 2014. Lyon, France: International Agency for Research on Cancer. World Health Organization; 2014.

[2] American Cancer Society. Cancer facts and figures 2015. Atlanta: American Cancer Society; 2015.

[3] Korean National Cancer Information Center. National registration statistics 2012. [cited July 8, 2015]. Available from: http://www.cancer.go.kr/mbs/cancer/subview.jsp?id=cancer_040101000000.

[4] Allard P, Bernard P, Fradet Y, Tetu B. The early clinical course of primary Ta and T1 bladder cancer: a proposed prognostic index. Br J Urol 1998;81:692−8.

[5] Burger M, Catto JW, Dalbagni G, Grossman HB, Herr H, Karakiewicz P, et al. Epidemiology and risk factors of urothelial bladder cancer. Eur Urol 2013;63:234−41.

[6] Raghavan D, Shipley WU, Garnick MB, Russell PJ, Richie JP. Biology and management of bladder cancer. N Engl J Med 1990;322:1129−38.

[7] Stein JP, Lieskovsky G, Cote R, Groshen S, Feng AC, Boyd S, et al. Radical cystectomy in the treatment of invasive bladder cancer: long-term results in 1,054 patients. J Clin Oncol 2001;19:666−75.

[8] Ghoneim MA, Abdel-Latif M, el-Mekresh M, Abol-Enein H, Mosbah A, Ashamallah A, et al. Radical cystectomy for carcinoma of the bladder: 2,720 consecutive cases 5 years later. J Urol 2008;180:121−7.

[9] Foxtrot Collaborative G. Feasibility of preoperative chemotherapy for locally advanced, operable colon cancer: the pilot phase of a randomised controlled trial. Lancet Oncol 2012;13:1152−60.

[10] Song WA, Zhou NK, Wang W, Chu XY, Liang CY, Tian XD, et al. Survival benefit of neoadjuvant chemotherapy in non-small cell lung cancer: an updated meta-analysis of 13 randomized control trials. J Thorac Oncol 2010;5:510−16.

[11] Robova H, Rob L, Halaska MJ, Pluta M, Skapa P, Strnad P, et al. High-dose density neoadjuvant chemotherapy in bulky IB cervical cancer. Gynec Oncol 2013;128:49−53.

[12] Tajima H, Ohta T, Kitagawa H, Okamoto K, Sakai S, Makino I, et al. Pilot study of neoadjuvant chemotherapy with gemcitabine and oral S-1 for resectable pancreatic cancer. Exp Ther Med 2012;3:787−92.

[13] Fisher B, Bryant J, Wolmark N, Mamounas E, Brown A, Fisher ER, et al. Effect of preoperative chemotherapy on the outcome of women with operable breast cancer. J Clin Oncol 1998;16:2672−85.

[14] Grossman HB, Natale RB, Tangen CM, Speights VO, Vogelzang NJ, Trump DL, et al. Neoadjuvant chemotherapy plus cystectomy compared with cystectomy alone for locally advanced bladder cancer. N Engl J Med 2003;349:859−66.

[15] Advanced Bladder Cancer (ABC) Meta-Analysis Collaboration. Neoadjuvant chemotherapy in invasive bladder cancer: update of a systematic review and meta-analysis of individual patient data advanced bladder cancer (ABC) meta-analysis collaboration. Eur Urol 2005;48:202−5. discussion 5−6.

[16] Stenzl A, Cowan NC, De Santis M, Kuczyk MA, Merseburger AS, Ribal MJ, et al. [Treatment of muscle-invasive and metastatic bladder cancer: update of the EAU guidelines]. Actas Urol Esp 2012;36:449−60.

[17] National Comprehensive Cancer Network. NCCN clinical practice guidelines in oncology: bladder cancer. Fort Washington, PA: NCCN; 2013.

[18] Balar AV, Milowsky MI. Neoadjuvant therapy in muscle-invasive bladder cancer: a model for rational accelerated drug development. Urol Clin North Am 2015;42:217−24. viii−ix.

[19] Calabro F, Sternberg CN. Neoadjuvant and adjuvant chemotherapy in muscle-invasive bladder cancer. Eur Urol 2009;55:348−58.

[20] Teramukai S, Nishiyama H, Matsui Y, Ogawa O, Fukushima M. Evaluation for surrogacy of end points by using data from observational studies: tumor downstaging for evaluating neoadjuvant chemotherapy in invasive bladder cancer. Clin Cancer Res 2006;12:139−43.

[21] Millikan R, Dinney C, Swanson D, Sweeney P, Ro JY, Smith TL, et al. Integrated therapy for locally advanced bladder cancer: final report of a randomized trial of cystectomy plus adjuvant M-VAC versus cystectomy with both preoperative and postoperative M-VAC. J Clin Oncol 2001;19:4005−13.

[22] Sledge GW, Neuberg D, Bernardo P, Ingle JN, Martino S, Rowinsky EK, et al. Phase III trial of doxorubicin, paclitaxel, and the combination of doxorubicin and paclitaxel as front-line chemotherapy for metastatic breast cancer: an intergroup trial (E1193). J Clin Oncol 2003;21:588−92.

[23] Cresta S, Grasselli G, Mansutti M, Martoni A, Lelli G, Capri G, et al. A randomized phase II study of combination, alternating and sequential regimens of doxorubicin and docetaxel as first-line chemotherapy for women with metastatic breast cancer. Ann Oncol 2004;15:433−9.

[24] Conte PF, Guarneri V, Bruzzi P, Prochilo T, Salvadori B, Bolognesi A, et al. Concomitant versus sequential administration of epirubicin and paclitaxel as first-line therapy in metastatic breast carcinoma: results for the Gruppo Oncologico Nord Ovest randomized trial. Cancer 2004;101:704−12.

[25] Alba E, Martin M, Ramos M, Adrover E, Balil A, Jara C, et al. Multicenter randomized trial comparing sequential with concomitant administration of doxorubicin and docetaxel as first-line treatment of metastatic breast cancer: a Spanish Breast Cancer Research Group (GEICAM-9903) phase III study. J Clin Oncol 2004;22:2587−93.

[26] Moreau LC, Rajan R, Thirlwell MP, Alcindor T. Response to chemotherapy in metastatic colorectal cancer after exposure to oxaliplatin in the adjuvant setting. Anticancer Res 2013;33:1765−8.

[27] von der Maase H, Hansen SW, Roberts JT, Dogliotti L, Oliver T, Moore MJ, et al. Gemcitabine and cisplatin versus methotrexate, vinblastine, doxorubicin, and cisplatin in advanced or metastatic bladder cancer: results of a large, randomized, multinational, multicenter, phase III study. J Clin Oncol 2000;18:3068−77.

[28] Yeshchina O, Badalato GM, Wosnitzer MS, Hruby G, RoyChoudhury A, Benson MC, et al. Relative efficacy of perioperative gemcitabine and cisplatin versus methotrexate, vinblastine, adriamycin, and cisplatin in the management of locally advanced urothelial carcinoma of the bladder. Urology 2012;79:384−90.

[29] Fairey AS, Daneshmand S, Quinn D, Dorff T, Dorin R, Lieskovsky G, et al. Neoadjuvant chemotherapy with gemcitabine/cisplatin vs. methotrexate/vinblastine/doxorubicin/cisplatin for muscle-invasive urothelial carcinoma of the bladder: a retrospective analysis from the University of Southern California. Urol Oncol 2013;31:1737−43.

[30] Zargar H, Espiritu PN, Fairey AS, Mertens LS, Dinney CP, Mir MC, et al. Multicenter assessment of neoadjuvant chemotherapy for muscle-invasive bladder cancer. Eur Urol 2015;67:241−9.

[31] Griffiths G, Hall R, Sylvester R, Raghavan D, Parmar MK. International phase III trial assessing neoadjuvant cisplatin, methotrexate, and vinblastine chemotherapy for muscle-invasive bladder cancer: long-term results of the BA06 30894 trial. J Clin Oncol 2011;29:2171−7.

[32] Wallace DM, Raghavan D, Kelly KA, Sandeman TF, Conn IG, Teriana N, et al. Neoadjuvant (pre-emptive) cisplatin therapy in invasive transitional cell carcinoma of the bladder. Br J Urol 1991;67:608−15.

[33] Martinez-Pineiro JA, Gonzalez Martin M, Arocena F, Flores N, Roncero CR, Portillo JA, et al. Neoadjuvant cisplatin chemotherapy before radical cystectomy in invasive transitional cell carcinoma of the bladder: a prospective randomized phase III study. J Urol 1995;153:964−73.

[34] Sengelov L, von der Maase H, Lundbeck F, Barlebo H, Colstrup H, Engelholm SA, et al. Neoadjuvant chemotherapy with cisplatin and methotrexate in patients with muscle-invasive bladder tumours. Acta Oncol 2002;41:447−56.

[35] Sherif A, Holmberg L, Rintala E, Mestad O, Nilsson J, Nilsson S, et al. Neoadjuvant cisplatinum based combination chemotherapy in patients with invasive bladder cancer: a combined analysis of two Nordic studies. Eur Urol 2004;45:297−303.

[36] Advanced Bladder Cancer Meta-analysis Collaboration. Neoadjuvant chemotherapy in invasive bladder cancer: a systematic review and meta-analysis. Lancet 2003;361:1927−34.

[37] Meeks JJ, Bellmunt J, Bochner BH, Clarke NW, Daneshmand S, Galsky MD, et al. A systematic review of neoadjuvant and adjuvant chemotherapy for muscle-invasive bladder cancer. Eur Urol 2012;62:523−33.

[38] Sonpavde G, Sternberg CN. Neoadjuvant chemotherapy for invasive bladder cancer. Curr Urol Rep 2012;13:136−46.

[39] Winquist E, Kirchner TS, Segal R, Chin J, Lukka H. Neoadjuvant chemotherapy for transitional cell carcinoma of the bladder: a systematic review and meta-analysis. J Urol 2004;171:561−9.

[40] National Comprehensive Cancer Network. NCCN clinical practice guidelines in oncology: bladder cancer. Fort Washington, PA: NCCN; 2016.

[41] Milowsky MI, Rumble RB, Booth CM, Gilligan T, Eapen LJ, Hauke RJ, et al. Guideline on muscle-invasive and metastatic bladder cancer (European Association of Urology Guideline): American Society of Clinical Oncology Clinical Practice Guideline Endorsement. J Clin Oncol 2016;34:1945−52.

[42] Pouessel D, Gauthier H, Serrate C, Pfister C, Culine S. Dose-dense methotrexate, vinblastine, doxorubicin, and cisplatin neoadjuvant chemotherapy in bladder cancer: ready for prime time? J Clin Oncol 2014;32:4168−9.

[43] Kassouf W, Spiess PE, Brown GA, Munsell MF, Grossman HB, Siefker-Radtke A, et al. P0 stage at radical cystectomy for bladder cancer is associated with improved outcome independent of traditional clinical risk factors. Eur Urol 2007;52:769−74.

[44] Rosenblatt R, Sherif A, Rintala E, Wahlqvist R, Ullen A, Nilsson S, et al. Pathologic downstaging is a surrogate marker for efficacy and increased survival following neoadjuvant chemotherapy and radical cystectomy for muscle-invasive urothelial bladder cancer. Eur Urol 2012;61:1229–38.

[45] Tilki D, Svatek RS, Novara G, Seitz M, Godoy G, Karakiewicz PI, et al. Stage pT0 at radical cystectomy confers improved survival: an international study of 4,430 patients. J Urol 2010;184:888–94.

[46] Palapattu GS, Shariat SF, Karakiewicz PI, Bastian PJ, Rogers CG, Amiel G, et al. Cancer specific outcomes in patients with pT0 disease following radical cystectomy. J Urol 2006;175:1645–9. discussion 9.

[47] Neoadjuvant cisplatin, methotrexate, and vinblastine chemotherapy for muscle-invasive bladder cancer: a randomised controlled trial. International collaboration of trialists. Lancet 1999;354:533–40.

[48] Sternberg CN, de Mulder P, Schornagel JH, Theodore C, Fossa SD, van Oosterom AT, et al. Seven year update of an EORTC phase III trial of high-dose intensity M-VAC chemotherapy and G-CSF versus classic M-VAC in advanced urothelial tract tumours. Eur J Cancer 2006;42:50–4.

[49] Sternberg CN, de Mulder PH, Schornagel JH, Theodore C, Fossa SD, van Oosterom AT, et al. Randomized phase III trial of high-dose-intensity methotrexate, vinblastine, doxorubicin, and cisplatin (MVAC) chemotherapy and recombinant human granulocyte colony-stimulating factor versus classic MVAC in advanced urothelial tract tumors: European Organization for Research and Treatment of Cancer Protocol no. 30924. J Clin Oncol 2001;19:2638–46.

[50] Choueiri TK, Jacobus S, Bellmunt J, Qu A, Appleman LJ, Tretter C, et al. Neoadjuvant dose-dense methotrexate, vinblastine, doxorubicin, and cisplatin with pegfilgrastim support in muscle-invasive urothelial cancer: pathologic, radiologic, and biomarker correlates. J Clin Oncol 2014;32:1889–94.

[51] Plimack ER, Hoffman-Censits JH, Viterbo R, Trabulsi EJ, Ross EA, Greenberg RE, et al. Accelerated methotrexate, vinblastine, doxorubicin, and cisplatin is safe, effective, and efficient neoadjuvant treatment for muscle-invasive bladder cancer: results of a multicenter phase II study with molecular correlates of response and toxicity. J Clin Oncol 2014;32:1895–901.

[52] Galsky MD, Pal SK, Chowdhury S, Harshman LC, Crabb SJ, Wong YN, et al. Comparative effectiveness of gemcitabine plus cisplatin versus methotrexate, vinblastine, doxorubicin, plus cisplatin as neoadjuvant therapy for muscle-invasive bladder cancer. Cancer 2015.

[53] Canter D, Viterbo R, Kutikov A, Wong YN, Plimack E, Zhu F, et al. Baseline renal function status limits patient eligibility to receive perioperative chemotherapy for invasive bladder cancer and is minimally affected by radical cystectomy. Urology 2011;77:160–5.

[54] Dash A, Galsky MD, Vickers AJ, Serio AM, Koppie TM, Dalbagni G, et al. Impact of renal impairment on eligibility for adjuvant cisplatin-based chemotherapy in patients with urothelial carcinoma of the bladder. Cancer 2006;107:506–13.

[55] Mertens LS, Meijer RP, Kerst JM, Bergman AM, van Tinteren H, van Rhijn BW, et al. Carboplatin based induction chemotherapy for nonorgan confined bladder cancer—a reasonable alternative for cisplatin unfit patients? J Urol 2012;188:1108–13.

[56] Raghavan D. Progress in the chemotherapy of metastatic cancer of the urinary tract. Cancer 2003;97:2050–5.

[57] Trump DL, Elson P, Madajewicz S, Dickman SH, Hahn RG, Harris JE, et al. Randomized phase II evaluation of carboplatin and CHIP in advanced transitional cell carcinoma of the urothelium. The Eastern Cooperative Oncology Group. J Urol 1990;144:1119–22.

[58] Raabe NK, Fossa SD, Paro G. Phase II study of carboplatin in locally advanced and metastatic transitional cell carcinoma of the urinary bladder. Br J Urol 1989;64:604–7.

[59] Hansen PV, Glavind K, Panduro J, Pedersen M. Paternity in patients with testicular germ cell cancer: pretreatment and post-treatment findings. Eur J Cancer 1991;27:1385–9.

[60] Skinner DG, Daniels JR, Russell CA, Lieskovsky G, Boyd SD, Nichols P, et al. The role of adjuvant chemotherapy following cystectomy for invasive bladder cancer: a prospective comparative trial. J Urol 1991;145:459–64. discussion 64–7.

[61] Stockle M, Meyenburg W, Wellek S, Voges G, Gertenbach U, Thuroff JW, et al. Advanced bladder cancer (stages pT3b, pT4a, pN1 and pN2): improved survival after radical cystectomy and 3 adjuvant cycles of chemotherapy. Results of a controlled prospective study. J Urol 1992;148:302–6. discussion 6–7.

[62] Logothetis CJ, Johnson DE, Chong C, Dexeus FH, Sella A, Ogden S, et al. Adjuvant cyclophosphamide, doxorubicin, and cisplatin chemotherapy for bladder cancer: an update. J Clin Oncol 1988;6:1590–6.

[63] Logothetis CJ, Johnson DE, Chong C, Dexeus FH, Ogden S, von Eschenbach A, et al. Adjuvant chemotherapy of bladder cancer: a preliminary report. J Urol 1988;139:1207–11.

[64] Wosnitzer MS, Hruby GW, Murphy AM, Barlow LJ, Cordon-Cardo C, Mansukhani M, et al. A comparison of the outcomes of neoadjuvant and adjuvant chemotherapy for clinical T2-T4aN0-N2M0 bladder cancer. Cancer 2012;118:358–64.

[65] Taneja SS. Management of high grade bladder cancer: a multidisciplinary approach. Urol Clin North Am 2015;42:xi–xii.

[66] Porter MP, Kerrigan MC, Donato BM, Ramsey SD. Patterns of use of systemic chemotherapy for Medicare beneficiaries with urothelial bladder cancer. Urol Oncol 2011;29:252–8.

[67] Miles BJ, Fairey AS, Eliasziw M, Estey EP, Venner P, Finch D, et al. Referral and treatment rates of neoadjuvant chemotherapy in muscle-invasive bladder cancer before and after publication of a clinical practice guideline. Can Urol Assoc J 2010;4:263–7.

[68] Raj GV, Karavadia S, Schlomer B, Arriaga Y, Lotan Y, Sagalowsky A, et al. Contemporary use of perioperative cisplatin-based chemotherapy in patients with muscle-invasive bladder cancer. Cancer 2011;117:276–82.

[69] David KA, Milowsky MI, Ritchey J, Carroll PR, Nanus DM. Low incidence of perioperative chemotherapy for stage III bladder cancer 1998 to 2003: a report from the National Cancer Data Base. J Urol 2007;178:451–4.

[70] Feifer A, Taylor JM, Shouery M, et al. Multi-institutional quality-of-care initiative for nonmetastatic, muscle-invasive, transitional cell carcinoma of the bladder [abstract 240]. J Clin Oncol 2011;29(Suppl 7).

[71] Kim SH, Seo HK, Shin HC, Chang SJ, Yun S, Joo J, et al. Trends in the use of chemotherapy before and after radical cystectomy in patients with muscle-invasive bladder cancer in Korea. J Korean Med Sci 2015;30(8):1150–6.

Chapter 23

Radical Cystectomy (RC) with Urinary Diversion

Chapter Outline

Chapter 23.1

Timing of Radical Cystectomy

Hong Koo Ha
Pusan National University Hospital, Busan, South Korea

INTRODUCTION

Nonmuscle-invasive bladder cancer (NMIBC) accounts for 75% of all newly diagnosed cases of urothelial carcinoma of the bladder [1]. The successful

Bladder Cancer. DOI: http://dx.doi.org/10.1016/B978-0-12-809939-1.00023-0
353

management of NMIBC is consisted of two principles, including complete transurethral resection (TUR) of the bladder tumor (TUR-B) and intravesical therapy. However, as high-grade NMIBC features the histopathological, clinical, and biological characteristics of invasive tumors, it often progresses to MIBC and requires radical cystectomy (RC) [2,3]. However, the timing of RC for patients with high-risk NMIBC is one of the most debated issues in urology, as RC for all high-risk NMIBC patients would clearly be an overtreatment. In addition to risk of overtreatment with early RC, the potential morbidity and mortality of the RC must be taken into consideration. The overall 90-day complication rates of RC have been reported to be as high as 59%−64% [4,5]. Furthermore, the decreased long-term renal function, particularly in older patients with comorbidities, after RC also should be consider [6]. In this article, we reviewed evidences and role of RC in high-risk NMIBC.

THE RISK GROUP STRATIFICATION OF NMIBC

To facilitate treatment recommendations, European Association of Urology (EAU) categorized patients into risk groups based on the prognostic factors and in particular data from the European Organization for Research and Treatment of Cancer (EORTC) risk table [2]. Table 23.1.1 shows a definition of three risk groups, which takes into account the EORTC risk tables' probabilities of recurrence and especially progression. The American Urological Association (AUA) also categorized patients into three risk groups [7]. Low risk was defined as Grade 1 or low grade. High risk included groups that had no Grade 1 (low grade) patients or were entirely Tis and/or T1.

TABLE 23.1.1 Risk Group Stratification of NMIBC

Risk Group	Characteristics
Low-risk tumors	Primary, solitary, Ta, G1[a] (PUNLMP, low grade), <3 cm, no CIS
Intermediate-risk tumors	All tumors not defined in the two adjacent categories (between the category of low and high risk)
High-risk tumors	Any of the following • T1 tumor • G3[b] (High grade) tumor • CIS • Multiple and recurrent and large (>3 cm) Ta G1G2 tumors (all conditions must be presented in this point)

PUNLMP, papillary urothelial neoplasms of low malignant potential.
[a]Low grade is mixture of G1 and G2.
[b]High grade is mixture of some G2 and all G3.
From EAU guideline 2016, http://www.uroweb.org/guidelines/, under permission of EAU guideline office.

THE PATHOLOGIC RESULTS OF RADICAL CYSTECTOMY IN NMIBC

Despite improvements in imaging technology, radical surgery still offers the most accurate staging modality. Unfortunately, the pathologic results of RC in NMIBC are disappointing. The reported staging accuracy for T1 tumors by TUR-B is low with 27%−51% of patients being upstaged to muscle-invasive tumor at RC [8−12]. A recent series from the University of Southern California (USC) including 114 clinical NMIBC patients undergoing RC with extended lymphadenectomy detected an upstaging to muscle invasive disease in 24% of patients and 7.9% were found to have lymph node (LN) metastases [13]. Furthermore, Fritsche et al. [9] reported that postoperative upstaging to muscle invasive disease occurred in 51% of patients and 16% were found to have LN metastases.

THE RESULTS OF IMMEDIATE OR EARLY VERSUS DELAYED CYSTECTOMY IN HIGH-RISK NMIBC

Interestingly, studies compared primary and progressive carcinoma invading bladder muscle concluded that patients with NMIBC who progress to MIBC have a worse prognosis after RC than patients who are initially diagnosed with MIBC at primary [14−17]. Disease progression of high-risk NMIBC could be prevented by adopting an immediate aggressive surgical approach at the time of first diagnosis. It seems that progression to MIBC and death in NMIBC patients is an early event mainly occurring within 48 months [9,18]. According to data from a meta-analysis ($n = 3088$), the rates of progression to muscle invasive disease and death in high-risk NMIBC patients are 21% and 14%, respectively [18]. Hautmann et al. [19] in their early versus delayed cystectomy series compared the presence of tumor upstaging in the cystectomy specimen (64% vs 29%), extravesical tumor extension and LN metastases (20% vs 9%), and were able to show a definite correlation with delay. These authors confirmed that the 10-year cancer-specific survival rate was in favor of early cystectomy (79% vs 65%). This result is in line with previous reports. In patients in whom RC is performed at the time of pathological NMIBC, the 5-year disease-free survival rate exceeds 80% [20−24]. Tumor-specific survival rates after immediate RC for carcinoma in situ (CIS) are excellent, but as many as 40%−50% of patients might be overtreated [25].

THE ROLE OF SECOND TRANSURETHRAL RESECTION OF BLADDER TUMOR

The EAU and National Comprehensive Cancer Network (NCCN) recommend a second TUR-B (within 6 weeks) in all T1 NMIBC [26,27]. The reported rate of persistent tumor after resection of T1 tumor is about 33%−55% [28−32].

As muscle-invasive disease is detected by second resection of initially T1 tumor ranges from 4% to 25% [33], the second TUR-B distinguishes the true nonmuscle-invasive tumors from cases of understaged disease and provides accurate staging. In addition, it has been demonstrated that a second TUR-B can increase recurrence-free survival [28,29] and improve outcomes after bacillus Calmette-Guerin (BCG) treatment [34]. However, it is important to note that the 78% of patients with residual T1 disease on second TUR-B eventually progressed to MIBC regardless of their original pathology, including many who responded initially to BCG therapy [1]. Therefore, patients with persistent NMIBC on second TUR-B require close follow-up and, in some cases, could be considered for early cystectomy [35].

THE EFFECT OF INTRAVESICAL BACILLUS CALMETTE-GUERIN TREATMENT ON TIMING OF RADICAL CYSTECTOMY

Adjuvant intravesical BCG is the first line treatment recommended for high-risk NMIBC by EAU and NCCN following TUR-B as well as a treatment option for intermediate-risk NMIBC [26,27]. Two meta-analyses have demonstrated that adjuvant intravesical BCG therapy significantly decreases recurrence and progression of NMIBC [36,37]. As compared with TUR-B alone or adjuvant intravesical chemotherapy, intravesical BCG therapy showed more effective in reducing the risk of progression in high-risk NMIBC patients [38,39]. Furthermore, the addition of maintenance intravesical BCG following the initial 6-week induction therapy showed more beneficial to prevent progression [36−38,40]. However, intravesical BCG treatment is exposed to two main risks: the first is the understaging of the initial tumor and the second is the non-BCG-response, which can lead to metastatic diffusion during the intravesical instillation period. Van den Bosch and Witjes [18] reviewed 19 trials on BCG therapy results. In more than 3000 patients, the progression risk was estimated at 21% and the 4-year cancer-specific survival after progression in this population of high-risk NMIBC at 35%. Interestingly, some patients die from progressive disease even when no cancer was found on the cystectomy specimen (pT0). As intravesical BCG treatment is only a local pure treatment, RC was definitively delayed for this population. Although RC should have been performed at the primary diagnosis in this population, unfortunately, there is no predictive factor to emphasize the BCG impact on the tumor. Furthermore, despite the proven efficacy of BCG, 30%−50% of patients experience disease recurrence and/or progression, and BCG is deemed to have failed [41,42]. Similarly, a recent evaluation of EORTC phase 3 trials in Ta−T1 NMIBC showed that patients with high-grade T1 disease had a progressing probability of 11.4% at 1 year and 19.8% at 5-year despite of recommended BCG maintenance schedules [43]. In this population, the immediate RC is urgently required. Because a delay in radical surgery might lead to decreased disease-specific survival, patients in whom BCG fails recommended RC as soon as the recurrence occurs during the first 6 months after the end of BCG courses [2,44].

THE SELECTION CRITERIA FOR EARLY RADICAL CYSTECTOMY IN HIGH-GRADE NMIBC: THE RISK-BASED PERFORMANCE OF RADICAL SURGERY

EORTC reported a scoring system to predict the prognosis in patients with NMIBC [2]. The EORTC scoring system was developed on the basis of the six most significant clinical and pathologic factors, such as number of tumors, tumor size, prior recurrence rate, tumor stage, and presence of concomitant CIS, and calculations using data from 2596 patients who did not have a second TUR or receive maintenance BCG therapy. The patients with recurrence scores of 10–17 are considered at risk of recurrence and those with progression scores of 7–23 as being at risk of progression [2,45]. On the contrary, NCCN considers all patients with T1, TaG3, and CIS NMIBC at risk of recurrence and progression [26].

The additional current clinicopathological factors to consider performing RC in NMIBC are listed at Table 23.1.2. The radical surgery is based on the individual risk of progression, which can be approximated according to the negative clinical and pathological factors. Among these factors, deep lamina propria involvement [51–53], residual high-grade (G3) tumor at second TUR [35,48], and patients failing BCG or alternative intravesical bladder preserving strategies [42,43] are considered to be one of the most critical factors for performing early RC in high-risk NMIBC.

In addition to the risk-based performance of radical surgery, cystectomy may also be considered in informed patients who wish to undergo immediate cystectomy. Furthermore, RC could be an option in patients with clinically extensive papillary Ta disease not amenable to endoscopic management and patients with severe functional bladder issues either primarily or as a consequence of repetitive TURs and/or instillation therapies.

NONUROTHELIAL BLADDER CANCERS

As micropapillary variant and nested variant have a poorer prognosis, radical approach should be considered at diagnosis [55,59]. Carcinosarcoma should also be treated with extensive radical surgery if possible [60]. In contrast, urothelial carcinoma exhibiting small-cell components should be treated with neoadjuvant chemotherapy, including cisplatin and etoposide, followed by RC or irradiation [61]. Muscle-invading urothelial cancers with squamous or adenocarcinomatous elements also recommended to treat with neoadjuvant cisplatin-based multidrug chemotherapy before surgery [62].

TABLE 23.1.2 Current Clinicopathological Factors to Consider Performing Radical Cystectomy in NMIBC

Multiple and/or large (> 3 cm) T1G3 tumors	[46]
T1G3 tumors (multiple) with concomitant CIS of the urinary bladder	[46]
T1G3 tumors with concomitant CIS of the prostatic urethra	[47]
Residual high-grade (G3) tumor at second TUR	[35,48]
Early recurrence (at the 3-month clinical evaluation)	[49]
Recurrent T1G3 tumors	[50]
Deep lamina propria involvement	[51−53]
Recurrent, treatment refractory CIS of the urinary bladder with upper tract and prostate excluded as site of recurrence origin	[45]
Tumors involving bladder diverticula	[54]
Micropapillary tumor differentiation	[55]
Primary adenocarcinoma, primary squamous cell carcinoma	[56,57]
Lymphovascular invasion	[58]
Patients failing BCG or alternative intravesical bladder preserving strategies	[42,43]

THE EFFECT OF TIME FROM DIAGNOSIS TO RADICAL CYSTECTOMY ON DISEASE PROGRESSION

In patients who meet the criteria for RC, surgery should not be withheld or delayed. Time from establishing indications for radical approach to surgery correlates with the change of diagnosis of an organ confined disease and affects recurrence-free, as well as overall survival [48,63]. A population-based study from the US Surveillance Epidemiology and End Results (SEER)—Medicare database suggests that 12 week is the outside limit beyond which there is a negative impact on outcome [64].

CONCLUSION

While cancer-specific survival rate was in favor of patients who undergo early RC for high-risk NMIBC, significant proportion of patients still would be overtreated. In addition, the potential morbidity and mortality of the RC must be taken into consideration. Therefore the careful follow-up strategies for bladder preservation, including second resection of bladder tumor and induction and maintenance of intravesical BCG treatment, should be firstly performed in high-risk NMIBC patients. However, as certainly a small proportion of high-risk NMIBC patients will eventually progressed to muscle-invasive disease, the presence of clinicopathological factors needs to be weighted the potential morbidities resulting from RC during bladder-sparing approach.

REFERENCES

[1] Herr HW. Role of repeat resection in non-muscle-invasive bladder cancer. J Natl Comprehen Cancer Netw 2015;13(8):1041−6.

[2] Sylvester RJ, van der Meijden AP, Oosterlinck W, Witjes JA, Bouffioux C, Denis L, et al. Predicting recurrence and progression in individual patients with stage Ta T1 bladder cancer using EORTC risk tables: a combined analysis of 2596 patients from seven EORTC trials. Eur Urol 2006;49(3):466-5; discussion 75-7.

[3] Cheng L, Weaver AL, Neumann RM, Scherer BG, Bostwick DG. Substaging of T1 bladder carcinoma based on the depth of invasion as measured by micrometer: a new proposal. Cancer 1999;86(6):1035−43.

[4] Novara G, Catto JW, Wilson T, Annerstedt M, Chan K, Murphy DG, et al. Systematic review and cumulative analysis of perioperative outcomes and complications after robot-assisted radical cystectomy. Eur Urol 2015;67(3):376−401.

[5] Shabsigh A, Korets R, Vora KC, Brooks CM, Cronin AM, Savage C, et al. Defining early morbidity of radical cystectomy for patients with bladder cancer using a standardized reporting methodology. Eur Urol 2009;55(1):164−74.

[6] Eisenberg MS, Thompson RH, Frank I, Kim SP, Cotter KJ, Tollefson MK, et al. Long-term renal function outcomes after radical cystectomy. J Urol 2014;191(3):619−25.

[7] Hall MC, Chang SS, Dalbagni G, Pruthi RS, Seigne JD, Skinner EC, et al. Guideline for the management of nonmuscle invasive bladder cancer (stages Ta, T1, and Tis): 2007 update. J Urol 2007;178(6):2314−30.

[8] Bianco Jr. FJ, Justa D, Grignon DJ, Sakr WA, Pontes JE, Wood Jr. DP. Management of clinical T1 bladder transitional cell carcinoma by radical cystectomy. Urol Oncol 2004;22 (4):290−4.

[9] Fritsche HM, Burger M, Svatek RS, Jeldres C, Karakiewicz PI, Novara G, et al. Characteristics and outcomes of patients with clinical T1 grade 3 urothelial carcinoma treated with radical cystectomy: results from an international cohort. Eur Urol 2010;57 (2):300−9.

[10] Huguet J, Crego M, Sabate S, Salvador J, Palou J, Villavicencio H. Cystectomy in patients with high risk superficial bladder tumors who fail intravesical BCG therapy: pre-cystectomy prostate involvement as a prognostic factor. Eur Urol 2005;48(1):53−9. discussion 9.

[11] May M, Bastian PJ, Brookman-May S, Burger M, Bolenz C, Trojan L, et al. Pathological upstaging detected in radical cystectomy procedures is associated with a significantly worse tumour-specific survival rate for patients with clinical T1 urothelial carcinoma of the urinary bladder. Scand J Urol Nephrol 2011;45(4):251−7.

[12] Turker P, Bostrom PJ, Wroclawski ML, van Rhijn B, Kortekangas H, Kuk C, et al. Upstaging of urothelial cancer at the time of radical cystectomy: factors associated with upstaging and its effect on outcome. BJU Int 2012;110(6):804−11.

[13] Bruins HM, Skinner EC, Dorin RP, Ahmadi H, Djaladat H, Miranda G, et al. Incidence and location of lymph node metastases in patients undergoing radical cystectomy for

clinical non-muscle invasive bladder cancer: results from a prospective lymph node mapping study. Urol Oncol 2014;32(1) 24.e13-9.

[14] Moschini M, Sharma V, Dell'oglio P, Cucchiara V, Gandaglia G, Cantiello F, et al. Comparing long-term outcomes of primary and progressive carcinoma invading bladder muscle after radical cystectomy. BJU Int 2016;117(4):604–10.

[15] Breau RH, Karnes RJ, Farmer SA, Thapa P, Cagiannos I, Morash C, et al. Progression to detrusor muscle invasion during urothelial carcinoma surveillance is associated with poor prognosis. BJU Int 2014;113(6):900–6.

[16] Ferreira U, Matheus WE, Nardi Pedro R, Levi D'Ancona CA, Reis LO, Stopiglia RM, et al. Primary invasive versus progressive invasive transitional cell bladder cancer: multicentric study of overall survival rate. Urol Int 2007;79(3):200–3.

[17] Schrier BP, Hollander MP, van Rhijn BW, Kiemeney LA, Witjes JA. Prognosis of muscle-invasive bladder cancer: difference between primary and progressive tumours and implications for therapy. Eur Urol 2004;45(3):292–6.

[18] van den Bosch S, Witjes JA. Long-term cancer-specific survival in patients with high-risk, non-muscle-invasive bladder cancer and tumour progression: a systematic review. Eur Urol 2011;60(3):493–500.

[19] Hautmann RE, Volkmer BG, Gust K. Quantification of the survival benefit of early versus deferred cystectomy in high-risk non-muscle invasive bladder cancer (T1 G3). World J Urol 2009;27(3):347–51.

[20] Stein JP, Lieskovsky G, Cote R, Groshen S, Feng AC, Boyd S, et al. Radical cystectomy in the treatment of invasive bladder cancer: long-term results in 1,054 patients. J Clin Oncol: Offic J Am Soc Clin Oncol 2001;19(3):666–75.

[21] Madersbacher S, Hochreiter W, Burkhard F, Thalmann GN, Danuser H, Markwalder R, et al. Radical cystectomy for bladder cancer today—a homogeneous series without neoadjuvant therapy. J Clin Oncol: Offic J Am Soc Clin Oncol 2003;21(4):690–6.

[22] Hautmann RE, Gschwend JE, de Petriconi RC, Kron M, Volkmer BG. Cystectomy for transitional cell carcinoma of the bladder: results of a surgery only series in the neobladder era. J Urol 2006;176(2):486–92. discussion 91-2.

[23] Shariat SF, Karakiewicz PI, Palapattu GS, Lotan Y, Rogers CG, Amiel GE, et al. Outcomes of radical cystectomy for transitional cell carcinoma of the bladder: a contemporary series from the Bladder Cancer Research Consortium. J Urol 2006;176(6 Pt 1): 2414–22. discussion 22.

[24] Shariat SF, Palapattu GS, Amiel GE, Karakiewicz PI, Rogers CG, Vazina A, et al. Characteristics and outcomes of patients with carcinoma in situ only at radical cystectomy. Urology 2006;68(3):538–42.

[25] Lamm DL. Carcinoma in situ. Urol Clin North Am 1992;19(3):499–508.

[26] Clark PE, Agarwal N, Biagioli MC, Eisenberger MA, Greenberg RE, Herr HW, et al. Bladder cancer. J Natl Comprehen Cancer Network 2013;11(4):446–75.

[27] Babjuk M, Bohle A, Burger M, Capoun O, Cohen D, Comperat EM, et al. EAU guidelines on non-muscle-invasive urothelial carcinoma of the bladder: update 2016. Eur Urol 2017;71:447–61.

[28] Grimm MO, Steinhoff C, Simon X, Spiegelhalder P, Ackermann R, Vogeli TA. Effect of routine repeat transurethral resection for superficial bladder cancer: a long-term observational study. J Urol 2003;170(2 Pt 1):433–7.

[29] Divrik RT, Yildirim U, Zorlu F, Ozen H. The effect of repeat transurethral resection on recurrence and progression rates in patients with T1 tumors of the bladder who received intravesical mitomycin: a prospective, randomized clinical trial. J Urol 2006;175(5):1641–4.

[30] Jahnson S, Wiklund F, Duchek M, Mestad O, Rintala E, Hellsten S, et al. Results of second-look resection after primary resection of T1 tumour of the urinary bladder. Scand J Urol Nephrol 2005;39(3):206−10.

[31] Lazica DA, Roth S, Brandt AS, Bottcher S, Mathers MJ, Ubrig B. Second transurethral resection after Ta high-grade bladder tumor: a 4.5-year period at a single university center. Urol Int 2014;92(2):131−5.

[32] Vasdev N, Dominguez-Escrig J, Paez E, Johnson MI, Durkan GC, Thorpe AC. The impact of early re-resection in patients with pT1 high-grade non-muscle invasive bladder cancer. Ecancermedicalscience 2012;6:269.

[33] Herr HW, Donat SM. Quality control in transurethral resection of bladder tumours. BJU Int 2008;102(9 Pt B):1242−6.

[34] Sfakianos JP, Kim PH, Hakimi AA, Herr HW. The effect of restaging transurethral resection on recurrence and progression rates in patients with nonmuscle invasive bladder cancer treated with intravesical bacillus Calmette-Guerin. J Urol 2014;191(2):341−5.

[35] Bishr M, Lattouf JB, Latour M, Saad F. Tumour stage on re-staging transurethral resection predicts recurrence and progression-free survival of patients with high-risk non-muscle invasive bladder cancer. Can Urol Assoc J 2014;8(5−6):E306−10.

[36] Bohle A, Bock PR. Intravesical bacille Calmette-Guerin versus mitomycin C in superficial bladder cancer: formal meta-analysis of comparative studies on tumor progression. Urology 2004;63(4):682−6. discussion 6-7.

[37] Sylvester RJ, van der MA, Lamm DL. Intravesical bacillus Calmette-Guerin reduces the risk of progression in patients with superficial bladder cancer: a meta-analysis of the published results of randomized clinical trials. J Urol 2002;168(5):1964−70.

[38] Sylvester RJ, van der Meijden AP, Witjes JA, Kurth K. Bacillus calmette-guerin versus chemotherapy for the intravesical treatment of patients with carcinoma in situ of the bladder: a meta-analysis of the published results of randomized clinical trials. J Urol 2005;174 (1):86−91. discussion -2.

[39] Witjes JA, Hendricksen K. Intravesical pharmacotherapy for non-muscle-invasive bladder cancer: a critical analysis of currently available drugs, treatment schedules, and long-term results. Eur Urol 2008;53(1):45−52.

[40] Lamm DL, Blumenstein BA, Crissman JD, Montie JE, Gottesman JE, Lowe BA, et al. Maintenance bacillus Calmette-Guerin immunotherapy for recurrent TA, T1 and carcinoma in situ transitional cell carcinoma of the bladder: a randomized Southwest Oncology Group Study. J Urol 2000;163(4):1124−9.

[41] Fernandez-Gomez J, Madero R, Solsona E, Unda M, Martinez-Pineiro L, Ojea A, et al. The EORTC tables overestimate the risk of recurrence and progression in patients with non-muscle-invasive bladder cancer treated with bacillus Calmette-Guerin: external validation of the EORTC risk tables. Eur Urol 2011;60(3):423−30.

[42] Yates DR, Brausi MA, Catto JW, Dalbagni G, Roupret M, Shariat SF, et al. Treatment options available for bacillus Calmette-Guerin failure in non-muscle-invasive bladder cancer. Eur Urol 2012;62(6):1088−96.

[43] Cambier S, Sylvester RJ, Collette L, Gontero P, Brausi MA, van Andel G, et al. EORTC nomograms and risk groups for predicting recurrence, progression, and disease-specific and overall survival in non-muscle-invasive stage Ta-T1 urothelial bladder cancer patients treated with 1-3 years of maintenance bacillus Calmette-Guerin. Eur Urol 2016;69(1):60−9.

[44] Brausi M, Witjes JA, Lamm D, Persad R, Palou J, Colombel M, et al. A review of current guidelines and best practice recommendations for the management of nonmuscle invasive bladder cancer by the International Bladder Cancer Group. J Urol 2011;186(6):2158−67.

[45] Babjuk M, Burger M, Zigeuner R, Shariat SF, van Rhijn BW, Comperat E, et al. EAU guidelines on non-muscle-invasive urothelial carcinoma of the bladder: update 2013. Eur Urol 2013;64(4):639−53.

[46] Millan-Rodriguez F, Chechile-Toniolo G, Salvador-Bayarri J, Palou J, Vicente-Rodriguez J. Multivariate analysis of the prognostic factors of primary superficial bladder cancer. J Urol 2000;163(1):73−8.

[47] Palou J, Sylvester RJ, Faba OR, Parada R, Pena JA, Algaba F, et al. Female gender and carcinoma in situ in the prostatic urethra are prognostic factors for recurrence, progression, and disease-specific mortality in T1G3 bladder cancer patients treated with bacillus Calmette-Guerin. Eur Urol 2012;62(1):118−25.

[48] Dalbagni G, Vora K, Kaag M, Cronin A, Bochner B, Donat SM, et al. Clinical outcome in a contemporary series of restaged patients with clinical T1 bladder cancer. Eur Urol 2009;56(6):903−10.

[49] Solsona E, Iborra I, Dumont R, Rubio-Briones J, Casanova J, Almenar S. The 3-month clinical response to intravesical therapy as a predictive factor for progression in patients with high risk superficial bladder cancer. J Urol 2000;164(3 Pt 1):685−9.

[50] Fernandez-Gomez J, Solsona E, Unda M, Martinez-Pineiro L, Gonzalez M, Hernandez R, et al. Prognostic factors in patients with non-muscle-invasive bladder cancer treated with bacillus Calmette-Guerin: multivariate analysis of data from four randomized CUETO trials. Eur Urol 2008;53(5):992−1001.

[51] Orsola A, Trias I, Raventos CX, Espanol I, Cecchini L, Bucar S, et al. Initial high-grade T1 urothelial cell carcinoma: feasibility and prognostic significance of lamina propria invasion microstaging (T1a/b/c) in BCG-treated and BCG-non-treated patients. Eur Urol 2005;48(2):231−8. discussion 8.

[52] Chang WC, Chang YH, Pan CC. Prognostic significance in substaging ofT1 urinary bladder urothelial carcinoma on transurethral resection. Am J Surg Pathol 2012;36(3):454−61.

[53] Martin-Doyle W, Leow JJ, Orsola A, Chang SL, Bellmunt J. Improving selection criteria for early cystectomy in high-grade t1 bladder cancer: a meta-analysis of 15,215 patients. J Clin Oncol: Offic J Am Soc Clin Oncol 2015;33(6):643−50.

[54] Golijanin D, Yossepowitch O, Beck SD, Sogani P, Dalbagni G. Carcinoma in a bladder diverticulum: presentation and treatment outcome. J Urol 2003;170(5):1761−4.

[55] Kamat AM, Dinney CP, Gee JR, Grossman HB, Siefker-Radtke AO, Tamboli P, et al. Micropapillary bladder cancer: a review of the University of Texas M. D. Anderson Cancer Center experience with 100 consecutive patients. Cancer 2007;110(1):62−7.

[56] Wasco MJ, Daignault S, Zhang Y, Kunju LP, Kinnaman M, Braun T, et al. Urothelial carcinoma with divergent histologic differentiation (mixed histologic features) predicts the presence of locally advanced bladder cancer when detected at transurethral resection. Urology 2007;70(1):69−74.

[57] Blochin EB, Park KJ, Tickoo SK, Reuter VE, Al-Ahmadie H. Urothelial carcinoma with prominent squamous differentiation in the setting of neurogenic bladder: role of human papillomavirus infection. Mod Pathol 2012;25(11):1534−42.

[58] Kim HS, Kim M, Jeong CW, Kwak C, Kim HH, Ku JH. Presence of lymphovascular invasion in urothelial bladder cancer specimens after transurethral resections correlates with risk of upstaging and survival: a systematic review and meta-analysis. Urol Oncol 2014;32(8):1191−9.

[59] Comperat E, Roupret M, Yaxley J, Reynolds J, Varinot J, Ouzaid I, et al. Micropapillary urothelial carcinoma of the urinary bladder: a clinicopathological analysis of 72 cases. Pathology 2010;42(7):650−4.

[60] Wang J, Wang FW, Lagrange CA, Hemstreet Iii GP, Kessinger A. Clinical features of sarcomatoid carcinoma (carcinosarcoma) of the urinary bladder: analysis of 221 cases. Sarcoma 2010;2010:454792.

[61] Siefker-Radtke AO, Gee J, Shen Y, Wen S, Daliani D, Millikan RE, et al. Multimodality management of urachal carcinoma: the M. D. Anderson Cancer Center experience. J Urol 2003;169(4):1295−8.

[62] Scosyrev E, Ely BW, Messing EM, Speights VO, Grossman HB, Wood DP, et al. Do mixed histological features affect survival benefit from neoadjuvant platinum-based combination chemotherapy in patients with locally advanced bladder cancer? A secondary analysis of Southwest Oncology Group-Directed Intergroup Study (S8710). BJU Int 2011;108(5):693−9.

[63] Lee CT, Madii R, Daignault S, Dunn RL, Zhang Y, Montie JE, et al. Cystectomy delay more than 3 months from initial bladder cancer diagnosis results in decreased disease specific and overall survival. J Urol 2006;175(4):1262−7. discussion 7.

[64] Gore JL, Lai J, Setodji CM, Litwin MS, Saigal CS. Mortality increases when radical cystectomy is delayed more than 12 weeks: results from a Surveillance, Epidemiology, and End Results-Medicare analysis. Cancer 2009;115(5):988−96.

Chapter 23.2

Indications

Min Chul Cho

Seoul Metropolitan Government − Seoul National University Borame Medical Center, Seoul, South Korea

INDICATIONS FOR RADICAL CYSTECTOMY

In patients fit and willing to undergo surgery, radical cystectomy (RC) with bilateral pelvic lymph node dissection (LND) and urinary diversion remains the gold standard therapy for MIBC T2-T4a, N0-Nx, and M0 [1,2]. Also, RC may be indicated in patients with high-risk or recurrent nonmuscle-invasive bladder cancer (NMIBC), bacillus Calmette-Guerin (BCG)-refractory carcinoma in situ (CIS), or high-grade NMIBC, as well as those with extensive tumors that cannot be controlled with transurethral resection (TUR) or intravesical therapy (Table 23.2.1) [1,3]. Because histologic variants of urothelial cancer (micropapillary urothelial carcinoma and nested variant) are more likely to be diagnosed at an advanced stage with extravesical disease and metastasis than conventional urothelial cancer, RC should be considered at diagnosis [2−6]. Also, in patients with sarcoma (leiomyosarcoma, etc.), and signet ring cell carcinoma, RC is recommended due to the aggressive

TABLE 23.2.1 Indications for RC

- MIBC T2-T4a, N0-Nx, M0

- T1 NMIBC at a high risk of progression (high grade, diffuse CIS, lymphovascular invasion, multifocality, large tumor size, etc.)

- Extensive tumors that cannot be controlled with TUR or intravesical therapy

- Salvage cystectomy for BCG-refractory high-grade NMIBC or recurrence after bladder-sparing treatments

- A palliative option for intractable symptoms such as hematuria and pain

MIBC, muscle-invasive bladder cancer; NMIBC, nonmuscle-invasive bladder cancer; CIS, carcinoma in situ; BCG, bacillus Calmette-Guérin; TUR, transurethral resection.

features of such conditions (Table 23.2.1) [2,4,5,7]. However, RC cannot be suitable for very frail patients or those with advanced age, those with serious medical comorbidites, or mentally impaired patients insufficient for recovery from RC. Recently, robot-assisted RC with urinary diversion is increasingly performed worldwide. Accumulated evidence suggests that robot-assisted RC seems to be similar to open RC in terms of operative, mid-term oncological, and functional outcomes [8]. Rather, robot-assisted RC can result in less blood loss or less rate of transfusion during surgery, faster recovery during the postoperative period, and faster discharge from hospital, compared with open RC. The indications for robot-assisted RC appear to be nearly identical to open RC. The robot-assisted RC is feasible even in selected patients who underwent prior lower intraabdominal surgery or pelvic irradiation, although the decision to proceed the robotic surgery is determined primarily by surgeons' experience and consultation with the patients [8]. Because contralateral LN involvement is relatively common in bladder cancer, a bilateral pelvic LND is necessary in patients who undergo RC [6]. Although the extent of pelvic LND remains to be determined, RC with pelvic LN dissection showed better oncologic outcomes than RC without LND [9].

SELECTION OF THE MOST APPROPRIATE URINARY DIVERSION

Appropriate patient selection is most important for successful urinary diversion that does not compromise the locoregional control of bladder cancer. During the past several decades, a variety of urinary diversion methods, including a conduit, cutaneous continent diversion, and an orthotopic neobladder, have been developed and technically refined [10–13]. Since cutaneous continent urinary diversion has been largely supplanted by use of an orthotopic neobladder, it has become a secondary option after orthotopic neobladder placement [10,14]. In this section, we briefly deal with the indications and contraindications of an orthotopic neobladder, cutaneous continent urinary diversion, and a conduit.

Orthotopic Neobladder

All patients who are eligible for RC can be considered potential candidates for orthotopic neobladder [10]. However, there are some prerequisites and contraindications to orthotopic neobladder that should be identified (Table 23.2.2). First, the absolute oncologic contraindication for orthotopic neobladder is the presence of urothelial carcinoma at the urethral margin on intraoperative frozen section at the time of RC [13]. Tumor involvement of the prostatic urethra in male patients and of the bladder neck in female patients is associated with a higher risk of subsequent urethral recurrence [10,13]. Second, impaired renal function is an important absolute contraindication for orthotopic neobladder [10,13]. Although the exact cut-off value of acceptable renal function for consideration of orthotopic neobladder remains to be determined, reabsorption of urinary constituents through the bowel mucosa leads to an increase in acid load, which must be processed by the kidneys [13,14]. As a general guide, orthotopic neobladder should be avoided in patients with a serum creatinine level >1.7 mg/dL or a glomerular filtration rate (GFR) <50 mL/min [14]. Third, severely impaired hepatic function is a contraindication to orthotopic neobladder since the reabsorption of ammonium through the bowel mucosa can result in hyperammonemia [10]. Fourth, patients' motivation and their ability for active participation is an important factor when considering orthotopic neobladder [14]. The patients should be willing and able to perform self-catheterization of the

---

TABLE 23.2.2 Contraindications for Orthotopic Neobladder

Absolute Contraindications

- Positive urethral margin on intraoperative frozen section
- Tumor involvement of the prostatic urethra in male patients and of the bladder neck or anterior vaginal wall in female patients
- Renal insufficiency (serum creatinine >1.7 mg/dL or GFR <50 mL/min)
- Severe hepatic dysfunction
- Severe inflammatory bowel disease such as Crohn's disease
- Physical or mental impairment (inability to do self-catheterization)

Relative Contraindications

- Prior pelvic radiation
- Advanced age and medical comorbidities

neobladder [13]. Also, they should have the intellectual and physical capacity to understand the voiding mechanism of the neobladder [10]. Fifth, severe urethral stricture disease is a contraindication for orthotopic neobladder [13]. Sixth, presence of a severe inflammatory bowel disease such as Crohn's disease is a contraindication for orthotopic neobladder [10]. Prior radiation therapy can be a relative contraindication, because patients with prior irradiation are at a high risk of complications, even with the conduit urinary diversion [10,13]. Meanwhile, chronologic age alone or locally advanced tumor stage is not an absolute contraindication for continent diversion and the options should be considered for each patient on the basis of other factors [13,14].

Cutaneous Continent Urinary Diversion

As cutaneous continent urinary diversion is accepted by both urologists and patients as an acceptable form of urinary diversion after RC, it should be considered in some appropriate patients. Cutaneous continent urinary diversion aims to provide a well-functioning reservoir with satisfactory daytime and nighttime continence for the majority of selected patients who undergo RC [15]. Cutaneous continent urinary diversion uses a low-pressure pouch constructed of detubularized bowel with a functional mechanism designed to prevent involuntary efflux of urine [11]. Over the past 35 years, an evolution and refinement have occurred in the techniques used to create antireflux and continence mechanisms to make them more effective and reliable [16]. However, even though cutaneous continent urinary diversion is appropriate in selected patients who undergo RC, the surgical procedures are technically more challenging with higher complication rates compared to incontinent urinary diversion [16]. Thus, the selection of patients appropriate for cutaneous continent urinary diversion is critical for its successful outcomes. Although the prerequisites and contraindications for cutaneous continent urinary diversion are generally similar to those for orthotopic neobladder substitution, it requires clean intermittent self-catheterization to empty the reservoir and irrigate retained mucus [11]. Also, cutaneous continent urinary diversion can be indicated when urethral removal is deemed necessary due to a high risk of recurrence of bladder cancer [14]. Patients with multiple sclerosis, quadriplegic individuals, and very frail or mentally impaired patients are considered as poor candidates of cutaneous continent urinary diversion, because they will require family or visiting nurses for basic care at some point in their lives [16].

Conduit Urinary Diversion

An indication for conduit diversion is the need for urinary diversion after RC. Although a conduit is constructed using the ileum, jejunum, or colon, ileal conduit has become the gold standard method for incontinent urinary diversion

[10]. Also, it remains the procedure of choice for patients with contraindications for orthotopic neobladder [10]. In general, ileal conduit is relatively easy and quick to construct, with a low rate of postoperative complications [11]. However, it is not recommended in patients with short bowel syndrome, severe inflammatory bowel disease, or prior extensive radiation therapy.

REFERENCES

[1] Witjes JA, Lebret T, Compérat EM, Cowan NC, De Santis M, Bruins HM, et al. Updated 2016 EAU Guidelines on muscle-invasive and metastatic bladder cancer. Eur Urol 2016 Jun 30; pii: S0302-2838(16)30290-1. doi: 10.1016/j.eururo.2016.06.020.

[2] Guzzo TJ, Vaughn DJ. Management of metastatic and invasive bladder cancer. In: Wein AJ, Kavoussi LR, Partin AW, Peters CA, editors. Campbell-Walsh urology. 11th ed. Philadelphia, PA: Elsevier; 2016. p. 2223−41.

[3] Gakis G, Efstathiou J, Lerner SP, Cookson MS, Keegan KA, Guru KA, et al. International Consultation on Urologic Disease-European Association of Urology Consultation on Bladder Cancer 2012. ICUD-EAU International Consultation on Bladder Cancer 2012: radical cystectomy and bladder preservation for muscle-invasive urothelial carcinoma of the bladder. Eur Urol 2013;63:45−57.

[4] Scosyrev E, Noyes K, Feng C, Messing E. Sex and racial differences in bladder cancer presentation and mortality in the US. Cancer 2009;115:68−74.

[5] Kamat AM, Dinney CP, Gee JR, Grossman HB, Siefker-Radtke AO, Tamboli P, et al. Micropapillary bladder cancer: a review of the University of Texas M. D. Anderson Cancer Center experience with 100 consecutive patients. Cancer 2007;110:62−7.

[6] Kamat AM, Hahn NM, Efstathiou JA, Lerner SP, Malmström PU, Choi W, et al. Bladder cancer. Lancet 2016 Jun 23; pii: S0140-6736(16)30512-8. doi: 10.1016/S0140-6736(16)30512-8.

[7] Terada T. Spindle cell carcinoma progressed from transitional cell carcinoma of the urinary bladder. Int J Clin Exp Pathol 2012;5:83−8.

[8] Wilson TG, Guru K, Rosen RC, Wiklund P, Annerstedt M, Bochner BH, et al. Pasadena Consensus Panel. Best practices in robot-assisted radical cystectomy and urinary reconstruction: recommendations of the Pasadena Consensus Panel. Eur Urol 2015;67:363−75.

[9] Bruins HM, Veskimae E, Hernandez V, Imamura M, Neuberger MM, Dahm P, et al. The impact of the extent of lymphadenectomy on oncologic outcomes in patients undergoing radical cystectomy for bladder cancer: a systematic review. Eur Urol 2014;66:1065−77.

[10] Minervini A, Serni S, Vittori G, Masieri L, Siena G, Lanciotti M, et al. Current indications and results of orthotopic ileal neobladder for bladder cancer. Expert Rev Anticancer Ther 2014;14:419−30.

[11] Lee RK, Abol-Enein H, Artibani W, Bochner B, Dalbagni G, Daneshmand S, et al. Urinary diversion after radical cystectomy for bladder cancer: options, patient selection, and outcomes. BJU Int 2014;113:11−23.

[12] Dahl DM. Use of intestinal segments in urinary diversion. In: Wein AJ, Kavoussi LR, Partin AW, Peters CA, editors. Campbell-Walsh urology. 11th ed. Philadelphia, PA: Elsevier; 2016. p. 2281−316.

[13] Skinner EC, Daneshmand S. Orthotopic urinary diversion. In: Wein AJ, Kavoussi LR, Partin AW, Peters CA, editors. Campbell-Walsh urology. 11th ed. Philadelphia, PA: Elsevier; 2016. p. 2344−68.

[14] Hautmann RE, Abol-Enein H, Davidsson T, Gudjonsson S, Hautmann SH, Holm HV, et al. International Consultation on Urologic Disease-European Association of Urology Consultation on Bladder Cancer 2012. ICUD-EAU International Consultation on Bladder Cancer 2012: urinary diversion. Eur Urol 2013;63:67−80.

[15] Wiesner C, Bonfig R, Stein R, Gerharz EW, Pahernik S, Riedmiller H, et al. Continent cutaneous urinary diversion: long-term follow-up of more than 800 patients with ileocecal reservoirs. World J Urol 2006;24:315−18.

[16] DeCastro GJ, McKiernan JM, Benson MC. Cutaneous continent urinary diversion. In: Wein AJ, Kavoussi LR, Partin AW, Peters CA, editors. Campbell-Walsh urology. 11th ed. Philadelphia, PA: Elsevier; 2016. p. 2317−43.

Chapter 24

Open Techniques and Extent (Including Pelvic Lymphadenectomy)

Chapter Outline

Bladder Cancer. DOI: http://dx.doi.org/10.1016/B978-0-12-809939-1.00024-2

Chapter 24.1

Radical Cystectomy

Jun Hyuk Hong

University of Ulsan, Asan Medical Center, Seoul, South Korea

PREOPERATIVE EVALUATION AND PREPARATION

As well as other cancer surgery, preoperative evaluation and staging should be performed before radical cystectomy. Staging work-up usually includes abdomen−pelvis computed tomographic (CT) scan of pre- and postcontrast imaging. CT of the chest and bone scan also should be performed to rule out metastasis to lung and bone. When renal function is impaired, magnetic resonance urography can be performed instead of CT scan.

After staging tests, a thorough medical evaluation and anesthetic consultation are necessary, considering the long operative time and the wide extent of this surgery.

Patient should undergo bowel preparation before surgery (Table 24.1.1). Oral antibiotics and a low residue diet are needed. Parenteral broad spectrum antibiotics are administered just before the operation.

POSITION AND INCISION

The patient is placed in the supine position with the bed extended to 10−15 degrees and with a Trendelenburg tilt. If a total urethrectomy is planned, the

TABLE 24.1.1 Preop Preparation (Asan Medical Center)

1. Preop Day 2

   Liquid diet (from lunch)

   Ciprofloxacin 1 g p.o. (7 p.m.)

   Magcorol solution 500 mL p.o. (7 p.m.)

   Intravenous hydration (DNK 1000 mL, 80 mL/hour) (7 p.m.)

2. Preop Day 1

   NPO

   Ciprofloxacin 1 g p.o. (2 p.m.)

   Magcorol solution 500 mL p.o. (2 p.m.)

   Intravenous hydration (DNK 1000 mL, 120 mL/hour) (2 p.m.)

   Fleet enema rectal (7 p.m.)

3. Op day

   Fleet enema rectal (7 am)

NPO, Nothing by mouth (nil per os) DNK, dextrose 50g (5%), NaCl 4.5g, KCl 2.2g in 1000ml.

patient is put in a lithotomy position for easy access to the perineum. The genital organs and the perineal area are prepared. In female patients, the vagina should be prepared. Surgical fields are draped and an 18 Fr Foley catheter is introduced into the bladder.

A midline incision is usually made extending from upper epigastrium to the level of the symphysis pubis. In some cases, a lower midline incision may be adequate. After the midline is identified, the fascia is divided and the space of Retzius is entered. The bladder is released from the pelvic sidewall by blunt dissection using sponge stick.

INITIAL EXPOSURE

The peritoneum is incised lateral to the medial umbilical ligaments bilaterally to the level of the internal inguinal rings. The vas deferens in men or the round ligaments in women are divided. The abdominal cavity and pelvis are inspected and palpated. When the bladder is explored, the size and consistency of the mass and its mobility should be determined, if possible.

Self-retaining retractor (Omni-tract retractor or Balfour abdominal retractor, etc.) can be installed. Small and large intestines are packed with large pad and retracted out of the pelvis. The peritoneal incision is extended along both sides of the urachal remnant. The urachal remnant is clamped with Kelly clamp and provides a convenient place for traction on the bladder.

CYSTECTOMY IN MEN

The peritoneal incision is extended along the external and common iliac vessels. The vas deferens of either side is ligated and divided near the internal ring. Both ureters are identified at the crossing of common iliac artery and are dissected distally for 4–5 cm preserving adequate ureteral adventitia tissue. Ureter is ligated and divided. The distal end of ureter is sent for frozen section analysis to rule out the presence of urothelial carcinoma or carcinoma in situ of ureter.

With a counter-traction using sponge stick on the prostate, endopelvic fascia of both sides are incised with Metzenbaum scissors. After opening the fascia, blunt dissection along the lateral side of prostate can be done with fingers.

The space between bladder, seminal vesicle, prostate, and the rectum is opened with blunt scissors. Traction of the bladder anteriorly with narrow Deaver retractor will help this part of dissection. The dissection is extended along the posterior side of prostate, and the apex of prostate can be palpated with fingertips. The dissection is extended laterally, and the posterior pedicles are identified and ligated with clips or ties, or Endo GIA Stapler.

The pubo-prostatic ligaments are identified and divided with sharp scissors. Traction on the prostate with sponge stick will be helpful for careful dissection. Dorsal vein complex is clamped with Babcock clamp over the prostate and is sutured with 2-0 vicryl over the apex. The dorsal vein complex is incised proximal to the sutures, and the incision is extended to the urethra until the Foley catheter can be seen. Foley catheter is withdrawn, and proximal urethra is clamped with Kelly and transected. The bladder specimen is removed. The distal end of urethra is suture ligated if necessary. If orthotopic bladder substitution is planned, you must be cautious to avoid damage to the urethra and periurethral tissues and adequate urethral length should be preserved. The urethral margin is sent for a frozen section.

After the control of bleeding vessels, one or two closed suction drains (Jackson-Pratt (JP) drain) are inserted into pelvic cavity.

CYSTECTOMY IN WOMEN

If the patient is postmenopausal, the fallopian tubes and ovaries are usually removed with the uterus, cervix, and anterior vagina. The gonadal veins and suspensory ligaments are ligated and divided. The ureters are identified and divided near the bladder. The arterial supply to the uterus and vagina are ligated and divided.

With the medial traction of the bladder with fingers, the superior vesical artery is identified and ligated. The lateral pedicle is also ligated using clips or ties, or Endo GIA Stapler.

In the rectovaginal cul-de-sac, the posterior peritoneum is incised. Blunt dissection is made along the posterior wall of vagina. A sponge stick is inserted into the vagina, and it elevates the apex of vagina. Vaginal apex is opened with Bovie cautery and incision is extended laterally.

If urethrectomy is planned, the venous plexus anterior to the urethra are ligated just as the dorsal vein complex in men. From perineal side, the labia are retracted laterally and inverted U incision is made around the urethra. Blunt dissection is made along the urethra until there is continuity between the perineum and the pelvis. The whole specimen now can be removed.

After the control of bleeding vessels, one or two closed suction drains (JP drain) are inserted into the pelvic cavity (Figs. 24.1.1–24.1.4).

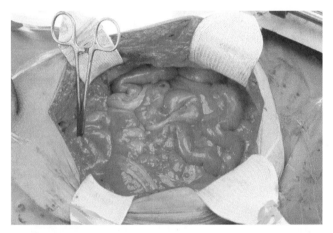

FIGURE 24.1.1 A long midline incision is made and Omni-tract retractor is installed.

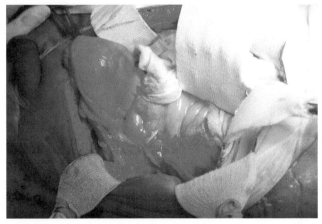

FIGURE 24.1.2 Left ureter is dissected and ligated at 4–5 cm distal to the crossing of Left common iliac artery with a Hem-o-lok clip.

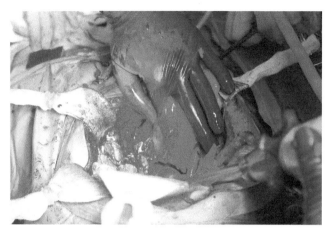

FIGURE 24.1.3 Left lateral vascular pedicle of bladder is ligated using Endo GIA Stapler.

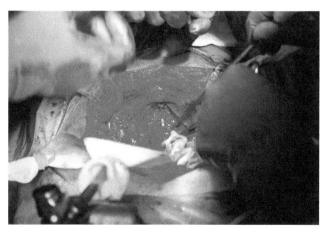

FIGURE 24.1.4 After the removal of bladder, any bleeders can be controlled with sutures or clips. The distal margin of urethra is seen with curved sound dilator in situ.

Chapter 24.2

Pelvic Lyphadenectomy

Gyeong E. Min and Seung H. Jeon
Kyung Hee University School of Medicine, Seoul, South Korea

THE ANATOMIC TEMPLATE OF PELVIC LYMPHADENECTOMY

The extent of lymph node dissection (LND) is categorized as follows (Fig. 24.2.1), limited LND, standard LND, extended LND (ELND), and super-extended LND (SELND) [2].

1. Limited LND

   Limited LND is defined as the removal of the obturator lymph nodes, bounded laterally by the external iliac vein and medially by the obturator nerve [3–8] (Fig. 24.2.2).
2. Standard LND

   Standard LND involves the resection of all lymphatic tissue including the internal iliac, presacral, obturator fossa, and external iliac nodes,

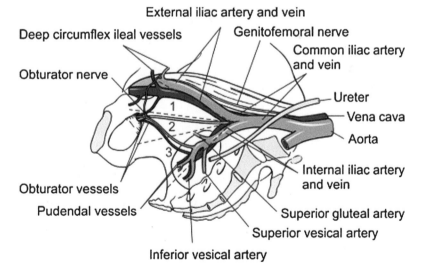

FIGURE 24.2.1 Field of PLND. *Source: Reprinted from Bader P, Burkhard FC, Markwalder R, Studer UE. Disease progression and survival of patients with positive lymph nodes after radical prostatectomy. Is there a chance of cure? J Urol 2003;169:849–54. Copyright (2003), with permission from Elsevier [1].*

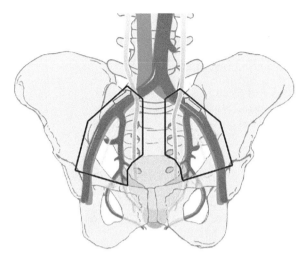

FIGURE 24.2.2 Template of standard LND. *Source: Reprinted from Zehnder P, Studer UE, Skinner EC, et al. Super extended versus extended pelvic lymph node dissection in patients undergoing radical cystectomy for bladder cancer: a comparative study. J Urol 2011;186:1261−8. Copyright (2011), with permission from Elsevier [9].*

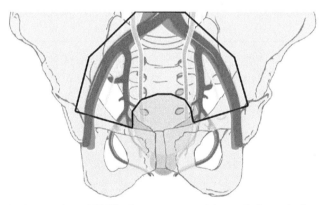

FIGURE 24.2.3 Template of ELND. *Source: Reprinted from Zehnder P, Studer UE, Skinner EC, et al. Super extended versus extended pelvic lymph node dissection in patients undergoing radical cystectomy for bladder cancer: a comparative study. J Urol 2011;186:1261−8. Copyright (2011), with permission from Elsevier [9].*

proximally up to the bifurcation of the common iliac vessels, laterally to the genitofemoral nerve, medially to the ureter, bladder, and internal iliac vessels, and distally to the circumflex iliac vein crossing over the external iliac artery and including the node of Cloquet [4−8,10,11] (Fig. 24.2.3).

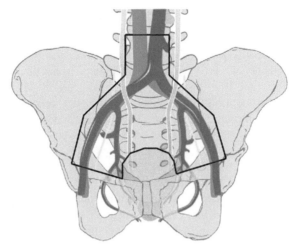

FIGURE 24.2.4 Template of SELND. *Source: Reprinted from Zehnder P, Studer UE, Skinner EC, et al. Super extended versus extended pelvic lymph node dissection in patients undergoing radical cystectomy for bladder cancer: a comparative study. J Urol 2011;186:1261−8. Copyright (2011), with permission from Elsevier [9].*

3. ELND

    ELND excises all LNs between the aortic bifurcation proximally, the genitofemoral nerves laterally, and the point where the circumflex iliac vein crosses over the external iliac artery distally, encompassing the node of Cloquet, internal iliac veins, obturator fossa, and presacral lymphatic tissue [5−7,10,12−14].

4. SELND

    SELND extends the template of ELND up to the level of the inferior mesenteric artery [9,15] (Fig. 24.2.4).

	Limited LND	Standard LND	ELND	SELND
Lymph node	Obturator node	Internal iliac, presacral, obturator fossa, and external iliac nodes	Internal iliac, presacral, obturator fossa, external and common iliac nodes	
Proximal border		Bifurcation of common iliac vessels	Aortic bifurcation	Inferior mesenteric artery
Distal border		Circumflex iliac vein	Circumflex iliac vein	Circumflex iliac vein
Lateral border	External iliac vein	Genitofemoral nerve	Genitofemoral nerve	Genitofemoral nerve
Medial border	Obturator nerve	Ureter, bladder and internal iliac vessels		

ONCOLOGIC OUTCOMES OF PELVIC LYMPHADENECTOMY TEMPLATES

1. LND versus No LND

Abdollah et al. [16] analyzed the data from the Surveillance, Epidemiology, and End Results database to compare the efficacy of LND against that of no LND in patients with bladder cancer. The 10-year cancer-specific mortality-free rates for patients undergoing pelvic lymphadenectomy (PLND) and those who did not were 80% vs 71.9% for pTa/is ($P = 0.02$), 81.7% vs 70.0% for pT1 ($P < 0.001$), 71.5% vs 56.1% for pT2 ($P = 0.001$), 43.7% vs 38.8% for pT3 ($P = 0.006$), and 35.1% vs 32.0% for pT4 ($P = 0.1$), respectively. On multivariate analyses, PLND omission was associated with higher cancer-specific mortality in patients with pTa/is, pT1, and pT2 disease ($P \le 0.01$ in all cases) but not in those with pT3 and pT4 disease. Omitting PLND predisposed to higher overall mortality across all tumor stages (all $P \le 0.03$).

All other studies comparing LND with no LND reported better oncological outcome for the node dissection group regardless of the template [17−20].

2. Limited LND versus standard LND

No study to date has compared limited LND and standard LND in terms of the oncological outcome.

3. Limited LND versus ELND

Jensen et al. [14] analyzed the survival benefit attributed to ELND compared with limited LND. In LN-negative patients there was no significant difference in terms of recurrence-free survival (RFS) or disease-specific survival (DSS) between the ELND and limited LND cohorts ($P = 0.8$ and 0.6, respectively); however, for LN-positive patients significantly better RFS (5-year RFS 29% vs 8%, $P = 0.03$) and DSS (5-year DSS 39% vs 14%, $P = 0.002$) were observed in the ELND cohort. For organ-confined disease (T1-2, N0-2) the prognosis was comparable for both the ELND and limited LND cohorts (RFS and DSS, $P = 0.9$ and 0.9, respectively), whereas a tendency towards better RFS (5-year RFS 61% vs 54%, $P = 0.09$) and significantly better DSS (5-year DSS 76% vs 62%, $P = 0.008$) was demonstrated for ELND in patients with non-organ-confined disease (T3-4, N0-2). The extent of LND (extended vs limited) was an independent determinant of OS but not of RFS or DSS on multivariate analysis.

Holmer et al. [13] compared 101 patients undergoing ELND with 69 patients undergoing limited LND. In non-organ-confined disease, patients who underwent ELND demonstrated significantly longer time to recurrence (hazard ratio (HR) 0.45, 95% confidence interval (CI) 0.22−0.93; $P = 0.032$). On multivariate analysis adjusting for tumor stage, lymph node status, age, sex, and adjuvant chemotherapy, ELND significantly improved survival (HR 0.47, 95% CI 0.25−0.88; $P = 0.018$) and time to recurrence (HR 0.42, 95% CI 0.23−0.79; $P = 0.007$).

4. Standard LND versus ELND

Simone et al. [12] analyzed the data from 933 patients treated either with standard or ELND, which revealed that ELND was a strong predictor of improved RFS (1-, 3-, and 5-year estimates for standard vs ELND: 71.2%, 49.4%, and 42.6% vs 86%, 68.6%, and 63.1 %, respectively) and cancer-specific survival (CSS) (1-, 3-, and 5-year estimates for standard vs ELND: 87.7%, 62%, and 50.9% vs. 93.5%, 78.5%, and 68.8 %, respectively). ELND was an independent determinant of DFS (HR 1.95, $P < 0.001$) and CSS (HR 1.80, $P < 0.001$), and its benefit on DFS and CSS was significant across all pT stages higher than pT2 and across all pN stages.

Similarly, Dhar et al. [5] compared recurrence patterns and survival of patients with urothelial bladder cancer undergoing radical cystectomy at two institutions (limited PLND at the Cleveland Clinic and extended PLND at the University of Bern). The 5-year RFS of patients with lymph node−positive disease was 7% and 35% after limited and extended PLND, respectively. The 5-year RFS for pT2pN0 disease was 67% and 77% after limited and extended PLND, respectively, and the respective percentages for pT3pN0 disease were 23% and 57% ($P < 0.0001$). The 5-year RFS for pT2pN0-2 disease was 63% and 71% for limited and extended PLND, respectively, and for pT3pN0-2 disease, the respective figures were 19% and 49% ($P < 0.0001$). Extended PLND has thus been shown to allow for more accurate staging and improved survival in patients with non-organ-confined and lymph node−positive disease.

Poulsen et al. [10] also assessed the influence of the extent of PLND through comparison of ELND and standard LND. Extended PLND substantially improved the 5-year RFS for tumors confined to the bladder wall (tumor stage $\leq$ pT3a) (85% vs 64% for standard LND, $P < 0.02$) and without lymph node metastasis (stage $\leq$ pT3a, pN0) (90% vs 71% for standard LND, $P < 0.02$). However, in this study, survival was similar for either template among patients with pT3b disease or greater.

5. ELND versus SELND

Two multi-institutional studies compared ELND and SELND [9,21]. Both studies reported no statistically significant difference in survival outcomes between ELND and SELND, irrespective of tumor stage or nodal status.

SUMMARY

PLND is a procedure that must be performed in conjunction with radical cystectomy in the surgical treatment of patients with muscle-invasive bladder cancer. Although several options exist with regard to the extent of PLND as mentioned earlier, extended PLND is the procedure recommended by recent studies based on the oncologic outcome. However, most of these studies are retrospective observational studies, suggesting the necessity of further validation through prospective randomized studies.

REFERENCES

[1] Bader P, Burkhard FC, Markwalder R, Studer UE. Disease progression and survival of patients with positive lymph nodes after radical prostatectomy. Is there a chance of cure? J Urol 2003;169(3):849−54, http://dx.doi.org/10.1097/01.ju.0000049032.38743.c7. PubMed PMID: 12576797.

[2] Bruins HM, Veskimae E, Hernandez V, Imamura M, Neuberger MM, Dahm P, et al. The impact of the extent of lymphadenectomy on oncologic outcomes in patients undergoing radical cystectomy for bladder cancer: a systematic review. Eur Urol 2014;66(6): 1065−77, http://dx.doi.org/10.1016/j.eururo.2014.05.031. PubMed PMID: 25074764.

[3] Brossner C, Pycha A, Toth A, Mian C, Kuber W. Does extended lymphadenectomy increase the morbidity of radical cystectomy? BJU Int 2004;93(1):64−6. PubMed PMID: 14678370.

[4] Herr HW, Faulkner JR, Grossman HB, Natale RB, deVere White R, Sarosdy MF, et al. Surgical factors influence bladder cancer outcomes: a cooperative group report. J Clin Oncol 2004;22(14):2781−9, http://dx.doi.org/10.1200/JCO.2004.11.024. PubMed PMID: 15199091.

[5] Dhar NB, Klein EA, Reuther AM, Thalmann GN, Madersbacher S, Studer UE. Outcome after radical cystectomy with limited or extended pelvic lymph node dissection. J Urol 2008;179(3):873−8, discussion 8. http://dx.doi.org/10.1016/j.juro.2007.10.076. PubMed PMID: 18221953.

[6] Dorin RP, Skinner EC. Extended lymphadenectomy in bladder cancer. Curr Opin Urol 2010; 20(5):414−20, http://dx.doi.org/10.1097/MOU.0b013e32833c9194. PubMed PMID: 20657290.

[7] Stein JP. The role of lymphadenectomy in patients undergoing radical cystectomy for bladder cancer. Curr Oncol Rep 2007;9(3):213−21. PubMed PMID: 17430693.

[8] Stein JP, Skinner DG. Surgical atlas. Radical cystectomy. BJU Int 2004;94(1):197−221, http://dx.doi.org/10.1111/j.1464-410X.2004.04981.x. PubMed PMID: 15217471.

[9] Zehnder P, Studer UE, Skinner EC, Dorin RP, Cai J, Roth B, et al. Super extended versus extended pelvic lymph node dissection in patients undergoing radical cystectomy for bladder cancer: a comparative study. J Urol 2011;186(4):1261−8, http://dx.doi.org/10.1016/j. juro.2011.06.004. PubMed PMID: 21849183.

[10] Poulsen AL, Horn T, Steven K. Radical cystectomy: extending the limits of pelvic lymph node dissection improves survival for patients with bladder cancer confined to the bladder wall. J Urol 1998;160(6 Pt 1):2015−19, discussion 20. PubMed PMID: 9817313.

[11] Mills RD, Fleischmann A, Studer UE. Radical cystectomy with an extended pelvic lymphadenectomy: rationale and results. Surg Oncol Clin N Am 2007;16(1):233−45, http://dx.doi.org/10.1016/j.soc.2006.10.001. PubMed PMID: 17336246.

[12] Simone G, Papalia R, Ferriero M, Guaglianone S, Castelli E, Collura D, et al. Stage-specific impact of extended versus standard pelvic lymph node dissection in radical cystectomy. Int J Urol 2013;20(4):390−7, http://dx.doi.org/10.1111/j.1442-2042.2012.03148.x. PubMed PMID: 22970939.

[13]   Holmer M, Bendahl PO, Davidsson T, Gudjonsson S, Mansson W, Liedberg F. Extended lymph node dissection in patients with urothelial cell carcinoma of the bladder: can it make a difference? World J Urol 2009;27(4):521−6, http://dx.doi.org/10.1007/s00345-008-0366-9. PubMed PMID: 19145436.

[14]   Jensen JB, Ulhoi BP, Jensen KM. Extended versus limited lymph node dissection in radical cystectomy: impact on recurrence pattern and survival. Int J Urol 2012;19(1):39−47, http://dx.doi.org/10.1007/s00345-008-0366-9. PubMed PMID: 22050425.

[15]   Zlotta AR. Limited, extended, superextended, megaextended pelvic lymph node dissection at the time of radical cystectomy: what should we perform? Eur Urol 2012;61(2):243−4, http://dx.doi.org/10.1016/j.eururo.2011.11.006. PubMed PMID: 22119158.

[16]   Abdollah F, Sun M, Schmitges J, Djahangirian O, Tian Z, Jeldres C, et al. Stage-specific impact of pelvic lymph node dissection on survival in patients with non-metastatic bladder cancer treated with radical cystectomy. BJU Int 2012;109(8):1147−54, http://dx.doi.org/10.1111/j.1464-410X.2011.10482.x. PubMed PMID: 21883849.

[17]   Isaka S, Okano T, Sato N, Shimazaki J, Matsuzaki O. [Pelvic lymph node dissection for invasive bladder cancer] [in Japanese]. Nihon Hinyokika Gakkai Zasshi 1989;80 (3):402−6. PubMed PMID: 2733302.

[18]   Miyakawa M, Oishi K, Okada Y, Takeuchi H, Okada K, Yoshida O. Results of the multidisciplinary treatment of invasive bladder cancer. Hinyokika Kiyo 1986;32(12):1931−9. PubMed PMID: 3825830.

[19]   Yuasa M, Yamamoto A, Kawanishi Y, Higa I, Numata A, Imagawa A. Clinical evaluation of total cystectomy for bladder carcinoma: a ten-year experience. Hinyokika Kiyo 1988;34(6):975−81. PubMed PMID: 3223462.

[20]   Zhang F, Wang F, Weng Z. Clinical significance of standard lymphadenectomy in radical cystectomy for bladder cancer. J Practical Oncol 2013;28:284−6.

[21]   Simone G, Abol Enein H, Ferriero M, et al. Extended versus superextended PLND during radical cystectomy: comparison of two prospective series. J Urol 2012;187(Suppl 4):e708.

Chapter 24.3

Laparoscopic/Robot-Assisted Radical Cystectomy

Jong H. Pyun[1] and Seok H. Kang[2]

[1]*Sungkyunkwan University School of Medicine, Seoul, South Korea,* [2]*Korea University College of Medicine, Seoul, South Korea*

INTRODUCTION

Open radical cystectomy (ORC) is associated with high morbidity and significant mortality; however, it remains the gold-standard therapy for muscle-invasive and high-risk non-muscle-invasive bladder cancer. Within urology, minimally invasive surgery has been encouraged as a replacement for many open procedures to decrease the morbidity of each operation [1–6]. Robot-assisted surgery offers the advantages of a minimally invasive approach, with greater technical ease and a shorter learning curve than pure laparoscopy [7]. Accordingly, Menon et al. reported the first series of robot-assisted radical cystectomy (RARC) and urinary diversion in 2003 [8], and RARC has subsequently emerged as a minimally invasive alternative to ORC, with the goal of reducing procedure-related morbidity. However, the results of a recent prospective randomized trial indicated that robotic technology holds promise in improving patient outcomes. Similar complication rates were observed between RARC and ORC; however, this report remains controversial for several reasons [9].

Recently, as surgical experience increases and ergonomics improve, intracorporeal urinary diversion (ICUD) has become the latest trend, primarily due to potential benefits that include decreased fluid loss from evaporation, reduced body cooling, reduced estimated blood loss (EBL), less pain, a smaller incision, and a faster return to bowel function. However, at present, only a limited number of studies have reported the benefits of ICUD when compared with extracorporeal urinary diversion (ECUD). In our tertiary referral hospital, we performed RARC over 100 cases, which included 50 cases of ICUD by a single surgeon. The goal of this chapter is to describe our techniques for both intracorporeal orthotopic neobladder and ileal conduit diversions, as well as to assess the current evidence by reviewing the literature and reporting the comparative outcomes of RARC over ORC.

TECHNIQUE

Step 1. Preoperative Preparation and Postoperative Care

There are no differences in patient evaluation between RARC and ORC. Before surgery, patient preparation should begin with an extensive discussion about the risks and benefits of RARC during both the perioperative and postoperative periods. It is particularly important for patients to receive counsel regarding the options for urinary diversion. Inclusion criteria for orthotopic neobladder are the same as those for ORC, with all suitable patients primarily considered for orthotopic neobladder. For those in whom a neobladder is contraindicated and for those who prefer, an ileal conduit should be chosen as an alternative [10]. Reconstruction for urinary diversion can be performed using either an intracorporeal or an extracorporeal method, depending on the experience of the surgeon.

Bowel preparation should not be recommended for urinary reconstruction, as it causes more adverse effects than benefits. It leads to dehydration and may cause electrolyte abnormalities, and in several randomized controlled trials, no statistically significant benefits were observed when mechanical bowel preparations or rectal enemas were used in colorectal surgery [11]. Based on this evidence, we no longer routinely use a mechanical bowel preparation, and patients are only required to be None Per Oral (NPO) after a soft diet on the morning of the day before the surgery. Postoperative care after RARC is identical to the care given after ORC according to the Enhanced Recovery After Surgery guidelines.

Step 2. Surgical Positioning and Port Placement

Proper positioning is critical to successful motion of the robotic arms, with safe and effective access to the bedside assistant port required (Fig. 24.3.1). The patient is placed in the dorsal lithotomy position with the legs in stirrups with minimal hip flexion and the knees flexed to a gentle 30 degrees. The arms are adducted in arm guard foam pads using the patient's draw sheet. It is important that positioning complications such as peripheral neuropraxia are encountered early in the learning curve. Care must be taken to cushion all pressure points with foam padding, and cotton padding must be taped over the

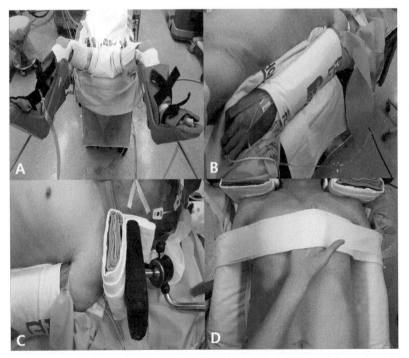

FIGURE 24.3.1 Patient positioning. (A) Minimal hip flexion and gentle 30-degree knee flexion. (B) The patient's arms are tucked into position using foam pads and a draw sheet. (C) All pressure points are cushioned with foam padding, and cephalad slipping in the steep Trendelenburg position is prevented. (D) Chest wall motion for ventilation must be confirmed.

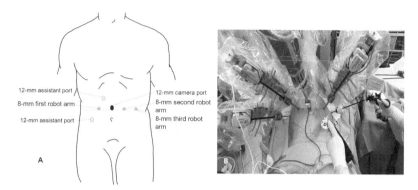

FIGURE 24.3.2 Port placement. (A, B) The robotic arm ports are placed on the same level as that of the camera port if extended PLND is to be performed.

patient's chest to prevent cephalad slipping in the steep Trendelenburg position; however, the tape should not be so tight as to prevent chest wall motion during surgery. The combined application of graduated compression stockings and intermittent pneumatic compressions during the operation is recommended for thromboprophylaxis.

The draping should be sterile and prepared from the subxiphoid region down to the mid-thigh region including the perineum. The urethral catheter is inserted, and the penis should be exposed in the field to allow for intraoperative manipulation. A six-port technique via a transperitoneal approach is used, with the camera port placed 4 cm above the umbilicus in the midline. The camera port is placed by performing a small mini laparotomy with a 12-mm Hasson trocar, and the other ports are placed in view of the camera. The first, second, and third 8-mm robotic arms are placed at the same level as that of the camera port on the left and right sides at 8-cm lateral intervals. One assistant port is placed at 8 cm lateral to the right robotic port at the level of the umbilicus, and the other assistant port is placed superior−lateral to the ipsilateral robotic port on the opposite side of the assistant port (Fig. 24.3.2). The two assistant ports are usually 12 mm, enabling laparoscopic stapling by the assistant. The major difference from robot-assisted radical prostatectomy (RARP) is that the ports are placed more cephalad to perform extended pelvic lymph node dissection (PLND) and to simplify the ICUD procedure. The preferred positioning is tilted at maximum Trendelenburg with the head down at approximately 30 degrees, similar to RARP. The robot is docked between the split legs.

Step 3. Ureteral Identification and Transection

Development of the periureteral space is initiated on the patient's left side by incising the avascular white line of Toldt. The posterior peritoneum

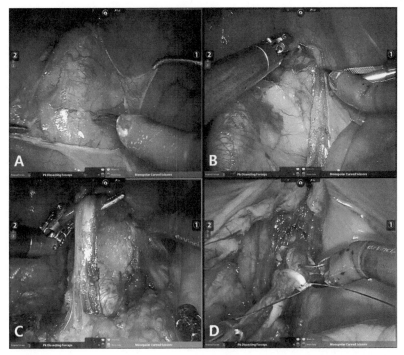

FIGURE 24.3.3 Ureteral mobilization. (A, B) Posterior peritoneum overlying the external iliac artery is opened lateral to the right colon. (C) Identification of ureter. (D) Ureter being clipped at bladder insertion.

overlying the external iliac artery is opened lateral to the right colon, and the colon should be released from the right side wall to expose the retroperitoneal space, allowing access to the right ureter, which crosses over the iliac vessels. The ureters should be free of periureteric tissue as cranially towards the bladder as possible to allow for maximal ureteral mobilization. The ureter can be divided distally with Hem-o-Lok clips, and the proximal clip on the ureter end should have a suture pretied to the clip (Fig. 24.3.3). This pretied clip facilitates later identification and orientation with no additional tagging and minimalizes manipulation of the ureter, which may result in ureteric trauma and devitalization, and may contribute to anastomotic stricture. The distal margin may be sent for frozen section analysis at this point. An identical dissection is performed on the left side.

Step 4. Division of Anterior Pedicle

The vas deferens is divided to open the space medial to the external iliac vessel. The anterior pedicle including the superior vesical artery and umbilical artery is clearly identified after the identification of the ureter between

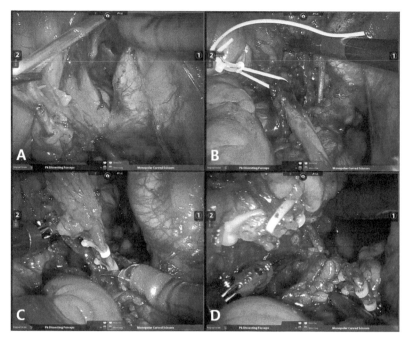

FIGURE 24.3.4 (A) Vas deferens transection. (B–D) Development of the anterior pedicle, shown on the patient's right side.

the pelvic sidewall and the lateral aspect of the bladder. These vessels should be visible just lateral to the insertion of the ureter into the bladder and can be clipped and divided using a Hem-o-Lok or metal clip to avoid electrocautery injury near the neurovascular bundle as a nerve-sparing technique (Fig. 24.3.4).

Step 5. Development of the Posterior Vesical Space

The posterior peritoneum between the bladder and the anterior sigmoid colon should be incised from the left to right. The plane of the posterior leaflet of Denonvilliers' fascia should be confirmed by performing a blunt cautery dissection as carefully as possible. When the dissection of this plane carried out to the level of the prostatic apex, the posterior pedicle of the bladder is developed (Fig. 24.3.5). It is necessary for the assistant to retract the bladder and its posterior structures anteriorly.

Step 6. Development of the Paravesical Space and Division of the Posterior Bladder and Prostatic Pedicles

Once the limits of dissection are reached along the posterior aspect of the bladder, the lateral attachment of the bladder can be divided. The paravesical

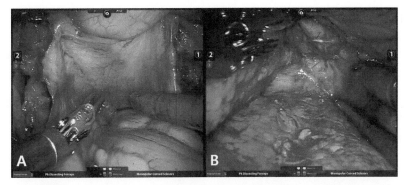

FIGURE 24.3.5 (A) Visualization of posterior peritoneum to be incised. (B) Posterior dissection to reveal vas deferens, seminal vesicles, and Denonvilliers' fascia.

space is developed by incising between the medial umbilical ligament and iliac vessels. Wide peritoneal wings are taken downward, and the median umbilical ligaments are divided. This dissection should be carried caudad through the endopelvic fascia with locking clips. The endopelvic fascia is identified and incised on each side, thereby completely mobilizing the bladder from its lateral attachment and the rectum at this point. This allows for the identification of the prostatic pedicles, which are divided by the bedside assistant using a Hem-o-Lok clip. The bladder and prostatic pedicles are carefully controlled as they come off the internal iliac artery using Hem-o-Lok clips or a stapler to prevent thermal injury to the neurovascular bundles (Fig. 24.3.6).

Step 7. Dropping of the Bladder

After the pedicles are completely divided, the only remaining bladder attachments should be at the median umbilical ligaments, anterior attachments, prostate, and urethra. The median umbilical ligaments are first divided just below the level of the umbilicus. The dissection and peritoneal incision is carried widely in an inferior direction until the pubic bone is exposed (Fig. 24.3.7). The space of Retzius is then completely dissected, thereby completing the apical dissection of the prostate.

Step 8. Division of the Dorsal Venous Complex, and Ligation and Division of the Urethra

The exposed dorsal venous complex (DVC) can be incised using electric cautery (if a non-nerve-sparing technique is performed) or using the scissors (if a nerve-sparing technique is performed) after suture ligation is performed with 2-0 Vicryl on a CT-1 needle passed underneath the DVC, distal to the

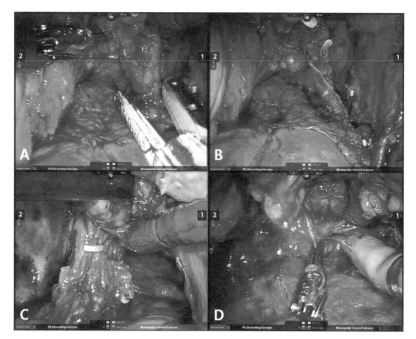

FIGURE 24.3.6 (A–C) Vesical and prostatic pedicles are controlled using Hem-o-Lok clips or a stapler. (D) Complete mobilization of the bladder is enabled from its lateral attachment and the rectum at this point.

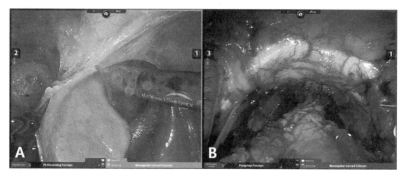

FIGURE 24.3.7 (A) The medial umbilical ligaments and urachus are divided via electrocautery. (B) The space of Retzius is completely dissected.

apex of the prostate. The urethra is exposed, and the indwelling Foley catheter is lifted upward. A Hem-o-lok clip is then placed over the catheter to prevent tumor spillage and divided distal to the clip leaving the balloon inflated, with the assistant pulling the cut catheter in a cranial direction. A frozen section can be taken from the proximal portion of the divided urethra if needed. The posterior urethra is divided, and minor remnants of the rectourethralis

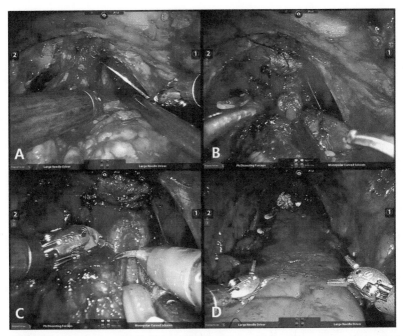

FIGURE 24.3.8 (A) Suture ligation with 2-0 Vicryl on a CT-1 needle passed underneath the DVC. (B) Urethra exposure (C) The indwelling Foley catheter is lifted upward. (D) Entrapped specimen was placed in the superior aspect of the abdomen.

are released (Fig. 24.3.8). The specimen including the bladder, prostate, and seminal vesicles is placed in a large Lap Bag and retraced into the superior aspect of the abdomen. It is necessary to determine whether there is any bleeding, thereby confirming that there is sufficient hemostasis around the pedicle. At this point, an extended PLND is performed.

Step 9. Extended PLND

Extended PLND has been considered to be an essential element of radical cystectomy that affects improved oncologic outcomes and acts as a surrogate indicator of the quality of the surgery. Contemporary RARC series have revealed lymph node (LN) yields comparable to ORC series through the enhanced vision and technological advances in the robot platform. Lymphadenectomy procedures at the external iliac zones, obturator zone, common iliac zones, presacral zone, inferior mesenteric artery, and aortic bifurcation suggest the necessity for dissection of the pelvic region, particularly for the purpose of staging.

The nodes are separately harvested after the dissection, and each resected nodal packet is individually extracted with the aid of a small Lap Bag via the 12-mm assistant port to minimize metastasis (Fig. 24.3.9).

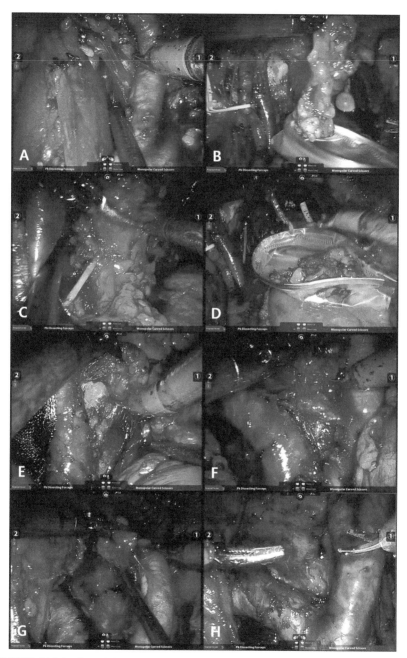

FIGURE 24.3.9 Extended PLND. (A, B) External iliac zone. (C, D) Obturator zone. (E, F) Aortic bifurcation zone. (G, H) Presacral and common iliac zones. Each resected nodal packet was individually retrieved with a small Lap Bag.

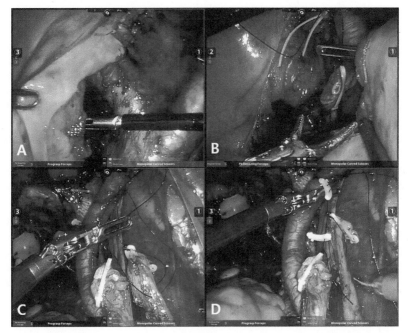

FIGURE 24.3.10 (A, B) The left ureter is passed through mesenteric window for transposition. (C, D) Locking clips are placed onto both ureteral tags.

Step 10. Transposition of the Left Ureter to the Right Side

After the completion of radical cystectomy and PLND, grasping forceps are passed the presacral area under the sigmoid colon by the assistant from the right side to the left side. The left ureter is grasped by the stay suture on the end of the left ureter and brought to the right side (Fig. 24.3.10).

Step 11. Urinary Diversion

Urinary reconstruction is the step that is most likely to vary in terms of operative time, and it also accounted for the longest operative time in a recent study [12]. The robot-assisted approach is implemented during cystectomy and bilateral PLND procedures, as well as for intracorporeal urethrovesical anastomotic stitches in cases of orthotopic neobladder reconstruction. In cases of ECUD using an orthotopic neobladder, after excision of the bladder, the robot is undocked, and urinary diversion is extracorporeally performed. The robot is then redocked into the pelvis for urethroneovesical anastomosis with robot assistance. In cases of ICUD, all procedures including urinary diversion are intracorporeally completed regardless of whether an ileal conduit or orthotopic neobladder is created. Intracorporeal bowel harvest is performed after the position of the patient is reduced to a 10- to 15-degree Trendelenburg position, and the bagged specimen is positioned into the pelvis to allow bowel manipulation.

Ileal Conduit

In cases of ECUD, the specimen is extracted via an infraumbilical midline incision and a bowel harvest procedure. A 15-cm segment of ileal loop that is 15 cm away from the ileocecal valve is isolated and harvested using 60-mm and 45-mm intestinal staplers (Endo-GIA; Covidien Corp., Dublin, Ireland). Bowel-to-bowel anastomosis is then performed, followed by extracorporeal urinary tract reconstruction including ureteroenteric anastomosis, similar to ORC.

It is important to keep a vascular supply for the small bowel segment, particularly for an ileal conduit, as the bowel segment is short. In cases of ICUD, transillumination by laparoscope is a useful technique for identifying the mesenteric blood supply. The intestine can be elevated to reveal the vascular structures using the third robotic arm and the long forceps of the left assistant. The overhead light from the portable lamp running through the right assistant trocar should also be helpful for visualizing the vascular supply to the small bowel.

An Endo GIA stapler is fired to divide the bowel and mesentery. Care is taken to fire the stapler perpendicular to the bowel into the mesentery. If necessary, the mesenteric window can be further developed using an additional stapler (45 mm; Fig. 24.3.11). The bowel continuity is then reestablished using the same stapler in a side-to-side fashion along the antimesenteric borders. The ends of the small bowel are secured together with stay sutures at the antimesenteric sites 5 cm from the stapled ends. The cutting hole of the distal staple line on the antimesenteric side is made using the robotic scissors. The 60-mm stapler is passed through each of these two holes to restore the continuity of the bowel. The additional 45-mm stapler can also be used sequentially to further extend the space. The bowel anastomosis is then completed by transverse firing of the stapler to close the open ends of the ileum.

Two separate openings in the proximal part where the ureters are to be implanted are created. The ureters are secured with the third robotic arm, and each end of the spatulated ureters is approximated at the bowel opening and placed with stay sutures. The anastomosis between the ureters and the conduit is carried out using 4-0 Vicryl running sutures on the posterior side of each ureter. Using the stay sutures, the opposite site is exposed, and before suturing, a double J catheter is inserted into the ureter. The robot is then undocked for creation of the stoma, and a drain is inserted through the third robotic arm port. The stoma is constructed at its approximately marked location.

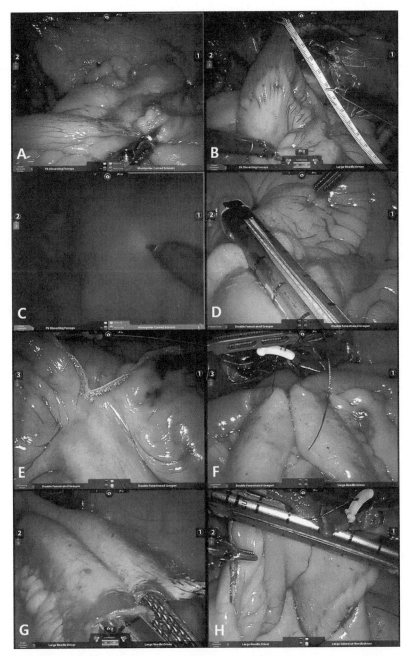

FIGURE 24.3.11 Bowel harvest. (A) Identification of the ileocecal valve. (B) Isolation of the bowel segment. (C) Visualization of the vascular supply to the small bowel using a portable lamp. (D—H) The ileum is isolated, and side-to-side anastomosis is performed to restore continuity using the 60-mm stapler (Endo-GIA; Covidien Corp., Dublin, Ireland).

Orthotopic Neobladder

In cases of ECUD, after excision of the bladder, the robot is undocked yet kept sterile, and urinary diversion is extracorporeally performed. Bowel harvest is performed similar to ORC through an infraumbilical small incision. The robot is then redocked into the pelvis for urethroneovesical anastomosis using robot assistance.

In cases of ICUD, all procedures including urinary diversion are completed intracorporeally. The orthotopic neobladder is fashioned based on the Studer technique, which requires a 45-cm segment of bowel identified 15 cm proximal to the ileocecal valve. All points (both ends, urethroileal anastomosis site, and afferent limb) are marked with stay sutures and ink. Bowel resection and continuity are achieved intracorporeally with the same maneuver in a side-to-side anastomosis. After restoration of bowel continuity, the specimen bag is delivered to the abdomen. The 15-cm section proximal to the projected distal aspect of the ileal segment, which reached the urethra in an inverted U-shape without tension, was selected. Using robotic scissors, a 20 F opening is created at the antimesenteric border, and the urethroileal anastomosis is then performed using a bidirectional barbed suture technique with Stratafix 3-0 (Ethicon Inc., Somerville, NJ, USA). It is necessary to have a urethral catheter placed during the procedure.

The distal 30-cm section of the isolated ileal segment, excluding a proximal 15-cm portion as an afferent limb, is detubularized along the antimesenteric border. The inner edges of the U-shape (the posterior part of the Studer pouch) are then closed with multiple running sutures using V-Loc 3-0. After completion of the posterior wall of the pouch, the neobladder is then folded over from the right-upper bottom, approximating to the left-limb mid-outer edges of the U-shape. The remaining part of the reservoir is sutured, using the same sutures as those used on the posterior wall. Although the proximal half of the anterior part of the reservoir can be left open to facilitate the passage of ureteral stents, an additional opening in the afferent limb may be used instead for ureteral stents (Fig. 24.3.12). The ureteroenteric anastomosis is performed using the Bricker technique with a 4-0 Vicryl suture. The seromuscular layer of the distal part of the afferent limb is opened at the site where the left ureter is to be implanted. Each end of the spatulated ureter is approximated at the bowel opening and placed with stay sutures. While the stay sutures are held by the third robotic arm and an assistant, running sutures are placed between the two stay sutures. Using the stay sutures, the opposite site is exposed, and before suturing, a single J catheter is inserted into the ureter through the assistant's right hand port. Each single J stent passed through the afferent limb comes into the opening made previously. After the ureteroileal anastomosis is completed, the catheters are taken out through a 4-mm incision in the midline just above the pubic symphysis and fixed to the skin. The opening in the afferent limb is then closed to fasten

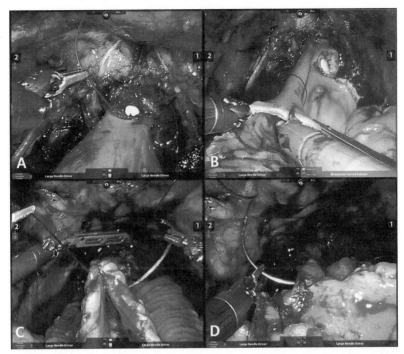

FIGURE 24.3.12 Orthotopic neobladder formation. (A) Ureteroileal anastomosis is performed using a bidirectional barbed suture technique with Stratafix 3-0 (Ethicon Inc., Somervile, NJ, USA). (B) The ileum is detubularized along the antimesenteric border. (C, D) The posterior part and remaining folded part of the reservoir are closed with multiple running sutures (3-0 V-Loc).

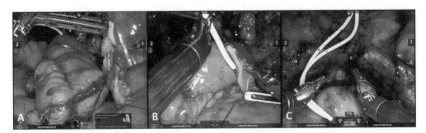

FIGURE 24.3.13 Ureter reimplantation. (A—C) Ureteroileal anastomosis is completed, and the single J catheter is then passed through the afferent limb, taken out through a 4-mm incision in the midline just above the pubic symphysis, and fixed to the skin.

the ureteral catheters using V-Loc 3-0 sutures. After inflating the balloon of the indwelling catheter, the neobladder is then filled with 50 mL of saline to check for leakage. If leakage is observed, extra sutures should be considered. A 21 F passive drain is placed in the small pelvis through the third robotic port and is secured to the skin with a silk suture (Fig. 24.3.13).

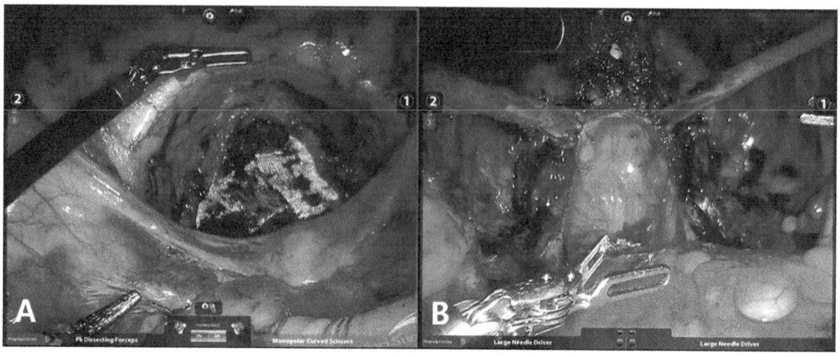

FIGURE 24.3.14 Female cystectomy. (A) Preservation of genital organs. (B) Suspension of the vaginal stump by preserving the round ligament.

FEMALE ROBOTIC CYSTECTOMY

Cystectomy in male and female patients differs with regard to the surgical approach. The classical technique in women is anterior pelvic exenteration, which involves en bloc removal of the bladder, uterus, fallopian tubes, ovaries, anterior vaginal wall, and urethra [13]. Recently, it was concluded that preservation of the gynecologic organs either partially or totally in the course of radical cystectomy and orthotopic neobladder substitution is possible in selected patients.

After ureteral mobilization, an inverted U-shaped incision is made in the peritoneum between the bladder and the uterus, and the cervix is then developed by blunt and sharp dissection. To identify the vaginal apex, a sponge stick or a vaginal manipulator is used. After transecting the round ligament, the vascular pedicles are divided using LigaSure or Hem-o-Lok. In cases of anterior exenteration, the anterior vaginal wall is resected along the bladder, and the vagina is closed with a V-Loc suture. For patients selected for both neobladder reconstruction and anterior pelvic exenteration, a surgical technique that preserves the round ligament can be readily attempted. It is used to suspend the vaginal stump and to help prevent urinary retention (Fig. 24.3.14).

In women who are candidates for neobladder reconstruction, preservation of the female organs to suspend the neobladder posterior wall is expected to reduce the incidence of urinary retention after radical cystectomy with orthotopic neobladder reconstruction.

OUTCOMES AND CONCLUSION

Cumulative analyses have demonstrated that LN yields and positive surgical margin (SM) rates serve as oncologic surrogate markers, and oncologic outcomes of ≤5 years have been shown to be similar between RARC and ORC

[3]. Recently, an International Robotic Cystectomy Consortium (IRCC) analysis reported that the largest multi-institutional cohort of RARC presented long-term oncologic outcomes that appear to be similar to historical ORC data: soft tissue SMs were positive in 8%, the median LN yield was 16, and 21% of patients had positive LNs. The 5-year recurrence-free survival, cancer-specific survival, and overall survival rates were 67%, 75%, and 50%, respectively, in pathologic organ-confined disease [14]. In a total of three randomized controlled trials of open versus robotic radical cystectomy, no differences in the positive SM rate and LN yield were found between the two groups [3,15,16]. These results from published studies demonstrate the oncologic safety and comparable efficacy of RARC compared to ORC.

Although functional outcomes are important factors for patients undergoing RARC, the available data for functional outcomes are very limited. Yuh et al. reported that the 12-month continence rates with continent diversion were 83%−100% in men for daytime continence and 66%−76% for nighttime continence in a systemic review and cumulative analysis. In one series, among 41 patients who underwent nerve-sparing RARC, potency was recovered in 26 patients (63%) with or without the use of PDE5-Is after 12 months [17].

The longer operative time of RARC is a critical issue regarding this complex procedure, as the longer anesthesia time may adversely affect perioperative morbidity and increase postoperative complications. A cumulative analysis in a systemic review demonstrated that the mean operative time of 385 minutes for RARC was shorter than the operative time for ORC [18]. However, the operative times reported in a contemporary RARC series should be examined with consideration of several factors, such as the mean yield and territory of PLND, the method of urinary diversion (ileal conduit vs orthotopic neobladder), and the surgeon experience relative to the learning curve. Atmaca et al. [19] reported a mean operative time of 586 minutes vs 552 minutes in their comparison study of RARC vs ORC. The urinary reconstructions in their study were all intracorporeal Studer diversions in both groups. Additionally, the mean LN yield was 25.4 vs 20.4, and 100% vs 71.4% of patients underwent extended PLND in the RARC and ORC groups, respectively. Canda et al. reported on their initial experience series of intracorporeal RARC a mean operative time of 594 minutes and a mean EBL of 429 mL for intracorporeal RARC, of which 92% of patients underwent orthotopic neobladder formation; in this series, the mean LN yield was 24.8, and 93% of patients (25 of 27) underwent extended PLND [20]. However, the analysis only included the console time. Bochner et al. reported a mean operative time of 464 minutes in their RARC cohort [9]. The urinary diversions in their study were performed extracorporeally, and 53% of patients (30 of 56) underwent orthotopic neobladder formation; additionally, the mean LN yield was 31.8, and the rate of patients who underwent extended PLND was 88%. In a study performed by our institution, the mean total operative time was 513 minutes, with a mean console time of 390 minutes and a mean EBL of 217 mL. The mean number of LNs harvested was 26.7, and the rate of patients who underwent extended PLND was 73.4%. Additionally, 41% (26 of 64) of the urinary diversions were constructed intracorporeally, and the rate of orthotopic neobladder urinary diversion was 41% [21]. Almost all of these cases for which the operative times were reported served as the surgeon's initial experience of intracorporeal urinary reconstruction, although robotic cystectomy was adopted by an experienced team. Intracorporeal bowel harvest and suturing for anastomosis accounted for a greater portion of the total operative time; therefore, the learning curve must be considered.

EBL and transfusion rates were significantly lower with RARC than with ORC in several studies [18]. Xia et al. reported that 10 studies including 1247 patients showed a shorter postoperative length of stay in the RARC group than in the ORC group in an updated systematic review and meta-analysis [22]. However, other studies reported similar results in both groups [19]. Complication rates were mostly similar between RARC and ORC or slightly better for RARC in comparison with laparoscopic radical cystectomy [18]. Conversely, other studies reported that the rates of overall and low-grade complications were significantly higher among RARC patients [23]. Furthermore, Bochner et al. reported that their prospective, randomized trial resulted in 62% and 66% 90-day postoperative complication rates for extra-corporeal RARC and ORC, respectively [9]. However, it is common knowledge that the main driver for radical cystectomy complications is the reconstructive urinary diversion [24]. It is important to consider that most series reporting on RARC involved ECUD. A robotic approach, particularly ICUD, has a theoretical advantage over ORC in terms of a faster return of bowel function, a shorter hospital stay, an earlier return to normal activities, and EBL and transfusion rates. However, it is true that controversy remains on whether to perform an ICUD or ECUD, as ECUD is a simpler and faster procedure than ICUD. Although limited, several series from high-volume centers have demonstrated the feasibility of ICUD. The IRCC published an analysis of 935 patients who underwent ICUD after RARC and were compared with ECUD patients; the results indicated that ICUD produced outcomes that were similar to ECUD, although with fewer complications [25]. If the learning curve can be overcome safely with a clearly defined training program and a standardized approach, ICUD will warrant positive impact with its theoretical advantage.

Robot-assisted surgery has been quickly adapted and is significantly positioned as a replacement for many open procedures within urology. To date, the current clinical trials of RARC versus ORC are incomplete, as both involve ECUD. In the future, further research may be necessary to compare intracorporeal RARC with ORC to confirm the superior aspects of a robotic system, as the reconstructive urinary diversion is the main driver for radical cystectomy complications.

REFERENCES

[1] Sohn W, Lee HJ, Ahlering TE. Robotic surgery: review of prostate and bladder cancer. Cancer J 2013;19(2):133−9.

[2] Hemal AK. Role of robot-assisted surgery for bladder cancer. Curr Opin Urol 2009;19(1): 69−75.

[3] Yuh B, Wilson T, Bochner B, Chan K, Palou J, Stenzl A, et al. Systematic review and cumulative analysis of oncologic and functional outcomes after robot-assisted radical cystectomy. Eur Urol 2015;67(3):402−22.

[4] Johar RS, Hayn MH, Stegemann AP, Ahmed K, Agarwal P, Balbay MD, et al. Complications after robot-assisted radical cystectomy: results from the International Robotic Cystectomy Consortium. Eur Urol 2013;64(1):52−7.

[5] Yuh BE, Nazmy M, Ruel NH, Jankowski JT, Menchaca AR, Torrey RR, et al. Standardized analysis of frequency and severity of complications after robot-assisted radical cystectomy. Eur Urol 2012;62(5):806−13.

[6] Stein JP, Skinner DG. Radical cystectomy for invasive bladder cancer: long-term results of a standard procedure. World J Urol 2006;24(3):296−304.

[7] Khosla A, Wagner AA. Robotic surgery of the kidney, bladder, and prostate. Surg Clin N Am 2016;96(3): 615- +.

[8] Menon M, Hemal AK, Tewari A, Shrivastava A, Shoma AM, El-Tabey NA, et al. Nerve-sparing robot-assisted radical cystoprostatectomy and urinary diversion. BJU Int 2003;92(3): 232−6.

[9] Bochner BH, Dalbagni G, Sjoberg DD, Silberstein J, Keren Paz GE, Donat SM, et al. Comparing open radical cystectomy and robot-assisted laparoscopic radical cystectomy: a randomized clinical trial. Eur Urol 2015;67(6):1042−50.

[10] Collins JW, Hosseini A, Sooriakumaran P, Nyberg T, Sanchez-Salas R, Adding C, et al. Tips and tricks for intracorporeal robot-assisted urinary diversion. Curr Urol Rep 2014; 15(11).

[11] Guenaga KF, Matos D, Wille-Jorgensen P. Mechanical bowel preparation for elective colorectal surgery. Cochrane Database Syst Rev 2011;(9):CD001544.

[12] Desai MM, de Abreu ALC, Goh AC, Fairey A, Berger A, Leslie S, et al. Robotic intracorporeal urinary diversion: technical details to improve time efficiency. J Endourol 2014; 28(11):1320−7.

[13] Stein JP, Lieskovsky G, Cote R, Groshen S, Feng AC, Boyd S, et al. Radical cystectomy in the treatment of invasive bladder cancer: long-term results in 1,054 patients. J Clin Oncol 2001;19(3):666−75.

[14] Raza SJ, Wilson T, Peabody JO, Wiklund P, Scherr DS, Al-Daghmin A, et al. Long-term oncologic outcomes following robot-assisted radical cystectomy: results from the International Robotic Cystectomy Consortium. Eur Urol 2015;68(4):721−8.

[15] Nix J, Smith A, Kurpad R, Nielsen ME, Wallen EM, Pruthi RS. Prospective randomized controlled trial of robotic versus open radical cystectomy for bladder cancer: perioperative and pathologic results. Eur Urol 2010;57(2):196−201.

[16] Parekh DJ, Messer J, Fitzgerald J, Ercole B, Svatek R. Perioperative outcomes and oncologic efficacy from a pilot prospective randomized clinical trial of open versus robotic assisted radical cystectomy. J Urol 2013;189(2):474−9.

[17] Tyritzis SI, Hosseini A, Collins J, Nyberg T, Jonsson MN, Laurin O, et al. Oncologic, functional, and complications outcomes of robot-assisted radical cystectomy with totally intracorporeal neobladder diversion. Eur Urol 2013;64(5):734−41.

[18] Novara G, Catto JW, Wilson T, Annerstedt M, Chan K, Murphy DG, et al. Systematic review and cumulative analysis of perioperative outcomes and complications after robot-assisted radical cystectomy. Eur Urol 2015;67(3):376−401.

[19] Atmaca AF, Canda AE, Gok B, Akbulut Z, Altinova S, Balbay MD. Open versus robotic radical cystectomy with intracorporeal Studer diversion. JSLS 2015;19(1): e2014 00193.

[20] Canda AE, Atmaca AF, Altinova S, Akbulut Z, Balbay MD. Robot-assisted nerve-sparing radical cystectomy with bilateral extended pelvic lymph node dissection (PLND) and intracorporeal urinary diversion for bladder cancer: initial experience in 27 cases. BJU Int 2012;110(3):434−44.

[21] Pyun JH, Kim HK, Cho S, Kang SG, Cheon J, Lee JG, et al. Robot-assisted radical cystectomy with total intracorporeal urinary diversion: comparative analysis with extracorporeal urinary diversion. J Laparoendosc Adv Surg Tech A 2016;26(5):349−55.

[22] Xia L, Wang X, Xu T, Zhang X, Zhu Z, Qin L, et al. Robotic versus open radical cystectomy: an updated systematic review and meta-analysis. PLoS One 2015;10(3):e0121032.

[23] Gandaglia G, Karl A, Novara G, de Groote R, Buchner A, D'Hondt F, et al. Perioperative and oncologic outcomes of robot-assisted vs. open radical cystectomy in bladder cancer patients: A comparison of two high-volume referral centers. Eur J Surg Oncol 2016.

[24] Desai MM, Gill IS. "The devil is in the details": randomized trial of robotic versus open radical cystectomy. Eur Urol 2015;67(6):1053−5.

[25] Ahmed K, Khan SA, Hayn MH, Agarwal PK, Badani KK, Balbay MD, et al. Analysis of intracorporeal compared with extracorporeal urinary diversion after robot-assisted radical cystectomy: results from the International Robotic Cystectomy Consortium. Eur Urol 2014;65(2):340−7.

Chapter 24.4

Methods for Urinary Diversion

Victor M. Schüttfort, Felix K.-H. Chun, Margit Fisch and Luis A. Kluth

University Medical Center Hamburg-Eppendorf, Hamburg, Germany

INTRODUCTION

Urinary diversion remains a challenging and ever changing field in modern urology. There are several forms of urinary diversion, each with its specific set of complications and advantages. Numerous modifications of continent and incontinent reconstruction have been described, and several times due to the large number of variations, good data are missing and comparison is not always possible. Various problems in the treatment of advanced bladder cancer result from to the need to divert urine. Many surgeons agree that urinary diversion is the most difficult part of cystectomy.

HISTORY

In 1851, John Simons performed the first documented urinary diversion, diverting urine to the intestine. In the absence of modern surgery and anesthesiological techniques, as well as essential medications like antibiotics, results of early attempts of urinary diversions were poor [1]. Problems like rupture or incontinence result from the natural high-pressure peaks while using bowel segments in diversion. It took until the 1970s when it was realized that detubularization prevents peristaltic movements, creating high-volume and low-pressure reservoirs and thus enabling high rates of continence [2].

OVERVIEW

Four main types of diversion can be distinguished: *ureterocutaneostomy* (UCN), conduit, continent cutaneous diversion (pouch), and orthotopic reconstruction (neobladder). Important characteristics by which these types of diversion distinguish themselves are continent and incontinent diversion, as well as between orthotopic and heterotopic diversion.

CHOICE OF DIVERSION—STANDARD OF CARE

Today, a patient expects a continent and safe solution, offering the maximum with regard to quality of life (QoL) [3]. Due to the obvious advantages in terms of body imaging nowadays and voiding function, today neobladders represent the standard of care and all patients should at least be considered for orthotopic reconstruction [4]. Still, there are numerous factors that have to be considered while choosing the type of urinary diversion. There is often a lack of consensus in which type of diversion should be preferred, and several times the best surgical option remains unclear [5,6]. Urinary diversion does not seem to have any impact on the oncological outcome [7].

QOL AFTER URINARY DIVERSION

The type of diversion does not seem to affect QoL; however, there is a lack of high-quality data [4]. Prospective studies showed a high rate of satisfaction for both conduit and continent diversion, whereas most patients would opt for the same type of diversion again [8]. In general, most studies comparing different forms of diversion are biased by different patient characteristics, as patients with incontinent diversion are usually significantly older.

DAY-TO-DAY PRACTICE

While in pioneering centers in the United States the majority of all patients receive a continent diversion, the overall rate of patients being diverted via ileal conduit is around 85% [9]. However, especially for younger and healthier patients, experts prefer orthotopic reconstruction [10]. This raises the question whether all advancements in the field of urinary diversion have made it into day-to-day practice. Outcome in respect to peri- and postoperative morbidity and mortality is known to be better in high-volume centers [11].

PATIENT SELECTION

All forms of urinary diversion remain imperfect, as they all have a specific set of complications. For the choice of diversion surgery time, preexisting medical conditions, need for catheterization, patient preference, and oncological safety have to be considered. The medical history has to be examined closely, especially with regard to recurrent urethral stricture or previous radiation therapy. Patients with chronic intestinal disorder like ulcerative colitis or Crohn's disease should not be considered for neobladders or pouches; however, it should be considered for patients with the risk of short bowel syndrome after multiple previous operations. If renal function is reduced (> 150 to 200 μmol/L), a continent diversion is contraindicated as the renal function is insufficient to compensate severe *electrolyte imbalances which can result if intestine is used for urinary diversion* [12].

ADVANTAGES AND DISADVANTAGES OF DIFFERENT BOWEL SEGMENTS

All different types of intestine have been used as means of diversion. Due to very tight intracellular junctions of the colon, this segment is regarded ideal for urinary diversion, as there is only a minimal loss of water [13]. The intracellular junctions are less tight in ileal segments, but there is adaptation of the epithelium after contact with urine, enhancing the status of ileum as a bladder substitute [13]. The process of degeneration of ileal mucosa greatly reduces the risk of metabolic complications [14].

Jejunum and gastric tissue have leaky junctions; however, bidirectional fluxes cancel out significant shift of electrolytes in the stomach. These fluxes are not available in jejunum, creating a high degree of electrolyte shifts. This can lead to a high degree of electrolyte imbalances (Table 24.4.1).

SPECIFIC COMPLICATIONS AFTER USE OF INTESTINE FOR URINARY DIVERSION

A high degree of compliance is needed if a continent diversion is to be performed. Pouches and neobladders require a lifelong follow-up, and patients will need to accept some degree of incontinence and in rare cases also the need for catheterization in neobladders. Due to the risk of metabolic acidosis, it is necessary to perform regular blood gas analysis postoperatively.

TABLE 24.4.1 Metabolic Changes of Different Bowel Segments in Use for Urinary Diversion

Bowel Segment	Examples	Specific Metabolic Changes	Specific Advantage and Disadvantages
Stomach	Gastric continent urinary reservoir	Metabolic alkalosis Hypochloremia Hypokalemia [13,15,16]	Higher risk for secondary malignancies [17] Higher chance of incontinence [18] Hematuria–dysuria syndrome Iron deficiency Megaloblastic anemia [19] High degree of electrolyte imbalances [20] Elevated aldosterone Hypergastrinemia
Jejunum	Jejunal conduit	Metabolic acidosis Hypochloremia Hyperkalemia Hyponatremia [13,15,16]	High metabolic complication rates [13] Salt loss syndrome Malabsorption of nutrients Elevated renin and angiotensin [21]
Ileum	Ileal conduit Neobladders T-Pouch Mansura Pouch	Metabolic acidosis Hyperchloremia Hypokalemia Hypocalcemia Hypomagnesemia Metabolic acidosis [13,15,16,22–24]	Unproblematic resection of larger amount of intestine possible Epithelium adapts very well to contact of urine [13] Possible vitamin B12 and fat-soluble vitamin deficiency (terminal ileum) [24] Higher risk for urinary calculi [13,24]
Ileocolic	Mainz Pouch I Indiana Pouch Lundiana Pouch	Metabolic acidosis Hyperchloremia Hypokalemia Hypomagnesemia [13,15,16,22–24]	Loss of ileocecus can lead to fasten transmit of stool, bacterial colonization of the small intestine (following possible deconjugation of bile acids with subsequent steatorrhea, chronic diarrhea, as well as compromised fat digestion and uptake of fat soluble vitamins) [13,24]

(Continued)

TABLE 24.4.1 (Continued)

Bowel Segment	Examples	Specific Metabolic Changes	Specific Advantage and Disadvantages
Colon	Colon Conduit Mainz Pouch III Florida Pouch Charleston Pouch	Metabolic acidosis Hyperchloremia Hypokalemia Hypocalcemia Hypomagnesemia [13,15,16,22−24]	Tight intercellular junctions; only minimal loss of water [13] High rate of hypokalemia [25] Higher excretion of bicarbonate [26] Higher risk for bone demineralization [27] Secondary malignancy [28,29] Higher rates of bacteriuria, pyuria, and UTI [29]
Sigma	Sigmoid Neobladder Mainz Pouch II	Metabolic acidosis Hyperchloremia Hypokalemia [24,30,31]	Secondary malignancy [29] Higher chance of incontinence [32] High degree of electrolytes imbalances [33] Higher rates of bacteriuria, pyuria, and UTI [29]
Rectum	Modified rectal Bladder	Metabolic acidosis Hyperchloremia Hypokalemia [24,30,31]	Secondary malignancy [29] High degree of electrolytes imbalances [33] Higher chance of incontinence [34] Higher rates of bacteriuria, pyuria, and UTI [29]

A voiding diary should be kept to detect functional problems. Especially for continent diversion, patient education is paramount in order to prevent treatment delay of possible complications (Fig. 24.4.1, Table 24.4.2).

PREOPERATIVE AND POSTOPERATIVE CARE OF URINARY DIVERSION

Routine bowel preparation does not improve outcomes and should only be performed in selected patients [82]. For safe urine drainage and the avoidance of urinoma, ureteral stents and transurethral catheter should be used [83]. Postoperative imaging using intravenous pyelogram and cystogram can be used to diagnose leakage. In patients with neobladders or pouches, proper voiding or clean intermittent catheterization (CIC) should be checked to avoid complications due to residual urine or improper catheter use. Patients will need to be taught that the known sensation of a full bladder does not exist after cystectomy. Especially in the beginning, timed voiding should be performed. If patients report daytime incontinence, pelvic floor exercises using biofeedback can be performed. To prevent mucus and stone formation, adequate fluid intake is necessary. If voiding protocols show a low reservoir capacity, careful reservoir training can be carried out. If the patient suffers

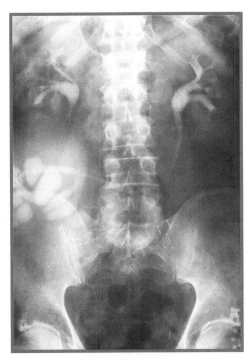

FIGURE 24.4.1   Urolithiasis in continent cutaneous diversion.

TABLE 24.4.2 Specific Complications After Use of Intestine for Urinary Diversion

Hyperchloremic metabolic acidosis	Ammonium ions of the urine can dissociate into ammonia and hydrogen, afterwards entering the epithelial cells while hydrogen ions are actively absorbed in exchange for sodium. In the intestinal mucosa, chloride is absorbed while in return bicarbonate is excreted. An increased amount of ammonium will lead to an increased absorption of chloride with an increased excretion of bicarbonate. This leads do hyperchloremic acidosis [13,35]. Up to 15% of all patients with ileal conduit are affected while the rate for continent urinary diversion is higher [36]. Especially patients with impaired renal function are at risk, as a healthy kidney can compensate these imbalances of electrolytes. Acute treatment includes catheter placement, correction of acidosis using bicarbonate ($NaHCO_3$), and treatment of any concurrent UTI. Treatment of chronic acidosis includes oral fluids with high salt diet, cessation of proton pump inhibitor or H_2-blocker agents (in order to prevent worsening of the acidosis due gastric acid retention) as well as bicarbonate orally [37]. Persistent acidosis can lead to further sequelae such as demineralization of the skeleton, and should therefore be treated, especially if pH is <7.2.
Hyperammonemia	As mentioned, ammonium can dissolve into the intestinal mucosa. This reabsorption can lead to hyperammonemia followed by encephalopathy and hepatic coma, if liver function is not sufficient to compensate higher amount of reabsorbed ammonium. In the case of UTI due to urea splitting organisms (klebsiella, proteus, pseudomonas, etc.), even patients with normal liver function are at risk of hyperammonemia [38]. Treatment includes oral nonabsorbable disaccharides to reduce ammonium reabsorption of the intestine. A high sodium diet can reduce the ammonium uptake [39]. Hyperammonemia usually does not affect patients with ileal conduits [13].
Electrolyte imbalances	All intestines used for diversions will continue to absorb and excrete electrolyte. While about 10% of all patients with conduits will be affected, for continent diversion, relevant imbalances will affect nearly every second patient due to the longer contact time of urine to the intestine [15,24,36]. General symptoms for electrolyte imbalances include dehydration, lethargy, seizures, respiratory distress, nausea/vomiting, weakness, polydipsia, and fatigue. Magnesium deficiency due to urinary diversion can lead to neuromuscular dysfunction with various symptoms (muscular weakness, tremor, neurological symptoms).

(Continued)

TABLE 24.4.2 (Continued)

Vitamin B12 deficiency	Vitamin B12 reabsorption takes place in the terminal ileum. If this part is used for urinary diversion, chronic vitamin B12 deficiency may follow. This can present in severe neurological and hematological dysfunctions [40,41]. Storage of vitamin B12 is sufficient for 3−5 years due to previously stored cobalamin and only then will symptoms occur [42]. Up to one-third of all patients may need vitamin supplementation [43].
Bone demineralization	Chronic acidosis can lead to extraction from calcium of the bones, as calcium and carbonate are used as buffers to take up hydrogen ions [44,45]. Acidosis can also impair the production of vitamin D of the kidney [46]. If large parts of intestine are used, the absorption of vitamin D and calcium may be significantly reduced [47]. Acidosis may also lead to activation of osteoclasts, resulting in increased breakdown of bone tissue [48]. Besides correction of acidosis via oral sodium bicarbonate, vitamin D and calcium supplementation are considered [49,50]. The extent to which bone density is compromised by urinary diversion is unclear [47,51,52]. Nevertheless, especially in patients with impaired renal function, this specific complication should always be kept in mind and long-term follow-up is necessary.
Bacteriuria and UTI	Bacteriuria is common for all types of urinary diversion. Clean intermittent catheterization and residual urine can increase the chance of bacteriuria, while its significance remains unclear [53]. Continent diversion, urine leakage, ureteral stricture, and residual urine are known risk factors for UTI [54,55]. Chronic UTI can lead to reduced renal function [56]. High rates of asymptomatic bacteriuria are frequent following diversion, suggesting that antibiotic treatment is not always necessary [57]. There seems to be no benefit from prophylactic antibiotic therapy [58].
Mucus production	Continent reservoirs can produce more than 30 g of mucus per day [59]. Especially in the early time after diversion, continuous irrigation using NaCl is necessary to prevent catheter blockage and damage to the reservoir due to increased intraluminal pressure [37]. Mucus retention occurs in up to 3% of all patients [60]. Especially patients with incomplete voiding and patients performing clean intermittent catheterization are in risk of mucus buildup. Mucus is known to be a secondary factor to stone formation and UTIs [61,62]. It seems that ileal mucosa tends to produce less mucus with time, in contrast to colonic mucosa [63,64]. N-acetylcysteine and urea are frequently prescribed to reduce complications of mucus buildup as they are known effective mucolytic agents [41,65]. However, the real benefit of mucolytic agents remains controversial [66].

(Continued)

TABLE 24.4.2 (Continued)

Formation of calculi	The risk for urolithiasis is 3%–4% for ileal conduits and up to 40% in reservoirs [67]. Risk factors include excess conduit length, dehydration, urine stasis, chronic UTI (especially with urea-splitting organism), hyperchloremic metabolic acidosis (as the loss of bicarbonate will lead to hypercalciuria), residual urine, and the presence of foreign bodies such as staples or sutures [67–69]. In patients where ileum has been used as means of urinary intestinal, there may be an increased absorption of oxalate, which can lead to the formation of oxalate calculi [13]. Furthermore, the bowel epithelium itself can lead to formation of stones in the reservoir [24].
Renal function	Renal function is known to decrease after urinary diversion. Over a 11-year period, a reduction in glomerular filtration rate of up to 25% has been described [70,71]. Some studies suggest a similar decrease of renal function for incontinent and continent diversion [72,73]. For low-pressure reservoirs, only a minimal reduction can be expected [74]. Risk factors include stenosis of the ureteral anastomosis, chronic UTI, and stone formation. Antirefluxive implantation techniques do not seem to have any benefit with respect to renal function [14,75,76].
Altered bowl function	30% of all patients after cystectomy report defecation disturbances, which can have a severe impact on the QoL [77]. Still, if less than 60 cm of the ileum is used, there are usually few postoperative side effects [37]. Malabsorption of nutrients is possible especially if jejunum is used. Many patients suffer from diarrhea due to loss of bile salts and fats as well as reduced water uptake [56].
Altered drug metabolism	Many drugs that are secreted over the kidney can be reabsorbed over the intestine used for urinary diversion [78,79]. Especially for drugs that are not altered after excretion, this can cause major adverse effects, as well as for toxic drugs like chemotherapy agents. Therefore the use of catheters during possible chemotherapy is recommended. Glucose can be absorbed in continent reservoirs, enhancing the risk of high blood sugar in patients with diabetes [80].
Secondary malignancies	Especially patients in whom gastric, sigma, or rectal segments have been used seem to be at risk for secondary malignancies [17,81]. Most tumors will be adenocarcinomas. In neobladders constructed from colon, there is a slightly higher risk for secondary tumors [28]. For ureterosigmoidostomy, there is a high risk for tumors at the ureterocolonic borderline. Regular endoscopic controls of ureterosigmoidostomies are recommended [81].

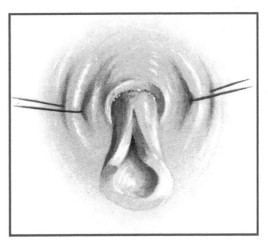

FIGURE 24.4.2   Direct ureter implantation 1.

primarily of nighttime incontinence, alcohol, diuretic, and hypnotic medications should be dismissed [37].

ANTIREFLUXIVE URETER IMPLANTATION TECHNIQUES

Reflux can damage the kidney due to higher intraluminal pressure and lead to an increased rate of upper urinary tract infections (UTIs) [84]. However, all antirefluxive ureter implantation techniques carry a high risk of anastomotic stricture and subsequent kidney damage compared to direct refluxing implantation. New data suggest that this risk outweighs the benefit [75]. In neobladders, antirefluxive techniques seem to double the risk of obstruction for nonrefluxing techniques and are therefore not generally recommended [14,76] (Figs. 24.4.2 and 24.4.3, Table 24.4.3).

LAPAROSCOPY AND ROBOTICS IN URINARY DIVERSION

The first laparoscopic cystectomy was performed in 1992 [102]. However, urinary diversion was mostly performed extracorporeally, minimizing the benefit of laparoscopy. The feasibility of robot-assisted cystectomy was first described in 2003, and today also for urinary diversion, a robotic approach seems feasible [103]. Still, robotic intracorporeal neobladder reconstruction is in the starting phase [104]. Even construction of pouches has been performed using a robotic intracorporeal approach [105].

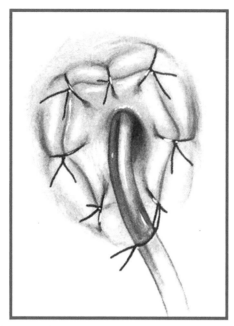

FIGURE 24.4.3   Direct ureter implantation 2.

TISSUE ENGINEERING AND ALLOPLASTIC REPLACEMENT

Several new concepts are arising which might offer different treatment options in the future. Regenerative medicine has been proven to work in different settings in reconstructive urology [106,107]. Tissue engineering in bladders may solve the dilemma of having to use intestine as means of diversion. However, despite all advances, this is not a feasible solution today [108]. Due to the risk of graft ischemia, fibrous contraction, and perforation, a complete replacement still does not seem possible [109]. Still, it remains a prospective solution to the many problems that the use of intestine creates in the field of urinary diversion [110].

The same is true for the use of artificial bladder replacement made of different sorts of plastic. The first artificial bladder was tried in 1960 in dogs. Various tests mostly using artificial bladders made of different sorts of plastic have followed, but none have made it into clinical trials. The problem seems to be a high rate of hydronephrosis due to fibrosis as well as connection problems at the anastomosis. Still, further research shows promising results [111,112].

TABLE 24.4.3 Overview of Ureter Implantation Techniques

	Technique	Details	Application	Rate of Stenosis
Refluxive				
Bricker [85]	Simple end-to-side anastomosis to the intestine	Basic form of ureterointestinal anastomosis	Conduit	2.9% (for ileal conduit) [86]
Nesbit [87]	Elliptic end-to-side technique, simple anastomosis of spatulated ureter, and intestinal mucosa	Various adaptations exist, also using the ileocecal valve as an antirefluxive mechanism	Conduit	3.4% (for ileal neobladder) [88] 4.2% (for ileal conduit)
Wallace [89]	Both ureters are spatulated and connected in a side-to-side manner, creating a ureteral plate, which is connected to the intestine	Easy to perform, low rate of stenosis; however, if revision is necessary, both ureters need to be reoperated	Conduit Neobladder	5.4% (for ileal neobladder) [90] 1.9% for ileal conduit [86]
Direct implantation of ureters to continent reservoir	Ureters are implanted without any form of antirefluxive technique	Very low rate of stenosis	Neobladder Pouch	1.7% (for Indiana Pouch or Neobladder) [91]
Antirefluxive				
LeDuc et al. [92]	Ureter is placed in a sulcus created of the ileal mucosa	High rate of stenosis	Neobladder Pouch	4.9% (for ileal neobladder) [93]
Goodwin et al. [94]	Ureter runs through a submucosal tunnel, either at the end of the intestine (open end technique) or through the wall (button hole technique)	The pressure inside the reservoir closes the intramural ureter, thus preventing reflux	For colon only	7.3% (for Mainz Pouch I) [95]

(Continued)

TABLE 24.4.3 (Continued)

	Technique	Details	Application	Rate of Stenosis
Abol-Enein and Ghoneim[96]	Ureter runs through a serous lined extramural tunnel	Especially for short or previously dilated ureters	Neobladder Pouch	4.1% (for Mainz Pouch I) [95]
Split Cuff Technique [97]	Ureter is spatulated (about 1–2 cm), and then pulled back and attached to itself, creating a cuff. This cuff is then pulled through the reservoir	Simple procedure, especially if a tunnel procedure is not possible	Neobladder Pouch	3.1% [98]
Kock nipple valve [99]	Ureter is implanted directly into an ileal segment. This is used to create an intussuscepted ileal valve	High incidence of afferent nipple valve malfunction [100]	Neobladder Pouch	4.3% [101]

INCONTINENT DIVERSION

Ureterocutaneostomy

Indication	Advantages	Disadvantages
Old/multimorbid patients with reduced life expectancy	No intestinal surgery	Stoma stenosis, usually requiring Mono-J usage (with need for frequent changes + UTIs)
Palliative treatment	Short surgery time	High postoperative morbidity
Contraindication of intestinal surgery (previous or planned radiotherapy, ulcerative colitis, and Crohn's disease)	Low perioperative morbidity	Skin irritation

History and Introduction

Ureterocutaneostomy (UCN) describes the technique of implanting both ureters to the skin after cystectomy (either as an end-to-end or end-to-side anastomosis of the ureters). It represents the oldest and simplest form of urinary diversion, while also being the least invasive form. A transperitoneal UCN as well as a retroperitoneal UCN is possible [113]. Laparoscopic and retroperitoneoscopic approaches exist, making it a very easy form of diversion in combination with laparoscopic cystectomy, as no further steps are necessary [114].

Indication

It should only be performed in selected patients with reduced life expectancy and reduced status of health, as there is a very high rate of stoma stenosis. Recent data suggest that cystectomy is still a good option in carefully selected older and multimorbid patients [115]. UCN is the preferable form of urinary diversion for those patients due to its simplicity [116].

Complications

There is a high postoperative complication rate; therefore, UCN is inappropriate for patients with a medium or longer life expectancy. A frequent problem is the occurrence of stoma stenosis, making many patients dependent on ureteral stenting [117]. This leads to a high rate of bacteriuria with an increased rate of UTI [118]. A rare complication is the development of uretero-aortic fistula [119]. Due to those serious complications, alternatives like percutaneous nephrostomy should be considered in very sick patients [120]. This accounts especially for patients with uremia and hydronephrosis and patients for whom cystectomy does not seem feasible due to reduced performance status (<1 year). Nevertheless, refined techniques for tubeless UCN have been described, offering significant lower rates of stenosis and independence of catheterization [121].

Conduit (Ileal, Jejunal, Colon, or Sigma Conduit)

Indication	Advantages	Disadvantages
Advanced tumors and older patients with shorter life expectancy	Short surgery time	High rate for postoperative morbidity including stoma stenosis and skin irritation
Malfunction of previous urinary diversion	Low perioperative morbidity	
	Only short segment of bowl needed, malabsorption is rare	Higher rate of reflux in comparison to other urinary diversions
		Cost of supplies for urostomy can be significant

History and Introduction

Introduced in 1950, the ileal conduit represents an easy to perform, yet safe and reliable method to divert urine [85,122]. Due to higher complexity of the earlier forms of continent cutaneous diversion, the conduit remained the gold standard in urinary diversion for many years and is still widely used today [9,123]. For the ileal conduit, about 15−20 cm of ileum is used, starting usually about 15 cm proximal of the ileocecal valve (Fig. 24.4.4).

Indication

Especially for patients with advanced tumors and older patients with shorter life expectancy, it should be considered the primary choice of diversion.

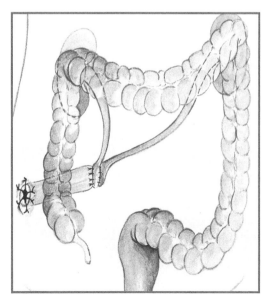

FIGURE 24.4.4 Ileal conduit.

After some time of accustomization, it offers a high QoL. Studies suggest a high rate of satisfaction without any clear advantage of continent forms diversion [4,8].

Complications

Long-term results show high rates of complications, especially concerning the upper urinary tract [4]. Ureteral obstruction and renal impairment have been described [124,125]. Up to 20% of all patients will develop a serious reduction in renal function over a 10-year period, while also higher rates of deterioration have been described [126,127]. Stoma problems including stoma stenosis, parastomal hernia, and skin conditions are frequent and increasing with time, often in need of surgery [128]. Stone formation and mucus production are further problems, however to a lesser degree than for continent diversion. Bacteriuria is a very common problem in conduits, leading to an increased rate of upper UTIs and urosepsis [126,129].

If jejunum is used, special respect should be paid to the "jejunal conduit syndrome" (hyperchloremia, hyponatremia, hyperkalemia, and acidosis). However, use of shorter segments seems feasible [127]. It offers the advantage of being easily feasible in radiated patients. For those patients, a conduit using transverse colon also seems feasible [130]. A sigma conduit is a good alternative if the stoma needs to be on left side of the abdomen (Figs. 24.4.5 and 24.4.6).

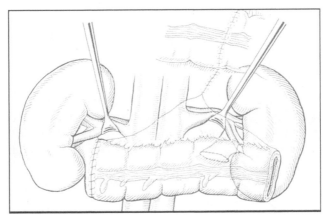

FIGURE 24.4.5 Transverse colon conduit 1.

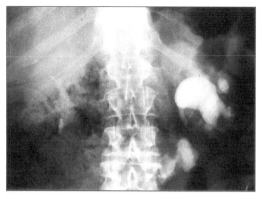

FIGURE 24.4.6 Transverse colon conduit 2.

CONTINENT DIVERSION

Orthotopic Reconstruction/Neobladder

Indication	Contraindication	Advantages	Disadvantages
Standard of care for all patients <75 years, if patient is compliant	Tumor distal prostatic urethra in man and bladder neck in woman	Best body imaging	Higher perioperative morbidity, more extensive surgery time
	Chronic bowl disease, multiple former bowl operations	Only low rate of CIC necessary	Requires large resection of intestine
	Reduced liver and kidney function	Normal voiding	Risk of local recurrence
	External sphincter dysfunction		Voiding dysfunction, nighttime incontinence
	Recurrent urethral stricture		High risk of ventral hernia (due to need of Valsalva maneuver for voiding)

History and Introduction

A neobladder refers to the formation of an orthotopic bladder replacement with connection of ureter and urethra. First experiences with orthotopic bladder reconstructions were made in the 1980s solely in men [131]. Voiding is performed using the Valsalva maneuver, while at the same time relaxing the pelvic floor musculature. Neobladders offer the best form of body imaging and are considered feasible in most patients [132] (Figs. 24.4.7 and 24.4.8).

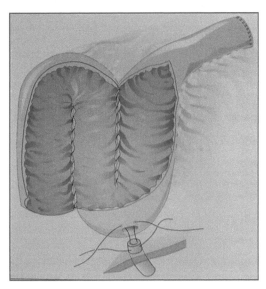

FIGURE 24.4.7 Neobladder.

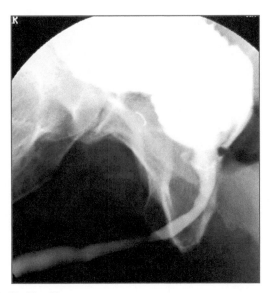

FIGURE 24.4.8 Neoblase X-ray.

Indication

Today, orthotopic reconstruction represents the standard of care and every patient should at least be considered for this urinary diversion [4]. After first experiences in men, some authors also suggest that neobladders can be performed in women [133–135]. Preoperative evaluation of the bladder neck and intraoperative frozen section analysis is paramount to avoid urethral recurrence. If in doubt, heterotopic reconstruction should be preferred. Still, the oncological outcome does not seem to be compromised [136]. The majority of all patients will be able to void without difficulties, still some patients will depend on CIC [137–139]. Increased experience with neobladders has extended the indication of orthotopic reconstruction. Leading experts in the field of urinary diversion now also describe orthotopic reconstruction as feasible in the elderly, lymph node metastases and locally advanced cancers [5]. If adjuvant chemotherapy seems likely, conduits should be preferred due to expected complications like prolonged wound healing. An advantage of the neobladder is that it may convince patients with high-risk cases of non-invasive bladder cancer to an earlier cystectomy, thus increasing overall survival [140].

Orthotopic Reconstruction/Neobladders in Female Patients

Some authors consider neobladders to be feasible in women. However, results with respect to incontinence, hypercontinence, and residual urine are worse than in male patients [4,138,141]. CIC is necessary in up to 43% of all women [142]. There is a higher rate of possible complications including the development of vesicovaginal fistulas, where surgical revision can be impossible [138]. If preservation of the sphincter seems uncertain, a continent cutaneous diversion should be preferred. These poorer results should be discussed with the patient beforehand, as some will opt for a different urinary diversion. Transformation of neobladders to pouches is possible, yet technically challenging.

Continence

Good daytime continence rates have been described for all kinds of different neobladders, with slightly poorer results concerning nighttime continence [143]. Continence usually improves significantly in the first year after surgery, as the reservoir capacity increases [144]. For women, continence rates seem to be lower compared to men [4,138]. The degree of incontinence is normally mild. Older patients and patients without nerve-sparing cystectomy seem to be affected more strongly [37].

Complications

Main complications include incisional hernia (6.4%), ileus or small bowel obstruction (3.6%), UTI (5.7%), and subneovesical obstruction (3.1%) [90]. The upper urinary tract is thought to be preserved after orthotopic reconstruction, as ureteroileal stenosis is rare (with respect to the different techniques of ureterointestinal anastomosis) and renal function is only decreased in patients with preoperative or postoperative ureteral obstruction [145].

High rates of residual urine (22%) and bacteriuria have been described [58,143]. More than one-third of patients will be able to have erections with the use of medical support.

Local Recurrence

A specific problem for all neobladders is the chance of local urethral recurrence as the urethra needs to remain intact to enable normal voiding. Local recurrence is thought to be under 5% [132]. Recent studies suggest low local rates of recurrence also in women, suggesting orthotopic reconstruction without urethrectomy a theoretically safe oncological procedure [146]. If the bladder neck is not infiltrated, a concurrent infiltration of the urethra is very unlikely [147]. If carcinoma in situ (CIS) is found, it represents an increased risk for recurrence at the anastomosis.

Variations

A variety of modifications using different bowel segments have been described. Some are widely used, while others are only performed at single institutions. Comparison of the different variations of orthotopic reconstruction is difficult, as high-quality, long-term, and comparative studies are still lacking. There seems to be no difference in respect to survival between the various forms of orthotopic replacement [148]. QoL does not seem to differ in respect to the form of orthotopic reconstruction [149,150]. Due the various possibilities, no clear recommendation can be given. Stomach, rectum, or sigmoid should only be used in special patients due to a higher chance of incontinence [4,151] (Table 24.4.4).

POUCHES (CONTINENT CUTANEOUS DIVERSION)

Indication	Contraindication	Advantages	Disadvantages
If continent diversion is aimed for, but orthotopic reconstruction seems impossible	Chronic bowl disease	No sphincter necessary (especially in women frequently no adequate continence)	Frequent need for revision
Excellent alternative especially in women	Former bowl operations	Continent diversion with safe oncological outcome even if the urethra is involved or previous irradiation of the pelvis is foregone	Requires large resection of intestine
	Reduced liver and kidney function	Continence	CIC necessary (costly)

TABLE 24.4.4 Overview Neobladders

Form of Neobladder	Description	Continence Day (%)	Continence Night (%)	Specific Problems
Gastric neobladder	Reservoir formed using gastric tissue	37	NA	Lower capacity with high incontinence rates, only recommended in very selected patients [18]
U-shape/Camey I and II [152]	Sixty centimeter of detubularized ileum, folded upon itself to form a transverse U-shaped reservoir, implantation using the Leduc–Camey technique	92.6	74.3	High rates of ureteral stenosis (10.5%) [152]
U-shape neobladder (Studer) [153]	Approximately 40 cm are opened antimesenterically formed to a sagitally folded U-shaped reservoir while a proximal segment remains unaltered for ureteral implantation	92	79	Low rate of ureteroileal stenosis (2.7%) [143]
S-shape neobladder (Schreiter) [154]	Approximately 45 cm of ileum are detubularized using an antimesenteric incision and afterwards placed in an S-shape manner. Another 15 cm of ileum are used to create the intussuscepted nipple valve, serving as the antireflux mechanism	93.8	×	High volume [155]
W-shape neobladder (Hautmann) [156]	Detubularized W-shaped reservoir with two nondetubularized chimneys, where the ureters are implanted in a refluxive manner	96.8	87.1	Low rate of anastomotic strictures for double chimney implantation technique (4%) [157,158]
Modified W-pouch [60]	W-shaped reservoir with serous lined extramural tunnel as an antirefluxive procedure	93.3	80	Antirefluxive technique with good preservation of the upper tract [60]

	Description			Comments
T-pouch [159]	Sagittally folded U-shaped with a serous lined extramural ileal flap valve technique	87	72 [142]	Comparable outcome but higher rate for secondary surgical procedures [75,101]
N-shaped pouch [56]	Ileum is used for the pouch formation in a N-shaped manner	96 (♂) 84.6 (♀)	60(♂) 66.7 (♀)	Rather high complication rates [160]
Padovana ileal neobladder [161]	A proximal loop of ileum is folded in a reverse S, ureteral implantation via two serous lined intestinal tunnels	NA	NA	Lack of long term data, promising results with slightly lower continence rates [162]
Le Bag neobladder [163]	Ileocolonic pouch of approximately 20 cm detubularized ileum and 20 cm cecum	91	80	Risk of hyperchloremic metabolic acidosis [164]
Right colon neobladder [165]	Detubularized, remodeled right colon and intact cecum	100	92	Very large capacity reservoir (more than 600 mL) few data available [166]
Sigmoid neobladder/ Reddy pouch [167]	Detubularized sigmoid neobladder (modification: Roux-Y-shaped)	74.6	57.1 [168]	Low nighttime continence due to small functional capacity [32]; very low rate of residual urine [148]
Rectal neobladder	Sigmoid colon is connected to anal sphincter while the bladder is connected to the urethra	NA	NA	High risk of sigmoid retraction, necrosis, and defecation incontinence (14%) [34]; only rarely used today

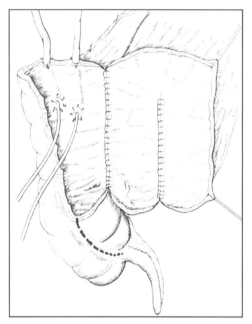

FIGURE 24.4.9 Mainz Pouch.

History and Introduction

A continent cutaneous diversion describes a large, low-pressure reservoir which is emptied via catheterization. Initial descriptions date back to the 1890s, but only after another century in the 1980s, due to improvements in surgical methods, the concept of pouches showed acceptable results [169,170]. After the development of orthotopic reconstruction, the rate of pouches significantly decreased. Today, the rate in the United States is under 10%, though there is a huge difference between pioneering centers and other institution [5]. Pouches are technically challenging, but long results in general are excellent and comparable with other forms of urinary diversion [171] (Fig. 24.4.9).

Indication

As high rates of complications can be expected after orthotopic reconstruction in women, pouches are an excellent alternative offering outstanding rates of continence and unaltered body imaging. They are also invaluable alternatives in complicated patients with an increased risk for incontinence or nonfunctional urethra. These include men who previously underwent radical prostatectomy before cystectomy, where results of neobladders are generally poorer [172]. Pouches are also good alternatives if urethrectomy seems necessary or high risk of local recurrence. This includes patients with tumor of the distal prostatic urethra in men and bladder neck in women. Pouches should be favored if widespread CIS is found or urethrectomy seems necessary [173]. The patient needs to be compliant as well as physically and mentally capable for catheterization. Other criteria are similar to neobladders, e.g., good renal function, good status of health, and patient compliance.

Continence rate

From the beginning, continence rates are excellent. Due to a higher capacity, continence rates seem to be superior to neobladders, especially with regard to nighttime continence. Still, due to the need for daily catheterization, there is a higher risk for hypercontinence due to nipple stenosis.

Complications

The construction of a pouch is an advanced surgery and the rate of late complications is known to be high. Still there seems to be no difference in terms of general complications between neobladders and pouches [4,170,173]. There is a high degree of revision surgery (up to 20%), but many of these surgeries are extraperitoneal and can be considered minor surgeries. The nipple is the critically part of the pouch construction, as it determines the level of continence, but is also under a high risk of stenosis due to the need of CIC [171,174]. General rates of poucholithiasis are between 5% and 10%. All pouches should be irrigated on a daily basis to preserve function and reduce the risk of UTI. If not emptied completely, there is a risk of acute urinary retention due to stored back mucus, which also increases the risk of UTI.

Afferent Limb

Similar to neobladders, there is controversy regarding the afferent limb and if an antireflux technique has to be applied. In analogy to orthotopic reconstruction, good results have been made using refluxing techniques [4,175]. The rate of ureterointestinal stenosis is described between 5% and 8.2% (see Table 24.4.5).

Pouch Nipple—Efferent Limb

Many different techniques for the construction of a continent efferent limb exist [176]. Due to the lack of randomized comparing data, no technique can be considered superior. The most common techniques either use nipple valve (e.g., intussuscepted ileal nipple valve) or flap valves (e.g., appendix stoma) as a continence mechanism [177]. The underlying principle in both is that through increased filling of the reservoir, the efferent limb is being compressed. For nipple valves, the tube is not attached to the lumen, whereas for flap valves the afferent limb usually is embedded in the wall [178]. Most complications present within the first year and stomal incontinence are rare

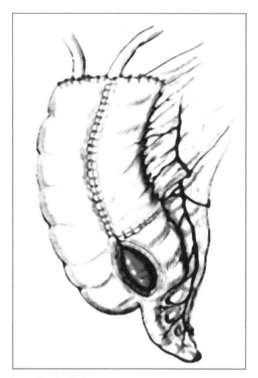

FIGURE 24.4.10   Appendix nipple 1.

[179]. The intussuscepted nipple valves show low rates of stenosis (15.3%) and good continence rates (92.8%), whereas the classic appendix stoma has slightly higher rates for stomal stenosis with excellent continence rates [95,175,180]. Artificial sphincter systems and tissue engineering have yet failed to show satisfactory results [178].

Management of stomal stenosis includes catheter insertion and careful dilation. In acute urinary retention, suprapubic catheter place is often necessary. Percutaneous drainage can enable previously impossible catheterization due to a lower intraluminal pressure. In many cases, surgical revision will be necessary (Figs. 24.4.10−24.4.12).

Variations

Over time, various types of pouches have been described. Many pouches that have been developed are not used any more due to various complications [123,181,182]. Similar to neobladders, there is very little data available of comparison between the different pouch types. Most pouches offer excellent continence rates, still for all the rate of revision surgery is high (Table 24.4.5).

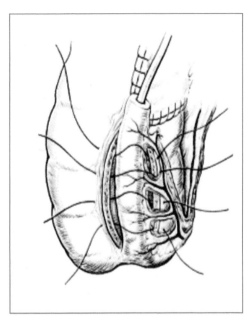

FIGURE 24.4.11 Appendix nipple 2.

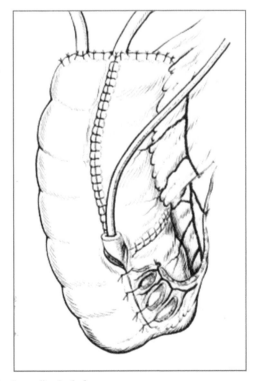

FIGURE 24.4.12 Appendix nipple 3.

TABLE 24.4.5 Overview Continent Cutaneous Diversion

Pouch	Bowl Segment	Detail	Continence Mechanism	Continence Rate (%)	Stoma/ Nipple Stenosis (%)
Lundiana Pouch [183,184]	Ascending colon	Ascending colon is detubularized while the ureters run through submucosal tunnels as an antirefluxive mechanism	Ileal nipple valve, which is usually constructed using staples and connected to the rectus muscle	93.7 [173]	7.1 [173]
Mainz Pouch I [185]	Ileocecal	After an antimesenteric incision of the ileocecum, a spherical reconfiguration is performed; the ureters are implanted in a submucosal fashion	Either intussuscepted terminal ileum or submucosal appendix in situ or intussuscepted ileal nipple [186]	Appendix: 96.0 Intussuscepted nipple: 89.5 [180]	Appendix: 23.5 Intussuscepted nipple: 15.3 [180]
Indiana Pouch [187,188]	Ileocecal	Pouch is formed using the ileocecum, while along the tenia libera the ureters connected to the reservoir	Usually a tapered ileal segment is used, in combination with the ileocecal valve and plication sutures	72.0 [189]	15.2 [189]
Florida Pouch [165]	Cecum and ascending colon	A reservoir is formed using cecum as well as ascending colon up to the colonic flexure The ureters are generally implanted in a refluxive manner or via the LeDuc technique	The ileocecal valve is used in combination with a double plication of the efferent segment	93.3 [190]	4.0 [190]

Miami Pouch [191]	Cecum and ascending colon	Cecum and ascending colon opened antimesenterically, formation of the reservoir in an U-shaped manner	Tapered ileum which is supported via special three proximal sutures	95.6 [192]	NA
Charleston Pouch [193]	Ileocecum	Detubularized reservoir formed out of terminal ileum and ascending colon	Usually a slightly altered appendix stoma is used	98 [194]	8.2 [194]
Mainz Pouch III [195]	Upper ascending or descending colon and colon transversum	The intestine is folded in a U-shaped which is placed upside down	The ureter is connected to a tailored bowel segment	83.8 [196]	4.2 [196]
Kock Pouch [197]	Ileum	Continent ileal reservoir, with the ileal segment reinforced by tapes	Intussuscepted ileal nipple for both the afferent and efferent segment	NA	10.4 [101]
Mansura Pouch [198]	Ileum	W-shaped ileal reservoir is detubularized while the ureters are implanted via two serosa lined extramural tunnels	Either tapered ileum or appendix	94.6 [198]	5.37 [198]

URETEROSIGMOIDEOSTOMY/MAINZ POUCH II

Indication	Contraindication	Advantages	Disadvantages
Rarely used in the western world	Sphincter failure, e.g., patients with neurogenic bladder (possible impaired of anal sphincter function)	Continent diversion with no need of further supplies	Frequent UTI
	Diverticulosis		Metabolic acidosis
	Radiation of the pelvis		Risk of secondary malignancy

Ureterosigmoideostomy represents a very old form of urinary diversion, in which the anal sphincter is used for the means of continence. A modern modification uses detubularization to form a low-pressure reservoir, increasing rates of continence as well as the capacity [199,200]. Preoperatively, the function of the anal sphincter has to be checked via intra rectal fluid application for 3 hours. Today, it is rarely performed in patients with bladder cancer due to high incidence of secondary malignancies at the ureterointestinal anastomosis (up to 15%) and fecal urinary incontinence [201]. Furthermore, metabolic changes are very frequent with a high degree of patients in need of therapy due hyperchloremic acidosis [202,203]. Still, it remains a simple and reproducible option in selected patients if orthotopic neobladder seems impossible and cost of necessities to support an urostoma cannot be paid. Due to the simplicity of the operation, it is able to be laparoscopically performed completely [204].

REFERENCES

[1]   Basic DT, Hadzi-Djokic J, Ignjatovic I. The history of urinary diversion. Acta Chir Iugosl 2007;54:9.

[2]   Hautmann RE. Ileal bladder substitute. Urologe A 2008;47:33.

[3]   Stein J, Skinner D. Orthotopic urinary diversion. In: Walsh PC, Retik, AB, Vaughan ED, Wein AJ, editors. Campbell's urology. 8th ed, vol. 4. Philadelphia: W.B. Saunders; 2002. p. 3835−67.

[4]   World Health Organization Consensus Conference on Bladder Cancer, Hautmann RE, Abol-Enein H, et al. Urinary diversion. Urology 2007;69:17.

[5]   Hautmann RE, Abol-Enein H, Lee CT, et al. Urinary diversion: how experts divert. Urology 2015;85:233.

[6]   Gerharz EW, Mansson A, Hunt S, et al. Quality of life after cystectomy and urinary diversion: an evidence based analysis. J Urol 2005;174:1729.

[7]   Madersbacher S, Studer UE. Contemporary cystectomy and urinary diversion. World J Urol 2002;20:151.

[8]   Hardt J, Filipas D, Hohenfellner R, et al. Quality of life in patients with bladder carcinoma after cystectomy: first results of a prospective study. Qual Life Res 2000;9:1.

[9]   Gore JL, Litwin MS, Urologic Diseases in America, P. Quality of care in bladder cancer: trends in urinary diversion following radical cystectomy. World J Urol 2009;27:45.

[10] Hautmann RE, Abol-Enein H, Davidsson T, et al. ICUD-EAU International Consultation on Bladder Cancer 2012: Urinary diversion. Eur Urol 2013;63:67.

[11] Kim SP, Boorjian SA, Shah ND, et al. Contemporary trends of in-hospital complications and mortality for radical cystectomy. BJU Int 2012;110:1163.

[12] Skinner D, Studer U, Okada K, et al. Which patients are suitable for continent diversion or bladder substitution following cystectomy or other definitive local treatment? Int J Urol 1995;105.

[13] Vasdev N, Moon A, Thorpe AC. Metabolic complications of urinary intestinal diversion. Indian J Urol 2013;29:310.

[14] Hautmann R. 15 years experience with the ileal neobladder. what have we learned? Urologe A 2001;40:360.

[15] Stein R, Ziesel C, Frees S, et al. Metabolic long-term complications after urinary diversion. Urologe A 2012;51:507.

[16] Stein R, Rubenwolf P. Metabolic consequences after urinary diversion. Front Pediatr 2014;2:15.

[17] Austen M, Kalble T. Secondary malignancies in different forms of urinary diversion using isolated gut. J Urol 2004;172:831.

[18] Lin DW, Santucci RA, Mayo ME, et al. Urodynamic evaluation and long-term results of the orthotopic gastric neobladder in men. J Urol 2000;164:356.

[19] Steiner MS, Morton RA. Nutritional and gastrointestinal complications of the use of bowel segments in the lower urinary tract. Urol Clin North Am 1991;18:743.

[20] Gosalbez Jr. R, Woodard JR, Broecker BH, et al. Metabolic complications of the use of stomach for urinary reconstruction. J Urol 1993;150:710.

[21] Golimbu M, Morales P. Jejunal conduits: technique and complications. J Urol 1975; 113:787.

[22] Dahl D, McDougal W. Use of intestinal segments in urinary diversion. In: Wein A, Kavoussi L, Novick A, et al., editors. Campbell-Walsh urology. Philadelphia: Saunders W.B; 2007. p. 2534−78.

[23] McDougal WS. Metabolic complications of urinary intestinal diversion. J Urol 1992; 147:1199.

[24] Van der Aa F, Joniau S, Van Den Branden M, et al. Metabolic changes after urinary diversion. Adv Urol 2011.

[25] Williams RE, Davenport TJ, Burkinshaw L, et al. Changes in whole body potassium associated with uretero-intestinal anastomoses. Br J Urol 1967;39:676.

[26] Koch MO, Gurevitch E, Hill DE, et al. Urinary solute transport by intestinal segments: a comparative study of ileum and colon in rats. J Urol 1990;143:1275.

[27] Mundy AR, Nurse DE. Calcium balance, growth and skeletal mineralisation in patients with cystoplasties. Br J Urol 1992;69:257.

[28] Kalble T, Hofmann I, Riedmiller H, et al. Tumor growth in urinary diversion: a multicenter analysis. Eur Urol 2011;60:1081.

[29] Shigemura K, Tanaka K, Arakawa S, et al. Postoperative bacteriuria, pyuria and urinary tract infection in patients with an orthotopic sigmoid colon neobladder replacement. J Antibiot (Tokyo) 2014;67:143.

[30] Stamey TA. The pathogenesis and implications of the electrolyte imbalance in ureterosigmoidostomy. Surg Gynecol Obstet 1956;103:736.

[31] Fisch M, Wammack R, Abol-Enein H, et al. Sodium absorption in the sigma-rectum pouch, augmented rectal bladder and ureterosigmoidostomy. Investig Urol (Berl) 1994; 5:124.

[32] Schrier BP, Laguna MP, van der Pal F, et al. Comparison of orthotopic sigmoid and ileal neobladders: continence and urodynamic parameters. Eur Urol 2005;47:679.

[33] Miyake H, Hara S, Eto H, et al. Significance of renal function in changes in acid-base metabolism after orthotopic bladder replacement: colon neobladder compared with ileal neobladder. Int J Urol 2004;11:83.

[34] Novak R, Kraus D. Rectal neobladder. A 25-year experience. Acta Urol Belg 1991;59:97.

[35] Ferris DO, Odel HM. Electrolyte pattern of the blood after bilateral ureterosigmoidostomy. J Am Med Assoc 1950;142:634.

[36] Kamidono S, Oda Y, Ogawa T. Clinical study of urinary diversion. II: Review of 41 ileocolic conduit cases, their complications and long term (6−9 years) follow-up. Nishinihon J Urol 1985;47:415.

[37] Varol C, Studer UE. Managing patients after an ileal orthotopic bladder substitution. BJU Int 2004;93:266.

[38] Albersen M, Joniau S, Van Poppel H, et al. Urea-splitting urinary tract infection contributing to hyperammonemic encephalopathy. Nat Clin Pract Urol 2007;4:455.

[39] Stampfer DS, McDougal WS. Inhibition of the sodium/hydrogen antiport by ammonium ion. J Urol 1997;157:362.

[40] Yakout H, Bissada NK. Intermediate effects of the ileocaecal urinary reservoir (Charleston pouch 1) on serum vitamin B12 concentrations: can vitamin B12 deficiency be prevented? BJU Int 2003;91:653.

[41] Gillon G, Mundy AR. The dissolution of urinary mucus after cystoplasty. Br J Urol 1989;63:372.

[42] Terai A, Okada Y, Shichiri Y, et al. Vitamin B12 deficiency in patients with urinary intestinal diversion. Int J Urol 1997;4:21.

[43] Pfitzenmaier J, Lotz J, Faldum A, et al. Metabolic evaluation of 94 patients 5 to 16 years after ileocecal pouch (Mainz pouch 1) continent urinary diversion. J Urol 2003;170:1884.

[44] Bettice JA, Gamble Jr. JL. Skeletal buffering of acute metabolic acidosis. Am J Physiol 1975;229:1618.

[45] McDougal WS, Koch MO, Shands III C, et al. Bony demineralization following urinary intestinal diversion. J Urol 1988;140:853.

[46] Lee SW, Russell J, Avioli LV. 25-hydroxycholecalciferol to 1,25-dihydroxycholecalciferol: conversion impaired by systemic metabolic acidosis. Science 1977;195:994.

[47] Kawakita M, Arai Y, Shigeno C, et al. Bone demineralization following urinary intestinal diversion assessed by urinary pyridinium cross-links and dual energy x-ray absorptiometry. J Urol 1996;156:355.

[48] Arnett TR, Dempster DW. Effect of pH on bone resorption by rat osteoclasts in vitro. Endocrinology 1986;119:119.

[49] Stein R, Fisch M, Beetz R, et al. Urinary diversion in children and young adults using the Mainz Pouch I technique. Br J Urol 1997;79:354.

[50] Perry W, Allen LN, Stamp TC, et al. Vitamin D resistance in osteomalacia after ureterosigmoidostomy. N Engl J Med 1977;297:1110.

[51] Poulsen AL, Overgaard K, Steven K. Bone metabolism following bladder substitution with the ileal urethral Kock reservoir. Br J Urol 1997;79:339.

[52] Roosen A, Gerharz EW, Roth S, et al. Bladder, bowel and bones—skeletal changes after intestinal urinary diversion. World J Urol 2004;22:200.

[53] Wullt B, Agace W, Mansson W. Bladder, bowel and bugs—bacteriuria in patients with intestinal urinary diversion. World J Urol 2004;22:186.

[54] Kim KH, Yoon HS, Yoon H, et al. Febrile urinary tract infection after radical cystectomy and ileal neobladder in patients with bladder cancer. J Korean Med Sci 2016;31:1100.

[55] Parker WP, Toussi A, Tollefson MK, et al. Risk factors and microbial distribution of urinary tract infections following radical cystectomy. Urology 2016;94:96.

[56] Joniau S, Benijts J, Van Kampen M, et al. Clinical experience with the N-shaped ileal neobladder: assessment of complications, voiding patterns, and quality of life in our series of 58 patients. Eur Urol 2005;47:666.

[57] Suriano F, Gallucci M, Flammia GP, et al. Bacteriuria in patients with an orthotopic ileal neobladder: urinary tract infection or asymptomatic bacteriuria? BJU Int 2008;101:1576.

[58] Wullt B, Holst E, Steven K, et al. Microbial flora in ileal and colonic neobladders. Eur Urol 2004;45:233.

[59] Bushman W, Howards SS. The use of urea for dissolution of urinary mucus in urinary tract reconstruction. J Urol 1994;151:1036.

[60] Abol-Enein H, Ghoneim MA. Functional results of orthotopic ileal neobladder with serous-lined extramural ureteral reimplantation: experience with 450 patients. J Urol 2001; 165:1427.

[61] Parra Muntaner L, Lopez Pacios JC, Vega Vega A, et al. Urinary stone in a Bricker's ileal conduit. Arch Esp Urol 2004;57:851.

[62] Keegan SJ, Graham C, Neal DE, et al. Characterization of Escherichia coli strains causing urinary tract infections in patients with transposed intestinal segments. J Urol 2003; 169:2382.

[63] Gatti R, Ferretti S, Bucci G, et al. Histological adaptation of orthotopic ileal neobladder mucosa: 4-year follow-up of 30 patients. Eur Urol 1999;36:588.

[64] Mansson W, Colleen S, Low K, et al. Immunoglobulins in urine from patients with ileal and colonic conduits and reservoirs. J Urol 1985;133:713.

[65] Sheffner AL. The reduction in vitro in viscosity of mucoprotein solutions by a new mucolytic agent, N-acetyl-L-cysteine. Ann N Y Acad Sci 1963;106:298.

[66] N'Dow J, Robson CN, Matthews JN, et al. Reducing mucus production after urinary reconstruction: a prospective randomized trial. J Urol 2001;165:1433.

[67] Terai A, Ueda T, Kakehi Y, et al. Urinary calculi as a late complication of the Indiana continent urinary diversion: comparison with the Kock pouch procedure. J Urol 1996; 155:66.

[68] Terai A, Arai Y, Kawakita M, et al. Effect of urinary intestinal diversion on urinary risk factors for urolithiasis. J Urol 1995;153:37.

[69] Turk TM, Koleski FC, Albala DM. Incidence of urolithiasis in cystectomy patients after intestinal conduit or continent urinary diversion. World J Urol 1999;17:305.

[70] Kristjansson A, Wallin L, Mansson W. Renal function up to 16 years after conduit (refluxing or anti-reflux anastomosis) or continent urinary diversion. 1. Glomerular filtration rate and patency of uretero-intestinal anastomosis. Br J Urol 1995;76:539.

[71] Kristjansson A, Bajc M, Wallin L, et al. Renal function up to 16 years after conduit (refluxing or anti-reflux anastomosis) or continent urinary diversion. 2. Renal scarring and location of bacteriuria. Br J Urol 1995;76:546.

[72] Eisenberg MS, Thompson RH, Frank I, et al. Long-term renal function outcomes after radical cystectomy. J Urol 2014;191:619.

[73] Al Hussein Al Awamlh B, Wang LC, Nguyen DP, et al. Is continent cutaneous urinary diversion a suitable alternative to orthotopic bladder substitute and ileal conduit after cystectomy? BJU Int 2015;116:805.

[74] Furrer MA, Roth B, Kiss B, et al. Patients with an orthotopic low pressure bladder substitute enjoy long-term good function. J Urol 2016;196:1172.

[75] Skinner EC, Fairey AS, Groshen S, et al. Randomized trial of studer pouch versus T-pouch orthotopic ileal neobladder in patients with bladder cancer. J Urol 2015;194:433.

[76] Studer UE, Danuser H, Thalmann GN, et al. Antireflux nipples or afferent tubular segments in 70 patients with ileal low pressure bladder substitutes: long-term results of a prospective randomized trial. J Urol 1996;156:1913.

[77] Thulin H, Kreicbergs U, Onelov E, et al. Defecation disturbances after cystectomy for urinary bladder cancer. BJU Int 2011;108:196.

[78] Davidsson T, Akerlund S, White T, et al. Mucosal permeability of ileal and colonic reservoirs for urine. Br J Urol 1996;78:64.

[79] Alhasso A, Bryden AA, Neilson D. Lithium toxicity after urinary diversion with ileal conduit. BMJ 2000;320:1037.

[80] Sridhar KN, Samuell CT, Woodhouse CR. Absorption of glucose from urinary conduits in diabetics and non-diabetics. Br Med J (Clin ResEd) 1983;287:1327.

[81] Kalble T, Hofmann I, Thuroff JW, et al. Secondary malignancies in urinary diversions. Urologe A 2012;51:500.

[82] Cerantola Y, Valerio M, Persson B, et al. Guidelines for perioperative care after radical cystectomy for bladder cancer: Enhanced Recovery After Surgery (ERAS((R))) society recommendations. Clin Nutr 2013;32:879.

[83] Mattei A, Birkhaeuser FD, Baermann C, et al. To stent or not to stent perioperatively the ureteroileal anastomosis of ileal orthotopic bladder substitutes and ileal conduits? Results of a prospective randomized trial. J Urol 2008;179:582.

[84] McGuire EJ, Woodside JR, Borden TA, et al. Prognostic value of urodynamic testing in myelodysplastic patients. J Urol 1981;126:205.

[85] Bricker EM. Bladder substitution after pelvic evisceration. Surg Clin North Am 1950;30:1511.

[86] Davis NF, Burke JP, McDermott T, et al. Bricker versus Wallace anastomosis: A meta-analysis of ureteroenteric stricture rates after ileal conduit urinary diversion. Can Urol Assoc J 2015;9:E284.

[87] Nesbit RM. Ureterosigmoid anastomosis by direct elliptical connection; a preliminary report. J Urol 1949;61:728.

[88] Minervini R, Pagni R, Mariani C, et al. Effects on renal function of obstructive and non-obstructive dilatation of the upper urinary tract in ileal neobladders with refluxing ureteroenteric anastomoses. Eur J Surg Oncol 2010;36:287.

[89] Wallace DM. Ureteric diversion using a conduit: a simplified technique. Br J Urol 1966;38:522.

[90] Hautmann RE, de Petriconi RC, Volkmer BG. 25 years of experience with 1,000 neobladders: long-term complications. J Urol 2011;185:2207.

[91] Pantuck AJ, Han KR, Perrotti M, et al. Ureteroenteric anastomosis in continent urinary diversion: long-term results and complications of direct versus nonrefluxing techniques. J Urol 2000;163:450.

[92] Le Duc A, Camey M, Teillac P. An original antireflux ureteroileal implantation technique: long-term followup. J Urol 1987;137:1156.

[93] Lugagne PM, Herve JM, Lebret T, et al. Ureteroileal implantation in orthotopic neobladder with the Le Duc-Camey mucosal-through technique: risk of stenosis and long-term follow-up. J Urol 1997;158:765.

[94] Goodwin WE, Harris AP, Kaufman JJ, et al. Open, transcolonic ureterointestinal anastomosis; a new approach. Surg Gynecol Obstet 1953;97:295.

[95]   Wiesner C, Pahernik S, Stein R, et al. Long-term follow-up of submucosal tunnel and serosa-lined extramural tunnel ureter implantation in ileocaecal continent cutaneous urinary diversion (Mainz pouch I). BJU Int 2007;100:633.

[96]   Abol-Enein H, Ghoneim MA. A novel uretero-ileal reimplantation technique: the serous lined extramural tunnel. A preliminary report. J Urol 1994;151:1193.

[97]   Warwick RT, Ashken MH. The functional results of partial, subtotal and total cystoplasty with special reference to ureterocaecocystoplasty, selective sphincterotomy and cystocystoplasty. Br J Urol 1967;39:3.

[98]   Sagalowsky AI. Further experience with split-cuff nipple ureteral reimplantation in urinary diversion. J Urol 1998;159:1843.

[99]   Kock NG. Intussuscepted ileal nipple valve—early experience. Scand J Urol Nephrol Suppl 1992;142:59.

[100]   Arai Y, Kawakita M, Terachi T, et al. Long-term followup of the Kock and Indiana pouch procedures. J Urol 1993;150:51.

[101]   Stein JP, Freeman JA, Esrig D, et al. Complications of the afferent antireflux valve mechanism in the Kock ileal reservoir. J Urol 1996;155:1579.

[102]   Parra RO, Andrus CH, Jones JP, et al. Laparoscopic cystectomy: initial report on a new treatment for the retained bladder. J Urol 1992;148:1140.

[103]   Menon M, Hemal AK, Tewari A, et al. Nerve-sparing robot-assisted radical cystoprostatectomy and urinary diversion. BJU Int 2003;92:232.

[104]   Fahmy O, Asri K, Schwentner C, et al. Current status of robotic assisted radical cystectomy with intracorporeal ileal neobladder for bladder cancer. J Surg Oncol 2015;112:427.

[105]   Goh AC, Aghazadeh MA, Krasnow RE, et al. Robotic intracorporeal continent cutaneous urinary diversion: primary description. J Endourol 2015;29:1217.

[106]   Peters KM, Dmochowski RR, Carr LK, et al. Autologous muscle derived cells for treatment of stress urinary incontinence in women. J Urol 2014;192:469.

[107]   Zhang F, Liao L. Tissue engineered cystoplasty augmentation for treatment of neurogenic bladder using small intestinal submucosa: an exploratory study. J Urol 2014; 192:544.

[108]   Atala A, Bauer SB, Soker S, et al. Tissue-engineered autologous bladders for patients needing cystoplasty. Lancet 2006;367:1241.

[109]   Alberti C. Whyever bladder tissue engineering clinical applications still remain unusual even though many intriguing technological advances have been reached? G Chir 2016; 37:6.

[110]   Alberti C. Outlines on nanotechnologies applied to bladder tissue engineering. G Chir 2012;33:234.

[111]   Rohrmann D, Albrecht D, Hannappel J, et al. Alloplastic replacement of the urinary bladder. J Urol 1996;156:2094.

[112]   Cosentino M, Gaya JM, Breda A, et al. Alloplastic bladder substitution: are we making progress? Int Urol Nephrol 2012;44:1295.

[113]   Furubayashi N, Negishi T, Kashiwagi E, et al. Clinical outcome of transperitoneal ureterocutaneostomy using the transverse mesocolon. Mol Clin Oncol 2013;1:721.

[114]   Yoshimura K, Ichioka K, Terada N, et al. Retroperitoneoscopic tubeless cutaneous ureterostomy. BJU Int 2002;89:964.

[115]   Wuethrich PY, Vidal A, Burkhard FC. There is a place for radical cystectomy and urinary diversion, including orthotopic bladder substitution, in patients aged 75 and older: results of a retrospective observational analysis from a high-volume center. Urol Oncol 2016;34:58 e19.

[116] Deliveliotis C, Papatsoris A, Chrisofos M, et al. Urinary diversion in high-risk elderly patients: modified cutaneous ureterostomy or ileal conduit?. Urology 2005;66:299.

[117] MacGregor PS, Montie JE, Straffon RA. Cutaneous ureterostomy as palliative diversion in adults with malignancy. Urology 1987;30:31.

[118] Matsuda S, Nagatani Y, Kanematsu M, et al. Study of urinary infection in tubeless cutaneous ureterostomy--pathognomonic meaning of bacterial flora in the renal pelvis and methods of collecting urine. Nihon Hinyokika Gakkai Zasshi 1987;78:76.

[119] De Wilde P, Oosterlinck W, De Sy WA. Uretero-aortic fistula: a severe complication of ureterocutaneostomy. Eur Urol 1990;17:262.

[120] Ekici S, Sahin A, Ozen H. Percutaneous nephrostomy in the management of malignant ureteral obstruction secondary to bladder cancer. J Endourol 2001;15:827.

[121] Kim CJ, Wakabayashi Y, Sakano Y, et al. Simple technique for improving tubeless cutaneous ureterostomy. Urology 2005;65:1221.

[122] Lee RK, Abol-Enein H, Artibani W, et al. Urinary diversion after radical cystectomy for bladder cancer: options, patient selection, and outcomes. BJU Int 2014;113:11.

[123] Gilchrist RK, Merricks JW, Hamlin HH, et al. Construction of a substitute bladder and urethra. Surg Gynecol Obstet 1950;90:752.

[124] Neal DE. Complications of ileal conduit diversion in adults with cancer followed up for at least five years. Br Med J (Clin Res Ed), 290. 1985. p. 1695.

[125] Gilbert SM, Lai J, Saigal CS, et al. Downstream complications following urinary diversion. J Urol 2013;190:916.

[126] Iborra I, Casanova J, Solsona E. Tolerance of external urinary diversion (bricker) followed for more than 10 years. Eur Urol Supp 2010;9:736.

[127] Fontaine E, Barthelemy Y, Houlgatte A, et al. Twenty-year experience with jejunal conduits. Urology 1997;50:207.

[128] Madersbacher S, Schmidt J, Eberle JM, et al. Long-term outcome of ileal conduit diversion. J Urol 2003;169:985.

[129] Bruce AW, Reid G, Chan RC, et al. Bacterial adherence in the human ileal conduit: a morphological and bacteriological study. J Urol 1984;132:184.

[130] Ravi R, Dewan AK, Pandey KK. Transverse colon conduit urinary diversion in patients treated with very high dose pelvic irradiation. Br J Urol 1994;73:51.

[131] Skinner DG, Boyd SD, Lieskovsky G, et al. Lower urinary tract reconstruction following cystectomy: experience and results in 126 patients using the Kock ileal reservoir with bilateral ureteroileal urethrostomy. J Urol 1991;146:756.

[132] Hautmann RE, Volkmer BG, Schumacher MC, et al. Long-term results of standard procedures in urology: the ileal neobladder. World J Urol 2006;24:305.

[133] Colleselli K, Stenzl A, Eder R, et al. The female urethral sphincter: a morphological and topographical study. J Urol 1998;160:49.

[134] Stein JP, Cote RJ, Freeman JA, et al. Indications for lower urinary tract reconstruction in women after cystectomy for bladder cancer: a pathological review of female cystectomy specimens. J Urol 1995;154:1329.

[135] Stein JP, Stenzl A, Esrig D, et al. Lower urinary tract reconstruction following cystectomy in women using the Kock ileal reservoir with bilateral ureteroileal urethrostomy: initial clinical experience. J Urol 1994;152:1404.

[136] Stein JP, Penson DF, Lee C, et al. Long-term oncological outcomes in women undergoing radical cystectomy and orthotopic diversion for bladder cancer. J Urol 2009;181:2052.

[137] Madersbacher S, Mohrle K, Burkhard F, et al. Long-term voiding pattern of patients with ileal orthotopic bladder substitutes. J Urol 2002;167:2052.

[138] Mills RD, Studer UE. Female orthotopic bladder substitution: a good operation in the right circumstances. J Urol 2000;163:1501.

[139] Ali-El-Dein B, Gomha M, Ghoneim MA. Critical evaluation of the problem of chronic urinary retention after orthotopic bladder substitution in women. J Urol 2002;168:587.

[140] Hautmann RE, Paiss T. Does the option of the ileal neobladder stimulate patient and physician decision toward earlier cystectomy? J Urol 1998;159:1845.

[141] Mills RD, Burkhard F, Studer UE. Bladder substitution in women. Int Urogynecol J Pelvic Floor Dysfunct 2000;11:246.

[142] Stein JP, Dunn MD, Quek ML, et al. The orthotopic T pouch ileal neobladder: experience with 209 patients. J Urol 2004;172:584.

[143] Studer UE, Burkhard FC, Schumacher M, et al. Twenty years experience with an ileal orthotopic low pressure bladder substitute--lessons to be learned. J Urol 2006;176:161.

[144] Sevin G, Soyupek S, Armagan A, et al. Ileal orthotopic neobladder (modified Hautmann) via a shorter detubularized ileal segment: experience and results. BJU Int 2004;94:355.

[145] Thoeny HC, Sonnenschein MJ, Madersbacher S, et al. Is ileal orthotopic bladder substitution with an afferent tubular segment detrimental to the upper urinary tract in the long term? J Urol 2002;168:2030.

[146] Chang SS, Cole E, Cookson MS, et al. Preservation of the anterior vaginal wall during female radical cystectomy with orthotopic urinary diversion: technique and results. J Urol 2002;168:1442.

[147] Stein JP, Esrig D, Freeman JA, et al. Prospective pathologic analysis of female cystectomy specimens: risk factors for orthotopic diversion in women. Urology 1998;51:951.

[148] Miyake H, Furukawa J, Takenaka A, et al. Experience with various types of orthotopic neobladder in Japanese men: long-term follow-up. Urol Int 2010;84:34.

[149] Minervini R, Morelli G, Fontana N, et al. Functional evaluation of different ileal neobladders and ureteral reimplantation techniques. Eur Urol 1998;34:198.

[150] Jerlstrom T, Andersson G, Carringer M. Functional outcome of orthotopic bladder substitution: a comparison between the S-shaped and U-shaped neobladder. Scand J Urol Nephrol 2010;44:197.

[151] Santucci RA, Park CH, Mayo ME, et al. Continence and urodynamic parameters of continent urinary reservoirs: comparison of gastric, ileal, ileocolic, right colon, and sigmoid segments. Urology 1999;54:252.

[152] Barre PH, Herve JM, Botto H, et al. Update on the Camey II procedure. World J Urol 1996;14:27.

[153] Studer UE, Ackermann D, Casanova GA, et al. A newer form of bladder substitute based on historical perspectives. Semin Urol 1988;6:57.

[154] Schreiter F, Noll F. The S-bladder, an ileal bladder substitution. Acta Urol Belg 1991; 59:251.

[155] Schreiter F, Noll F. Kock pouch and S bladder: 2 different ways of lower urinary tract reconstruction. J Urol 1989;142:1197.

[156] Hautmann RE, Egghart G, Frohneberg D, et al. The ileal neobladder. J Urol 1988;139:39.

[157] Ballouhey Q, Thoulouzan M, Lunardi P, et al. Prospective study of the results of uretero-intestinal anastomosis in 100 patients after the Hautmann ileal neobladder with double chimney. Prog Urol 2012;22:255.

[158] Belot PY, Fassi-Fehri H, Colombel M, et al. The W-shaped ileal neobladder: Long term functional outcomes and health-related quality of life. Prog Urol 2016;26:367.

[159] Stein JP, Lieskovsky G, Ginsberg DA, et al. The T pouch: an orthotopic ileal neobladder incorporating a serosal lined ileal antireflux technique. J Urol 1998;159:1836.

[160] De Sutter T, Akand M, Albersen M, et al. The N-shaped orthotopic ileal neobladder: functional outcomes and complication rates in 119 patients. Springerplus 2016;5:646.

[161] Pagano F, Artibani W, Ligato P, et al. Vescica ileale Padovana: a technique for total bladder replacement. Eur Urol 1990;17:149.

[162] Novara G, Ficarra V, Minja A, et al. Functional results following vescica ileale Padovana (VIP) neobladder: midterm follow-up analysis with validated questionnaires. Eur Urol 2010;57:1045.

[163] Light JK, Scardino PT. Radical cystectomy with preservation of sexual and urinary function. Use of the ileocolonic pouch ("Le Bag"). Urol Clin North Am 1986;13:261.

[164] Kolettis PN, Klein EA, Novick AC, et al. The Le Bag orthotopic urinary diversion. J Urol 1996;156:926.

[165] Lockhart JL. Remodeled right colon: an alternative urinary reservoir. J Urol 1987; 138:730.

[166] D'Orazio OR, Lambert OL, Vallati JC, et al. Total and immediate daytime and nighttime continence with a right colonic neobladder—what makes it possible? An 11-year followup. J Urol 2005;174:1882.

[167] Reddy PK. The colonic neobladder. Urol Clin North Am 1991;18:609.

[168] Xu K, Liu CX, Zheng SB, et al. Orthotopic detaenial sigmoid neobladder after radical cystectomy: technical considerations, complications and functional outcomes. J Urol 2013;190:928.

[169] Rink M, Kluth L, Eichelberg E, et al. Continent catheterizable pouches for urinary diversion. European Urology Supplements 2010;9:754.

[170] Large MC, Katz MH, Shikanov S, et al. Orthotopic neobladder versus Indiana pouch in women: a comparison of health related quality of life outcomes. J Urol 2010;183:201.

[171] Fisch M, Thuroff JW. Continent cutaneous diversion. BJU Int 2008;102:1314.

[172] Huang EY, Skinner EC, Boyd SD, et al. Radical cystectomy with orthotopic neobladder reconstruction following prior radical prostatectomy. World J Urol 2012;30:741.

[173] Mansson W, Davidsson T, Konyves J, et al. Continent urinary tract reconstruction—the Lund experience. BJU Int 2003;92:271.

[174] Bailey S, Kamel MH, Eltahawy EA, et al. Review of continent urinary diversion in contemporary urology. Surgeon 2012;10:33.

[175] Skinner EC. Continent cutaneous diversion. Curr Opin Urol 2015;25:555.

[176] Benson MC, Olsson CA. Continent urinary diversion. Urol Clin North Am 1999;26:125.

[177] Mitrofanoff P. Trans-appendicular continent cystostomy in the management of the neurogenic bladder. Chir Pediatr 1980;21:297.

[178] Ardelt PU, Woodhouse CR, Riedmiller H, et al. The efferent segment in continent cutaneous urinary diversion: a comprehensive review of the literature. BJU Int 2012;109:288.

[179] Thomas JC, Dietrich MS, Trusler L, et al. Continent catheterizable channels and the timing of their complications. J Urol 2006;176:1816.

[180] Wiesner C, Bonfig R, Stein R, et al. Continent cutaneous urinary diversion: long-term follow-up of more than 800 patients with ileocecal reservoirs. World J Urol 2006; 24:315.

[181] Verhoogen J. Neostomie uretero-cecale. Formation d'une poche vesicale et d'un noveau uretre. Assoc Franc d'Urol 1908;12:352.

[182] Makkas M. Zur Behandlung der Blasenekstrophie: Umwandlung des ausgeschalteten Zokums zur Blase und der Appendix zur Urethra. Zentralbl Chir 1910;37:1073.

[183] Mansson W, Sundin T. Experience with a continent caecal reservoir in urinary diversion. Scand J Urol Nephrol 1978;48.

[184] Mansson W, Davidsson T, Colleen S. The detubularized right colonic segment as urinary reservoir: evolution of technique for continent diversion. J Urol 1990;144:1359.

[185] Thuroff JW, Alken P, Riedmiller H, et al. The Mainz pouch (mixed augmentation ileum and cecum) for bladder augmentation and continent diversion. J Urol 1986;136:17.

[186] Riedmiller H, Burger R, Muller S, et al. Continent appendix stoma: a modification of the Mainz pouch technique. J Urol 1990;143:1115.

[187] Rowland R, Mitchell M, Bihrle R. The cecoileal continent urinary reservoir. World J Urol 1985;3:185.

[188] Rowland RG, Mitchell ME, Bihrle R, et al. Indiana continent urinary reservoir. J Urol 1987;137:1136.

[189] Holmes DG, Thrasher JB, Park GY, et al. Long-term complications related to the modified Indiana pouch. Urology 2002;60:603.

[190] Webster C, Bukkapatnam R, Seigne JD, et al. Continent colonic urinary reservoir (Florida pouch): long-term surgical complications (greater than 11 years). J Urol 2003; 169:174.

[191] Bejany DE, Politano VA. Stapled and nonstapled tapered distal ileum for construction of a continent colonic urinary reservoir. J Urol 1988;140:491.

[192] Sanchez-Valdivieso E, Gonzalez Enciso A, Herrera Gomez A, et al. Preliminary experience with the Miami type ileocolonic urinary reservoir in the practice of oncologic gynecology. Arch Esp Urol 2001;54:327.

[193] Bissada NK. New continent ileocolonic urinary reservoir: Charleston pouch with minimally altered in situ appendix stoma. Urology 1993;41:524.

[194] Bochner BH, Karanikolas N, Barakat RR, et al. Ureteroileocecal appendicostomy based urinary reservoir in irradiated and nonirradiated patients. J Urol 2009;182:2376.

[195] Leissner J, Black P, Fisch M, et al. Colon pouch (Mainz pouch III) for continent urinary diversion after pelvic irradiation. Urology 2000;56:798.

[196] Stolzenburg JU, Schwalenberg T, Liatsikos EN, et al. Colon pouch (Mainz III) for continent urinary diversion. BJU Int 2007;99:1473.

[197] Kock NG, Nilson AE, Nilsson LO, et al. Urinary diversion via a continent ileal reservoir: clinical results in 12 patients. J Urol 1982;128:469.

[198] Abol-Enein H, Salem M, Mesbah A, et al. Continent cutaneous ileal pouch using the serous lined extramural valves. The Mansoura experience in more than 100 patients. J Urol 2004;172:588.

[199] Fisch M, Wammack R, Muller SC, et al. The Mainz pouch II (sigma rectum pouch). J Urol 1993;149:258.

[200] D'Elia G, Pahernik S, Fisch M, et al. Mainz Pouch II technique: 10 years' experience. BJU Int 2004;93:1037.

[201] Azimuddin K, Khubchandani IT, Stasik JJ, et al. Neoplasia after ureterosigmoidostomy. Dis Colon Rectum 1999;42:1632.

[202] Ignjatovic I, Basic D. Modified Mainz pouch II (Sigma Rectum pouch) urinary diversion: 12 years experience. Acta Chir Iugosl 2007;54:73.

[203] Hadzi-Djokic JB, Basic DT. A modified sigma-rectum pouch (Mainz pouch II) technique: analysis of outcomes and complications on 220 patients. BJU Int 2006;97:587.

[204] Turk I, Deger S, Winkelmann B, et al. Complete laparoscopic approach for radical cystectomy and continent urinary diversion (sigma rectum pouch). Tech Urol 2001;7:2.

Chapter 25

Morbidity, Mortality, and Survival for Radical Cystectomy

Juhyun Park and Hyeon Jeong
Seoul National University, Seoul, South Korea

Chapter Outline

INTRODUCTION

To date, radical cystectomy and urinary diversion have been the standard treatment for muscle-invasive bladder cancer. However, radical cystectomy procedures are complicated, involving simultaneous surgery on the genitourinary tract, gastrointestinal tract, and pelvic organs. Consequently, surgery-related complications frequently occur during the perioperative period and even after successful discharge.

According to several reports, the incidence of postoperative morbidity varies widely (from 20% to 60%) [1,2]. Large differences in the morbidity rate cannot be attributed to attempts to conceal or underestimate lapses in radical cystectomy patient management, but instead to the absence of an organized systematic reporting system with which to document surgical complications. However, the recently upgraded, modified Clavien–Dindo classification is assisting with the objective and systematic classification of surgical morbidities in study subjects (Table 25.1) [3,4].

A large difference in surgery-related mortality and survival after radical cystectomy has been reported in different studies. Therefore, clinicians need to carefully compare the different study variables. Clinical outcomes can be affected depending on patient age, gender, comorbidities, and ethnicity [5–7]. Surgical techniques, including diversion methods, are also important

Bladder Cancer. DOI: http://dx.doi.org/10.1016/B978-0-12-809939-1.00025-4

TABLE 25.1 Clavien–Dindo Classification for the Surgical Complication

Grade	Definition	Examples
Grade I	Any deviation from the normal postoperative course without the need for pharmacological treatment or surgical, endoscopic, and radiological interventions. Acceptable therapeutic regimens are drugs such as antiemetics, antipyretics, analgesics, diuretics, and electrolytes, and physiotherapy. This grade also includes wound infections opened at the bedside	Atelectasis requiring physiotherapy Postoperative pain requiring analgesics
Grade II	Requiring pharmacological treatment with drugs other than those allowed for Grade I complications. Blood transfusions and total parenteral nutrition are also included	Pneumonia, urinary tract infection, and infectious diarrhea requiring antibiotics Transient ischemic accident requiring anticoagulants
Grade III	Requiring surgical, endoscopic, or radiological intervention	
Grade IIIa	Intervention not under general anesthesia	Ureteroenteric site stenosis requiring PCN insertion Wound dehiscence requiring surgical repair under local anesthesia
Grade IIIb	Intervention under general anesthesia	Postoperative bleeding, anastomostic site leakage requiring reoperation
Grade IV	Life-threatening complication (including CNS complications: brain hemorrhage, ischemic stroke, subarachnoid bleeding, but excluding transient ischemic attacks) requiring IC/ICU management	
Grade IVa	Single organ dysfunction (including dialysis)	Heart failure, ischemic stroke requiring ICU management, and renal insufficiency requiring dialysis
Grade IVb	Multiorgan dysfunction	Two or more condition of Grade IVa
Grade V	Death of a patient	
Suffix "d"	If the patient suffers from a complication at the time of discharge the suffix "d" (for disability) is added to the respective grade of complication. This label indicates the need for a follow-up to evaluate the complication fully	

CNS, central nervous system; ICU, intensive care unit; PCN, percutaneous nephrostomy.
Source: Adapted from Dindo D, Demartines N, Clavien PA. Classification of surgical complications: a new proposal with evaluation in a cohort of 6336 patients and results of a survey. Ann Surg 2004;240:205–13, Copyright©2004, with permission from Wolters Kluwer Health, Inc.

and especially very recently. Satisfactory results, when compared with those obtained using open radical cystectomy, have been published on robotic-assisted radical cystectomy in several studies. There is a need to systematically review the accumulated survival data on robotic-assisted radical cystectomy [8−10].

This chapter focuses on morbidity, mortality, and survival following radical cystectomy, together with the latest reports on the worldwide spread of minimally invasive surgery and especially robotic-assisted radical cystectomy

MORBIDITY AFTER RADICAL CYSTECTOMY

As mentioned previously, radical cystectomy extensively deals with the genitourinary tract, gastrointestinal tract, pelvic organs, and lymph nodes. It involves the simultaneous use of resection surgery and reconstructive procedures. Therefore, the risk of complications is relatively higher compared to the use of other urological surgery.

Perioperative significant blood loss and transfusion are common complications during radical cystectomy. The percentage of patients who received a perioperative transfusion was estimated to be from 40% to 63% in several, recent retrospective studies. Some researchers reported that blood loss and massive blood transfusion were associated with other major complications and tumor recurrence via the immunomodulatory pathway. The relevant evidence is gradually accumulating [11−13]. Therefore, intraoperative fluid restriction and meticulous hemostasis are of high priority during radical cystectomy. It is also essential that surgeons apply strict criteria for perioperative blood transfusions [12].

Bowel obstruction, for example, postoperative ileus, is a common complication and reported to affect 23%−38% of early convalescent patients after radical cystectomy [14,15]. More aggressive action during each recovery stage is recommended by the recently proposed Enhanced Recovery After Surgery (ERAS) program, in contrast to former recommendations of conservative management. The program defines the preoperative, intraoperative, and postoperative steps required for the early restoration of normal bowel function and for the prevention of bowel obstruction [16].

Acute pyelonephritis is included as a common infectious complication, occurring in roughly 20%−25% of patients after radical cystectomy [14,15]. Leakage from the ureteroenteric anastomosis site can give rise to infection, while urinoma or abdominal abscesses have resulted in some cases. It was reported in a prospective study by Mattei et al. that perioperative ureteral stenting indwelling prevented urinary leakage and reduced complication rates. However, there were an insufficient number of subjects in their study. This made it difficult to determine differences between the urinary diversion methods. Thus, it is necessary to interpret the results carefully [17].

The incidence of wound dehiscence or hernia, classified as wound-related complications, is reported to occur in 15%−18% of patients [14,15]. Wound complications are the main independent contributing risk factor to increased hospitalization, advancing age, a higher body mass index, and underlying comorbidities [18]. Gupta et al. concluded that an interrupted suture (as opposed to a continuous suture) in the fascia layer could lower the risk of wound dehiscence by half, following a meta-analysis of 23 randomized controlled trials [19].

There is a lower risk of wound dehiscence with robotic radical cystectomy. However, complications relating to an access port, such as a trocar site hernia, were tailed by up to 6.7%. Surgeons have to pay special attention when closing port sites in robotic radical cystectomy because more access ports are needed and have to be maintained for longer (when compared to other robotic surgery), while additional incision is required for extraction of the specimen [20]. Meanwhile, several convenient laparoscopic port-site closure instruments, including the classical Carter−Thomason Needle-Point Suture Passer, are currently on the market to reduce port-site challenges [21].

Postoperative deep vein thrombosis and pulmonary embolism are life-threatening conditions that account for 3.5%−8.0% of complications following radical cystectomy [14,15]. The ERAS program recommends the prophylactic management of venous thromboembolism by using a low-molecular weight heparin for 19−21 consecutive days after radical cystectomy. The use of intermittent pneumatic compression or a compression stocking and early ambulation after surgery is preferred and encouraged in the event of persistent postoperative bleeding or a high risk of bleeding [16].

Postoperative acute myocardial infarction occurs less frequently but is included as a fatal complication, so clinicians need to aware of it. Conducting in-depth preoperative interviews with patients and being familiar with their angina or arrhythmia medical history is essential to effectively evaluate preoperative risk. If needed, an examination, such as echocardiography or cardiac angiography, and consultation with cardiologists, are helpful when choosing appropriate surgical candidates for radical cystectomy [22].

Extended lymphadenectomy occasionally leads to complications, such as the formation of lymphoceles or lymphedema [14,15]. Nevertheless, recent studies have shown survival gains from extended lymphadenectomy; there is a focus on the procedures and these apply to all bladder cancer patients. Consequently, the risk of lymphoceles or lymphedema is increased. Thus, surgeons should take care to minimize injury to the adjunct tissue and ensure proper ligation or clipping of the lymphatic vessel to prevent lymphadenectomy-related complications [23,24].

The incidence of overall complication rates after radical cystectomy is ≥60%, and major (Grade 3−5) complications are high, with an incidence of 10%. Radical cystectomy is one of the most challenging, complicated examples of urological surgery [14,15]. Therefore, a detailed preoperative checkup and risk evaluation can help to predict and prevent potential intraoperative and postoperative complications [1].

Robotic radical cystectomy is now commanding considerable attention and has spread worldwide as a comparable surgical technique to open radical cystectomy [25]. It has several advantages, including less blood loss, a shorter hospital stay, and equivalent complication rates. However, the longer operating time and having to overcome the learning curve are disadvantages. A totally intracorporeal approach may be preferable to extracorporeal urinary diversion to reduce postoperative complication rates [26]. A comparison between the two is necessary because it has been reported that robotic radical cystectomy is a safer surgical option than open radical cystectomy [8].

MORTALITY AFTER RADICAL CYSTECTOMY

Discrepancies in the mortality rate after radical cystectomy have been shown in different studies and have depended on patient characteristics or the surgical techniques used. Mortality rates vary from 1.9% to 9.0% [8,14,15,22,26–29].

Thirty-day mortality rates (inhospital mortality) were reported previously. However, 30- and 90-day mortality reports are preferred currently. Recent advances in medical technology, including quality improvements in the intensive care unit and the accumulation of experience and knowledge with regard to radical cystectomy patient management, meant that a 90-day mortality rate was more applicable to surgery-related deaths in a recent radical cystectomy series [30].

The main causes of death involved acute cardiopulmonary events, such as myocardial infarction or pulmonary embolism. Sepsis following an infectious condition, originating from intestinal anastomotic or urinary leakage, was also associated with mortality [15,27].

In addition to the patients and surgical methods used, hospital volumes and the level of surgeon competence can affect mortality rates following radical cystectomy. It was concluded in a study in which the National Cancer Database was used to analyze 35,055 radical cystectomy cases, that a low volume hospital, i.e., ≤10 radical cystectomy cases, was associated with a 1.5-fold risk of 30-day mortality and a 1.2-fold risk of 90-day mortality, compared to a high-volume hospital of ≥20 cases [31]. In another study in which healthcare data from the Canadian Quebec region were used, high-volume hospitals and surgeons were shown to be critical factors in lowering the overall mortality rate following radical cystectomy [32].

This tendency was also observed with respect to several other high-risk cancer operations. The ability to improve patient management quality, for example by standardizing surgical procedures, can easily be achieved with high-volume cancer. Also, the accumulation of experience and knowledge in relation to postoperative morbidity ultimately helps to lower the mortality rate in high-volume centers [33] (Table 25.2).

TABLE 25.2 Summary of Mortality and Morbidity in Recent Radical Cystectomy Series

Selected Series	No. of Patients	Features	Morbidity and Mortality
Shabsigh et al., 2009 [15]	1142	Prospective database Single center Open radical cystectomy Continent diversion 37%	Overall complication 64% Grade 1−2 in 51% Grade 3−5 in 13% 30-day mortality 1.5% 90-day mortality 2.7%
Yuh et al., 2012 [26]	196	Prospective database Single center Robot radical cystectomy Continent diversion 68% Extracorporeal diversion 100%	Overall complication 80% Grade 1−2 in 55% Grade 3−5 in 35% 30-day mortality 2% 90-day mortality 4.1%
Johar et al., 2013 [29]	939	Prospective database Multicenter Robot radical cystectomy Continent diversion 32% Intracorporeal diversion 23%	Overall complication 48% Grade 1−2 in 29% Grade 3−5 in 19% 30-days mortality 1.3% 90-days mortality 4.2%
Shiavinia et al., 2013 [27]	404	Retrospective database Single center Open radical cystectomy Continent diversion 37%	Overall complication 52% Grade 1−2 in 34.4% Grade 3−4 in 17.3% 30-day mortality 3.2% 90-day mortality 4.5%
Kim et al., 2014 [14]	308	Retrospective database Single center Open radical cystectomy Continent diversion 47.7%	Overall complication 49% Grade 1−2 in 29% Grade 3−4 in 20% 30-day mortality 2.2% 90-day mortality 6.6%

SURVIVAL AFTER RADICAL CYSTECTOMY

Survival after radical cystectomy are mainly determined by postoperative features, inter alia, pathological tumor stage and lymph node status are the most valuable predictors of survival outcomes following cystectomy [5,34−41].

When the survival rate was analyzed by T stage, patients with pT0 or residual noninvasive disease had excellent outcomes, with 5-year cancer-specific survival rates approaching 90% on final pathology. Five-year cancer-specific survival rates ranging from 58% to 85% were observed in patients with pT2 tumors. The presence of non-organ-confined disease (>pT2) were related to a poorer survival outcome. Five-year, cancer-specific survival rates ranging from 36% to 60% were reported in patients with T3 disease [5,35,36,38,40].

The presence of lymph node metastasis appears to be the most important predictor of survival outcome. Node-positive disease confers a poor prognosis, with 5-year disease-specific survival rates ranging from 22% to 56% [5,35,36,38,40].

The surgical margin status is also an important predictor of recurrence following radical cystectomy. An overall soft tissue positive margin rate of 6.3% was reported in a multicenter, retrospective study on 4410 radical cystectomy patients. A positive soft tissue margin was associated with a significantly increased risk of recurrence [hazard ratio (HR) = 1.52, $P < 0.001$] and cancer-specific mortality (HR = 1.51, $P < 0.001$) [42].

Additional several variables have been proposed as having prognostic value following radical cystectomy. The presence of lymphovascular invasion was the representative pathological finding. Shariat et al. reported that because lymphovascular invasion was a major prognostic factor in lymph node–negative patients treated with radical cystectomy, assessment of a lymphovascular invasion could help with the selection of patients with survival gain from adjuvant therapy following radical cystectomy [35].

Cell cycle- and proliferation-related molecular markers, such as p53, p21, p27, cyclin E, and Ki-67 expression, are believed to be prognostic factors. Patients with more than two altered markers were at risk of unfavorable clinical outcomes [43] Ku et al. did not use a special biological marker but reported on a systematic inflammatory response according to the pretreatment status of albumin, lymphocyte count, and platelet count, all of which have prognostic value [44].

Body composition is also known to be a prognostic factor in bladder cancer patients who underwent radical cystectomy. Smith et al. reported that sarcopenia in women was a predictor of major complications and poorer 2-year survival after radical cystectomy [45].

Advanced age has been reported to be a poor prognostic factor. However, the aggressive surgical management of bladder cancer in older patients may improve survival [46,47].

As mentioned previously, the proficiency of the surgeon and hospital volume also relate to survival outcomes [31,32]. However, recurrence and the mortality rate with respect to bladder cancer tend to decrease steadily, regardless of hospital volume and region. According to nationwide statistics from the United States from 1973 to 2009 on 5-year survival and mortality rates for 148,315 bladder cancer patients, stage-specific 5-year survival rate increased for all stages, except for metastatic disease [48] (Table 25.3).

TABLE 25.3 Percentage of 5-Year Cancer-Specific Survival According to the Pathologic Features of the Cystectomy Specimen

Selected Series	No. of Patients	T-stage			N-stage		Resection Margin	
		T ≤ 1	T2	T3—4	LN—	LN+	R—	R+
Shariat et al., 2006 [35]	888	87	79	43	80	35		
Ghoneim et al., 2008 [36]	2720	82	58	36	62	27		
Hautmann et al., 2012 [38]	1100	93	74	60	81	22		
Ploussard et al., 2014 [5]	8141	88	74	49	77	37	70	32
Raza et al., 2015 [40]	702	93	85	53	87	56	82	65

REFERENCES

[1] Liedberg F. Early complications and morbidity of radical cystectomy. Eur Urol 2010;9:25—30.

[2] Collins JW, Wiklund NP. Totally intracorporeal robot-assisted radical cystectomy: optimizing total outcomes. BJU Int 2014;114:326—33.

[3] Mitropoulos D, Artibani W, Graefen M, Remzi M, Roupret M, Truss M. Reporting and grading of complications after urologic surgical procedures: an ad hoc EAU guidelines panel assessment and recommendations. Eur Urol 2012;61:341—9.

[4] Dindo D, Demartines N, Clavien PA. Classification of surgical complications: a new proposal with evaluation in a cohort of 6336 patients and results of a survey. Ann Surg 2004;240:205—13.

[5] Ploussard G, Shariat SF, Dragomir A, Kluth LA, Xylinas E, Masson-Lecomte A, et al. Conditional survival after radical cystectomy for bladder cancer: evidence for a patient changing risk profile over time. Eur Urol 2014;66:361—70.

[6] Psutka SP, Boorjian SA, Moynagh MR, Schmit GD, Frank I, Carrasco A, et al. Mortality after radical cystectomy: impact of obesity versus adiposity after adjusting for skeletal muscle wasting. J Urol 2015;193:1507—13.

[7] Novotny V, Froehner M, Koch R, Zastrow S, Heberling U, Leike S, et al. Age, American Society of Anesthesiologists physical status classification and Charlson score are independent predictors of 90-day mortality after radical cystectomy. World J Urol 2016;34 (8):1123—9. <http://dx.doi.org/10.1007/s00345-015-1744-8>.

[8]   Ishii H, Rai BP, Stolzenburg JU, Bose P, Chlosta PL, Somani BK, et al. Robotic or open radical cystectomy, which is safer? A systematic review and meta-analysis of comparative studies. J Endourol 2014;28:1215−23.

[9]   Koupparis A, Villeda-Sandoval C, Weale N, El-Mahdy M, Gillatt D, Rowe E. Robot-assisted radical cystectomy with intracorporeal urinary diversion: impact on an established enhanced recovery protocol. BJU Int 2015;116:924−31.

[10] Yuh B, Wilson T, Bochner B, Chan K, Palou J, Stenzl A, et al. Systematic review and cumulative analysis of oncologic and functional outcomes after robot-assisted radical cystectomy. Eur Urol 2015;67:402−22.

[11] Linder BJ, Frank I, Cheville JC, Tollefson MK, Thompson RH, Tarrell RF, et al. The impact of perioperative blood transfusion on cancer recurrence and survival following radical cystectomy. Eur Urol 2013;63:839−45.

[12] Lee JS, Kim HS, Jeong CW, Kwak C, Kim HH, Ku JH. The prognostic impact of perioperative blood transfusion on survival in patients with bladder urothelial carcinoma treated with radical cystectomy. Korean J Urol 2015;56:295−304.

[13] Morgan TM, Barocas DA, Chang SS, Phillips SE, Salem S, Clark PE, et al. The relationship between perioperative blood transfusion and overall mortality in patients undergoing radical cystectomy for bladder cancer. Urol Oncol 2013;31:871−7.

[14] Kim SH, Yu A, Jung JH, Lee YJ, Lee ES. Incidence and risk factors of 30-day early and 90-day late morbidity and mortality of radical cystectomy during a 13-year follow-up: a comparative propensity-score matched analysis of complications between neobladder and ileal conduit. Jpn J Clin Oncol 2014;44:677−85.

[15] Shabsigh A, Korets R, Vora KC, Brooks CM, Cronin AM, Savage C, et al. Defining early morbidity of radical cystectomy for patients with bladder cancer using a standardized reporting methodology. Eur Urol 2009;55:164−74.

[16] Azhar RA, Bochner B, Catto J, Goh AC, Kelly J, Patel HD, et al. Enhanced recovery after urological surgery: a contemporary systematic review of outcomes, key elements, and research needs. Eur Urol 2016;70(1):176−87. <http://dx.doi.org/10.1016/j.eururo.2016.02.051>.

[17] Mattei A, Birkhaeuser FD, Baermann C, Warncke SH, Studer UE. To stent or not to stent perioperatively the ureteroileal anastomosis of ileal orthotopic bladder substitutes and ileal conduits? Results of a prospective randomized trial. J Urol 2008;179:582−6.

[18] Spiliotis J, Tsiveriotis K, Datsis AD, Vaxevanidou A, Zacharis G, Giafis K, et al. Wound dehiscence: is still a problem in the 21th century: a retrospective study. World J Emerg Surg 2009;4:12.

[19] Gupta H, Srivastava A, Menon GR, Agrawal CS, Chumber S, Kumar S. Comparison of interrupted versus continuous closure in abdominal wound repair: a meta-analysis of 23 trials. Asian J Surg 2008;31:104−14.

[20] Christie MC, Manger JP, Khiyami AM, Ornan AA, Wheeler KM, Schenkman NS. Occult radiographically evident port-site hernia after robot-assisted urologic surgery: incidence and risk factors. J Endourol 2016;30:92−6.

[21] del Junco M, Okhunov Z, Juncal S, Yoon R, Landman J. Evaluation of a novel trocar-site closure and comparison with a standard Carter-Thomason closure device. J Endourol 2014;28:814−18.

[22] Quek ML, Stein JP, Daneshmand S, Miranda G, Thangathurai D, Roffey P, et al. A critical analysis of perioperative mortality from radical cystectomy. J Urol 2006;175:886−9, discussion 9−90.

[23] Moschini M, Karnes RJ, Gandaglia G, Luzzago S, Dell'Oglio P, Rossi MS, et al. Preoperative favorable characteristics in bladder cancer patients cannot substitute the

necessity of extended lymphadenectomy during radical cystectomy: a sensitivity curve analysis. Urology 2016;88:97–103.

[24] Abdollah F, Sun M, Schmitges J, Djahangirian O, Tian Z, Jeldres C, et al. Stage-specific impact of pelvic lymph node dissection on survival in patients with non-metastatic bladder cancer treated with radical cystectomy. BJU Int 2012;109:1147–54.

[25] Kurpad R, Woods M, Pruthi R. Current status of robot-assisted radical cystectomy and intracorporeal urinary diversion. Curr Urol Rep 2016;17:42.

[26] Yuh BE, Nazmy M, Ruel NH, Jankowski JT, Menchaca AR, Torrey RR, et al. Standardized analysis of frequency and severity of complications after robot-assisted radical cystectomy. Eur Urol 2012;62:806–13.

[27] Schiavina R, Borghesi M, Guidi M, Vagnoni V, Zukerman Z, Pultrone C, et al. Perioperative complications and mortality after radical cystectomy when using a standardized reporting methodology. Clin Genitourin Cancer 2013;11:189–97.

[28] Aziz A, May M, Burger M, Palisaar RJ, Trinh QD, Fritsche HM, et al. Prediction of 90-day mortality after radical cystectomy for bladder cancer in a prospective European multicenter cohort. Eur Urol 2014;66:156–63.

[29] Johar RS, Hayn MH, Stegemann AP, Ahmed K, Agarwal P, Balbay MD, et al. Complications after robot-assisted radical cystectomy: results from the International Robotic Cystectomy Consortium. Eur Urol 2013;64:52–7.

[30] Isbarn H, Jeldres C, Zini L, Perrotte P, Baillargeon-Gagne S, Capitanio U, et al. A population based assessment of perioperative mortality after cystectomy for bladder cancer. J Urol 2009;182:70–7.

[31] Nielsen ME, Mallin K, Weaver MA, Palis B, Stewart A, Winchester DP, et al. Association of hospital volume with conditional 90-day mortality after cystectomy: an analysis of the National Cancer Data Base. BJU International 2014;114:46–55.

[32] Santos F, Zakaria AS, Kassouf W, Tanguay S, Aprikian A. High hospital and surgeon volume and its impact on overall survival after radical cystectomy among patients with bladder cancer in Quebec. World J Urol 2015;33:1323–30.

[33] Finks JF, Osborne NH, Birkmeyer JD. Trends in hospital volume and operative mortality for high-risk surgery. N Engl J Med 2011;364:2128–37.

[34] Hautmann RE, Gschwend JE, de Petriconi RC, Kron M, Volkmer BG. Cystectomy for transitional cell carcinoma of the bladder: results of a surgery only series in the neobladder era. J Urol 2006;176:486–92, discussion 91–2.

[35] Shariat SF, Karakiewicz PI, Palapattu GS, Lotan Y, Rogers CG, Amiel GE, et al. Outcomes of radical cystectomy for transitional cell carcinoma of the bladder: a contemporary series from the Bladder Cancer Research Consortium. J Urol 2006;176:2414–22, discussion 22.

[36] Ghoneim MA, Abdel-Latif M, el-Mekresh M, Abol-Enein H, Mosbah A, Ashamallah A, et al. Radical cystectomy for carcinoma of the bladder: 2,720 consecutive cases 5 years later. J Urol 2008;180:121–7.

[37] Manoharan M, Ayyathurai R, Soloway MS. Radical cystectomy for urothelial carcinoma of the bladder: an analysis of perioperative and survival outcome. BJU Int 2009;104:1227–32.

[38] Hautmann RE, de Petriconi RC, Pfeiffer C, Volkmer BG. Radical cystectomy for urothelial carcinoma of the bladder without neoadjuvant or adjuvant therapy: long-term results in 1100 patients. Eur Urol 2012;61:1039–47.

[39] Patel MI, Bang A, Gillatt D, Smith DP. Contemporary radical cystectomy outcomes in patients with invasive bladder cancer: a population-based study. BJU Int 2015;116(Suppl 3): 18–25.

[40] Raza SJ, Wilson T, Peabody JO, Wiklund P, Scherr DS, Al-Daghmin A, et al. Long-term oncologic outcomes following robot-assisted radical cystectomy: results from the International Robotic Cystectomy Consortium. Eur Urol 2015;68:721−8.

[41] Moschini M, Sharma V, Dell'oglio P, Cucchiara V, Gandaglia G, Cantiello F, et al. Comparing long-term outcomes of primary and progressive carcinoma invading bladder muscle after radical cystectomy. BJU Int 2016;117:604−10.

[42] Novara G, Svatek RS, Karakiewicz PI, Skinner E, Ficarra V, Fradet Y, et al. Soft tissue surgical margin status is a powerful predictor of outcomes after radical cystectomy: a multicenter study of more than 4,400 patients. J Urol 2010;183:2165−70.

[43] Shariat SF, Passoni N, Bagrodia A, Rachakonda V, Xylinas E, Robinson B, et al. Prospective evaluation of a preoperative biomarker panel for prediction of upstaging at radical cystectomy. BJU Int 2014;113:70−6.

[44] Ku JH, Kang M, Kim HS, Jeong CW, Kwak C, Kim HH. The prognostic value of pretreatment of systemic inflammatory responses in patients with urothelial carcinoma undergoing radical cystectomy. Br J Cancer 2015;112:461−7.

[45] Smith AB, Deal AM, Yu H, Boyd B, Matthews J, Wallen EM, et al. Sarcopenia as a predictor of complications and survival following radical cystectomy. J Urol 2014;191:1714−20.

[46] Nielsen ME, Shariat SF, Karakiewicz PI, Lotan Y, Rogers CG, Amiel GE, et al. Advanced age is associated with poorer bladder cancer-specific survival in patients treated with radical cystectomy. Eur Urol 2007;51:699−706, discussion-8.

[47] Hollenbeck BK, Miller DC, Taub D, Dunn RL, Underwood III W, Montie JE, et al. Aggressive treatment for bladder cancer is associated with improved overall survival among patients 80 years old or older. Urology 2004;64:292−7.

[48] Abdollah F, Gandaglia G, Thuret R, Schmitges J, Tian Z, Jeldres C, et al. Incidence, survival and mortality rates of stage-specific bladder cancer in United States: a trend analysis. Cancer Epidemiol 2013;37:219−25.

Chapter 26

Adjuvant Chemotherapy

Jong Jin Oh

Seoul National University Bundang Hospital, Seongnam, South Korea

Chapter Outline

INTRODUCTION

According to reports from annual surveys, it is estimated that approximately 380,000 patients are newly diagnosed with bladder cancer worldwide each year. Additionally, approximately 150,000 bladder cancer-related deaths occur each year [1,2]. Although most patients have non-muscle-invasive bladder cancer, 10%−20% of these patients eventually progress to muscle-invasive bladder cancer (MIBC). In addition, nearly 30% of newly diagnosed cases have muscle invasion at the time of diagnosis [3].

Until recently, radical cystectomy (RC) was considered the gold standard of treatment for MIBC; however, the 5-year survival rate for all stages of MIBC ranges from 48% to 66% [4,5]. In particular, the 5-year survival rate for patients with a higher pathologic stage ($\geq$T3) N0 was 47% after RC; patients with lymph node metastases had an overall 5-year survival rate of $\leq$31% after RC [4,6]. Therefore, recurrence is believed to be due mainly to systemic disease not apparent at the time of RC. This problem can be addressed by the use of either neoadjuvant or adjuvant systemic chemotherapy [7].

Bladder Cancer. DOI: http://dx.doi.org/10.1016/B978-0-12-809939-1.00026-6
© 2018 Elsevier Inc. All rights reserved.

RATIONALE FOR ADJUVANT CHEMOTHERAPY

Adjuvant chemotherapy after localized treatment has led to increased survival in patients with many different types of solid tumors [8]. The main advantage of this approach is that cystectomy can be performed immediately with no delay in definitive treatment and that the pathological pT/pN categories can be assessed. Stage and lymph node status are known prognostic factors for progression and survival [4]. High-risk patients who might benefit the most could then be selected to receive adjuvant chemotherapy. Although the majority of patients with pT2N0 bladder cancer may be cured by surgery alone, only a minority of patients with pT3 or higher remain cancer free. Combination cisplatin-containing chemotherapy regimens for metastatic bladder can produce a response in up to 70% of patients [9]. Three or four cycles of adjuvant chemotherapy after cystectomy aim to delay recurrence and extend survival in patients with MIBC or those with regional lymph node metastases.

RESULTS FROM CLINICAL TRIALS

Randomized controlled studies of adjuvant chemotherapy among patients after RC have been conducted. However, most of them were closed prematurely for several reasons. The summarized results of clinical trials for adjuvant chemotherapy after RC are shown in Table 26.1.

Historically, in 1988 Logothetis et al. [10] reported results from patients who underwent adjuvant chemotherapy CISCA (cisplatin, cyclophosphamide, and adriamycin) after RC. A total of 71 patients with extravesical tumor extension, lymphovascular invasion or pelvic visceral invasion were enrolled. These patients were compared in a nonrandomized fashion to 62 high-risk patients and 206 low-risk patients who did not receive adjuvant chemotherapy. The authors concluded that adjuvant CISCA conferred a 2-year disease-free survival (DFS) advantage to patients with unfavorable pathological findings (70% vs 30%; $P = 0.00012$).

Stockle et al. [11,12] randomized patients with pT3, pT4, and/or pelvic lymph nodes to three cycles of MVAC (methotrexate, vinblastine, doxorubicin, and cisplatin) or MVEC (methotrexate, vinblastine, epirubicin, and cisplatin) versus observation. Although the authors planned to enroll 100 patients, the study was closed after an interim analysis of 49 randomized patients revealed a significant advantage in relapse-free survival with chemotherapy ($P = 0.0015$).

Lehmann et al. [13] reported on the long-term follow-up of patients with locally advanced bladder cancer treated with adjuvant-combined chemotherapy. Between May 1987 and December 1990, 49 patients undergoing RC for locally advanced bladder cancer were randomized to observation only or adjuvant systemic chemotherapy with three cycles of methotrexate,

TABLE 26.1 Results From Clinical Trials of Adjuvant Chemotherapy for MIBC After Radical Cystectomy

| Clinical Trials | Report Year | Enrolled Number of Patients | | Inclusion | Regimen | Results (5-year DFS, OS) | | Notes |
		Adjuvant	Control			DFS (AC vs CT)	OS (AC vs CT)	
Logothetis et al.	1988	71	268	T3–4, N1	CISCA	70% vs 30% ($P = 0.00012$) (2-year DFS)		
Bono et al.	1989	35	48	T2–T4a, N0M0	CIS+ MTX	51% vs 56% ($P = 0.663$)	51% vs 62% ($P = 0.313$)	
Skinner et al.	1991	44	47	T3–T4, N+, M0	CISCA	70% vs 46% ($P < 0.001$) (3-year DFS)	71% vs 50% ($P = 0.027$) (3-year OS)	Stopped early
Stockle et al.	1992	26	23	T3b–T4a	MVA(E)C	66% vs 15% ($P = 0.021$) (3-year DFS)	58% vs 15% ($P = 0.048$) (3-year OS)	Stopped early
Studer et al.	1994	37	40	T1G2–T4a	CIS		57% vs 54% ($P = 0.877$)	Stopped early
Freiha et al.	1996	25	25	T3b–T4	CMV	37 months vs 12 months ($P = 0.002$)	63 months vs 36 months ($P = 0.152$)	Stopped early
Otto et al.	2003	55	53	T3N1–2M0	MVAC	44% vs 40% 4-year DFS		Not significant
Lehmann et al.	2006	26	23	T3–4a, N+	MVA(E)C	43.7% vs 13.0% ($P = 0.002$) 10-year DFS	26.9% vs 17.4% ($P = 0.069$) 10-year OS	Stopped early

(Continued)

TABLE 26.1 (Continued)

| Clinical Trials | Report Year | Enrolled Number of Patients | | Inclusion | Regimen | Results (5-year DFS, OS) | | Notes |
		Adjuvant	Control			DFS (AC vs CT)	OS (AC vs CT)	
Paz-Ares et al. (SOGUG 99/01)	2010	68	74	T3–4, N+	PGC		60% vs 31% ($P < 0.0009$)	Stopped early
Stadler et al.	2011	58	56	T1–2 (p53 +)	MVAC		Almost 40% ($P = 0.89$)	Stopped early
Cognetti et al.	2012	102	92	T2G3; T3–4, N+	GC	37.2% vs 42.3% ($P = 0.70$)	43.4% vs 53.7% ($P = 0.24$)	Stopped early
Sternberg et al. (EORTC 30994)	2015	141	143	T3–4, N+	GC, MVAC	47.6% vs 31.8% ($P < 0.0001$)	53.6% vs 47.7% ($P = 0.13$)	Stopped early

AC, adjuvant chemotherapy; CT, control; CIS, cisplatin; CMV, cisplatin, methotrexate, and vinblastine; MTX, methotrexate; SOGUG, Spanish Oncology Genitourinary Group; PGC, paclitaxel, gemcitabine, and cisplatin; GC, gemcitabine and cisplatin.

vinblastine, doxorubicin/epirubicin, and cisplatin (MVAC/MVEC). This trial intended to enroll 100 patients but was stopped after an interim analysis showed a marked difference in progression-free survival among the first 49 patients randomized to treatment. The 10-year progression-free survival was estimated to be 13.0% (control) vs 43.7% (adjuvant chemotherapy), and hazard ratios (HRs) with 95% confidence intervals (CIs) were 2.84 (95% CI: 1.46−5.54; $P = 0.002$). The 10-year overall survival (OS) was estimated 17.4% (control) vs 26.9% (adjuvant chemotherapy), and HR was 2.84 (95% CI: 1.46−5.54; $P = 0.002$) (Fig. 26.1). The authors concluded that adjuvant-combined chemotherapy with cisplatin-based regimens after RC for locally advanced bladder cancer significantly improves progression-free and tumor-specific survival.

The Spanish Oncology Genitourinary Group opened the 99/01 trial comparing four cycles of paclitaxel, cisplatin, and gemcitabine (PCG) compared to observation only [14]. The adjuvant 99/01 trial enrolled patients with pT3−4 and/or lymph node−positive bladder cancer with a creatinine clearance >50 mL/min and mandated chemotherapy commencement within 8 weeks of cystectomy, whereas prior studies had allowed up to 12 weeks after surgery. The trial enrolled 142 patients between July 2000 and July 2007, when it was closed prematurely due to poor enrollment. At a median follow-up of 30 months, OS was significantly prolonged in the PCG arm (median not reached; 5-year OS: 60%) compared to observation only (median: 26 months; 5-year OS: 31%; $P < 0.0009$). DFS ($P < 0.0001$) and disease-specific survival ($P < 0.0002$) were also superior in the PCG arm.

Another study by Stadler et al. [15] used p53 status by immunohistochemistry as a prognostic biomarker for recurrence and to identify candidates for adjuvant MVAC. In this study, 499 patients underwent p53 assessment. Of these, 272 were positive and 114 were randomized to receive

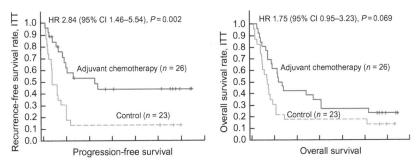

FIGURE 26.1 Disease-free progression survival rates and OS rates between patients with adjuvant chemotherapy and controls. *ITT*, intention-to-treat. *Source: Adapted from Lehmann J, Franzaring L, Thuroff J, Wellek S, Stockle M. Complete long-term survival data from a trial of adjuvant chemotherapy vs control after radical cystectomy for locally advanced bladder cancer. BJU Int 2006;97(1):42−7, permitted by John Wiley and Sons.*

three cycles of adjuvant MVAC or placebo. p53-negative patients were observed; but after the first 110 patients of the planned 190 were randomized, the study was closed due to futility. There was no difference in recurrence risk based on p53 status, and there was no difference in outcomes between the randomized patients.

More recently, Cognetti et al. [16] reported the results of a Phase III Italian multicenter randomized trial. One hundred and ninety-four patients with pT2G3, pT3–4, or N0–2 transitional cell bladder cancer were randomly allocated to control (92 patients) or to four courses of adjuvant chemotherapy (102 patients). These latter patients were further randomly assigned to receive gemcitabine 1000 mg/m^2 on days 1, 8, and 15 and cisplatin 70 mg/m^2 on Day 2 or gemcitabine as above plus cisplatin 70 mg/m^2 on Day 15, every 28 days (GC regimen). At the median follow-up time of 35 months, the 5-year OS was 43.4% in the adjuvant chemotherapy group and 53.7% in the control group (HR: 1.29; 95% CI: 0.84–1.99; $P = 0.24$); there was no significant difference between the two groups (Fig. 26.2). The control and adjuvant chemotherapy arms had comparable DFS (5-year DFS: 42.3% and 37.2%, respectively; HR: 1.08; 95% CI: 0.73–1.59; $P = 0.70$). Only 62% of patients received the planned cycles. Unfortunately, due to the low accrual rate, the trial was also prematurely closed, and the final analysis was carried out in July 2009. The authors, therefore, concluded that this study was underpowered in its ability to demonstrate that adjuvant chemotherapy with GC improves OS and DFS in patients with MIBC.

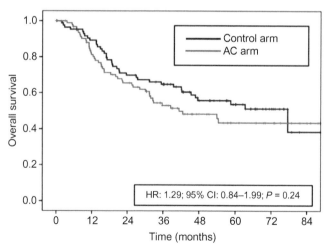

FIGURE 26.2 OS between patients with adjuvant chemotherapy (*AC*) and control. *Source: Adapted from Cognetti F, Ruggeri EM, Felici A, Gallucci M, Muto G, et al. Adjuvant chemotherapy with cisplatin and gemcitabine versus chemotherapy at relapse in patients with muscle-invasive bladder cancer submitted to radical cystectomy: an Italian, multicenter, randomized phase III trial. Ann Oncol 2012;23(3):695–700, permitted by Oxford University Press.*

Most recently, a randomized trial was published by Sternberg et al. [7]. The EORTC 30994 trial aimed to compare immediate versus deferred cisplatin-based combination chemotherapy after RC in patients with pT3−pT4 or N+ M0 urothelial carcinoma of the bladder. This intergroup open-label randomized Phase 3 trial recruited patients from hospitals across Europe and Canada. Eligible patients had histologically proven urothelial bladder cancer, pT3−pT4 disease, or node-positive (pN1−3) M0 disease after RC and bilateral lymphadenectomy with no evidence of any microscopic residual disease. Patients were assigned to two groups within 90 days of RC—an immediate chemotherapy group (adjuvant) (four cycles of GC, high-dose of MVAC/MVEC) or a delayed chemotherapy group (salvage) (six cycles at relapse). This trial was also closed early after recruiting 284 of the planned 660 patients. After a median follow-up of 7 years, 66 (47%) of 141 patients in the immediate treatment group had died, compared with 82 (57%) of 143 patients in the deferred treatment group. No significant improvement in OS was noted with immediate treatment when compared with deferred treatment (HR: 0.78; 95% CI: 0.56−1.08; $P = 0.13$). Immediate treatment significantly prolonged DFS compared with deferred treatment (HR: 0.54; 95% CI: 0.4−0.73; $P < 0.0001$), with a 5-year DFS rate of 47.6% in the immediate treatment group and 31.8% in the deferred treatment group. The authors concluded that the data did not show a significant improvement in OS with immediate versus deferred chemotherapy after RC (Fig. 26.3).

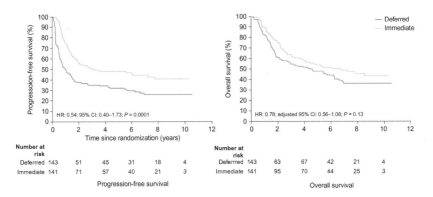

FIGURE 26.3 Progression-free survival and OS between patients with adjuvant chemotherapy and salvage chemotherapy. *Source: Adapted from Sternberg CN, Skoneczna I, Kerst JM, Albers P, Fossa SD, et al. Immediate versus deferred chemotherapy after radical cystectomy in patients with pT3-pT4 or N+ M0 urothelial carcinoma of the bladder (EORTC 30994): an intergroup, open-label, randomised phase 3 trial. Lancet Oncol 2015;16(1):76−86, permitted by Elsevier.*

RESULTS FROM META-ANALYSES

Despite multiple randomized clinical trials, the role of adjuvant chemotherapy in bladder cancer has remained controversial because most studies had no confirmed results for adjuvant chemotherapy after RC. The Advanced Bladder Cancer Meta-Analysis Collaboration conducted a meta-analysis in 2005 [17] based on 491 patients from six trials [11,18−22], representing 90% of all patients randomized in cisplatin-based combination chemotherapy trials and 66% of patients from all eligible trials. Four of the six trials (293/493 patients) were stopped early; three were stopped because the results of interim analyses favored chemotherapy [11,18,21] The fourth study by Studer et al. [20] was stopped due to interim results showing less benefit of chemotherapy than had been anticipated. Nevertheless, the results from this meta-analysis showed that the overall HR for survival was 0.75 (95% CI: 0.60−0.96, $P = 0.019$), suggesting a 25% relative reduction in the risk of death for chemotherapy compared to that of controls (Figs. 26.4 and 26.5).

Data on overall DFS was supplied for five trials including 383 patients and 239 events. The overall HR was 0.68 (95% CI: 0.53−0.89), representing a 32% relative decrease in the risk of recurrence or death with chemotherapy compared to that of controls ($P = 0.004$). This is equivalent to a 12% absolute improvement in DFS at 3 years. However, the authors warned of bias resulting from trials stopping early; the impact of patients not receiving allocated treatments or not receiving salvage chemotherapy is less clear. Additionally, the authors concluded that this meta-analysis provides the best evidence currently available on the role of adjuvant chemotherapy for

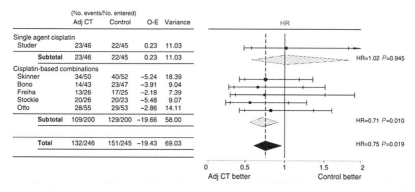

FIGURE 26.4 Results from a meta-analysis. The overall HR for survival was 0.75 (95% CI: 0.60−0.96; $P = 0.019$). *Adj. CT*, adjuvant chemotherapy. *Source: From Advanced Bladder Cancer (ABC) Meta-analysis Collaboration. Adjuvant chemotherapy in invasive bladder cancer: a systematic review and meta-analysis of individual patient data Advanced Bladder Cancer (ABC) Meta-analysis Collaboration Eur Urol 2005;48(2):189−99; discussion 199−201, permitted by Elsevier.*

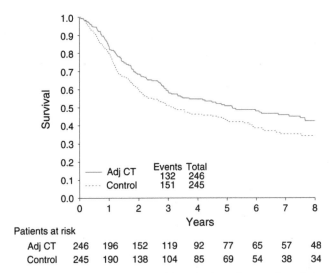

FIGURE 26.5 Kaplan—Meier analysis for OS. *Adj. CT,* adjuvant chemotherapy. *Source: Adapted from Advanced Bladder Cancer (ABC) Meta-analysis Collaboration. Adjuvant chemotherapy in invasive bladder cancer: a systematic review and meta-analysis of individual patient data Advanced Bladder Cancer (ABC) Meta-analysis Collaboration Eur Urol 2005;48(2):189—99; discussion 199—201, permitted by Elsevier.*

MIBC. However, at present, there is insufficient evidence from which to reliably base treatment decisions.

In 2006, Ruggeri and colleagues performed a composite analysis based on published data from all Phase 3 published studies of adjuvant chemotherapy [23]. In their analysis, five trials were used [11,18−21]. All patients were evaluable for OS (350 patients), and four of these patients were also evaluable for DFS (273 patients). A significant benefit from adjuvant chemotherapy was noted both in OS (Relative ratio (RR): 0.74; 95% CI: 0.62−0.88; $P = 0.001$) and DFS (RR: 0.65; CI: 0.54−0.78; $P = 0.001$) (Fig. 26.6).

This meta-analysis showed favorable results of adjuvant chemotherapy; however, the authors also warned that some studies were stopped early; therefore, future large-scale randomized studies are necessary.

A more recently conducted meta-analysis by Leow et al. [24] analyzed results from nine randomized clinical trials [13−16,18−22]. The updated 2013 meta-analysis reported a 23% risk reduction in mortality with adjuvant chemotherapy. All trials involved cisplatin-based regimens. The 2013 update by Leow et al. [24] added three trials and updated one trial to the original six trials included in the 2005 meta-analysis by the Advanced Bladder Cancer Meta-Analysis Corporation [17]. A total of 945 patients included in nine randomized trials were examined. For OS, the pooled HR across all nine trials was 0.77 (95% CI: 0.59−0.99; $P = 0.049$) (Fig. 26.7). For DFS,

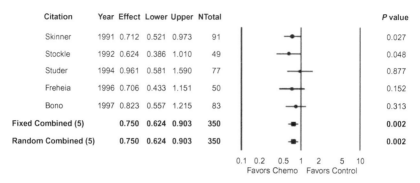

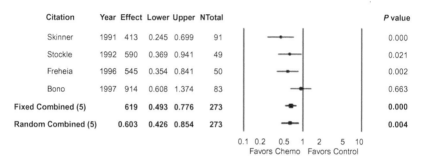

FIGURE 26.6 Relative risk ratio for the OS and DFS between a cohort of adjuvant chemotherapy after radical cystectomy and controls (upper figure: OS, lower figure: DFS). *Source: Adapted from Ruggeri EM, Giannarelli D, Bria E, Carlini P, Felici A, et al. Adjuvant chemotherapy in muscle-invasive bladder carcinoma: a pooled analysis from phase III studies. Cancer 2006;106(4):783–88, permitted by John Wiley and Sons.*

the pooled HR across seven trials reporting this outcome was 0.66 (95% CI, 0.45–0.91; $P = 0.014$) (Fig. 26.8). This DFS benefit was more apparent among those with positive nodal involvement ($P = 0.010$) (Fig. 26.9).

RESULTS FROM LARGE RETROSPECTIVE COHORT STUDIES

Recent large-scale multicenter retrospective studies show more favorable results for adjuvant chemotherapy for MIBC. In 2010, Svatek et al. [25] reported on a collaborative effort among 11 major centers that has yielded an international cohort analysis of off-trial adjuvant chemotherapy. The cohort consisted of 3947 patients undergoing RC and lymph node dissection between 1979 and 2008. Of these, 932 (23.6%) patients received adjuvant chemotherapy. Adjuvant chemotherapy was independently associated with improved OS (HR: 0.83; 95% CI: 0.72–0.97; $P = 0.017$). The risk group significantly predicted the survival impact of chemotherapy on outcomes.

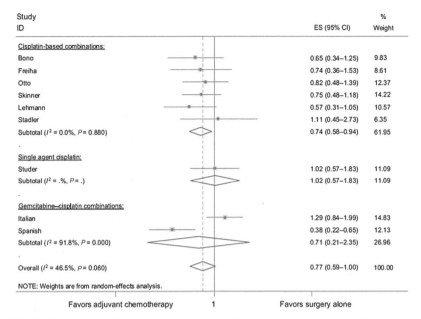

Study ID — ES (95% CI) — % Weight

Cisplatin-based combinations:
Bono — 0.65 (0.34–1.25) — 9.83
Freiha — 0.74 (0.36–1.53) — 8.61
Otto — 0.82 (0.48–1.39) — 12.37
Skinner — 0.75 (0.48–1.18) — 14.22
Lehmann — 0.57 (0.31–1.05) — 10.57
Stadler — 1.11 (0.45–2.73) — 6.35
Subtotal ($I^2 = 0.0\%$, $P = 0.880$) — 0.74 (0.58–0.94) — 61.95

Single agent cisplatin:
Studer — 1.02 (0.57–1.83) — 11.09
Subtotal ($I^2 = .\%$, $P = .$) — 1.02 (0.57–1.83) — 11.09

Gemcitabine–cisplatin combinations:
Italian — 1.29 (0.84–1.99) — 14.83
Spanish — 0.38 (0.22–0.65) — 12.13
Subtotal ($I^2 = 91.8\%$, $P = 0.000$) — 0.71 (0.21–2.35) — 26.96

Overall ($I^2 = 46.5\%$, $P = 0.060$) — 0.77 (0.59–1.00) — 100.00

NOTE: Weights are from random-effects analysis.

Favors adjuvant chemotherapy   1   Favors surgery alone

FIGURE 26.7 Pooled HRs between a cohort of adjuvant chemotherapy after radical cystectomy and controls (HR = 0.77; 95% CI: 0.59−0.99; $P = 0.049$). *ES*, effect size. *Source: Adapted from Leow JJ, Martin-Doyle W, Rajagopal PS, Patel CG, Anderson EM, et al. Adjuvant chemotherapy for invasive bladder cancer: a 2013 updated systematic review and meta-analysis of randomized trials. Eur Urol 2014;66(1):42−54, permitted by Elsevier.*

Increased benefit from adjuvant chemotherapy was observed across higher risk subgroups ($P < 0.001$), particularly in those with extravesical extension or nodal involvement. There was a significant improvement in survival between the treated and untreated patients in the highest risk quintile (HR: 0.75; 95% CI, 0.62−0.90; $P = 0.002$). This group was characterized by an estimated 32.8% 5-year probability of cancer-specific survival (CSS), with 86.6% of patients having both stage T3 or greater along with node metastasis.

More recently, Froehner et al. [26] showed that adjuvant chemotherapy decreased both OS and CSS after RC. A total of 798 patients who underwent RC between 1993 and 2011 for high-risk superficial, MIBC, or undifferentiated bladder cancer were included. The use of adjuvant chemotherapy was an independent predictor of decreased overall mortality (HR: 0.50; 95% CI, 0.38−0.66; $P < 0.0001$) and bladder cancer−specific mortality (HR: 0.71; 95% CI, 0.52−0.97; $P = 0.0321$). Adjuvant chemotherapy was particularly effective among patients with T3−4 N0 (HR = 0.37; 95% CI: 0.16−0.83; $P = 0.0113$).

A recent population-based study by Galsky et al. using the National Cancer Database suggested a benefit from using adjuvant chemotherapy [27].

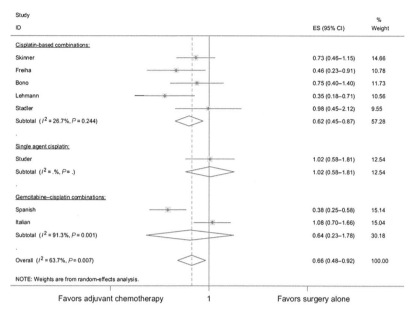

FIGURE 26.8 DFS between a cohort of adjuvant chemotherapy after radical cystectomy and controls (HR = 0.66; 95% CI: 0.45–0.91; $P = 0.014$). *ES*, effect size. *Source: Adapted from Leow JJ, Martin-Doyle W, Rajagopal PS, Patel CG, Anderson EM, et al. Adjuvant chemotherapy for invasive bladder cancer: a 2013 updated systematic review and meta-analysis of randomized trials. Eur Urol 2014;66(1):42−54, permitted by Elsevier.*

This study included cTany NI-3 M0 bladder cancer patients from the National Cancer Data Base (2003−12). Among 1739 patients who were lymph node−positive, 1104 underwent RC. Of the cystectomy patients, 328 received adjuvant chemotherapy. The crude 5-year OS for chemotherapy alone, cystectomy alone, preoperative chemotherapy followed by cystectomy, and cystectomy followed by adjuvant chemotherapy was 14%, 19%, 31%, and 26%, respectively (Fig. 26.10). Adjuvant chemotherapy was associated with a significant improvement in survival compared with cystectomy alone (HR: 0.68; 95% CI: 0.56−0.83).

RECOMMENDATIONS FROM SEVERAL GUIDELINES

According to the European Association of Urology (EAU) 2016 guidelines, adjuvant chemotherapy has limited evidence for the routine use of adjuvant chemotherapy from adequately conducted and accrued randomized Phase III trials. However, the result from meta-analyses and retrospective cohort studies showed an OS benefit. As a result, EAU guidelines state:

"Offer adjuvant cisplatin-based combination chemotherapy to patients with pT3/4 and/or pN+ disease if no neoadjuvant chemotherapy has been

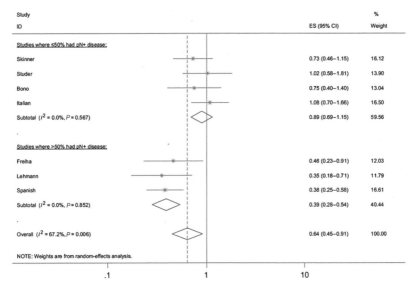

FIGURE 26.9   DFS according to node involvement. The HR for DFS associated with adjuvant cisplatin-based chemotherapy in studies with higher nodal involvement was 0.39 (95% CI: 0.28−0.54), compared with an HR of 0.89 (95% CI: 0.69−1.15) in studies with less nodal involvement. *ES*, effect size. *Source: Adapted from Leow JJ, Martin-Doyle W, Rajagopal PS, Patel CG, Anderson EM, et al. Adjuvant chemotherapy for invasive bladder cancer: a 2013 updated systematic review and meta-analysis of randomized trials. Eur Urol 2014;66(1):42−54, permitted by Elsevier.*

given."—Grade of recommendation C (Made despite the absence of directly applicable clinical studies of good quality)

In the summary article of the second international consultation on bladder cancer recommendations on chemotherapy for the treatment of blood cancer, for patients who did not receive neoadjuvant chemotherapy, we suggest considering adjuvant chemotherapy after RC with a cisplatin-based regimen for patients who have perivesical tumor extension (stage T3 or higher) and/or regional lymph node metastasis (Level of Evidence 2, Grade of recommendation C) [9].

In the National Comprehensive Cancer Network (NCCN) guidelines, if the pathologic T3−4 or node-positive patients who do not receive neoadjuvant chemotherapy, they should be considered for adjuvant chemotherapy (category 2B—based on lower level evidence, there is NCCN consensus that the intervention is appropriate).

CONCLUSIONS

Traditionally, MIBC has been associated with poor survival and limited treatment options. Although treatments and outcomes for bladder cancer

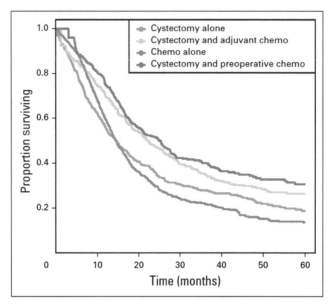

FIGURE 26.10 OS according to treatment scenarios. *Source: Adapted from Galsky MD, Stensland K, Sfakianos JP, Mehrazin R, Diefenbach M, et al. Comparative effectiveness of treatment strategies for bladder cancer with clinical evidence of regional lymph node involvement. J Clin Oncol 2016;34(22):2627−35, permitted by American Society of Clinical Oncology.*

have been largely unchanged over the last few decades, the landscape is evolving. Although clear evidence now exists supporting the use of neoadjuvant chemotherapy, adjuvant chemotherapy's evidence is still weak due to the failure of several previous randomized clinical trials. According to results of meta-analyses and large-scale cohort studies, we considered the recommendation to provide adjuvant chemotherapy to pT3−4 and/or node-positive bladder cancer patients after RC. Future research will need to focus on the adjuvant setting after RC. Targeted therapies and immunotherapy in adjuvant settings could also be promising.

REFERENCES

[1] Ferlay J, Shin HR, Bray F, Forman D, Mathers C, et al. Estimates of worldwide burden of cancer in 2008: GLOBOCAN 2008. Int J Cancer 2010;127(12):2893−917.

[2] Chavan S, Bray F, Lortet-Tieulent J, Goodman M, Jemal A. International variations in bladder cancer incidence and mortality. Eur Urol 2014;66(1):59−73.

[3] Grossman HB, Natale RB, Tangen CM, Speights VO, Vogelzang NJ, et al. Neoadjuvant chemotherapy plus cystectomy compared with cystectomy alone for locally advanced bladder cancer. N Engl J Med 2003;349(9):859−66.

[4] Stein JP, Lieskovsky G, Cote R, Groshen S, Feng AC, et al. Radical cystectomy in the treatment of invasive bladder cancer: long-term results in 1,054 patients. J Clin Oncol 2001;19(3):666–75.

[5] Madersbacher S, Hochreiter W, Burkhard F, Thalmann GN, Danuser H, et al. Radical cystectomy for bladder cancer today—a homogeneous series without neoadjuvant therapy. J Clin Oncol 2003;21(4):690–6.

[6] Frank I, Cheville JC, Blute ML, Lohse CM, Nehra A, et al. Transitional cell carcinoma of the urinary bladder with regional lymph node involvement treated by cystectomy: clinico-pathologic features associated with outcome. Cancer 2003;97(10):2425–31.

[7] Sternberg CN, Skoneczna I, Kerst JM, Albers P, Fossa SD, et al. Immediate versus deferred chemotherapy after radical cystectomy in patients with pT3-pT4 or N+ M0 urothelial carcinoma of the bladder (EORTC 30994): an intergroup, open-label, rando-mised phase 3 trial. Lancet Oncol 2015;16(1):76–86.

[8] Muss HB, Biganzoli L, Sargent DJ, Aapro M. Adjuvant therapy in the elderly: making the right decision. J Clin Oncol 2007;25(14):1870–5.

[9] Sternberg CN, Bellmunt J, Sonpavde G, Siefker-Radtke AO, Stadler WM, et al. ICUD-EAU International Consultation on Bladder Cancer 2012: chemotherapy for urothelial carcinoma-neoadjuvant and adjuvant settings. Eur Urol 2013;63(1):58–66.

[10] Logothetis CJ, Johnson DE, Chong C, Dexeus FH, Sella A, et al. Adjuvant cyclophospha-mide, doxorubicin, and cisplatin chemotherapy for bladder cancer: an update. J Clin Oncol 1988;6(10):1590–6.

[11] Stockle M, Meyenburg W, Wellek S, Voges G, Gertenbach U, et al. Advanced bladder cancer (stages pT3b, pT4a, pN1 and pN2): improved survival after radical cystectomy and 3 adjuvant cycles of chemotherapy. Results of a controlled prospective study. J Urol 1992;148(2 Pt 1):302–6, discussion 306–307.

[12] Stockle M, Meyenburg W, Wellek S, Voges GE, Rossmann M, et al. Adjuvant polyche-motherapy of nonorgan-confined bladder cancer after radical cystectomy revisited: long-term results of a controlled prospective study and further clinical experience. J Urol 1995;153(1):47–52.

[13] Lehmann J, Franzaring L, Thuroff J, Wellek S, Stockle M. Complete long-term survival data from a trial of adjuvant chemotherapy vs control after radical cystectomy for locally advanced bladder cancer. BJU Int 2006;97(1):42–7.

[14] Paz-Ares L, Solsona E, Esteban E, Saez A, Gonzalez-Larriba J, et al., editors. Randomized phase III trial comparing adjuvant paclitaxel/gemcitabine/cisplatin (PGC) to observation in patients with resected invasive bladder cancer: results of the Spanish Oncology Genitourinary Group (SOGUG) 99/01 study. ASCO annual meeting proceed-ings; 2010.

[15] Stadler WM, Lerner SP, Groshen S, Stein JP, Shi SR, et al. Phase III study of molecularly targeted adjuvant therapy in locally advanced urothelial cancer of the bladder based on p53 status. J Clin Oncol 2011;29(25):3443–9.

[16] Cognetti F, Ruggeri EM, Felici A, Gallucci M, Muto G, et al. Adjuvant chemotherapy with cisplatin and gemcitabine versus chemotherapy at relapse in patients with muscle-invasive bladder cancer submitted to radical cystectomy: an Italian, multicenter, random-ized phase III trial. Ann Oncol 2012;23(3):695–700.

[17] Advanced Bladder Cancer (ABC) Meta-analysis Collaboration. Adjuvant chemotherapy in invasive bladder cancer: a systematic review and meta-analysis of individual patient data Advanced Bladder Cancer (ABC) Meta-analysis Collaboration. Eur Urol 2005;48 (2):189–99, discussion 199–201.

[18] Skinner DG, Daniels JR, Russell CA, Lieskovsky G, Boyd SD, et al. The role of adjuvant chemotherapy following cystectomy for invasive bladder cancer: a prospective comparative trial. J Urol 1991;145(3):459–64, discussion 464–457.

[19] Bono AV, Benvenuti C, Reali L, Pozzi E, Gibba A, et al. Adjuvant chemotherapy in advanced bladder cancer. Italian Uro-Oncologic Cooperative Group. Prog Clin Biol Res 1989;303:533–40.

[20] Studer UE, Bacchi M, Biedermann C, Jaeger P, Kraft R, et al. Adjuvant cisplatin chemotherapy following cystectomy for bladder cancer: results of a prospective randomized trial. J Urol 1994;152(1):81–4.

[21] Freiha F, Reese J, Torti FM. A randomized trial of radical cystectomy versus radical cystectomy plus cisplatin, vinblastine and methotrexate chemotherapy for muscle invasive bladder cancer. J Urol 1996;155(2):495–9, discussion 499–500.

[22] Otto T, Goebell PJ, Rubben H. Perioperative chemotherapy in advanced bladder cancer—part II: adjuvant treatment. Onkologie 2003;26(5):484–8.

[23] Ruggeri EM, Giannarelli D, Bria E, Carlini P, Felici A, et al. Adjuvant chemotherapy in muscle-invasive bladder carcinoma: a pooled analysis from phase III studies. Cancer 2006;106(4):783–8.

[24] Leow JJ, Martin-Doyle W, Rajagopal PS, Patel CG, Anderson EM, et al. Adjuvant chemotherapy for invasive bladder cancer: a 2013 updated systematic review and meta-analysis of randomized trials. Eur Urol 2014;66(1):42–54.

[25] Svatek RS, Shariat SF, Lasky RE, Skinner EC, Novara G, et al. The effectiveness of off-protocol adjuvant chemotherapy for patients with urothelial carcinoma of the urinary bladder. Clin Cancer Res 2010;16(17):4461–7.

[26] Froehner M, Koch R, Heberling U, Novotny V, Oehlschlaeger S, et al. Decreased overall and bladder cancer-specific mortality with adjuvant chemotherapy after radical cystectomy: multivariable competing risk analysis. Eur Urol 2016;69(6):984–7.

[27] Galsky MD, Stensland K, Sfakianos JP, Mehrazin R, Diefenbach M, et al. Comparative effectiveness of treatment strategies for bladder cancer with clinical evidence of regional lymph node involvement. J Clin Oncol 2016;34(22):2627–35.

Chapter 27

Bladder-Sparing Treatments

Chapter Outline

Bladder Cancer. DOI: http://dx.doi.org/10.1016/B978-0-12-809939-1.00027-8

Chapter 27.1

Radical TURBT: Radical Transurethral Resection of the Bladder Tumor

Kang Su Cho

Yonsei University College of Medicine, Seoul, South Korea

Although organ preservation has emerged as a fundamental goal in the modern oncologic treatment of several malignancies, radical cystectomy is still regarded as standard therapy for locally confined MIBC or high-risk non-muscle-invasive bladder cancer (NMIBC) [1]. It is because bladder cancer differs from many other malignancies in its biologic behavior, and it arises as a field defect that can affect several different locations of the urothelium including the upper tracts [2]. Therefore, organ-sparing protocols for bladder cancer have been less progressive than those for other malignancies. Bladder-sparing protocols have been developed in an attempt to improve the patient's quality of life as well as to provide treatment alternatives for patients who are not surgical candidates.

Interest in transurethral resection of the bladder tumor (TURBT) monotherapy for MIBC arises from two factors. The first is the morbidity of radical cystectomy. Although greatly improved over early reports of radical cystectomy, recent results still demonstrate morbidity and mortality rates of approximately 20% and 2%, respectively, with rates especially high among older individuals [3,4]. In addition, the rate of pathologic T0 stage (pT0) disease seen in patients undergoing post-TURBT radical cystectomy is approximately 10%, confirming that TURBT alone can eradicate the tumor completely in some patients, especially in minimally muscle-invasive disease [1,5−7].

Prior to radical cystectomy, TURBT is performed to confirm the histologic diagnosis. Sometimes, no residual tumor can be found in the cystectomy specimen; this is defined as pT0 stage. The rate of pT0 cystectomy specimens ranges from approximately 6% to 20% [1,5−7]. Recent reported data suggest that pT0 cystectomy specimens indicate a curative therapy [5,7−9]. Pathological T0 cystectomy specimens can be explained by several reasons, including successful neoadjuvant therapy, residual tumors too small to detect in cystectomy specimens, misdiagnosis in previous TURBT, and complete resection throughout the previous TURBT [10,11]. Accordingly, pT0 cystectomy specimen does not necessarily mean the absolute absence of tumor, but these results have raised the question whether radical cystectomy is really necessary in all MIBC.

Several authors have reported studies on the feasibility of TURBT alone for MIBC, and the representative studies are summarized at Table 27.1.1. In 1987, Herr first reported results of his prospective series on the fate of patients with conservatively treated MIBC and subsequently demonstrated 10-year outcomes of patients with MIBC treated by TURBT alone at Memorial Sloan Kettering Cancer Center in 2001 [13,17]. He found that 10-year disease-specific survival was 76% in 99 patients who received TURBT as definitive therapy (57% with bladder preserved) compared with 71% in 52 patients who had immediate cystectomy ($P = 0.3$). Of the 99 patients treated with TURBT, 82% of 73 with T0 on restaging TURBT survived versus 57% of the 26 patients with residual T1 tumor on restaging TURBT ($P = 0.003$). Herr maintains that complete resection of the invasive cancer is critical to success of TURBT as a bladder-sparing strategy and stresses the importance of restaging. The study by Solsona and colleagues is the only other published prospective study that also involves aggressive radical transurethral resection [16,19]. Of 308 patients with muscle-infiltrating disease, 59 (19%) met the inclusion criteria of negative bimanual examination after TURBT and negative biopsies of the base and periphery of the lesion. With a minimum follow-up of more than 15 years, cancer-specific survival rates at 5, 10, and 15 years were 81.9%, 79.5%, and 76.7, respectively; progression-free rates with bladder preserved at 5, 10, and 15 years were 75.5%, 64.9%, and 57.8%, respectively.

All other series using TURBT as a monotherapy are retrospective, but still yield valuable information [14,18,20,21]. Leibovici et al. introduced their experiences of TURBT monotherapy for 27 MIBC patients, when no tumor in restaging TURBT; there was no MIBC recurrence in 66.6% with a median follow-up of 29.4 months [18]. Henry et al. reported a 63% 5-year survival rate for T2a tumors and 38% for T2b disease [14]. These figures were actually superior to those of patients treated with radical cystectomy during the same time interval at their institution. The authors noted that patients treated with TURBT alone were more likely to be older and have significant comorbidities. Other large series show similar results of approximately 50% overall survival (OS) [20,21]. However, not all investigators have demonstrated successful outcomes of TURBT alone for MIBC as previously described [12,15]. Roosen et al. reported that the survival rate was only 37% in patients receiving TURBT monotherapy, and Barnes et al. reported only 31% survival in their study [12,15]. Such studies imply that TURBT monotherapy should not be offered to all patients with muscle-invasive cancer.

Radical treatment means vigorous treatment that aims at the complete cure of a disease rather than the mere relief of symptoms. Accordingly, if TURBT monotherapy for MIBC can be "Radical TURBT," at least two criteria should be met.

TABLE 27.1.1 Contemporary Series of TURBT Monotherapy for the Treatment of MIBC

Author	Year	Study Design	N	Enrollment Criteria	Re-TURBT	Follow-up	Outcomes
Barnes et al. [12]	1977	Retrospective	75	Stage B	ND	A minimum follow-up of more than 5 years	5-year survival: 23/75 (31%) 10-year survival: 10/58 (17%) 15-year survival: 7/45 (16%) 20-year survival: 3/30 (10%)
Herr [13]	1987	Prospective Nonrandomized	45	MIBC	T0 in 20; CIS in 17; T1 in 4; T2 in 4	Median: 5.1 years Range: 3–7 years	Survival rate: 82% (37/45) Patients with functioning bladder: 67% (30/45)
Henry et al. [14]	1988	Retrospective	43	Stage B	ND	Not specified	5-year survival rate in B1: 63% 5-year survival rate in B2: 38%
Roosen et al. [15]	1997	Retrospective	90	All stages, complete TURBT	ND	A median of seven cystoscopies (range 1–41)	Median crude survival: 37 months Median survival in T1: 67 months Median survival in T2: 19 months Median survival in T3: 9 months Median survival in T4: 2 months
Solsona et al. [16]	1998	Prospective Nonrandomized	133	MIBC, complete TURBT, and negative biopsy of tumor bed	ND	Mean: 81.6 months Range: 11–183 months	CSS at 5 and 10 years: 80.59% and 74.5% Bladder preserved at 5 and 10 years: 82.7% Progression: 37 patients (27.8%) Died of disease: 26 patients (19.5%)
Herr [17]	2001	Prospective Nonrandomized	99	MIBC No tumor or NMIBC on Re-TURBT	T0 in 73 T1 in 26	Range: 10–20 years	10-year survival rate: 76% MIBC recurrence: 34 patients Salvage cystectomy: 18 patients Died of disease: 16 patients

Leibovici, et al. [18]	2007	Retrospective	27	MIBC No tumor on Re-TURBT	T0 in all subjects	Median: 29.4 months Range: 3.8–93.2 months	No recurrence: 12 patients (44.4%) NMIBC recurrence: 6 patients (22.2%) Progression: 9 patients (33.3%) Delayed cystectomy: 8 patients (29.6%) Died of disease: 2 patients (7.4%)
Solsona et al. [19]	2010	Prospective Nonrandomized	133	MIBC, complete TURBT, and negative biopsy of tumor bed	ND	A minimum follow-up of more than 15 years	CSS at 5, 10, and 15 years: 81.9%, 79.5%, and 76.7%, respectively Progression-free with bladder preserved at 5, 10, and 15 years: 75.5%, 64.9%, and 57.8%, respectively

CIS, carcinoma in situ; CSS, cancer-specific survival; ND, not done; Re-TURBT, restaging transurethral resection of the bladder tumor.

First, complete endoscopic tumor removal and proper patient selection are essential for successful bladder preservation with TURBT alone. Frequently, tumors may be present beyond the limits of resection, and the established risk of understaging is 30%−50% [3]. Kolozsy reported a series of patients undergoing "differential" TURBT, in which additional tissue was resected at the base and periphery of the lesion after all visible tumor had been resected [22]. Approximately one-third of the lesions had residual tumor in the base and periphery, even after the surgeon resected all visible tumor. Therefore, determining the completeness of TURBT is paramount. Herr used bladder preservation only in patients with superficial disease or no evidence of tumor in restaging TURBT, and he stresses the need for restaging TURBT 2−3 weeks after the original procedure [13,17]. Conversely, Solsona et al. did not perform routine restaging TURBT. They performed bimanual examination and biopsies of the periphery and depth of the tumor bed at the time of initial TURBT [16]. It is still uncertain which method is a more appropriate strategy among restaging TURBT and concomitant biopsies of tumor bed and periphery.

Second, the adequate candidates for radical TURBT are believed to be minimally muscle-invasive disease. It is because superficial muscle-invasive disease (T2a) might have a higher chance of complete tumor removal than deep muscle-invasive disease (T2b) obviously. In addition, the role of lymphadenectomy in radical cystectomy should be taken into the consideration; some retrospective studies have reported associations between extended lymphadenectomy and improved clinical outcomes in patients treated with radical cystectomy [23]. Indeed, the rate of LN metastasis increases from a low of 5%−10% in NMIBC to 15%−20% in pT2a, to 25%−30% in pT2b, and to >40% in pT3−4 [24]. Therefore, if radical TURBT is chosen for MIBC, especially for pT2b disease, the chance of cure throughout the pelvic lymphadenectomy might be missed regardless of endoscopic complete tumor removal.

Meanwhile, surgical proficiency of transurethral operation is the essential point to achieve the own aims of radical TURBT. As previously mentioned, complete endoscopic tumor removal should be confirmed either via biopsies of the periphery and depth of the tumor bed or restaging TURBT. I prefer serial resection biopsies of the tumor bed at initial operation, similar to the technique by Solsona and colleagues, rather than routine restaging TURBT. These resections should be performed layer by layer, and it would not be easy for a beginning surgeon. My techniques are shown in Fig. 27.1.1. First, the gross tumor area is completely removed. Then, tumor bed resection is performed; usually the superficial muscle layer is included in this section. Next, additional resection of muscle layers below the tumor bed is performed until perivesical adipose tissue is exposed. Although I do not perform restaging TURBT routinely, I do also perform restaging TURBT if there is any suspicion for the completeness of TURBT.

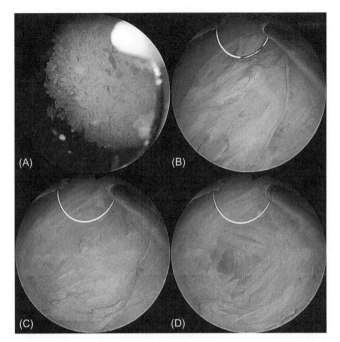

FIGURE 27.1.1 The representative images of radical transurethral resection of the bladder. (A) About three sized papillary mass, (B) complete resection of the gross tumor area, (C) tumor bed resection for superficial muscle layer, and (D) additional resection for deep muscle layer at tumor bed (usually perivesical adipose tissue is exposed).

Currently, radical TURBT can be a feasible option in selected MIBC patients. Endoscopic complete removal and subsequent determining of completeness of TURBT, either via restaging TURBT or biopsies for the tumor bed, should be achieved. Surgical proficiency is also very important factor for successful outcomes. Minimally muscle-invasive disease is regarded as the adequate candidate for radical TURBT. Although some series have shown that radical TURBT can be a viable modality for bladder preservation with favorable outcomes, it cannot be the evidence to justify bladder preservation in deep MIBC with TURBT alone. Notably, physicians should keep in mind that the chance of cure throughout radical cystectomy and the pelvic lymphadenectomy might be missed when selecting radical TURBT in MIBC patients and discuss with patients about these issues.

REFERENCES

[1] Stein JP, Lieskovsky G, Cote R, Groshen S, Feng AC, Boyd S, et al. Radical cystectomy in the treatment of invasive bladder cancer: long-term results in 1,054 patients. J Clin Oncol 2001;19:666−75.

[2] Bradley BA, Wajsman Z. The role of chemotherapy and radiation in organ-preservation strategies for muscle-invasive bladder cancer. World J Urol 2002;20:167−74.

[3] Pagano F, Bassi P, Galetti TP, Meneghini A, Milani C, Artibani W, et al. Results of contemporary radical cystectomy for invasive bladder cancer: a clinicopathological study with an emphasis on the inadequacy of the tumor, nodes and metastases classification. J Urol 1991;145:45−50.

[4] Stroumbakis N, Herr HW, Cookson MS, Fair WR. Radical cystectomy in the octogenarian. J Urol 1997;158:2113−17.

[5] Palapattu GS, Shariat SF, Karakiewicz PI, Bastian PJ, Rogers CG, Amiel G, et al. Cancer specific outcomes in patients with pT0 disease following radical cystectomy. J Urol 2006;175:1645−9. discussion 9.

[6] Thrasher JB, Frazier HA, Robertson JE, Paulson DF. Does of stage pT0 cystectomy specimen confer a survival advantage in patients with minimally invasive bladder cancer? J Urol 1994;152:393−6.

[7] Volkmer BG, Kuefer R, Bartsch Jr. G, Straub M, de Petriconi R, Gschwend JE, et al. Effect of a pT0 cystectomy specimen without neoadjuvant therapy on survival. Cancer 2005;104:2384−91.

[8] Lee SE, Jeong IG, Ku JH, Kwak C, Lee E, Jeong JS. Impact of transurethral resection of bladder tumor: analysis of cystectomy specimens to evaluate for residual tumor. Urology 2004;63:873−7. discussion 7.

[9] Kassouf W, Spiess PE, Brown GA, Munsell MF, Grossman HB, Siefker-Radtke A, et al. P0 stage at radical cystectomy for bladder cancer is associated with improved outcome independent of traditional clinical risk factors. Eur Urol 2007;52(3):769−74.

[10] Coblentz TR, Mills SE, Theodorescu D. Impact of second opinion pathology in the definitive management of patients with bladder carcinoma. Cancer 2001;91:1284−90.

[11] Jones EC. Urinary bladder. Mimics of neoplasia and new pathologic entities. Urol Clin North Am 1999;26:509−34. vi.

[12] Barnes RW, Dick AL, Hadley HL, Johnston OL. Survival following transurethral resection of bladder carcinoma. Cancer Res 1977;37:2895−7.

[13] Herr HW. Conservative management of muscle-infiltrating bladder cancer: prospective experience. J Urol 1987;138:1162−3.

[14] Henry K, Miller J, Mori M, Loening S, Fallon B. Comparison of transurethral resection to radical therapies for stage B bladder tumors. J Urol 1988;140:964−7.

[15] Roosen JU, Geertsen U, Jahn H, Weinreich J, Nissen HM. Invasive, high grade transitional cell carcinoma of the bladder treated with transurethral resection. A survival analysis focusing on TUR as monotherapy. Scand J Urol Nephrol 1997;31:39−42.

[16] Solsona E, Iborra I, Ricos JV, Monros JL, Casanova J, Calabuig C. Feasibility of transurethral resection for muscle infiltrating carcinoma of the bladder: long-term follow-up of a prospective study. J Urol 1998;159:95−8. discussion 8−9.

[17] Herr HW. Transurethral resection of muscle-invasive bladder cancer: 10-year outcome. J Clin Oncol 2001;19:89−93.

[18] Leibovici D, Kassouf W, Pisters LL, Pettaway CA, Wu X, Dinney CP, et al. Organ preservation for muscle-invasive bladder cancer by transurethral resection. Urology 2007;70:473−6.

[19] Solsona E, Climent MA, Iborra I, Collado A, Rubio J, Ricos JV, et al. Bladder preservation in selected patients with muscle-invasive bladder cancer by complete transurethral resection of the bladder plus systemic chemotherapy: long-term follow-up of a phase 2 nonrandomized comparative trial with radical cystectomy. Eur Urol 2009;55:911−19.

[20] Flocks RH. Treatment of patients with carcinoma of the bladder. J Am Med Assoc 1951;145:295—301.

[21] O'Flynn JD, Smith JM, Hanson JS. Transurethral resection for the assessment and treatment of vesical neoplasms: a review of 840 consecutive cases. Eur Urol 1975;1:38—40.

[22] Kolozsy Z. Histopathological "self control" in transurethral resection of bladder tumours. Br J Urol 1991;67:162—4.

[23] Cha EK, Donahue TF, Bochner BH. Radical transurethral resection alone, robotic or partial cystectomy, or extended lymphadenectomy: can we select patients with muscle invasion for less or more surgery? Urol Clin North Am 2015;42:189—99. viii.

[24] Shariat SF, Ehdaie B, Rink M, Cha EK, Svatek RS, Chromecki TF, et al. Clinical nodal staging scores for bladder cancer: a proposal for preoperative risk assessment. Eur Urol 2012;61:237—42.

Chapter 27.2

Partial Cystectomy

Sung-Hoo Hong
Seoul St. Mary's Hospital, Seoul, South Korea

INTRODUCTION

Radical cystectomy remains the gold-standard treatment for muscle-invasive bladder cancer (MIBC). However, morbidity and mortality associated with radical cystectomy and its effect on quality of life (QOL) make bladder preservation strategies an appealing alternative in highly selected patients. Partial cystectomy for the treatment of MIBC has historically been maligned after several series reported high recurrence rates and poor oncologic outcomes [1—3]. However, several studies demonstrated favorable results without compromising survival compared with radical cystectomy in carefully selected patients [4—7].

Partial cystectomy has several advantages over radical cystectomy. It offers maintenance of an intact bladder and voiding function, preservation of sexual function in male patients, and the lack of upper tract deterioration. In addition, perioperative morbidity and postoperative complications are minimal compared with radical cystectomy with urinary diversion. Disadvantage of partial cystectomy is the high recurrence of the tumor in the remained bladder. Local recurrence rates range from 40% to 70% after partial cystectomy [1]. Despite vigilant follow-up, 5%—10% of these patients will eventually require a radical cystectomy for disease progression.

PATIENT SELECTION

Selection criteria for partial cystectomy are a subject of continued debate. Traditionally, partial cystectomy has been indicated in two distinctly separate groups of patients: those who are unable or unwilling to undergo radical cystectomy and those with limited disease such as urachal adenocarcinoma and isolated urothelial carcinoma in diverticulum (Table 27.2.1). Patient selection for partial cystectomy can be challenging. Candidates for partial cystectomy include no history of previous urothelial cancer, solitary tumor in favorable locations without coexisting carcinoma in situ (CIS), and tumor amenable to complete resection with a negative margin. Patients must have a bladder volume that allows for resection of the diseased site with an adjacent 2-cm margin while still maintaining adequate functional capacity with normal compliance. Multifocal disease and CIS are at high risk for new development of tumor.

Age should be not the indication for partial cystectomy. Some authors insisted that partial cystectomy should be avoided if ureteral reimplantation would be required [5,8]. Although there are limited evidences to exclude these patients, it helped to minimize the chance of selecting patients who would be at increased risk to have less than 2-cm surgical margin of normal bladder if ureteral implantation was not performed as intended.

Urachal carcinoma is a tumor occurring most often at the junction of the urachal ligament and bladder dome. It accounts for less than 1% of bladder

TABLE 27.2.1 Indications and Contraindications of Partial Cystectomy

Indications

Solitary tumor in favorable location

Tumor in vesical diverticulum

Urachal tumor

En bloc resection for tumor invasion from other organ into bladder

Contraindications

Multiple tumors

Coexisting CIS

Recurrent tumors

History of bladder cancer

Inability to obtain a 2-cm surgical margin

Tumor located at the trigone or bladder neck

Resulting reduction of bladder capacity by >50%

cancers and approximately 40% of vesical adenocarcinomas [9,10]. The surgical approach has leaned more towards bladder sparing because the published reports do not seem to support a survival advantage with radical surgery [11−13].

Tumors that present within a vesical diverticulum are associated poor risk. Typically, there is no detrusor muscle overlying these tumors, and they can metastasize much easier. Transurethral resection has the increased risk of tumor spillage caused by perforation of the diverticulum. Partial cystectomy appears to give adequate local disease control for tumors in a diverticulum. Five-year survival is less than 10% in patients treated with either radical or partial cystectomy alone [14].

Preoperative evaluation before partial cystectomy should include cystoscopic examination of the tumor and biopsy should be obtained from the lesion and adjacent mucosa to identify the presence of CIS.

SURGICAL TECHNIQUES

Either a transperitoneal or an extraperitoneal approach can be used. The transperitoneal approach is recommended for posterior tumors, and the extraperitoneal approach is possible for dome or anterior tumors.

Open Technique

The patient is placed in a supine position and in the Trendelenburg position to allow displacement of the peritoneal contents cephalad. Foley catheter is inserted after draping of the patient. A lower midline incision is made from below the umbilicus to the symphysis pubis. Once the anterior rectus fascia has been incised and the rectus muscles have been separated in the midline, the transversalis fascia is incised and the Retzius space is developed bluntly. Pelvic lymphadenectomy is performed from the bifurcation of the common iliac artery down to the obturator fossa. After the bladder dissection is complete, the bladder is drained. Tumor is palpated within the bladder, and the bladder is opened through a midline cystostomy directed between two stay sutures. Suction is used to remove the residual fluid in the bladder. Electrocautery is used to incise the mucosa circumferentially around the tumor with 2-cm margin. It is then used to complete the excision of the tumor. Bladder is closed in two layers with absorbable sutures. The wound is irrigated copiously with sterile water to reduce any tumor cells. A closed drain is left in the space of Retzius and should not be placed directly adjacent to the cystostomy closure to minimize fistula formation.

Laparoscopic/Robotic Technique

Although open surgical excision has been the treatment of choice for many years, the laparoscopic or robotic approach has become an attractive alternative because of its association with less postoperative pain, better cosmesis, and rapid convalescence. The patient is placed in the Trendelenburg position. The transperitoneal approach is used with three to five ports in a fan shape. The tumor is inspected, and the peritoneal and preperitoneal tissue between the medial umbilical ligaments is dissected free of the transversalis fascia using a diathermy scissors. Dissection is carried out along the preperitoneal plane toward the umbilicus. The urachus and medial umbilical ligaments are detached just caudal to the umbilicus, maximizing the resection margin cephalad to the urachus. The bladder is distended with 200 mL normal saline to facilitate the mobilization and dissection. The space of the Retzius is entered, and the anterior wall of the bladder is mobilized to the level of the prostatovesical junction to allow subsequent tension-free reconstruction. The bladder is inflated and deflated repeatedly to demarcate the margin of the tumor. A small cystostomy is made using diathermy scissors, 2 cm away from the tumor margin after the bladder is deflated to minimize the tumor spillage. Once it is open, the bladder is distended with gas with the urethral stent clamped. Diathermy scissors are used to incise the mucosa circumferentially around the tumor with a 2-cm safety margin under the direct laparoscopic vision. The specimen is placed within a laparoscopic bag that is clipped to minimize tumor spillage immediately. Frozen biopsies are obtained from the bladder margins if suspected of remnant tumor. Bladder is closed in two layers with absorbable sutures. Watertight closure is confirmed by filling the bladder with 200 mL of normal saline. The wound is irrigated copiously with sterile water to reduce any tumor cells. A closed drain is left in the space of Retzius and should not be placed directly adjacent to the cystostomy closure to minimize fistula formation. The whole specimen is removed through the extended incision of the supraumbilical port.

Novel Techniques

Kim et al. [15] described a technique using cystoscopic tattooing to assist in locating tumor and determine appropriate resection margins during laparoscopic partial cystectomy. Under cystoscopic guidance, a fine needle and India ink are used to mark the lesion at 1 cm away from the outer margin of the lesion with adequate depth into the deep muscle layer. Laparoscopic partial cystectomy is then performed via a transperitoneal approach. After identifying the tattooed area around the mass, the bladder wall was incised by using monopolar electrocautery or ultrasonic shears following tattooing in the deflated state of the bladder.

Hockenberry et al. [16] described a technique using near-infrared fluorescence imaging without contrast agents, like indocyanine green, to identify otherwise obscured intraluminal areas of interest during robot-assisted laparoscopic surgery marked by the white light of endoscopic instruments. By filtering light wavelengths below near infrared, near-infrared fluorescence imaging causes the white light of the endoscopes to illuminate green while allowing simultaneous vision of the surrounding tissues. Cystoscopic illumination of the tumor during robot-assisted laparoscopic partial cystectomy enables more precise identification of important areas and successful completion of partial cystectomy.

ONCOLOGIC RESULTS OF PARTIAL CYSTECTOMY

In properly selected patients, partial cystectomy appears to yield survival rates equivalent to those of radical cystectomy (Table 27.2.2). Retrospective case series from Memorial Sloan Kettering Cancer Center [4] and MD Anderson Cancer Center [5] demonstrated 5-year recurrence-free survival ranging from 39% to 67%. A matched case–control study using the Surveillance Epidemiology and End Results database by Capitanio et al. [6] demonstrated similar overall and cancer-specific survival between partial cystectomy and radical cystectomy for MIBC. A more recent series from the Mayo clinic compared 86 partial and 167 radical cystectomy patients among a cohort matched according to patient's age, sex, pathologic tumor stage, and receipt of neoadjuvant chemotherapy [7]. They found no difference in the 10-year metastasis-free survival (61% vs. 66%; $P = 0.63$) or cancer-specific survival (58% vs. 63%; $P = 0.67$) for both groups suggesting that partial cystectomy for the appropriately selected patient does not compromise oncologic outcomes.

Although recent evidences demonstrating partial cystectomy can achieve cancer control comparable to radical cystectomy in properly selected patients, there remains a need to identify factors affecting recurrence and survival after partial cystectomy. Kassouf et al. [5] reported that patients with history of urothelial carcinoma and higher pathological stage had higher recurrence rates and lower survival rates compared with those with primary bladder cancer.

Ma et al. [8] reviewed 101 cases that received partial cystectomy for MIBC retrospectively. The multivariate analysis showed that history of urothelial carcinoma was associated with both cancer-specific survival and recurrence-free survival and weakly associated with overall survival (OS); lymphovascular invasion and ureteral reimplantation were associated with OS, cancer-specific survival, and recurrence-free survival. The authors concluded that history of urothelial carcinoma and ureteral reimplantation should be considered as contraindications for partial cystectomy, and lymphovascular invasion (LVI) is predictive of poor outcomes after partial cystectomy.

TABLE 27.2.2 Outcomes of Partial Cystectomy

Study	No. of Patients	Tumor Stage	Follow-up (Months)	Intravesical Recurrence (%)	Subsequent Radical Cystectomy (%)	5-Year Recurrence-Specific Survival (%)	5-Year Cancer-Specific Survival (%)	5-Year Overall Survival (%)
Holzbeierlein et al. (2004)	58	cTa–4	33.4	19	6.8	NR	NR	69
Kassouf et al. (2006)	37	cT2–3	72.6	24	16.2	39	87	67
Smaldone et al. (2008)	25	cT1–2	45.3	32	32	62	84	70
Capitanio et al. (2009)[a]	1573	pT1-4N1-2M0	64	NR	NR	NR	76.4	57.2
Fahmy et al. (2010)	714		5.2 years	NR	23.7	40.3	NR	49.8
Knoedler et al. (2012)	86	pT1-4N0-1Mx	6.2 years	38	19		58 at 10 years	36 at 10 years
Golombos et al. (2016)[b]	29	cTa–2	37	10	3.4	68	NR	79

NR = not reported.
[a]Surveillance Epidemiology and End Results (SEER) database.
[b]Robot-assisted partial cystectomy.

RECURRENCE FOLLOWING PARTIAL CYSTECTOMY

The major limitations of partial cystectomy are the risk of recurrence and the need for secondary therapies. The reported local recurrence rates following partial cystectomy ranged between 38% and 78% [17], varying significantly among published series due to varied patient selection. Whereas partial cystectomy will address the primary tumor, it will not address metachronous tumors in the remaining urothelium, which represents an at-risk site for recurrence. Kassouf et al. [5] reported 24% 5-year rate of intravesical superficial tumor recurrence and 65% 5-year rate of patient survival with an intact bladder. Knoedler et al. [7] reported that 38% of partial cystectomy patients experienced intravesical recurrence and 19% of patients eventually underwent salvage radical cystectomy. The authors noted a significantly higher rate of extravesical pelvic tumor recurrence after radical cystectomy than after partial cystectomy. Despite this difference, patients treated with radical cystectomy did not have a corresponding increase in the risk of distant recurrence or death from bladder cancer compared with those treated with partial cystectomy. Whereas some patients will recur following partial cystectomy, the lack of survival difference between partial and radical cystectomy may be due to the performance of an extended pelvic lymph node dissection at the time of partial cystectomy [18]. The same surgical principle should be followed for patients undergoing partial cystectomy.

Bruins et al. [19] reported series of 72 patients who underwent salvage radical cystectomy following partial cystectomy. They found that the median time from partial cystectomy to salvage radical cystectomy was 1.6 years. After salvage radical cystectomy, 61.2% had pathologically organ-confined disease, whereas 19.4% had extravesical disease and 19.4% had lymph node−positive disease. Five-year recurrence-free survival and OS following salvage radical cystectomy were 56% and 41%, respectively. On multivariable analysis, the presence of pathological tumor stage $\geq$ pT3a (hazard ratio 6.86, $P < 0.001$) and the presence of lymph node metastases (hazard ratio 8.78, $P < 0.001$) were associated with increased risk of recurrence after salvage radical cystectomy.

Appropriate patient selection for partial cystectomy is essential to decrease the risk of recurrence. Because of the high recurrence rate, lifelong cystoscopy and repeated abdominal and pelvic imaging should be performed. Early detection of organ-confined recurrence results in excellent ability to salvage patients with radical cystectomy [19].

COMPLICATIONS OF PARTIAL CYSTECTOMY

Although perioperative morbidity and postoperative complications are minimal compared with radical cystectomy, little literature exists regarding postop complications of partial cystectomy. Kates et al. [20] utilized the nationwide inpatient sample to examine over 10,000 patients who underwent partial cystectomy for bladder cancer between 2002 and 2008. They found that 15.8% of patients experienced a complication, with a mortality rate of 1.8%. Nonetheless, a complication rate of 15.8% is markedly decreased when compared to radical cystectomy as the 2009 series by Shabsigh et al. [21] found that 67% of radical cystectomy patients experienced an in-hospital complication and 13% had Clavien Grade 3−5 complications. Specific complications for partial cystectomy include reduced bladder capacity and urinary leakage. Tumor spillage during the resection is a concerned complication. Taking care during manipulation of the tumor and irrigating the wound with sterile water before closure may reduce the risk of tumor implantation. The use of a short course of preoperative radiotherapy may be considered to minimize the risk of tumor spillage [22].

PARTIAL CYSTECTOMY AS PART OF A BLADDER PRESERVATION PROTOCOL

Growing evidence suggests that bladder preservation treatments may lead to acceptable oncologic outcomes in carefully selected patients while offering improved QOL through preservation of a functioning bladder [23,24]. The trimodality bladder preservation protocol contributes to the improvement of QOL in MIBC patients, but one of its limitations is recurrence in the preserved bladder; the incidence has increased up to 30% at 5 years in a large series with a long-term follow-up; most of these recurrences develop in the original cancer sites. Several surgical treatment modalities have been described ranging from radical or serial transurethral resection to partial cystectomy with or without chemotherapy. Partial cystectomy as part of bladder preservation protocol has the advantages of allowing for accurate staging through full-thickness examination of the primary tumor and the ability to perform a concomitant bilateral pelvic lymphadenectomy.

A protocol that incorporates partial cystectomy as part of a bladder preservation protocol following an induction course of low-dose chemotherapy and radiation has been described in 183 rigorously selected patients [23]. These patients included those with solitary tumors or well-circumscribed multiple tumors encompassing less than 25% of the bladder surface (excluding the bladder neck or trigone). All patients were appropriately restaged, and 25% underwent partial cystectomy. In all, 5-year cancer-specific survival was 71%. For the 46 patients who underwent chemoradiation followed by partial cystectomy, 5-year cancer-specific and recurrence-free survival was 100% suggesting that this protocol may have great benefit in carefully selected patients.

CONCLUSION

Partial cystectomy can be offered as an equally efficacious alternative to radical cystectomy in highly selected patients. Lifelong follow-up with cystoscopy, urine biomarker, and abdominal imaging is recommended to detect recurrence.

REFERENCES

[1] Resnick MI, O'Conor Jr. VJ. Segmental resection for carcinoma of the bladder: review of 102 patients. J Urol 1973;109:1007−10.

[2] Novick AC, Stewart BH. Partial cystectomy in the treatment of primary and secondary carcinoma of the bladder. J Urol 1976;116:570−4.

[3] Schoborg TW, Sapolsky JL, Lewis Jr. CW. Carcinoma of the bladder treated by segmental resection. J Urol 1979;122:473−5.

[4] Holzbeierlein JM, Lopez-Corona E, Bochner BH, Herr HW, Donat SM, Russo P, et al. Partial cystectomy: a contemporary review of the Memorial Sloan-Kettering Cancer Center experience and recommendations for patient selection. J Urol 2004;172:878−81.

[5] Kassouf W, Swanson D, Kamat AM, Leibovici D, Siefker-Radtke A, Munsell MF, et al. Partial cystectomy for muscle invasive urothelial carcinoma of the bladder: a contemporary review of the M. D. Anderson Cancer Center experience. J Urol 2006;175:2058−62.

[6] Capitanio U, Isbarn H, Shariat SF, Jeldres C, Zini L, Saad F, et al. Partial cystectomy does not undermine cancer control in appropriately selected patients with urothelial carcinoma of the bladder: a population-based matched analysis. Urology 2009;74:858−64.

[7] Knoedler JJ, Boorjian SA, Kim SP, Weight CJ, Thapa P, Tarrell RF, et al. Does partial cystectomy compromise oncologic outcomes for patients with bladder cancer compared to radical cystectomy? A matched case-control analysis. J Urol 2012;188:1115−19.

[8] Ma B, Li H, Zhang C, Yang K, Qiao B, Zhang Z, et al. Lymphovascular invasion, ureteral reimplantation and prior history of urothelial carcinoma are associated with poor prognosis after partial cystectomy for muscle-invasive bladder cancer with negative pelvic lymph nodes. Eur J Surg Oncol 2013;39:1150−6.

[9] von Garrelts B, Moberg A, Ohman U. Carcinoma of the urachus: review of literature and report of two cases. Scand J Urol Nephrol 1971;5:91−3.

[10] el-Mekresh MM, el-Baz MA, Abol-Enein H, Ghoneim MA. Primary adenocarcinoma of the urinary bladder: report of 185 cases. Br Urol 1998;82:206−12.

[11] Santucci RA, True LD, Lange PH. Is partial cystectomy the treatment of choice for mucinous adenocarcinoma of the urachus? Urology 1997;49:536−40.

[12] D'Addessi A, Racioppi M, Fanasca A, La Rocca LM, Alcini E. Adenocarcinoma of the urachus: radical or conservative surgery? A report of a case and a review of the literature. Eur J Surg Oncol 1998;24:131−3.

[13] Ashley RA, Inman BA, Sebo TJ, Leibovich BC, Blute ML, Kwon ED, et al. Urachal carcinoma: clinicopathologic features and long-term outcomes of an aggressive malignancy. Cancer 2006;107:712−20.

[14] Garzotto M, Tewari A, Wajsman Z. Multimodal therapy for tumors in a vesical diverticulum. J Surg Oncol 1996;62:46−8.

[15] Kim BK, Song MH, Yang HJ, Kim DS, Lee NK, Jeon YS, et al. Use of cystoscopic tattooing in laparoscopic partial cystectomy. Korean J Urol 2012;53:401−4.

[16] Hockenberry MS, Smith ZL, Mucksavage P. A novel use of near-infrared fluorescence imaging during robotic surgery without contrast agents. J Endo Urol 2014;28:509−12.

[17] Sweeney PKE, Resnik MI. Partial cystectomy. Urologic Clinics of North America 1992;19:701−11.

[18] Knoedler J, Frank I. Organ-sparing surgery in urology: partial cystectomy. Curr Opin Urol 2015 Mar;25(2):111−15.

[19] Bruins HM, Wopat R, Mitra AP, Cai J, Miranda G, Skinner EC, et al. Long-term outcomes of salvage radical cystectomy for recurrent urothelial carcinoma of the bladder following partial cystectomy. BJU Int 2013;111:E37−42.

[20] Kates M, Gorin MA, Deibert CM, Pierorazio PM, Schoenberg MP, McKiernan JM, et al. In-hospital death and hospital-acquired complications among patients undergoing partial cystectomy for bladder cancer in the United States. Urol Oncol 2014;32. 53.e9-e14.

[21] Shabsigh A, Korets R, Vora KC, Brooks CM, Cronin AM, Savage C, et al. Defining early morbidity of radical cystectomy for patients with bladder cancer using a standardized reporting methodology. Eur Urol 2009;55:164−76.

[22] van der Werf-Messing B. Carcinoma of the bladder treated by suprapubic radium implants. The value of additional external irradiation. Eur J Cancer 1969;5:227−85.

[23] Zietman AL, Sacco D, Skowronski U, Gomery P, Kaufman DS, Clark JA, et al. Organ conservation in invasive bladder cancer by transurethral resection, chemotherapy and radiation: results of a urodynamic and quality of life study on long-term survivors. J Urol 2003;170:1772−6.

[24] Koga F, Kihara K, Yoshida S, Yokoyama M, Saito K, Masuda H, et al. Selective bladder-sparing protocol consisting of induction low-dose chemoradiotherapy plus partial cystectomy with pelvic lymph node dissection against muscle-invasive bladder cancer: oncological outcomes of the initial 46 patients. BJU Int 2012;109:860−6.

Chapter 27.3

Chemotherapy

Joo Yong Lee

Yonsei University College of Medicine, Seoul, South Korea

BLADDER PRESERVATION RATIONALE IN MUSCLE-INVASIVE BLADDER CANCER (MIBC)

In the treatment of MIBC, bladder preservation strategies do not produce outstanding cancer-related outcomes compared to radical cystectomy. However, too few randomized studies have been performed to adequately support this claim. Additionally, radical cystectomy also results in high morbidity. According to some studies at large-scale centers, readmission and mortality rates were 32% and 6%, respectively, within 90 days after radical cystectomy [1]. Goodney et al. found that the readmission rate within 30 days after radical cystectomy is 21%, which was the second highest among high-risk surgeries (after mitral valve replacement, 22%) [2].

Therefore, the focus is turning to treatment methods that can preserve the bladder in MIBC patients while achieving outcomes comparable to radical cystectomy. Bladder preservation strategies could be applied to T2 and T3a urothelial carcinoma patients [3]. They might be reasonable alternatives for patients who cannot undergo surgery because of medical problems or who seek a different treatment method. Bladder preservation strategies could be especially appealing for older, high-risk patients with an increased risk of surgical complications. Bladder preservation strategies must consider tumor location, depth of invasiveness, tumor size, condition of nonmalignant urothelium, and patient condition (e.g., bladder capacity, bladder function, and associated diseases). Generally, these strategies are not appropriate for multiple tumors, tumors larger than 5 cm, or tumors accompanied by carcinoma in situ (CIS), hydronephrosis, or pelvic lymph node metastases [4]. Previously investigated bladder preservation protocols include radical transurethral resection of bladder tumor (TURBT) or partial cystectomy, alone or in combination with chemotherapy, radiation therapy, or concurrent chemoradiotherapy [5].

CHEMOTHERAPY ALONE IN MIBC

It is difficult to achieve stable, complete remission using chemotherapy alone; consequently, the European Association of Urology guidelines do not recommend chemotherapy alone [6]. This recommendation is based on the research showing that the pathological complete remission rate after neoadjuvant chemotherapy alone is only 38% [7]. Chemotherapy alone is inferior to radiotherapy with concurrent radiosensitizing chemotherapy. Currently, chemotherapy is not useful for MIBC treatment without either concurrent radiation therapy or radical cystectomy. However, future developments in chemotherapy agents are expected to improve their ability to achieve effective bladder preservation.

CHEMOTHERAPY WITH BLADDER-SPARING OPERATION

Patients with complete response (CR) on restaging TURBT combined with neoadjuvant chemotherapy could be good candidates for bladder preservation strategies or delay of radical cystectomy. One prospective study treated 104 MIBC patients based on their response to three cycles of neoadjuvant MVAC chemotherapy (methotrexate, vinblastine, doxorubicin, and cisplatin) using TURBT alone (52 patients), partial cystectomy (3 patients), or radical cystectomy (39 patients) [8]. Among the 52 patients who underwent TURBT, 56% either showed CR (pT0) or superficial disease (pTa, T1, or CIS), 44% achieved long-term bladder-intact survival, and the 5-year survival rate was 67%. In a study of 111 T2–T3 MIBC patients considered radical cystectomy candidates who underwent neoadjuvant MVAC chemotherapy, 60 patients achieved CR (T0) on restaging TURBT. A total of 47 patients were selected for bladder-sparing surgery and 17 for radical cystectomy. The 10-year survival was 74% for bladder-sparing surgery patients, while 65% of patients who underwent radical cystectomy survived. Of the bladder-sparing group, 58% maintained intact bladder function.

However, restaging TURBT has limited accuracy in evaluating the extent of bladder cancer. In the Southwest Oncology Group Trial S0219 [9], restaging TURBT was performed in T2–T4a bladder cancer patients after three cycles of chemotherapy including paclitaxel, carboplatin, and gemcitabine. Of 74 patients, 46% showed CR on restaging TURBT. However, 10 received immediate cystectomy and 6 showed persistent tumors in cystectomy specimens. The authors stated that even when patients who completed chemotherapy achieve cT0 status, definitive local therapy must be considered before surveillance.

CHEMORADIATION

Concurrent cisplatin-based chemotherapy and radiotherapy is the most popular and widely used chemoradiation method because cisplatin is radioactivity sensitive. After complete TURBT, external beam radiotherapy is generally performed in doses of 40 Gy in four fields. Cisplatin is given in the first and fourth weeks, at varying doses. If remaining bladder cancer tissue is detected during cystoscopic reevaluation, radical cystectomy is recommended. If CR is observed, additional cisplatin and 25 Gy of external beam radiotherapy are administered, and progress is monitored by urine cytology and cystoscopy.

Several prospective clinical research results proved the validity of this method. The RTOG 89-03 study investigated 123 cT2–T4a MIBC patients undergoing radiotherapy and concurrent cisplatin, with or without MCV (methotrexate, cisplatin, and vinblastine) chemotherapy prior to radiation, and the 5-year survival rates of the two groups were both approximately 49% [10]. In RTOG 95-06, 34 patients were treated with radiotherapy twice a day and concurrent 5-FU and cisplatin, and the 3-year survival rate was 83% [11]. In RTOG 97-06, 47 TURBT patients were treated with radiotherapy twice a day and concurrent cisplatin before adjuvant chemotherapy with MCV, and the 3-year survival rate was 61% [12]. In RTOG 99-06, 80 TURBT patients were treated with an induction therapy of cisplatin and paclitaxel concurrent with radiotherapy, followed by additional adjuvant cisplatin and gemcitabine, and the 5-year survival rate was 56% [13]. Additionally, the complete remission rate was 59%–81%. Performing radiotherapy twice a day while simultaneously administering cisplatin and paclitaxel or 5-FU appears to be an effective alternative treatment. Cisplatin, cisplatin and 5-FU, 5-FU and mitomycin C, or cisplatin and paclitaxel are radiosensitizing therapies appropriate for use in bladder-preserving chemoradiation after TURBT [14].

CONCLUSION

Bladder preservation strategies are considered effective methods to replace radical cystectomy for selected MIBC patients. Among bladder preservation strategies, chemotherapy alone is not generally recommended, but there is an expectation of future developments in chemotherapy agents that may change this. Combining chemotherapy with a bladder-sparing operation (e.g., TURBT or partial cystectomy), concurrent radiotherapy, or both is effective, but large-scale randomized studies must confirm this. To achieve CR to treatment while maintaining bladder structure and function, it is important that urologists, medical oncologists, and radiation oncologists cooperate to implement a multimodal approach.

REFERENCES

[1] Aghazadeh MA, Barocas DA, Salem S, Clark PE, Cookson MS, Davis R, et al. Determining factors for hospital discharge status after radical cystectomy in a large contemporary cohort. J Urol 2011;185:85−9.

[2] Goodney PP, Stukel TA, Lucas FL, Finlayson EV, Birkmeyer JD. Hospital volume, length of stay, and readmission rates in high-risk surgery. Ann Surg 2003;238:161−7.

[3] Mak RH, Zietman AL, Heney NM, Kaufman DS, Shipley WU. Bladder preservation: optimizing radiotherapy and integrated treatment strategies. BJU Int 2008;102:1345−53.

[4] Balar A, Bajorin DF, Milowsky MI. Management of invasive bladder cancer in patients who are not candidates for or decline cystectomy. Ther Adv Urol 2011;3:107−17.

[5] Yafi FA, Cury FL, Kassouf W. Organ-sparing strategies in the management of invasive bladder cancer. Expert Rev Anticancer Ther 2009;9:1765−75.

[6] Witjes JA, Comperat E, Cowan NC, De Santis M, Gakis G, Lebret T, et al. EAU guidelines on muscle-invasive and metastatic bladder cancer: summary of the 2013 guidelines. Eur Urol 2014;65:778−92.

[7] Grossman HB, Natale RB, Tangen CM, Speights VO, Vogelzang NJ, Trump DL, et al. Neoadjuvant chemotherapy plus cystectomy compared with cystectomy alone for locally advanced bladder cancer. N Engl J Med 2003;349:859−66.

[8] Sternberg CN, Pansadoro V, Calabro F, Schnetzer S, Giannarelli D, Emiliozzi P, et al. Can patient selection for bladder preservation be based on response to chemotherapy? Cancer 2003;97:1644−52.

[9] deVere White RW, Lara Jr. PN, Goldman B, Tangen CM, Smith DC, Wood Jr. DP, et al. A sequential treatment approach to myoinvasive urothelial cancer: a phase II Southwest Oncology Group trial (S0219). J Urol 2009;181:2476−80. discussion 80−1.

[10] Shipley WU, Winter KA, Kaufman DS, Lee WR, Heney NM, Tester WR, et al. Phase III trial of neoadjuvant chemotherapy in patients with invasive bladder cancer treated with selective bladder preservation by combined radiation therapy and chemotherapy: initial results of Radiation Therapy Oncology Group 89-03. J Clin Oncol 1998;16:3576−83.

[11]   Kaufman DS, Winter KA, Shipley WU, Heney NM, Chetner MP, Souhami L, et al. The initial results in muscle-invading bladder cancer of RTOG 95-06: phase I/II trial of transurethral surgery plus radiation therapy with concurrent cisplatin and 5-fluorouracil followed by selective bladder preservation or cystectomy depending on the initial response. Oncologist 2000;5:471−6.

[12]   Hagan MP, Winter KA, Kaufman DS, Wajsman Z, Zietman AL, Heney NM, et al. RTOG 97-06: initial report of a phase I-II trial of selective bladder conservation using TURBT, twice-daily accelerated irradiation sensitized with cisplatin, and adjuvant MCV combination chemotherapy. Int J Radiat Oncol Biol Phys 2003;57:665−72.

[13]   Kaufman DS, Winter KA, Shipley WU, Heney NM, Wallace III HJ, Toonkel LM, et al. Phase I-II RTOG study (99-06) of patients with muscle-invasive bladder cancer undergoing transurethral surgery, paclitaxel, cisplatin, and twice-daily radiotherapy followed by selective bladder preservation or radical cystectomy and adjuvant chemotherapy. Urology 2009;73:833−7.

[14]   Mitin T, Hunt D, Shipley WU, Kaufman DS, Uzzo R, Wu CL, et al. Transurethral surgery and twice-daily radiation plus paclitaxel-cisplatin or fluorouracil-cisplatin with selective bladder preservation and adjuvant chemotherapy for patients with muscle invasive bladder cancer (RTOG 0233): a randomised multicentre phase 2 trial. Lancet Oncol 2013;14:863−72.

FURTHER READING

Herr HW, Faulkner JR, Grossman HB, Natale RB, deVere White R, Sarosdy MF, et al. Surgical factors influence bladder cancer outcomes: a cooperative group report. J Clin Oncol 2004;22:2781−9.

Chapter 27.4

Multimodality Therapy in Bladder-Sparing Treatment of Muscle-Invasive Bladder Cancer

Richard J. Lee
Harvard Medical School and Massachusetts General Hospital Cancer Center, Boston, MA, United States

INTRODUCTION

The past five decades have witnessed the embrace of organ-preserving therapies for a variety of cancers including anal carcinoma, laryngeal carcinoma, esophageal carcinoma, breast carcinoma, and limb sarcomas. Trimodality therapy (TMT) for definitive treatment of localized MIBC is an established alternative to radical cystectomy. TMT includes the use of chemotherapy, radiation therapy, and limited surgery (transurethral resection of bladder tumor, or TURBT). As such, the coordination of care is best achieved in a multidisciplinary setting with oncology specialists from urology, radiation oncology, and medical oncology. Together, that group must determine the answers to the first key questions:

1. Is the patient's bladder function adequate to warrant preservation?
2. Is the patient's disease appropriate for TMT?
3. Is surgical extirpation a possibility for salvage therapy if TMT is not successful?

Modern TMT and bladder preservation has benefited from improved radiation techniques and refinements in chemotherapy regimens. For appropriately selected patients, TMT offers 5-year overall survival (OS) rates that are comparable to contemporary cystectomy series. The adoption of TMT in the United States remains limited, potentially due to the requisite coordination of care among the involved medical disciplines.

AN UNMET MEDICAL NEED IN MIBC

MIBC is frequently undertreated in the United States. An evaluation of the National Cancer Database included over 28,000 patients with localized T2–T4a MIBC initiating treatment between 2004 and 2008 and revealed that nearly half did not receive "aggressive therapy" [1]. Aggressive therapy was defined as potentially curative therapy in the form of radical or partial cystectomy, or definitive radiation therapy with or without chemotherapy, to a total dose ≥ 50 Gy. In this analysis, 52.5% of patients received aggressive therapy, including 44.9% having surgery and 7.6% having radiation therapy. One-fourth of patients had observation only. Multivariate analyses indicated that patient factors associated with nonreceipt of aggressive therapy included advanced age, lower socioeconomic status, black race, lack of access to high-volume centers, higher Charlson comorbidity score, and the presence of hydronephrosis or hydroureter. Treatment with observation occurred in over 25% of patients aged 70–79 years and nearly 40% of patients aged 80–89 years.

Access to health care and management of MIBC in patients who are considered "unfit" due to age or comorbid conditions represents clear unmet medical needs. With broader uptake of selective bladder preservation, TMT could bridge this important gap in the care of MIBC patients.

OVERVIEW OF TMT APPROACHES

There are two general approaches that have garnered the most clinical experience and published reports (Fig. 27.4.1). A North American contemporary TMT bladder-sparing therapy algorithm consists of [2,3]:

1. maximal safe TURBT,
2. "induction" external beam radiation therapy (target dose: 40 Gy) with concurrent radiosensitizing chemotherapy,
3. cystoscopic assessment of treatment response with prompt cystectomy for nonresponders,
4. "consolidation" external beam radiation therapy (to a total dose of 64−66 Gy) with concurrent chemotherapy for responders,
5. adjuvant chemotherapy, and
6. long-term, active cystoscopic surveillance with salvage cystectomy for muscle-invasive recurrence and standard intravesical management for non-muscle-invasive recurrence.

This approach is truly trimodal and requires the coordination of urologic evaluations, radiation therapy, and radiation-sensitizing chemotherapy. For patients to enter this algorithm, they must be considered reasonable candidates for salvage cystectomy. Additionally, patients should be counseled in advance that if they require cystectomy, the prior pelvic radiation would make an ileal conduit their lone urinary diversion option, given the complications of creating a neobladder in a previously irradiated pelvis.

The second approach is an alternative for patients who are medically unfit for cystectomy, which will hereby be referred to as "definitive chemoradiation." There is no break in chemoradiation for cystoscopic evaluation of response to induction therapy; instead, chemoradiation is given in a defined 6- to 7-week course of daily radiation. A variety of chemoradiation protocols have been described. The published clinical experience with these approaches is further described below.

PATIENT SELECTION

The clinical experience to date has informed the appropriate selection of TMT for MIBC. As per the Introduction section, the key questions are as follows:

1. Is the patient's bladder function adequate to warrant preservation?
2. Is the patient's disease appropriate for TMT?
3. Is surgical extirpation a possibility for salvage therapy if TMT is not successful?

The first question for organ preservation strategies for any malignancy is whether the organ's *function* deserves preservation. Some extensive bladder

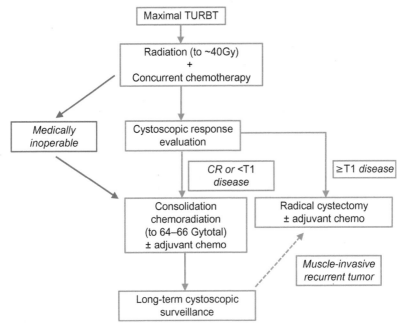

FIGURE 27.4.1   Schema for selective bladder-preserving trimodality therapy. Patients undergo the maximally safe TURBT. For patients who are medically unfit for cystectomy, the path on the left indicates that definitive chemoradiation is prescribed, without a break for cystoscopic response evaluation. For patients who may be fit for salvage cystectomy if needed, a break in chemoradiation after approximately 40 Gy of radiation allows for an evaluation by the urologist to assess for residual disease. Patients with CRs, Ta disease, or CIS may proceed on to consolidation chemoradiation, whereas patients with T1 disease or worse will move to prompt radical cystectomy. For patients with intact bladders after chemoradiation, long-term cystoscopic surveillance is prescribed, with intravesical therapies for non-muscle-invasive bladder recurrence or radical cystectomy for muscle-invasive recurrence.

tumors restrict the bladder's capacity such that the patient cannot hold a sufficient amount of urine, and therefore their quality of life (QOL) may be significantly diminished due to urinary frequency, urgency, or even incontinence. Despite maximal tumor resection and definitive therapy, such patients with poor pretreatment function are unlikely to enjoy a dramatic improvement in bladder function posttherapy and are therefore probably best managed with radical cystectomy.

Successful TMT is associated with several pretreatment features on multivariate analysis (Table 27.4.1) [4]. Older age, higher clinical stage, hydronephrosis, and tumor-associated carcinoma in situ (CIS) are associated with worse OS. Age, however, is not associated with disease-specific survival (DSS; see below). A visibly complete resection at TURBT is associated with the ability to preserve the bladder (bladder-intact DSS).

TABLE 27.4.1 Multivariate Analyses for OS, DSS, and Bladder-Intact DSS

Covariate	Comparison	OS			DSS			Bladder-Intact DSS		
		HR	P-value	95% CI	HR	P-value	95% CI	HR	P-value	95% CI
Age at diagnosis	Continuous	1.03	<0.001	1.01–1.04						
Clinical T stage	T2 vs T3/T4a	0.57	<0.001	0.44–0.75	0.51	<0.001	0.36–0.73			
Response to chemoradiation	Complete vs incomplete	0.61	0.001	0.46–0.81	0.49	<0.001	0.34–0.71	0.16	<0.001	0.12–0.21
Hydronephrosis	Presence vs absence	1.51	0.02	1.06–2.15				1.89	<0.001	1.33–2.63
Tumor-associated CIS	Presence vs absence	1.56	0.002	1.17–2.08	1.50	0.03	1.03–2.17			
TURBT	Complete vs incomplete							0.72	0.02	0.55–0.96

CI, confidence interval.

Source: Reproduced from table 4 of Giacalone NJ, Shipley WU, Clayman RH, Niemierko A, Drumm M, Heney NM, et al. Long-term outcomes after bladder-preserving tri-modality therapy for patients with muscle-invasive bladder cancer: an updated analysis of the Massachusetts General Hospital experience. Eur Urol 2017;71(6):952–60; permission may be required.

Salvage therapy for MIBC disease recurrence is an important consideration for selection of a specific TMT approach. Patients who are unfit for cystectomy either as upfront treatment of MIBC or as salvage therapy for recurrence after TMT are best served with definitive chemoradiation.

At our institution, our general approach for MIBC is as follows. If the bladder tumor is locally advanced (T4) or associated with hydronephrosis, extensive CIS, or poor overall function (and QOL), those patients will not benefit from bladder preservation and therefore are offered radical cystectomy with or without neoadjuvant chemotherapy. The remaining patients may be considered for TMT. If the patient is fit for cystectomy, we consider the North American approach with induction chemoradiation, with early salvage cystectomy if there is incomplete response to induction therapy or evidence of MIBC recurrence after completion of TMT. For patients who are unfit for cystectomy, we use the definitive chemoradiation approach. Prognostic nomograms have been developed to predict complete response (CR), DSS, and bladder-intact DSS, using clinical T stage, presence of hydronephrosis, possibility of a visibly complete TURBT, age, gender, and tumor grade [5].

DOES CHEMOTHERAPY MATTER?

When evaluating a patient for bladder preservation, given the older age and comorbidities commonly seen in the bladder cancer patient cohort, the medical team must judge whether the patient can tolerate chemotherapy. Considerations commonly include performance status, renal function, presence of baseline neuropathy, and hematopoietic function among others. What, then, is the benefit of chemotherapy? The German experience from the University of Erlangen and the University of Halle indicates a substantial improvement in CR rate when chemotherapy is added to radiation therapy [6]. The CR rate for radiation alone was 57%, but addition of carboplatin had 64% CR rate, cisplatin had 81% CR rate, and combined cisplatin with 5-fluorouracil (5-FU) had 87% CR rate. In addition to demonstrating the benefit of chemotherapy with radiation, these data suggest the superiority of cisplatin-based treatment over carboplatin. Additionally, these data, combined with studies from the United States and the United Kingdom summarized below, illustrate that successful TMT for bladder preservation is not restricted to a single institution's or country's experience.

TMT: THE RTOG/MGH EXPERIENCE

The North American experience with TMT has largely been shaped by a series of protocols run through the Radiation Therapy Oncology Group (RTOG, which was incorporated into a larger cooperative group known as NRG in 2014). Most of the patient accrual and protocol development occurred at the Massachusetts General Hospital (MGH). The MGH experience with 475 patients enrolled on protocols between 1986 and 2013 was recently updated with a median follow-up of 7.21 years for surviving patients [4]. This update summarizes the successive protocols that incorporated improvements in radiation, chemotherapy, and surgery, as well as patient selection. Notably, when evaluating patients treated among different eras (1986−95, 1996−2004, 2005−13), rates of CR to chemoradiation, OS, DSS, and bladder-intact DSS all significantly improved, while rates of salvage cystectomy fell (Table 27.4.2).

Iterative TMT protocols evaluated neoadjuvant chemotherapy, adjuvant chemotherapy, different schedules of radiation (daily or twice daily), and different regimens of radiation-sensitizing chemotherapy (cisplatin monotherapy, cisplatin with 5-FU, cisplatin with paclitaxel, and gemcitabine monotherapy). The maximum dose of radiation to the tumor was 64−66 Gy.

TABLE 27.4.2 Evolving Rates of CR, Survival, and Salvage Cystectomy Among Different Treatment Eras on RTOG/MGH Protocols

Time Period	1986−95	1996−2004	2005−13	P-value
n	208	158	109	
Response to Chemoradiation, n (%)				<0.001
Complete	132 (66)	128 (81)	96 (88)	
Incomplete	68 (34)	30 (19)	13 (12)	
OS (%)				<0.001
5-year	53	53	75	
10-year	35	35		
DSS (%)				<0.001
5-year	60	64	84	
10-year	54	56		
Risk of Salvage Cystectomy (%)				<0.001
5-year	42	21	16	
10-year	43	21		
Bladder-Intact DSS (%)				<0.001
5-year	40	53	75	
10-year	37	49		

Source: Reproduced from the top portion of table 3 of Giacalone NJ, Shipley WU, Clayman RH, Niemierko A, Drumm M, Heney NM, et al. Long-term outcomes after bladder-preserving trimodality therapy for patients with muscle-invasive bladder cancer: an updated analysis of the Massachusetts General Hospital experience. Eur Urol 2017;71(6):952−60; permission may be required.

In general, patients underwent concurrent cisplatin-based chemotherapy and radiation therapy after maximal TURBT. Repeat biopsy was performed after 40 Gy, with initial tumor response guiding subsequent therapy. Patients with CR (or Ta or CIS) then received consolidation with additional chemotherapy and radiation for a total dose of 64−65 Gy. Patients were then followed with close cystoscopic surveillance, with prompt salvage cystectomy for tumor persistence or an invasive recurrence. While two protocols incorporated neoadjuvant chemotherapy, the most recent protocols (RTOG 9706, 9906, 0233, and 0712) used adjuvant chemotherapy for all patients, primarily with combined cisplatin and gemcitabine for four cycles [4].

At present, for patients treated according to the RTOG/MGH experience, our current standard (which comprises the control arm for randomized trials comparing other TMT approaches) involves maximal TURBT followed by "induction" twice-daily radiation to 40.3 Gy over 26 fractions along with cis-platin (15 mg/m^2 on Days 1−3, 8−10, 15−17) and continuous infusion 5-FU (400 mg/m^2 on Days 1−3, 15−17). Patients with postinduction TURBT downstaging to T0 (CR), CIS, or Ta disease proceed on to "consolidation" twice-daily radiation to a total of 64.3 Gy (8 additional treatment days) with the same chemotherapy as in induction. If postconsolidation TURBT again shows no evidence of MIBC, patients then receive adjuvant chemotherapy with four cycles of cisplatin (70 mg/m^2 on Day 1 of 21-day cycles) and gem-citabine (1000 mg/m^2 on Days 1 and 8 of 21-day cycles) [7].

In the most recent update, 75% of patients achieved CR to induction ther-apy [4]. One hundred twenty-nine patients (27%) underwent salvage radical cystectomy, with 65 for incomplete response after induction chemoradiation and 64 for recurrent invasive tumors on posttreatment surveillance. Of note, 5-, 10-, and 15-year DSS rates were 66%, 59%, and 56%, and OS rates were 57%, 39%, and 25%, respectively (Fig. 27.4.2); and 5-, 10-, and 15-year bladder-intact DSS rates were 52%, 46%, and 40%, respectively.

Multivariate analyses identified disease features and patient factors that were associated with OS, DSS, and bladder-intact DSS (Table 27.4.1). The iterative analyses leading to improvements of these successive protocols undoubtedly led to improved patient selection and results. The importance of a visibly complete TURBT, previously shown by single institutions in the United States [8] and Europe [9], and later supported by RTOG data [10], was again demonstrated in this publication; among patients who had visibly complete TURBT, only 24% required cystectomy, in contrast with 43% with incomplete TURBT ($P < 0.001$) [4].

Thus, in long-term follow-up, *selective* bladder-preserving TMT is associ-ated with a high rate (71% at 5 years) of bladder preservation and OS that is comparable to contemporary radical cystectomy series (Table 27.4.3). In addition, DSS was not significantly different between patients older or youn-ger than 75 years ($P = 0.84$) [3], providing evidence that TMT may be a

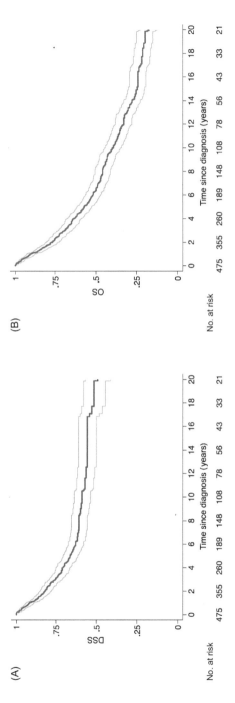

FIGURE 27.4.2 Kaplan–Meier plots of (A) DSS and (B) OS from a cohort of 475 patients treated with TMT on RTOG/MGH protocols between 1986 and 2013 [4]. *Source: Reproduced from figure 1 of Giacalone NJ, Shipley WU, Clayman RH, Niemierko A, Drumm M, Heney NM, et al. Long-term outcomes after bladder-preserving tri-modality therapy for patients with muscle-invasive bladder cancer: an updated analysis of the Massachusetts General Hospital experience. Eur Urol 2017;71(6):952–60; permission may be required.*

TABLE 27.4.3 MIBC: Survival Outcomes Following Curative-Intent Therapy in Contemporary Series

	Stage	N	5-Year OS	10-Year OS
Radical Cystectomy				
USC, 2001 [11]	pT2−4a	633	48%	32%
MSKCC, 2001 [12]	pT2−4a	181	36%	27%
SWOG/ECOG/CALGB,[a,b] 2003 [13]	cT2−3	303	49%	34%
Trimodality Therapy				
RTOG,[a] 1998 [10]	cT2−4a	123	49%	
Erlangen,[a] 2002 [6,9]	cT2−4	326	45%	29%
BC2001,[a] 2012 [14]	cT2−4a	182	48%	
RTOG pooled,[a] 2014 [3]	cT2−4a	468	57%	36%
MGH,[a] 2017 [4]	cT2−4a	475	57%	39%

[a]These series include all patients by their intention to treat.
[b]50% of patients were randomly assigned to receive three cycles of neoadjuvant chemotherapy (MVAC).

suitable alternative for patients whose age or comorbidities preclude radical cystectomy.

DEFINITIVE CHEMORADIATION

As described in the introduction, definitive chemoradiation is an alternative bladder-sparing approach for patients who are medically unfit for cystectomy and who would not therefore be eligible for the RTOG/MGH TMT approach described earlier. In this approach, chemoradiation is given in a defined 6- to 7-week course of daily radiation.

One advantage to definitive chemoradiation may be the relative simplicity of a defined course of daily radiation, as opposed to the required coordination of care for twice-daily radiation sessions surrounding cisplatin-based chemotherapy and requisite hydration, in addition to coordination of interim cystoscopic evaluations. A second advantage is that several published definitive chemoradiation regimens do not use cisplatin, which is an important consideration for patients with impaired renal function or poor performance status. Alternative approaches can allow for tailoring of TMT for such patients.

One standard approach was defined by the multicenter Bladder Cancer 2001 (BC2001) study from the United Kingdom [14]. BC2001 was a Phase III study that randomized 360 patients with MIBC with a median age of 72 years to undergo radiotherapy alone (either 55 Gy in 20 fractions or 64 Gy in 32 fractions) or with concurrent chemotherapy, consisting of 5-FU (500 mg/m^2 on Days 1−5 and 22−26) and mitomycin C (12 mg/m^2 only given on Day 1). In this study, 55% of patients underwent a complete TURBT and 33% received neoadjuvant chemotherapy. With a median follow-up of 69.9 months, the 5-year OS rate was 48% in the chemoradiation arm compared with 35% in the radiation-only arm (hazard ratio (HR), 0.82; $P = 0.16$). The primary endpoint of 2-year locoregional disease-free survival (survival free of recurrence in pelvic lymph nodes or bladder) was significantly improved with chemoradiation compared with radiation only, at 67% vs 54%, respectively (HR, 0.68; $P = 0.03$). Fifty-one of 360 patients (14%) underwent cystectomy, with 47 performed for recurrent disease and 4 performed due to late toxicity of radiation therapy. Patients tolerated the combined therapy well, with 36% of patients experiencing Acute Grade 3−4 toxicities, compared with 28% in the radiation-only group. The main toxicities were gastrointestinal (GI), with 9.6% acute and 8.3% Late Grade 3−4 GI toxicities. Although this study did not compare 5-FU and mitomycin C to cisplatin-based chemoradiation, these data established an alternative, effective, and tolerable radiosensitization regimen.

Other less-extensively studied chemoradiation regimens have been described. Definitive chemoradiation for MIBC with twice-weekly paclitaxel (25−35 mg/m^2) and 45−60 Gy is associated with durable local control [15]. Definitive chemoradiation with gemcitabine and 60 Gy over 30 fractions demonstrated that a twice-weekly dose of 27 mg/m^2 is the maximum tolerated dose of gemcitabine, given its potency as a radiation sensitizer, with 5-year OS of 76% in a study of 23 patients [16,17]. The most recent RTOG 0712 trial comparing gemcitabine vs the cisplatin and 5-FU regimen has been accrued but not yet reported.

At the University of Tsukuba, 77 patients with clinical T2−3N0M0 bladder cancer were treated by TURBT, three cycles of intra-arterial chemotherapy consisting of cisplatin at 50 mg/m^2 and methotrexate at 30 mg/m^2 and concurrent radiation therapy to a small pelvic field to a dose of 41.4 Gy (in 23 fractions) [18]. Intra-arterial chemotherapy was delivered by embolization of the superior gluteal arteries bilaterally and infusion of the chemotherapy through the right and the left internal iliac arteries over a period of 2 hours. Patients with CR then received a radiation boost to either 19.8 Gy with photons or 36.3 GyE with protons. Others were offered immediate salvage cystectomy. With a median follow-up of 38.5 months, 22% of patients experienced intravesical recurrence and 6.5% had systemic disease progression. Intra-arterial chemotherapy with radiation offers high rates of local control, although the technical aspect of this type of chemotherapy delivery is likely to limit the appeal of this approach.

SALVAGE CYSTECTOMY AFTER FAILURE OF TMT FOR MIBC

A concern among urologists is that salvage cystectomy is difficult to perform and tolerate in patients in whom bladder preservation therapy fails. Healing of surgical incisions and anastamoses is often cited as a reason to avoid bladder-sparing TMT. Ninety-one patients who underwent salvage cystectomy at the MGH were followed for a median of 12 years and evaluated for surgical complications and long-term survival [19]. The 91 patients included 50 who underwent immediate salvage cystectomy for persistent disease and 41 who underwent delayed salvage cystectomy for a subsequent invasive recurrence. The 90-day operative mortality rate was 2.2% (2 of 91). Fifteen patients (16%) experienced major complications within 90 days. Cardiovascular or hematological complications (pulmonary embolism, myocardial infarction, deep venous thrombosis, or transfusion) were more common in the immediate cystectomy group (37% vs 15%, $P = 0.02$), whereas tissue healing complications (facial dehiscence, wound infection, ureteral stricture, anastomotic stricture, stoma, or loop revision) were more common in the delayed group (35% vs 12%, $P = 0.05$). These surgical complication rates were believed to be acceptable although slightly higher than the rates with cystectomy alone.

A second concern raised by urologists is the general reluctance to construct orthotopic neobladders after pelvic radiation. The majority of patients who require salvage cystectomy undergo a loop diversion. Appropriate patient selection and counseling about the high rate of bladder preservation are critical for optimal success with TMT. It is not known whether 40 Gy of induction chemoradiation will impact the healing and function of neobladders.

QOL AFTER TMT FOR MIBC

Concerns about the impact of chemoradiation on QOL, including bladder function, sexual function, and GI toxicity, among others, have also been cited as reasons to avoid TMT for MIBC. Evaluations to date indicate that these concerns may be overstated. The instruments to assess QOL have been well established for prostate and gynecologic cancers, and have been adapted for patients with bladder cancer.

Long-term bowel and bladder toxicity after chemoradiation was investigated in patients enrolled in prospective RTOG trials [20]. Among 157 patients who underwent TMT for MIBC with a median follow-up of 5.4 years, only 7% experienced late (≥ 180 days after the start of consolidation chemoradiation) Grade 3 pelvic toxicity, 5.7% genitourinary (urinary urgency/frequency, hematuria), and 1.9% GI (sigmoid obstruction, proctitis). There were no late Grade 4 toxicities and no treatment-related deaths.

In a QOL analysis including urodynamic studies (UDS) in 49 TMT patients who responded to a survey of bladder function, the median age of respondents at the time of evaluation was 68.9 years, with a median follow-up of 6.3 years [21]. Of the 32 patients who underwent UDS, 75% (24 of 32) had normal functioning bladders. Reduced bladder compliance was seen in 22% of patients, with only one-third of these patients reporting "distressing" bladder symptoms. Of all female patients evaluated, 11% required wearing pads. Bowel symptoms occurred in 22% of patients and caused any level of distress in 14% of patients. Regarding sexual function, 36% of male patients reported normal erections and another 18% less firm erections, but sufficient for intercourse. A total of 54% were capable of orgasm and 50% of ejaculation. Only 8% of male patients reported being dissatisfied with their sexual function. Only two women completed the sexual function portion of the survey.

In a study that compared QOL in 64 patients who received TMT with 109 patients who underwent radical cystectomy (82% ileal conduit, 18% neobladder), six validated QOL questionnaires were employed [22]. Patients were from high-volume academic medical centers and disease free for ≥ 2 years, with median follow-up of 5.6 years. While both TMT and cystectomy were associated with good long-term QOL outcomes, the areas in which TMT scored markedly favorable compared with radical cystectomy included better sexual QOL, better informed decision-making, less concern about appearance, and less life interference from cancer or cancer treatment.

COMPARISON OF SURVIVAL FOLLOWING CYSTECTOMY VS BLADDER-PRESERVING TMT

A prospective, randomized trial comparing cystectomy and bladder-preserving TMT has not been performed. Comparing results of TMT to those of radical cystectomy series is difficult. One issue is the difference between clinical staging (TURBT) and pathological (cystectomy) staging. Gray et al. analyzed 16,953 patients with bladder cancer in the National Cancer Database [23]. At the time of radical cystectomy, 41.9% of patients were upstaged, with only 5.9% downstaged (with many downstaged patients having received neoadjuvant chemotherapy). Nevertheless, as seen in Table 27.4.3, there is a remarkable similarity in OS rates among surgical series and TMT series.

The TMT patients were all *clinically* staged, and the outcome analyses included all entered patients, not omitting those who did not complete the intended treatment. The similar OS rates may reflect, in part, the prompt use of cystectomy in nonresponders to TMT. However, it should also be acknowledged that patients treated on bladder-preserving TMT protocols are rigorously selected; thus, this population might not be comparable to patients undergoing cystectomies.

THE FUTURE OF TMT FOR MIBC

Based on comparisons of long-term outcomes in contemporary series, TMT in selected patients demonstrates similar disease control and OS compared with radical cystectomy for MIBC. Recent studies of long-term follow-up allay fears of significant rates of late tumor recurrences and of poor bladder function [4,20−22]. For many patients and clinicians, TMT may be an acceptable alternative to radical cystectomy. The European Association of Urology (EAU) and the US National Comprehensive Cancer Network (NCCN) accept bladder preservation for select patients with MIBC, reflecting the growing evidence supporting the use of TMT for MIBC [24,25]. Some health care systems have embraced bladder-sparing treatment modalities; for example, in the United Kingdom, 60% of eligible patients receive multimodality therapy, with surgery reserved for salvage therapy. At the same time, in other countries, such as the United States, only a minority of patients have been offered this strategy, due to historical management, clinician bias, and access and inertia to engage multidisciplinary care, among many other potential reasons.

Further improvements in delivery of treatment and selection of candidates could increase the rate of native bladder retention among patients selected for TMT. For example, intrafraction motion and bladder filling is a concern if the treatment time is long. Improvements in technology, such as faster cone-beam computer tomography (CT) reconstruction times and increased treatment automation could reduce the duration of radiation treatment. Daily CT-guided setup for radiation therapy in MIBC patients has been shown to be superior to daily positioning based on skin tattoos or bony anatomy, allowing for smaller margins [26]. These technology advances will significantly reduce the volume of irradiated small bowel, which could decrease treatment-related toxicity.

Predictive biomarkers of response to TMT would also shape the selection of patients. Retrospective evaluation of RTOG studies identified vascular endothelial growth factor B (VEGF-B) as a potential biomarker [27]. Higher levels of cytoplasmic VEGF-B in pretreatment TURBT specimens were associated with higher rates of distant metastasis and shorter survival. Similarly, overexpression of HER2 (ERB-B2) in bladder cancer cells was associated with reduced CR rate to TMT [28].

A potential predictive marker of radiation sensitivity is MRE11, a DNA damage-signaling protein. MRE11 expression was evaluated in MIBC patients treated with definitive radiation therapy or with cystectomy [29]. High tumor expression of MRE11 predicted for improved outcome with radiation therapy but not by cystectomy. In a cohort of patients undergoing TMT or radical cystectomy, MRE11 and other potential predictive biomarkers were evaluated [30]. Elevated expression of tat-interactive protein 60 kDa (TIP60) was significantly correlated with DSS in the cystectomy cohort but not the radiation cohort. Stratification based on combination of TIP60 and MRE11 staining resulted in significant differences in DSS between cystectomy and radiotherapy cohorts. Cystectomy was associated with better DSS compared with radiotherapy (HR 0.3; $P = 0.01$) in patients whose bladder cancers have low expression of MRE11 and high expression of TIP60, but with worse DSS (HR = 3.58; $P = 0.012$) in patients whose cancers exhibit high expression of MRE11 and low expression of TIP60. These findings require confirmation in prospective trials but may offer a pair of predictive markers to guide treatment decisions of clinicians and patients.

CONCLUSIONS

In selected patients with MIBC, bladder-preserving TMT that reserves cystectomy for tumor recurrence represents a safe and effective alternative to immediate radical cystectomy. The cumulative published data with long-term follow-up of more than 1000 patients in international, single-, and multi-institution cooperative group trials clearly demonstrate that TMT results in excellent local control in 70% of patients, with good preservation of bladder, GI, and sexual function, and no evident compromise of long-term survival.

For appropriate patients who are cystectomy candidates, our preferred TMT approach at MGH uses induction chemoradiation with the possibility of early salvage cystectomy for nonresponders. For patients who are not cystectomy candidates or cannot receive cisplatin, our approach typically employs definitive chemoradiation with 5-FU and mitomycin C.

The critical role of the urologist performing a visibly complete TURBT at entry for TMT consideration, as well as long-term posttreatment cystoscopic surveillance, cannot be overstated. The close coordination of care among urology, radiation oncology, and medical oncology is a common barrier to TMT therapy that needs to be overcome to provide this highly sought alternative to radical surgery for MIBC patients.

The TMT approach can further fill the gap for curative therapy in the nearly 50% of patients who do not receive "aggressive therapy" due to age, comorbidities, and socioeconomic factors [1]. Patients older than 75 years have comparable DSS to younger patients with TMT [3], highlighting the value of TMT to bridge the treatment gap for elderly patients. The incorporation of TMT in high-risk non-muscle-invasive bladder cancer is the subject of ongoing clinical trials. Research efforts are focused on improved selection of patients, greater effectiveness of treatment based on new biomarkers, and improved radiation-based therapy.

REFERENCES

[1] Gray PJ, Fedewa SA, Shipley WU, Efstathiou JA, Lin CC, Zietman AL, et al. Use of potentially curative therapies for muscle-invasive bladder cancer in the United States: results from the National Cancer Data Base. Eur Urol 2013;63(5):823−9. <http://dx.doi.org/10.1016/j.eururo.2012.11.015>.

[2] Housset M, Maulard C, Chretien Y, Dufour B, Delanian S, Huart J, et al. Combined radiation and chemotherapy for invasive transitional-cell carcinoma of the bladder: a prospective study. J Clin Oncol 1993;11(11):2150−7. <http://dx.doi.org/10.1200/jco.1993.11.11.2150>. PubMed PMID: 8229129.

[3] Mak RH, Hunt D, Shipley WU, Efstathiou JA, Tester WJ, Hagan MP, et al. Long-term outcomes in patients with muscle-invasive bladder cancer after selective bladder-preserving combined-modality therapy: a pooled analysis of Radiation Therapy Oncology Group Protocols 8802, 8903, 9506, 9706, 9906, and 0233. J Clin Oncol 2014;32(34):3801−9. <http://dx.doi.org/10.1200/jco.2014.57.5548>. PubMed PMID: 25366678.

[4] Giacalone NJ, Shipley WU, Clayman RH, Niemierko A, Drumm M, Heney NM, et al. Long-term outcomes after bladder-preserving tri-modality therapy for patients with muscle-invasive bladder cancer: an updated analysis of the Massachusetts General Hospital experience. Eur Urol 2017;71(6):952−60. <http://dx.doi.org/10.1016/j.eururo.2016.12.020>.

[5] Coen JJ, Paly JJ, Niemierko A, Kaufman DS, Heney NM, Spiegel DY, et al. Nomograms predicting response to therapy and outcomes after bladder-preserving trimodality therapy for muscle-invasive bladder cancer. Int J Radiat Oncol Biol Phys 2013;86(2):311−16. <http://dx.doi.org/10.1016/j.ijrobp.2013.01.020>.

[6] Rödel C, Grabenbauer GG, Kühn R, Papadopoulos T, Dunst J, Meyer M, et al. Combined-modality treatment and selective organ preservation in invasive bladder cancer: long-term results. J Clin Oncol 2002;20(14):3061−71. <http://dx.doi.org/10.1200/jco.2002.11.027>. PubMed PMID: 12118019.

[7] Mitin T, Hunt D, Shipley WU, Kaufman DS, Uzzo R, Wu C-L, et al. Transurethral surgery and twice-daily radiation plus paclitaxel-cisplatin or fluorouracil-cisplatin with selective bladder preservation and adjuvant chemotherapy for patients with muscle invasive bladder cancer (RTOG 0233): a randomised multicentre phase 2 trial. Lancet Oncol 2013;14(9):863−72. doi: 10.1016/S1470-2045(13)70255-9.

[8] Shipley WU, Prout Jr. GR, Kaufman SD, Perrone TL. Invasive bladder carcinoma. The importance of initial transurethral surgery and other significant prognostic factors for improved survival with full-dose irradiation. Cancer 1987;60(3 Suppl):514−20. Epub 1987/08/01. PubMed PMID: 3297285.

[9] Dunst J, Sauer R, Schrott KM, Kühn R, Wittekind C, Altendorf-Hofmann A. Organ-sparing treatment of advanced bladder cancer: a 10-year experience. Int J Radiat Oncol Biol Phys 1994;30(2):261−6. <http://dx.doi.org/10.1016/0360-3016(94)90003-5>.

[10] Shipley WU, Winter KA, Kaufman DS, Lee WR, Heney NM, Tester WR, et al. Phase III trial of neoadjuvant chemotherapy in patients with invasive bladder cancer treated with selective bladder preservation by combined radiation therapy and chemotherapy: initial results of Radiation Therapy Oncology Group 89-03. J Clin Oncol 1998;16(11):3576−83. <http://dx.doi.org/10.1200/jco.1998.16.11.3576>. PubMed PMID: 9817278.

[11] Stein JP, Lieskovsky G, Cote R, Groshen S, Feng A-C, Boyd S, et al. Radical cystectomy in the treatment of invasive bladder cancer: long-term results in 1,054 patients. J Clin

Oncol 2001;19(3):666−75. <http://dx.doi.org/10.1200/jco.2001.19.3.666>. PubMed PMID: 11157016.

[12] Dalbagni G, Genega E, Hashibe MIA, Zhang Z-F, Russo P, Herr H, et al. Cystectomy for bladder cancer: A contemporary series. J Urol 2001;165(4):1111−16.

[13] Grossman HB, Natale RB, Tangen CM, Speights VO, Vogelzang NJ, Trump DL, et al. Neoadjuvant chemotherapy plus cystectomy compared with cystectomy alone for locally advanced bladder cancer. N Engl J Med 2003;349(9):859−66. <http://dx.doi.org/10.1056/NEJMoa022148>.

[14] James ND, Hussain SA, Hall E, Jenkins P, Tremlett J, Rawlings C, et al. Radiotherapy with or without chemotherapy in muscle-invasive bladder cancer. N Engl J Med 2012;366(16):1477−88. <http://dx.doi.org/10.1056/NEJMoa1106106>. PubMed PMID: 22512481.

[15] Müller A-C, Diestelhorst A, Kuhnt T, Kühn R, Fornara P, Scholz H-J, et al. Organ-sparing treatment of advanced bladder cancer: paclitaxel as a radiosensitizer. Strahlentherapie und Onkologie 2007;183(4):177−83. <http://dx.doi.org/10.1007/s00066-007-1651-z>.

[16] Kent E, Sandler H, Montie J, Lee C, Herman J, Esper P, et al. Combined-modality therapy with gemcitabine and radiotherapy as a bladder preservation strategy: results of a phase I trial. J Clin Oncol 2004;22(13):2540−5. <http://dx.doi.org/10.1200/jco.2004.10.070>. PubMed PMID: 15226322.

[17] Oh KS, Soto DE, Smith DC, Montie JE, Lee CT, Sandler HM. Combined-modality therapy with gemcitabine and radiation therapy as a bladder preservation strategy: long-term results of a phase I trial. Int J Radiat Oncol Biol Phys 2009;74(2):511−17. <http://dx.doi.org/10.1016/j.ijrobp.2008.08.021>.

[18] Onozawa M, Miyanaga N, Hinotsu S, Miyazaki J, Oikawa T, Kimura T, et al. Analysis of intravesical recurrence after bladder-preserving therapy for muscle-invasive bladder cancer. Jpn J Clin Oncol 2012;42(9):825−30. <http://dx.doi.org/10.1093/jjco/hys105>.

[19] Eswara JR, Efstathiou JA, Heney NM, Paly J, Kaufman DS, McDougal WS, et al. Complications and long-term results of salvage cystectomy after failed bladder sparing therapy for muscle invasive bladder cancer. J Urol 2012;187(2):463−8. <http://dx.doi.org/10.1016/j.juro.2011.09.159>.

[20] Efstathiou JA, Bae K, Shipley WU, Kaufman DS, Hagan MP, Heney NM, et al. Late pelvic toxicity after bladder-sparing therapy in patients with invasive bladder cancer: RTOG 89-03, 95-06, 97-06, 99-06. J Clin Oncol 2009;27(25):4055−61. <http://dx.doi.org/10.1200/jco.2008.19.5776>. PubMed PMID: 19636019.

[21] Zietman AL, Sacco D, Skowronski URI, Gomery P, Kaufman DS, Clark JA, et al. Organ conservation in invasive bladder cancer by transurethral resection, chemotherapy and radiation: results of a urodynamic and quality of life study on long-term survivors. J Urol 2003;170(5):1772−6.

[22] Mak KS, Smith AB, Eidelman A, Clayman R, Niemierko A, Cheng J-S, et al. Quality of life in long-term survivors of muscle-invasive bladder cancer. Int J Radiat Oncol Biol Phys 2016;96(5):1028−36. <http://dx.doi.org/10.1016/j.ijrobp.2016.08.023>.

[23] Gray PJ, Lin CC, Jemal A, Shipley WU, Fedewa SA, Kibel AS, et al. Clinical-pathologic stage discrepancy in bladder cancer patients treated with radical cystectomy: results from the National Cancer Data Base.. Int J Radiat Oncol Biol Phys 2014;88(5):1048−56. <http://dx.doi.org/10.1016/j.ijrobp.2014.01.001>.

[24] Gakis G, Efstathiou J, Lerner SP, Cookson MS, Keegan KA, Guru KA, et al. ICUD-EAU International Consultation on Bladder Cancer 2012: radical cystectomy and bladder preservation

for muscle-invasive urothelial carcinoma of the bladder. Eur Urol 2013;63(1):45−57. <http://dx.doi.org/10.1016/j.eururo.2012.08.009>.

[25] Clark PE, Spiess PE, Agarwal N, Bangs R, Boorjian SA, Buyyounouski MK, et al. NCCN guidelines insights: bladder cancer, version 2.2016. J Natl Compr Canc Netw 2016;14(10):1213−24. <http://dx.doi.org/10.6004/jnccn.2016.0131>.

[26] Foroudi F, Pham D, Bressel M, Wong J, Rolfo A, Roxby P, et al. Bladder cancer radiotherapy margins: a comparison of daily alignment using skin, bone or soft tissue. Clin Oncol 2012;24(10):673−81. <http://dx.doi.org/10.1016/j.clon.2012.06.012>.

[27] Lautenschlaeger T, George A, Klimowicz AC, Efstathiou JA, Wu C-L, Sandler H, et al. Bladder preservation therapy for muscle-invading bladder cancers on Radiation Therapy Oncology Group Trials 8802, 8903, 9506, and 9706: vascular endothelial growth factor b overexpression predicts for increased distant metastasis and shorter survival. Oncologist 2013;18(6):685−6. <http://dx.doi.org/10.1634/theoncologist.2012-0461>.

[28] Chakravarti A, Winter K, Wu C-L, Kaufman D, Hammond E, Parliament M, et al. Expression of the epidermal growth factor receptor and Her-2 are predictors of favorable outcome and reduced complete response rates, respectively, in patients with muscle-invading bladder cancers treated by concurrent radiation and cisplatin-based chemotherapy: a report from the Radiation Therapy Oncology Group. Int J Radiat Oncol Biol Phys 2005;62(2):309−17. <http://dx.doi.org/10.1016/j.ijrobp.2004.09.047>.

[29] Choudhury A, Nelson LD, Teo MTW, Chilka S, Bhattarai S, Johnston CF, et al. MRE11 expression is predictive of cause-specific survival following radical radiotherapy for muscle-invasive bladder cancer. Cancer Res 2010;70(18):7017−26. <http://dx.doi.org/10.1158/0008-5472.can-10-1202>.

[30] Laurberg JR, Brems-Eskildsen AS, Nordentoft I, Fristrup N, Schepeler T, Ulhøi BP, et al. Expression of TIP60 (tat-interactive protein) and MRE11 (meiotic recombination 11 homolog) predict treatment-specific outcome of localised invasive bladder cancer. BJU Int 2012;110(11c):E1228−36. <http://dx.doi.org/10.1111/j.1464-410X.2012.11564.x>.

Chapter 28

Quality of Life in Bladder Cancer Patients

Chang Wook Jeong
Seoul National University Hospital, Seoul, South Korea

Chapter Outline

INTRODUCTION

Bladder cancer is the ninth most common cancer, worldwide, with an estimated 430,000 new cases diagnosed in 2012 [1]. In the United States, it is the fourth most common cancer, with 76,960 new cases estimated to be diagnosed during 2016 [2]. Because more than 70% of patients with bladder cancer are initially diagnosed with non-muscle-invasive cancer, there are many bladder cancer survivors. An estimated 765,950 bladder cancer survivors live in the United States [3].

For non-muscle-invasive bladder cancers, transurethral resection of the bladder tumor (TURBT), followed by intravesical chemotherapy (22%) or immunotherapy with bacillus Calmette−Guerin (BCG, 29%), is the most common treatment [3]. After surgery, surveillance, including regular cystoscopy, is crucial due to the high recurrence rate of non-muscle-invasive bladder cancers. For muscle-invasive disease, a combination of radical cystectomy, chemotherapy, and radiation therapy is a common treatment option. Such treatments can

Bladder Cancer. DOI: http://dx.doi.org/10.1016/B978-0-12-809939-1.00028-X

induce serious complications and greatly impact the patient's body image and quality of life (QoL). For metastatic bladder cancers, chemotherapy is a potential therapy option; however, curative treatment is very rare and its efficacy is limited. For all cancer stages, combined, the 5-year overall survival rate is 77%. For in situ urinary bladder cancer, which accounts for 51% of cases, the 5-year relative survival rate is 96%. The 5-year survival rate is 70% (81% for those with non-muscle-invasive disease and 47% for those with muscle-invasive disease).

Based on epidemiologic and treatment characteristics, QoL issues are noted to be very important for patients with bladder cancer. These issues can be summarized as follows: (1) surgical treatment varies from minimally invasive endoscopic surgery to complex radical cystectomy, which is associated with a substantial rate of serious complications; (2) the frequent recurrence of bladder cancer and the necessity of stringent surveillance might influence QoL; and (3) survival outcomes vary markedly, according to disease stage. Thus, preventing progression is very important.

The clinician should consider not only the impact of the possible treatments but also their impact on the patient's disease status and QoL. The ultimate treatment choice should be thoroughly discussed with the patient to ensure shared decision-making for this type of complex treatment scenario. However, QoL research among patients with bladder cancer has been minimal. In this review, we discuss QoL measurements, the impact of related conditions, and QoL comparisons for specific situations associated with bladder cancer.

HEALTH-RELATED QoL MEASUREMENT

The World Health Organization defines health-related quality of life (HRQOL) as an individual's perception of their position in life, within the context of their culture and value system and in relation to their goals, expectations, standards, and concerns [4]. HRQOL is a multidimensional concept that incorporates both the individual's functional status and their perception of their health. HRQOL measurements are important patient-centered outcome parameters. However, a consensus does not exist regarding the measurement of QoL in patients with bladder cancer. This lack of consensus makes interstudy comparisons difficult.

Questionnaires used to assess QoL in patients with bladder cancer can be categorized as general instruments, surgery-specific instruments, cancer-specific instruments, or bladder cancer–specific instruments. General measures are intended to be relevant to a wide range of patient groups and are deliberately broad in their scope of assessed domains. Surgery-specific instruments measure postsurgical convalescence and its impact on QoL [5]; relatively short-term QoL measures can be evaluated and compared following various surgical techniques. Cancer-specific instruments have the advantage of addressing problems that are specific to a given cancer patient population and may permit cross-study comparisons. Bladder cancer—specific instruments have recently become available; however, they have not been tested as extensively as other more generally applicable cancer-specific instruments. Additionally, almost all clinical QoL studies involving patients with bladder cancer have used ad hoc questionnaires with untested validity and reliability.

The Functional Assessment of Cancer Therapy (FACT)—Bladder Cancer (FACT-BL) instrument consists of the FACT-general version (FACT-G) plus 12 bladder cancer—specific items (including incontinence, diarrhea, body image, sexual function, and stoma care) [6]. The FACT-Vanderbilt Cystectomy Index (FACT-VCI) was developed for patients following radical cystectomy [7]. It contains the FACT-G, with an additional 17 bladder cancer- and treatment-related items (including incontinence, diarrhea, body image, sexual function, and perception of patient status). The Bladder Cancer Index (BCI) instrument is applicable to all bladder cancer patients, independent of tumor course or treatment [8]. It assesses 36 items across three (urinary, bowel, and sexual) domains. The European Organization for Research and Treatment of Cancer (EORTC) developed two bladder cancer modules, a 24-item questionnaire (EORTC QLQ-NMIBC24) for patients with non-muscle-invasive bladder cancer (Ta, T1, carcinoma in situ) and a 30-item questionnaire (EORTC QLQ-BLM30) for patients with muscle-invasive bladder cancer (T2, T3, T4a, and T4b) [9]. The two modules share a number of common items and scales, including those assessing urinary and bowel symptoms and sexual functioning. The EORTC QLQ-NMIBC24 contains items assessing the side effects of intravesical treatment (fever, malaise, and the convenience and worry caused by repeated cystoscopies). The EORTC QLQ-BLM30 contains items assessing problems associated with urostomy, catheter use, and body image.

The currently available QoL instruments for patients with bladder cancer are listed in Table 28.1. In many HRQOL studies, a combination of bladder cancer—specific and general and/or cancer-specific instruments are usually used. The purpose, number of questions, and validation of both the original and translated versions should be considered when selecting an instrument.

UTILITIES AND DISUTILITIES ASSOCIATED WITH BLADDER CANCER—RELATED CONDITIONS

Utilities represent a quantification of QoL adjustments, with perfect health assigned a value of 1.0 and death equal to 0. They represent the strength of a person's preference for a health-related outcome, which is based on both the health state and survival duration. Utilities are clearly different from descriptive HRQOL measurements. HRQOL instruments are often summarized into scores representing several different domains, whereas a utility reflects how

TABLE 28.1 Available HRQOL Instruments for Use in Bladder Cancer

Instruments	No. of Items
General	
EuroQol (EQ) Five Dimensions Questionnaire (5D) and Visual Analog Scale (VAS)	5
RAND Short Form (36) Health Survey (SF-36)	36
Nottingham Health Profile (NHP)	38
Sickness Impact Profile (SIP)	136
Quality of well-being scale	18
Hospital Anxiety and Depression (HAD) scale	14
Beck Depression Inventory (BDI)	13
Profile of Mood States (POMS)	6
Psychosocial Adjustment to Illness Scale (PAIS)	45
Surgery-Specific	
Convalescence and Recovery Evaluation (CARE)	27
Cancer-Specific	
Functional Assessment of Cancer Therapy-general version (FACT-G)	28
European Organization for Research and Treatment of Cancer Quality of Life Core Questionnaire (EORTC QLQ-C30)	30
Functional Living Index-Cancer (FLIC)	22
Cancer Inventory Problem Scale (CIPS)	145
Rotterdam Symptoms Checklist (RSCL)	34
Cancer Rehabilitation Evaluation System (CARES)	139
Cancer Rehabilitation Evaluation System-short form (CARES-SF)	59
Bladder Cancer–Specific	
Functional Assessment of Cancer Therapy-Bladder Cancer (FACT-BL)	39
FACT-Vanderbilt Cystectomy Index (FACT-VCI) 30	45
Bladder Cancer Index (BCI)	36
EORTC-QLQ-NMIBC24 (non-muscle-invasive bladder cancer–specific)	24
EORTC-QLQ-BLM30 (muscle-invasive bladder cancer–specific)	30

a respondent values a health state, not just the characteristics of that health state. Thus, a utility is a summarized, weighted value of the HRQOL for a certain health state.

A utility is used to calculate quality-adjusted life years (QALYs), which are composite outcomes of survival and HRQOLs [10]. QALYs combine quality and quantity of life and the answer to the "How long a person lives, how well?" question. QALYs are fundamental outcomes for various quality-adjusted survival and medical decision analyses, such as clinical decision analyses, cost—utility analyses, and cost—effectiveness analyses.

A utility value can be indirectly calculated using general, multiattribute utility instruments, such as EQ-5D, or converted using mapping formulae from disease-specific QoL instruments. However, a direct measurement would be more appropriate. Common methods for this include the standard gamble, time tradeoff, and visual analog rating scale [11].

Because of the lack of QoL-related studies in patients with bladder cancer, some utilities have been extrapolated from studies involving patients with similar conditions and complications. Table 28.2 presents published examples of bladder cancer—related utility or disutility values used for QoL outcome research.

IMPACT OF BLADDER CANCER DIAGNOSIS ON HRQOL

A cross-sectional study, from the United States, compared patient HRQOL measures before and after receiving a bladder cancer diagnosis [17]. Using the Surveillance, Epidemiology, and End Results (SEER)—Medical Health Outcome Survey linkage database, between 1998 and 2007, 1476 patients with bladder cancer, 65 years or older, were selected. The study assessed differences in physical and mental component summary scores, before and after the bladder cancer diagnosis. The results showed statistically significant differences in physical and mental scores between the pre- and postdiagnosis scores. In patients with non-muscle-invasive bladder cancer, the physical and mental score differences were -1.9 ($P < 0.01$) and -1.4 ($P = 0.01$), respectively. In those with muscle-invasive bladder cancer, there was a significant difference in the physical (-5.3; $P < 0.01$) but not the mental score (-2.7; $P = 0.07$). This physical domain difference continued for 10 years after the diagnosis of muscle-invasive bladder cancer. Patients with bladder cancer, in addition to ≥ 4 comorbid medical conditions and ≥ 1 daily living activity deficit, were most at risk for low physical component summary scores.

NON-MUSCLE-INVASIVE BLADDER CANCER

HRQOL studies involving patients with non-muscle-invasive bladder cancer are very rare. One prospective cohort study addressed HRQOL in this patient group [18]. A total of 244 patients from seven hospitals were followed for 1

TABLE 28.2 Utility or Disutility Values Related to Bladder Cancer

Reference	Condition	Utility or Disutility
Stevenson et al. [12]	Cystectomy (short term)	0.8
	Post cystectomy (urinary diversion) state	0.96
	TURBT	0.90
	Chemotherapy	0.64
	Disease recurrence or progression	0.62
	Complications: prolonged ileus	0.65
	Complications: small bowel obstruction with conservative management	0.65
	Complications: small bowel obstruction with surgical intervention	0.55
	Complications: total peripheral nutrition	0.65
	Complications: atrial fibrillation/arrhythmia	0.99
	Complications: delirium	0.51
	Complications: urinary tract infection	0.73
	Complications: fluid collection/abscess with conservative management	0.64
	Complications: fluid collection/abscess with surgical intervention	0.64
	Complications: fever not otherwise specified	0.64
	Complications: pneumonia	0.85
	Complications: urinary obstruction requiring percutaneous nephrostomy tube or stent	0.75
	Complications: deep vein thrombosis	0.67
	Complications: pulmonary embolism	0.62
	Complications: impotence	0.9
	Complications: incontinence	0.76
	Complications: neutropenia	0.64
	Complications: acute illness (cellulitis, line infection, wound infection)	0.64
	Complications: severe illness and hospitalization (bacteremia, endocarditis, osteomyelitis, and septic shock)	0.53
	Complications: acute sepsis	0.47

(Continued)

TABLE 28.2 (Continued)

Reference	Condition	Utility or Disutility
	Complications: kidney infections	0.66
	Complications: urinary or fecal fistula	0.68
Green et al. [13]	TURBT	−0.1
	Cystoscopy	0.997
	Fulguration	−0.05
Kulkarni et al. [14,15]	Cystectomy	0.8
	GI complication after cystectomy	0.97
	GU complication after cystectomy	0.93
	Impotence after cystectomy	0.91
	Metastases responsive to chemotherapy	0.62
	Metastases unresponsive to chemotherapy	0.3
	Surveillance cystoscopy	0.997
	Postcystectomy state	0.96
	Cystectomy complication	−0.3
	Chemotherapy	−0.36
	Chemotherapy complication	−0.54
	BCG therapy—induction	−0.02
	BCG complication	−0.2
	TURBT	−0.10
	TURBT for low risk Ta lesions	−0.06
Feenstra et al. [16]	Bladder cancer in women	0.89
	Bladder cancer in men	0.91

year using both a general instrument, the RAND Short Form-36 (SF-36), and a bladder cancer-specific instrument, the BCI. Physical health, measured using the SF-36, was comparable to the age-referenced US population group at baseline and during a 12-month follow-up. Mental health was significantly worse than the SF-36 reference values at the time of diagnosis (mean,

49.7 vs. 53.3; 95% confidence interval [CI], 52.5−54.2). The urinary domain improved significantly after diagnosis (mean, 85.2; 95% CI, 82.9−87.4) to the 12-month evaluation (mean, 90.2; 95% CI, 87.7−92.8), whereas the sexual domain showed deterioration from a mean value of 56.4 (95% CI, 52.8−59.9) to 53.7 (95% CI, 50.0−57.4). The adjusted HRQOL score from baseline to the 12-month follow-up, estimated using generalized estimating equation models, showed improvement in the following parameters: urinary domain after TURBT with or without intravesical therapy (mean, 3.9; 95% CI, 0.1−7.7), bowel domain following TURBT and BCG therapy (mean, 7.0; 95% CI, 2.4−11.5), and sexual domain following TURBT and mitomycin C treatment (mean, 13.1; 95% CI, 5.9−20.2).

A prospective, longitudinal, pilot study measured the HRQOL in 30 patients with non-muscle-invasive bladder cancer using the modified Munich Life Dimension List before, during, and after intravesical BCG therapy [19]. The results showed that although side effects occurred, QoL was not impaired. In a similar setting, Mack and Frick [20] attempted to determine the impact of BCG intravesical therapy on the physical, psychological, and social well-being of patients with non-muscle-invasive bladder cancer during the initial treatment cycle and during maintenance therapy. Although most patients had an acute QoL deterioration during induction, maintenance therapy was better tolerated. A Japanese multicenter research group performed a randomized controlled trial to compare efficacy, safety, and QoL outcomes following low-dose (40 mg) or standard-dose (80 mg) BCG instillation and induction therapy (weekly, eight times) [21]. They measured QoL using the European Organization for Research and Treatment of Cancer Quality of Life Core Questionnaire (EORTC QLQ-C30). The noninferiority of low-dose BCG was not proven. However, low-dose BCG instillation was associated with lower toxicity and higher QoL compared with the standard dose. Another multicenter, prospective, randomized, Phase II study compared HRQOL measures in patients with non-muscle-invasive bladder cancer receiving adjuvant intravesical gemcitabine or one-third dose BCG [22]. The HRQOL-related effects were measured using the EORTC QLQ-C30 and QLQ-NMIBC24 questionnaires. Local and systemic side effects were more frequently reported in the BCG arm. However, multivariate analyses showed no significant differences between the two groups in any QoL dimension. Furthermore, no significant changes, over time, in the QoL domains were detected for patients on BCG and gemcitabine, except for physical functioning, which decreased significantly in both groups.

Cost-effectiveness comparisons between office-based fulgurations and TURBT, with or without perioperative intravesical chemotherapy, for non-muscle-invasive bladder cancer have been reported [13]. The study used a Markov state-transition model with 20 cycles, which is equivalent to 5 years of follow-up after the initial TURBT. The perioperative intravesical therapy with fulguration strategy showed the best QALY (14.50) and TURBT without intravesical therapy rendered the worst QALY (14.34). Fulguration without perioperative intravesical therapy was the most cost-effective strategy in this setting. The limitation of the study was its lack of direct utility data for TURBT and an oversimplification of the Markov model. Al Hussein Al Awamlh et al. reported a similar analysis comparing office-based fulguration with operating room−based TURBT [23]. The results were similar; fulguration was both more effective (QALYs of 14.94 or 14.91, respectively) as well as less expensive ($17,494 vs $18,005, respectively) than TURBT.

High-grade T1 bladder cancer carries a poor prognosis and higher incidences of recurrence and progression than other non-muscle-invasive bladder cancers. Thus, controversy continues to exist regarding whether a conservative or an aggressive treatment strategy is better. The conservative option involves intravesical instillation of BCG after TURBT. Patients who respond to BCG can preserve their bladders; however, they may also have worse oncologic outcomes. In fact, the 3-year recurrence and/or tumor progression rates are 80% and 35%−48%, respectively [24]. By contrast, early cystectomy offers the highest probability of disease-specific and overall survival but may be associated with worse QoL outcomes than the conservative management strategy. One clinical decision analysis addressed this issue using a base case of a 60-year-old man [14]. The mean QALYs for the early cystectomy and BCG treatment were 12.32 and 11.97, respectively. Worsening patient comorbidity diminished the benefit of early cystectomy but altered the QALY-based preferred treatment for patients older than 65 years. A sensitivity analysis showed that elderly (>70 years) patients and those strongly averse to the loss of sexual function, gastrointestinal dysfunction, or life without a bladder had higher QALYs following BCG intravesical therapy. Thus, the authors concluded that the decision should be based on discussions that consider patient age, comorbid status, and the individual's preferences.

The same research team expanded this issue to include a cost-effectiveness analysis [15]. Early cystectomies in average patients with T1 high-grade bladder cancer demonstrated better QALYs and lower costs than BCG treatment. Early cystectomy was the dominant therapy for patients younger than 60 years, whereas BCG intravesical treatment was dominant for patients older than 75 years, in terms of cost-effectiveness. With increasing comorbidity, BCG treatment was more effective at lower age thresholds.

RADICAL CYSTECTOMY FOR MUSCLE-INVASIVE BLADDER CANCER

QoL outcomes, following treatment for muscle invasive bladder cancer, have not been comprehensively studied, despite improved treatment outcomes. The majority of the published studies are retrospective with low levels of evidence.

The most widely studied issue in muscle-invasive bladder cancer is QoL outcomes following radical cystectomy and urinary diversion. Because of its high complication rate and impacts on body image and sexual function, radical cystectomies may result in poorer QoL outcomes than many other cancer operations. The type of urinary diversion can also affect the patient's postsurgical QoL. The ileal conduit has remained the most commonly performed urinary diversion technique; however, a variety of continent urinary diversions have been developed to provide better body image and QoL outcomes. Over the past decade, the orthotopic neobladder has become a clinically accepted alternative to the ileal conduit. Of course, both have advantages and disadvantages. The ileal conduit procedure usually has a lower complication rate, shorter operating time, and a reduced hospital stay than orthotopic neobladder surgery. However, patients undergoing an ileal conduit procedure, after cystectomy, may be psychologically affected due to body image concerns associated with the stoma.

A Cochrane review of randomized or quasi-randomized controlled trials on this issue did not find any evidence that bladder replacement was better than the use of an ileal conduit [25]. Only five studies met the inclusion criteria, involving a total of 355 patients. These were small, moderate, or poor quality studies, and they reported few of the preselected outcome measures. A more recent systematic review and meta-analysis compared the QoL after continent versus incontinent urinary diversion in radical cystectomy patients [26]. Twenty-nine studies, involving 3754 patients, were selected for review. The patients reported poor postsurgical urinary and sexual functioning, compared with the general population. However, the overall QoL outcomes were similar between the two groups. A subgroup analysis demonstrated a greater improvement in physical health associated with incontinent, compared to continent diversions but no differences in mental and social health. Qualitative analyses showed that patients with orthotopic neobladders had superior emotional functioning and body image, compared with those undergoing cutaneous diversions. The authors concluded that the patient's preference should be a key factor in the diversion type selection.

A prospective cohort study evaluated QoL and body image for patients with bladder cancer undergoing radical cystectomy [27]. The EORTC QLQ-C30 and the Satisfaction with Life Scale (SWLS) questionnaires were administered before and 9−12 months after surgery. There was no significant change in the overall QoL evident with either the EORTC QLQ-C30 or the SWLS. Family, relationships, health, and finance were the most important determinants of QoL, whereas body image was not mentioned. Thus, the authors suggested that health and body image may not be important QoL considerations for patients undergoing cystectomy.

One cross-sectional survey study assessed QoL predictors after ileal conduit surgery [28]. Poor sexual life satisfaction was common among responders.

Social support and stoma self-management were associated with improved QoL measures. Female gender, younger age (<60 years), continuing to work, higher family income, longer postoperative periods, and the absence of stoma complications were predictors of better QoL outcomes.

BLADDER PRESERVATION THERAPY AND ROBOTIC SURGERY FOR MUSCLE-INVASIVE BLADDER CANCER

A multimodal strategy, using radical TURBT, chemotherapy, and radiation, may be an alternative to radical cystectomy in selected patients. Some patients may experience disease progression, but many remain disease-free with intact bladders. Thus, this approach is claimed to provide favorable HRQOL outcomes; however, only a small number of retrospective studies have been reported, to date [29−31]. The overall HRQOL in the bladder preservation group was reported to be higher than in the radical cystectomy group [29,30]. However, patients undergoing this treatment had lower QoL scores than did patients with non-muscle-invasive bladder cancer who underwent TURBT [31].

Robot-assisted radical cystectomy (RARC) is another modality that is gaining traction as a surgical approach for patients with muscle-invasive bladder cancer. However, only one retrospective study has evaluated HRQOL impacts and short-term convalescence among patients undergoing open radical cystectomy and RARC [32]. For the HRQOL assessment, the BCI instrument was used and short-term convalescence was evaluated using a surgery-specific instrument, the CARE questionnaire. Within 1 postsurgical year, the HRQOL score recoveries, across all BCI domains, were comparable, with scores returning to near baseline for all patients. The CARE scores at 4 weeks revealed that patients treated with open surgery had better pain (29.1 vs 20.0, $P = 0.02$) domain scores compared with patients undergoing RARC; these differences abated by Week 6. The authors concluded that QoL recovery and short-term convalescence were similar in these cohorts, following RARC and open radical cystectomy. The high rate of ileal conduit use was noted as one of the study's limitations. More than 75% of the patients in the RARC group and almost 70% of the patients in the open surgery group underwent ileal conduit procedures. Furthermore, all of the diversions in the RARC group were performed using an extracorporeal approach, whereas a completely intracorporeal approach may be necessary to realize the full benefits of the minimally invasive RARC.

CHEMOTHERAPY FOR ADVANCED OR METASTATIC BLADDER CANCER

Radical cystectomy is the standard treatment for patients with muscle-invasive bladder cancer. However, it only provides a 5-year survival of approximately 50% [33]. To improve this unsatisfactory oncologic result, neoadjuvant chemotherapy has been adopted. Platinum-based neoadjuvant chemotherapy, before radical cystectomy, has been shown to improve survival outcomes in these patients [34–36]. Only one cost-effectiveness analysis addressed a QoL comparison between neoadjuvant chemotherapy, before cystectomy, and cystectomy alone for muscle-invasive bladder cancer [12]. The study retrospectively examined data from a single institution to compare QALYs and cost-effectiveness. A total of 119 patients (65.4%) underwent radical cystectomy alone, and 63 (34.6%) also received neoadjuvant chemotherapy. The median overall survival times were 26.6 and 46.2 months, respectively; the median quality-adjusted life months (QALM) were 21.9 and 40.4 months, respectively. The additional cost, per QALM gained by neoadjuvant chemotherapy, was approximately $6000. The study concluded that neoadjuvant chemotherapy improves QoL and is cost-effective.

For decades, systemic chemotherapy with methotrexate, vinblastine, adriamycin, and cisplatin (MVAC) has been a standard treatment for advanced or metastatic bladder cancer [33]. However, because the report of a Phase III trial comparing a new combination therapy using gemcitabine plus cisplatin (GC) with MVAC [37], GC chemotherapy has been replacing MVAC as the treatment of choice for advanced or metastatic bladder cancer. The overall survival of patients treated with GC (median, 13.8 months; 95% CI, 12.3–15.8) was comparable to that for patients assigned to the MVAC group (median, 14.8 months; 95% CI, 13.2–16.8); however, GC was better tolerated than MVAC. In the GC arm, 63% of cycles were administered without dose adjustment compared with only 37% in the MVAC arm, indicating that GC has less treatment-related toxicity than MVAC. Patients in the MVAC arm experienced more Grade 3 or 4 neutropenia (MVAC, 82%; GC, 71%), significantly more neutropenic fever (MVAC, 14%; GC, 2%; $P < 0.001$), and significantly more neutropenic sepsis (MVAC, 12%; GC, 1%; $P < 0.001$) than did those in the GC arm. Grade 3 or 4 mucositis was also significantly more common in the MVAC arm (22%) than in the GC arm (1%, $P < 0.001$). Furthermore, patients in the GC arm gained significantly more weight after treatment than did patients in the MVAC arm. In addition, a higher percentage of patients in the GC arm showed a performance status improvement of ≥ 10 points over a period of at least 4 weeks, compared with those receiving MVAC (GC: 5, 37%; MVAC: 5, 31%). The investigators measured QoL using the EORTC QLQ-C30 instrument. Overall, the QoL profiles were similar in both arms, with the exception of fatigue. Ad hoc analysis of this Phase III trial showed that HRQOL parameters, such as physical and role functioning and anorexia, were the significant and independent prognostic factors for advanced or metastatic bladder cancer [38].

QoL IN LONG-TERM SURVIVORS

A population-based survey evaluated HRQOL among long-term survivors following a diagnosis of bladder cancer [39]. The study identified a cohort of bladder cancer (either non-muscle invasive or muscle invasive) patients from the Iowa data registry of the SEER program. The median time since diagnosis for the participants was 99.8 months. They used a validated bladder cancer—specific instrument, FACT-BL, in the study. There were no significant differences in general QoL scores between patients undergoing radical cystectomy and those with intact bladders. However, patients undergoing radical cystectomy had worse sexual function scores. Of the patients undergoing radical cystectomy, the QoL scores were not significantly different between those with ileal conduits or orthotopic neobladders. Of the patients with intact bladders, the QoL scores tended to decrease with increasing age. The presence of comorbidities also lowered the HRQOL scores.

CONCLUSION

Increased awareness of QoL may increase our understanding of the impact of bladder cancer and may help to choose the treatment option. However, bladder cancer QoL research is relatively inactive. Therefore, high-level evidence is very limited in across all bladder cancer stages and treatments. However, many dedicated researchers have established the foundation for HRQOL studies through efforts such as the development of bladder cancer—specific QoL questionnaires. It is the time now to perform well-designed, prospective, comparative QoL studies among bladder cancer patients. We also need high-quality studies to determine utility values for various bladder cancer situations. Furthermore, quality-adjusted bladder cancer survival analyses will support many medical decision analyses, including clinical decision analyses, cost—utility analyses, and cost—effectiveness analyses.

REFERENCES

[1] Antoni S, Ferlay J, Soerjomataram I, Znaor A, Jemal A, Bray F. Bladder cancer incidence and mortality: a global overview and recent trends. Eur Urol 2017;71(1):96—108.

[2] Siegel RL, Miller KD, Jemal A. Cancer statistics, 2016. CA Cancer J Clin 2016;66 (1):7—30.

[3] Miller KD, Siegel RL, Lin CC, Mariotto AB, Kramer JL, Rowland JH, et al. Cancer treatment and survivorship statistics, 2016. CA Cancer J Clin 2016;66(4):271—89.

[4] The World Health Organization Quality of Life assessment (WHOQOL): position paper from the World Health Organization. Soc Sci Med 1995;41(10):1403—09.

[5] Hollenbeck BK, Dunn RL, Wolf Jr. JS, Sanda MG, Wood DP, Gilbert SM, et al. Development and validation of the convalescence and recovery evaluation (CARE) for measuring quality of life after surgery. Qual Life Res 2008;17(6):915—26.

[6] Mansson A, Davidsson T, Hunt S, Mansson W. The quality of life in men after radical cystectomy with a continent cutaneous diversion or orthotopic bladder substitution: is there a difference? BJU Int 2002;90(4):386–90.

[7] Cookson MS, Dutta SC, Chang SS, Clark T, Smith Jr. JA, Wells N. Health related quality of life in patients treated with radical cystectomy and urinary diversion for urothelial carcinoma of the bladder: development and validation of a new disease specific questionnaire. J Urol 2003;170(5):1926–30.

[8] Gilbert SM, Dunn RL, Hollenbeck BK, Montie JE, Lee CT, Wood DP, et al. Development and validation of the Bladder Cancer Index: a comprehensive, disease specific measure of health related quality of life in patients with localized bladder cancer. J Urol 2010;183(5):1764–9.

[9] Blazeby JM, Hall E, Aaronson NK, Lloyd L, Waters R, Kelly JD, et al. Validation and reliability testing of the EORTC QLQ-NMIBC24 questionnaire module to assess patient-reported outcomes in non-muscle-invasive bladder cancer. Eur Urol 2014;66(6):1148–56.

[10] Drummond M, Brixner D, Gold M, Kind P, McGuire A, Nord E, et al. Toward a consensus on the QALY. Value Health 2009;12(Suppl 1):S31–5.

[11] Hunter RM, Baio G, Butt T, Morris S, Round J, Freemantle N. An educational review of the statistical issues in analysing utility data for cost-utility analysis. Pharmacoeconomics 2015;33(4):355–66.

[12] Stevenson SM, Danzig MR, Ghandour RA, Deibert CM, Decastro GJ, Benson MC, et al. Cost-effectiveness of neoadjuvant chemotherapy before radical cystectomy for muscle-invasive bladder cancer. Urol Oncol 2014;32(8):1172–7.

[13] Green DA, Rink M, Cha EK, Xylinas E, Chughtai B, Scherr DS, et al. Cost-effective treatment of low-risk carcinoma not invading bladder muscle. BJU Int 2013;111(3 Pt B): E78–84.

[14] Kulkarni GS, Finelli A, Fleshner NE, Jewett MA, Lopushinsky SR, Alibhai SM. Optimal management of high-risk T1G3 bladder cancer: a decision analysis. PLoS Med 2007;4(9): e284.

[15] Kulkarni GS, Alibhai SM, Finelli A, Fleshner NE, Jewett MA, Lopushinsky SR, et al. Cost-effectiveness analysis of immediate radical cystectomy versus intravesical Bacillus Calmette-Guerin therapy for high-risk, high-grade (T1G3) bladder cancer. Cancer 2009;115(23):5450–9.

[16] Feenstra TL, Hamberg-van Reenen HH, Hoogenveen RT, Rutten-van Molken MP. Cost-effectiveness of face-to-face smoking cessation interventions: a dynamic modeling study. Value Health 2005;8(3):178–90.

[17] Fung C, Pandya C, Guancial E, Noyes K, Sahasrabudhe DM, Messing EM, et al. Impact of bladder cancer on health related quality of life in 1,476 older Americans: a cross-sectional study. J Urol 2014;192(3):690–5.

[18] Schmidt S, Frances A, Lorente Garin JA, Juanpere N, Lloreta Trull J, Bonfill X, et al. Quality of life in patients with non-muscle-invasive bladder cancer: one-year results of a multicentre prospective cohort study. Urol Oncol 2015;33(1): 19.e17–19.e15.

[19] Bohle A, Balck F, von Weitersheim J, Jocham D. The quality of life during intravesical bacillus Calmette-Guerin therapy. J Urol 1996;155(4):1221–6.

[20] Mack D, Frick J. Quality of life in patients undergoing bacille Calmette-Guerin therapy for superficial bladder cancer. Br J Urol 1996;78(3):369–71.

[21] Yokomizo A, Kanimoto Y, Okamura T, Ozono S, Koga H, Iwamura M, et al. Randomized controlled study of the efficacy, safety and quality of life with low dose

bacillus Calmette-Guerin instillation therapy for nonmuscle invasive bladder cancer. J Urol 2016;195(1):41−6.

[22] Gontero P, Oderda M, Mehnert A, Gurioli A, Marson F, Lucca I, et al. The impact of intravesical gemcitabine and 1/3 dose bacillus Calmette-Guerin instillation therapy on the quality of life in patients with nonmuscle invasive bladder cancer: results of a prospective, randomized, phase II trial. J Urol 2013;190(3):857−62.

[23] Al Hussein Al Awamlh B, Lee R, Chughtai B, Donat SM, Sandhu JS, Herr HW. A cost-effectiveness analysis of management of low-risk non-muscle-invasive bladder cancer using office-based fulguration. Urology 2015;85(2):381−6.

[24] Cookson MS, Herr HW, Zhang ZF, Soloway S, Sogani PC, Fair WR. The treated natural history of high risk superficial bladder cancer: 15-year outcome. J Urol 1997;158 (1):62−7.

[25] Cody JD, Nabi G, Dublin N, McClinton S, Neal DE, Pickard R, et al. Urinary diversion and bladder reconstruction/replacement using intestinal segments for intractable incontinence or following cystectomy. Cochrane Database Syst Rev 2012; (2): CD003306.

[26] Yang LS, Shan BL, Shan LL, Chin P, Murray S, Ahmadi N, et al. A systematic review and meta-analysis of quality of life outcomes after radical cystectomy for bladder cancer. Surg Oncol 2016;25(3):281−97.

[27] Somani BK, Gimlin D, Fayers P, N'Dow J. Quality of life and body image for bladder cancer patients undergoing radical cystectomy and urinary diversion—a prospective cohort study with a systematic review of literature. Urology 2009;74(5):1138−43.

[28] Liu C, Ren H, Li J, Li X, Dai Y, Liu L, et al. Predictors for quality of life of bladder cancer patients with ileal conduit: a cross-sectional survey. Eur J Oncol Nurs 2016;21: 168−73.

[29] Caffo O, Fellin G, Graffer U, Luciani L. Assessment of quality of life after cystectomy or conservative therapy for patients with infiltrating bladder carcinoma. A survey by a self-administered questionnaire. Cancer 1996;78(5):1089−97.

[30] Zietman AL, Sacco D, Skowronski U, Gomery P, Kaufman DS, Clark JA, et al. Organ conservation in invasive bladder cancer by transurethral resection, chemotherapy and radiation: results of a urodynamic and quality of life study on long-term survivors. J Urol 2003;170(5):1772−6.

[31] Hashine K, Miura N, Numata K, Shirato A, Sumiyoshi Y, Kataoka M. Health-related quality of life after bladder preservation therapy for muscle invasive bladder cancer. Int J Urol 2008;15(5):403−6.

[32] Li AY, Filson CP, Hollingsworth JM, He C, Weizer AZ, Hollenbeck BK, et al. Patient-reported convalescence and quality of life recovery: a comparison of open and robotic-assisted radical cystectomy. Surg Innov 2016;23(6):598−605.

[33] Stenzl A, Cowan NC, De Santis M, Kuczyk MA, Merseburger AS, Ribal MJ, et al. Treatment of muscle-invasive and metastatic bladder cancer: update of the EAU guidelines. Eur Urol 2011;59(6):1009−18.

[34] Grossman HB, Natale RB, Tangen CM, Speights VO, Vogelzang NJ, Trump DL, et al. Neoadjuvant chemotherapy plus cystectomy compared with cystectomy alone for locally advanced bladder cancer. N Engl J Med 2003;349(9):859−66.

[35] Sherif A, Holmberg L, Rintala E, Mestad O, Nilsson J, Nilsson S, et al. Neoadjuvant cisplatinum based combination chemotherapy in patients with invasive bladder cancer: a combined analysis of two Nordic studies. Eur Urol 2004;45(3):297−303.

[36] Yin M, Joshi M, Meijer RP, Glantz M, Holder S, Harvey HA, et al. Neoadjuvant chemotherapy for muscle-invasive bladder cancer: a systematic review and two-step meta-analysis. Oncologist 2016;21(6):708–15.

[37] von der Maase H, Hansen SW, Roberts JT, Dogliotti L, Oliver T, Moore MJ, et al. Gemcitabine and cisplatin versus methotrexate, vinblastine, doxorubicin, and cisplatin in advanced or metastatic bladder cancer: results of a large, randomized, multinational, multicenter, phase III study. J Clin Oncol 2000;18(17):3068–77.

[38] Roychowdhury DF, Hayden A, Liepa AM. Health-related quality-of-life parameters as independent prognostic factors in advanced or metastatic bladder cancer. J Clin Oncol 2003;21(4):673–8.

[39] Allareddy V, Kennedy J, West MM, Konety BR. Quality of life in long-term survivors of bladder cancer. Cancer 2006;106(11):2355–62.

Section VI

Chemotherapy for Metastatic Bladder Cancer

Bhumsuk Keam

Seoul National University Hospital, Seoul, Korea

Section Outline

INTRODUCTION

The majority of patients with bladder cancer present with noninvasive bladder cancer, but 20%−40% of patients present with advanced stages and muscle-invasive disease or metastatic disease [1]. Systemic chemotherapy is widely used for inoperable, locally advanced cancer and metastatic bladder cancer. Typically, bladder cancer spreads first to regional lymph nodes, then disseminates to distant organs. The involvement of visceral organs, such as lung, liver, and bone, is a poor prognostic factor for bladder cancer [2].

Initial response rates to combination chemotherapy are high, but the median survival with combination chemotherapy is only approximately 12−15 months and the 5-year survival rate is roughly 15% [3,4]. Despite the fact that bladder cancer is relatively chemo-sensitive, the prognosis of patients with metastatic bladder cancer remains poor.

Systemic chemotherapy options for metastatic urothelial carcinoma of the renal pelvis or ureter are based on results from trials composed primarily of patients with urothelial carcinoma of the bladder. Systemic chemotherapy options for nonurothelial bladder cancer are distinct from those for urothelial bladder cancer. This chapter reviews systemic palliative chemotherapy for metastatic bladder cancer, including urothelial carcinoma of the renal pelvis or ureter, and nonurothelial bladder cancer.

MEDICAL FITNESS FOR CHEMOTHERAPY

Before considering palliative chemotherapy for metastatic bladder cancer, all patients should be evaluated for medical fitness for chemotherapy. The assessment should incorporate medical and physiologic considerations and include evaluation of renal and cardiac function, as well as performance status. A medical fitness assessment stratifies patients into medically "fit" or "unfit" patients, and this classification is used to determine treatment options.

Cisplatin-based combination chemotherapy is regarded as the standard regimen for metastatic bladder cancer. Cisplatin is cleared by the kidneys and is potentially nephrotoxic, and preexisting renal impairment is a risk factor for the nephrotoxic effects of cisplatin. As such, precise evaluation of a patient's renal function is important to predict his or her tolerance of cisplatin. Old age, urinary tract obstruction related to bladder cancer, prior nephronureterectomy, and smoking-related vascular disease are associated with high rates of renal impairment in patients with metastatic bladder cancer [5]. Reversible causes of renal impairment (e.g., urinary tract obstruction related to bladder cancer) should be identified and treated prior to initiation of cisplatin-based therapy. A working group consensus defined patients with metastatic urothelial carcinoma who are unfit to receive cisplatin-based chemotherapy [6]. The following criteria render a patient unfit for cisplatin-based therapy: Eastern Cooperative Oncology Group (ECOG) performance status of 2 or greater (Table 1) or a Karnofsky performance status of 60%−70% or lower (Table 2); creatinine clearance of less than 60 mL/min; a hearing loss (measured at audiometry) of 25 dB at two contiguous frequencies; grade 2 or greater peripheral neuropathy (e.g., sensory alteration or paresthesia, including tingling, that does not interfere with activities of daily living); and New York Heart Association class III or greater heart failure.

Patients are considered medically fit for chemotherapy if they do not meet any of the above criteria, and cisplatin-based combination chemotherapy can be recommended. For patients who are unable to receive cisplatin, other alternative treatment options can be considered, such as a carboplatin-based regimen (i.e., carboplatin plus gemcitabine), a nonplatinum-based combination (e.g., paclitaxel plus gemcitabine), or single-agent chemotherapy. A decision regarding a patient's ability to tolerate chemotherapy should take into account the patient's performance status and the clinician's medical judgment.

TABLE 1 Eastern Cooperative Oncology Group Performance Status Definitions

Performance Status	Definition
0	Fully active; no performance restrictions
1	Strenuous physical activity restricted; fully ambulatory and able to carry out light work
2	Capable of all self-care but unable to carry out any work activities; up and about at least 50% of waking hours
3	Capable of only limited self-care; confined to bed or chair at least 50% of waking hours
4	Completely disabled; cannot carry out any self-care; totally confined to bed or chair

TABLE 2 Karnofsky Performance Status Scale

Percentage of Functional Capacity	General Performance Status	Criteria
100	Normal, no complaints, no evidence of disease	Able to carry on normal activity and to work; no special care needed
90	Able to carry on normal activity, minor signs or symptoms of disease	
80	Normal activity with effort, some signs or symptoms of disease	
70	Cares for self; unable to carry on normal activity or to do active work	Unable to work; able to live at home and care for most personal needs; various degrees of assistance needed
60	Requires occasional assistance but is able to care for most needs	
50	Requires considerable assistance and frequent medical care	

(Continued)

TABLE 2 (Continued)

Percentage of Functional Capacity	General Performance Status	Criteria
40	Disabled; requires special care and assistance	Unable to care for self; requires equivalent of institutional or hospital care; disease may be progressing rapidly
30	Severely disabled; hospitalization is indicated although death is not imminent	
20	Hospitalization is necessary; very sick; active supportive treatment necessary	
10	Moribund; fatal processes progressing rapidly	
0	Dead	

FIRST-LINE CHEMOTHERAPY

A cisplatin-based combination chemotherapy regimen is the preferred initial approach for palliative chemotherapy for patients with metastatic urothelial cancer of the bladder and urinary tract who are able to tolerate cisplatin. The following combinations are commonly used cisplatin-based regimens for first-line chemotherapy:

- MVAC: methotrexate (30 mg/m^2 on days 1, 15, and 22), vinblastine (3 mg/m^2 on days 2, 15, and 22), doxorubicin (30 mg/m^2 on day 2), and cisplatin (70 mg/m^2), every 28 days.
- GC: gemcitabine (1000 mg/m^2 on days 1, 8, and 15) plus cisplatin (70 mg/m^2 on day 2), every 28 days.
- CMV: cisplatin (70 mg/m^2 on day 2), methotrexate (30 mg/m^2 on days 1 and 8), and vinblastine (4 mg/m^2 on days 1 and 8), every 21 days.
- PGC: paclitaxel (80 mg/m^2 on days 1 and 8), gemcitabine (1000 mg/m^2 on days 1 and 8), and cisplatin (70 mg/m^2 on day 1), every 21 days.

Methotrexate, Vinblastine, Doxorubicin, and Cisplatin

Of the various cisplatin-based combination chemotherapy regimens, GC and MVAC are the most widely used. Several decades ago, MVAC became the first standard regimen for bladder cancer on the basis of results of two phase III, randomized clinical trials that demonstrated improved survival outcomes

TABLE 3 Key Phase III Trial Results of Cisplatin-Based Combination Chemotherapy

Regimen	Complete Response (%)	Response Rate (%)	Medial Progression-Free Survival (Months)	Median Overall Survival (Months)	References
MVAC	12–35	39–65	7.4–10.0	12.5–14.8	[2,3,7,8]
GC	12	49	7.4	13.8	[3]
CMV	10	36	NA	7.0	[9]
PGC	13.5	55.5	8.3	15.8	[10]

(Table 3) [2,7]. MVAC demonstrated superiority in progression-free survival (PFS) and overall survival (OS) compared with single-agent cisplatin and combination cisplatin, cyclophosphamide, and doxorubicin [2,7].

The importance of both a combination approach to chemotherapy and dose intensity has been noted, and investigators have evaluated increasing the dose intensity of MVAC and administering granulocyte-colony stimulating factor every 2 weeks as supportive care. High-dose (HD)-intensity MVAC was compared with standard MVAC in a large randomized phase III trial [11]. Compared with standard MVAC, HD-MVAC showed a better complete response (CR) rate (21% vs. 9%), response rate (62% vs. 50%), and PFS (9.1 months vs. 8.2 months). Long-term data [12] that included 7.3 years of follow-up revealed that the OS rates were 21.8% in the HD-MVAC group and 13.5% in the standard MVAC group. Median survival was higher in the HD-MVAC group, with borderline statistical significance (median OS: HD-MVAC, 15.1 months vs. standard MVAC, 14.9 months). However, HD-MVAC does not offer clinically meaningful differences in OS. Still, on the basis of the phase III results, National Comprehensive Cancer Network (NCCN) guidelines include HD-MVAC instead of standard MVAC as a category 1 recommendation for first-line chemotherapy.

MVAC is associated with substantial toxicity, which is a major concern with MVAC therapy, particularly since many patients with bladder cancer are elderly or have multiple comorbidities. Most patients require dose adjustment at some point in their treatments. Myelosuppression, neutropenic fever, sepsis, mucositis, and nausea and vomiting are common. Notable numbers of patients experience toxic effects of MVAC, including neutropenia, anemia, thrombocytopenia, stomatitis, nausea, and fatigue. The rate of chemotherapy-induced fatality among patients with metastatic disease [13] may be as high as 3%, most often due to neutropenic sepsis [3]. In one study, 54% of patients were hospitalized due to toxicity [13]. The use of hematopoietic growth factor support may ameliorate some of these toxicities, especially myelosuppression and mucositis [14,15]. Despite the NCCN recommendation, some experts prefer standard MVAC over HD-MVAC due to the toxicities related to treatment.

Gemcitabine and Cisplatin

GC showed encouraging results in phase II studies, with response rates of 42%−66% and CR rates of 18%−28% [16,17]. In general, toxicity related to treatment was easily managed. On the basis of these phase II results, GC was compared with MVAC in a phase III study [3,4]. GC was administered in a 28-day cycle with gemcitabine 1000 mg/m^2 (days 1, 8, and 15) and cisplatin 70 mg/m^2 (day 2); GC showed similar efficacy to MVAC. Median survival rates of 14 months with GC and 15.2 months with MVAC were not significantly different [3,4]. However, GC had significantly less toxicity and improved tolerability compared with MVAC: GC showed less grade 3/4 toxicity, including neutropenia (71% vs. 82%), neutropenic sepsis (2% vs. 14%), and mucositis (1% vs. 22%) [3]. Patients who received GC gained more weight, reported less fatigue, and had better performance status than patients who received MVAC. This phase III trial was initially designed to demonstrate the superiority of GC compared with MVAC, and it was not powered to demonstrate equivalency between the two regimens. However, given the similar efficacy and lower toxicity, many consider GC rather than MVAC as a first-line regimen for patients with metastatic urothelial carcinoma of the bladder. Alternative 3-weekly dosing schedules of the GC regimen have investigated [17−19] and the results appear to be similar to the 28 days regimens.

Paclitaxel, Gemcitabine, and Cisplatin

The PGC triplet combination is another option for patients with metastatic urothelial carcinoma. The EORTC 30987 trial [10] enrolled 626 patients with advanced urothelial carcinoma and compared GC and PGC for a maximum of six cycles. The OS rate was 55.5% with PGC and 43.6% with GC ($P = 0.003$). Trends toward improved PFS (median, 8.3 months with PGC vs. 7.6 months with GC; $P = 0.11$) and longer OS (median, 15.8 months with PGC vs. 12.7 months with GC; $P = 0.075$) were observed with PGC. The addition of paclitaxel to GC provided a higher response rate and a 3.1-month survival benefit, but these results did not reach the statistical significance. Increased incidences of serious (grade ¾) toxicities, including neutropenia (65% vs. 51%), fatigue (15% vs. 11%), and infections (18% vs. 14%), were observed in the PGC group compared with the GC group. These results suggest that PGC is a treatment option for patients with metastatic urothelial carcinoma; it should be used for patients with the bladder as the primary origin of the cancer.

Chemotherapy for Cisplatin-Ineligible Patients

For patients who are not eligible to receive cisplatin but are otherwise candidates for chemotherapy, several alternative regimens can be considered. Gemcitabine plus carboplatin (GCb) is the preferred regimen for cisplatin-ineligible patients. The benefit of carboplatin-based therapy was demonstrated in the EORTC 30986 trial [20]. In this trial, 238 chemotherapy-naïve patients with impaired renal function (glomerular filtration rate between 30 mL/min and 60 mL/min) and/or poor performance status (ECOG ≥ 2) were randomly assigned to treatment with GCb or methotrexate, carboplatin, and vinblastine (M-CAVI). GCb showed a higher overall response rate (41.2% vs. 30.3%, $P = 0.08$), but the difference was not statistically significant. OS (median OS, 9.3 months vs. 8.1 months; $P = 0.64$) and PFS (median PFS, 5.8 months vs. 4.2 months; $P = 0.78$) were not different between the two regimens. The toxicity profile was better in the GCb group than in the M-CAVI group. GCb is as effective as M-CAVI with a better toxicity profile; these findings support its use in patients with impaired renal function or poor performance status (ECOG ≥ 2) who are otherwise candidates for the combination chemotherapy.

Other nonplatinum regimens such as paclitaxel plus gemcitabine or docetaxel plus gemcitabine have been evaluated and the results are encouraging. Paclitaxel plus gemcitabine showed an objective response rate (ORR) of 54%−69% and a median OS of 13−16 months [21,22]. Responses to single-agent chemotherapy are generally low, and single-agent chemotherapy has not shown consistent improvements in survival.

SECOND-LINE CHEMOTHERAPY

Despite the response rates of 40%−60% achieved with cisplatin-based first-line chemotherapy such as GC or MVAC, most patients experience disease progression a median 8−10 months or longer after first-line chemotherapy. Generally, impaired renal function, poor performance status, advanced age, and comorbidities of patients have limited trial design, feasibility, and patient accrual, particularly in the setting of second-line chemotherapy options [23]. To date, no standard second-line chemotherapy regimen exists for patients with metastatic bladder cancer who have disease progression after standard first-line platinum-based treatment with MVAC or GC. Comparisons of second-line trial results are fundamentally limited for several reasons: the lack of a generally accepted definition of second-line chemotherapy, different primary tumor sites (e.g., bladder or upper tract urothelial carcinoma), and missing risk-group stratification according to established prognostic parameters result in highly heterogeneous study populations [24].

Second-Line Chemotherapy Versus Best Supportive Care

One phase III trial [25] randomized 370 patients with advanced urothelial carcinoma who had received prior first-line platinum-based chemotherapy (in a 2:1 ratio) to received vinflunine plus best supportive care (BSC) or BSC only. The overall response rate, disease control, and PFS all significantly favored vinflunine over BSC only. Median OS also favored the vinflunine group (6.9 months with vinflunine vs. 4.6 months with BCS; $P = 0.287$). Imbalances in prognostic factors may have accounted for the lack of statistical significance in the primary analysis, with more patients in the BCS arm than in the vinflunine arm having a good performance status (ECOG = 0 in 38.5% of BSC group vs. 28.5% of the vinflunine group). A multivariate Cox analysis adjusted for prognostic factors; the results indicated that vinflunine significantly affected OS ($P = 0.036$) and reduced the risk of death by 23%. For that reason, vinflunine is approved in Europe as a second-line treatment for urothelial cancer. However, vinflunine is not approved in the United States because of the lack of statistically significant benefit in the OS. Therefore BSC remains a feasible approach in the second-line setting, especially in patients with poor performance status. However, in practice, treatment beyond first-line chemotherapy is usually administered to patients with good performance status. Second-line chemotherapy typically employs doublet regimens, single-agent chemotherapy, or clinical trials, if available.

Rechallenging Cisplatin as Second-Line Chemotherapy

For selected patients whose disease progresses after first-line cisplatin-based chemotherapy and is still eligible for cisplatin treatment, rechallenge with cisplatin-containing chemotherapy is feasible, depending on the initial response. A small phase II study [26] reported the outcomes of MVAC in patients who failed first-line GC. The overall response rate was 30%, with a 6.7% CR rate. Seven out of sixteen patients who previously responded to GC responded to MVAC, and 2 out of 14 patients who did not respond to GC responded to MVAC. Median PFS was 5.3 months and median OS was 10.9 months with MVAC. Response to first-line GC and age were independent predictors of PFS in patients who received second-line MVAC [27].

Nonplatinum Agents as Second-Line Chemotherapy

Several phase II results of second-line single agents, including pemetrexed, vinflunine, paclitaxel, docetaxel, gemcitabine, ifosfamide, and oxaliplatin,

TABLE 4 Phase II and Phase III Trials of Second-Line Chemotherapy for Urothelial Carcinoma

Agents	Phase	Year	N	ORR (%)	PFS (Months)	OS (Months)	References
Vinflunine	II	2006	51	18	3.0	6.6	[29]
Vinflunine	II	2009	151	15	2.8	8.2	[34]
Vinflunine	III	2009	253	9	3.0	6.9	[25]
Pemetrexed	II	2006	47	28	2.9	9.6	[30]
Pemetrexed	II	2007	13	8	NR	NR	[31]
Paclitaxel	II	1997	14	7	NR	NR	[33]
Paclitaxel (weekly)	II	2002	31	10	2.2	7.2	[32]
Docetaxel	II	1997	30	13	NR	9.0	[35]
Gemcitabine	II	2002	30	11	4.9	8.7	[36]
Gemcitabine	II	2007	46	25	3.1	12.6	[37]
Ifosfamide	II	1997	56	20	2.4	5.5	[38]

NR, not reported.

have been reported (Table 4). However, second-line single agents have only shown marginal benefit, with an overall response rate of 5%−20% and a median PFS of 3−4 months. Moreover, there is almost no evidence that second-line chemotherapy substantially improves OS or quality of life [28]. Neither single agent has been approved for use in patients with metastatic urothelial carcinoma nor has the activities of any single agent been validated in phase III clinical trials. Patients with advanced bladder cancer who have failed first-line chemotherapy should be encouraged to participate in clinical trials whenever possible.

Vinflunine. It, a third-generation vinca alkaloid, achieved an ORR of 18%, a disease control rate of 67%, and a median PFS of 3 months in a phase II trial [29]. Subsequently, in the first randomized phase III trial [25] in the second-line setting, vinflunine showed an ORR of 9% and a PFS of 3 months.

Pemetrexed. It, a multitargeted antifolate, has shown activity in previously treated patients. The initial phase II trial [30] showed a promising ORR of 28%, including a CR rate of 6%, a median PFS of 2.9 months, and a median OS of 9.6 months. The toxicity profile of pemetrexed without folate supplementation was favorable, with grade 3/4 thrombocytopenia occurring in 9% of 47 patients, neutropenia in 9%, and diarrhea in 4%. However, a subsequent phase II trial [31] of 13 patients failed, reporting an ORR of only 8%.

Paclitaxel. Taxanes, including paclitaxel, are commonly used as second-line chemotherapy agents. Taxanes have only a modest ORR of approximately 10%, but their good tolerability and lack of nephrotoxicity are advantageous. Single-agent paclitaxel demonstrated limited efficacy in two phase II trials [32,33] with ORRs of 7%−10%. Metronomic treatment with paclitaxel 80 mg/m^2 weekly [32] was tolerable.

Combination chemotherapy regimens have also been evaluated in the second-line setting. Generally, multidrug combinations achieved better response rates but also increased toxicity and did not necessarily improve survival outcomes [24]. Therefore combinations of conventional chemotherapeutic agents are usually not administered as second-line therapy, and standard combinations of second-line treatment are lacking.

NOVEL CHEMOTHERAPEUTIC AGENTS

Molecular Targeted Agents

Therapies targeting alterations of genetic pathways have demonstrated efficacy for several solid cancers. Urothelial carcinoma harbors numerous genomic aberrations and aberrant protein expressions that could potentially serve as drug targets. Recently, the Cancer Genome Atlas analysis found that 69% of 131 urothelial bladder cancer tissue samples harbored genetic alterations that can be targeted by drugs already approved for use in other indications or in clinical trials [39]. However, to date, the majority of clinical trials of targeted therapies as a single agent or as part of a combination with conventional chemotherapy have been unsatisfactory in urothelial carcinoma, primarily because most previous trials of molecular targeted agents did not assess the mutational status of actionable mutations. The following genetic alterations in urothelial carcinoma are potential drug targets: mutations in the receptor tyrosine kinases RAS and RAF, phosphoinositide 3-kinase/AKT/ mammalian target of rapamycin pathways, regulators of G1-S cell cycle progression such as TP53 and RB1, fibroblast growth factor receptor (FGFR)-3 mutations and translocations, and amplifications in FGFR1, CCND1, and MDM2 genes.

Immune Checkpoint Blocking Agents

Recently, immunomodulatory therapies have led to important advances in the treatment of cancer using immune checkpoint inhibition. Immune checkpoint blocking agents that target programmed death (PD)-1, PD ligand 1 (PD-L1), or cytotoxic T lymphocyte-associated antigen 4 have shown a great deal of promise in treating certain types of cancer. The interaction between

PD-1 of a cytotoxic T cell and PD-L1 of a tumor cell is thought to be a key mechanism of immune escape from cancer that is specific to the cytotoxic T cell. The PD-1 receptor and PD-L1 are prevalent in urothelial carcinoma. Anti-PD-1/PD-L1 antibodies enhance CD8 T-cell function of attacking cancer cells by blocking the PD-1/PD-L1 axis. Immune checkpoint inhibitors—anti-PD-1/PD-L1 antibodies—have shown promising results in urothelial carcinoma.

Atezolizumab. Atezolizumab (MPDL3280A) is an engineered humanized monoclonal immunoglobulin G1 antibody that binds selectively to PD-L1 and prevents its interaction with PD-1. An expanded phase I study [40] provided the initial evidence of the safety and efficacy of atezolizumab; the results showed higher response rates in patients with higher levels of PD-L1 expression on tumor-infiltrating immune cells than in patients with lower PD-L1 expression. These results were expanded in a phase II study [41] that included two different cohorts. The results of cohort 2, in which 310 patients with metastatic urothelial cancer were treated with atezolizumab, have been reported. All patients in this cohort had experienced disease progression during or after platinum-based chemotherapy. The ORR was 15%, including a CR rate of 5% among all patients. The ORR was higher in patients with more expression of PD-L1 on infiltrating immune cells, and objective responses were sometimes observed in patients with no expression of PD-L1. Immune checkpoint inhibitors are a promising approach to treatment, not only because of response rates but also because of the long duration of response (i.e., 1−2 years or more) in responders. Furthermore, the safety profile of immune checkpoint inhibitors is good, with the exception of some autoimmune adverse events. Atezolizumab showed durable activity and good tolerability, and this agent received a breakthrough therapy designation from the U.S. Food and Drug Administration in May 2016. Based on the promising phase II results with atezolizumab, several phase III trials comparing anti-PD-1/PD-L1 and standard chemotherapy in first-line and second-line settings are ongoing.

Other PD-1/PD-L1 inhibitors. Other PD-1 or PD-L1 inhibitors, including pembrolizumab, nivolumab, and durvalumab, have demonstrated some activity in early clinical studies and are currently being evaluated in randomized clinical trials in patients with urothelial carcinoma. These include trials of first-line and second-line therapy, as well as adjuvant therapy.

CHEMOTHERAPY FOR NONUROTHELIAL BLADDER CANCER

Nonurothelial bladder cancer accounts for less than 5% of all bladder tumors [42]. A majority of nonurothelial cancers are epithelial in origin, including squamous cell carcinomas, adenocarcinomas, and small cell tumors. Nonepithelial cancers are rare and include sarcoma, carcinosarcoma, paraganglioma, melanoma, and lymphoma. There is little data to recommend treatments for nonurothelial bladder cancer. Treatment is usually extrapolated from the approach to patients with urothelial bladder cancers. For patients who present with localized disease, the primary treatment is cystectomy. For patients with advanced nonurothelial bladder cancer who are not candidates for surgery, including those with metastatic disease, treatment options include palliative care, radiation therapy, or chemotherapy. The role of chemotherapy or radiation therapy is not clear for unresectable, metastatic squamous cell carcinoma or adenocarcinoma types of bladder cancer. One prospective study of ifosfamide, paclitaxel, and cisplatin in advanced nonurothelial bladder cancer (11 of 20 with adenocarcinoma, including 6 with urachal adenocarcinoma) reported a response rate of 36% and a median survival of 25 months [43]. For patients with nonepithelial nonurothelial bladder cancer, such as lymphoma or sarcoma, treatment should be given according to tumor type.

CONCLUSION

Systemic chemotherapy plays a central role in the management of metastatic bladder cancer. Before considering palliative systemic chemotherapy, medical fitness for chemotherapy should be determined. For patients with good performance status and adequate renal function who can tolerate cisplatin, cisplatin-based combination chemotherapy such as MVAC or GC is recommended. Cisplatin-based combination chemotherapy has led to substantial increases in survival rates in bladder cancer. A choice among regimens is individualized on the basis of a patient's performance status and ability to tolerate chemotherapy, as well as physicians' preferences. For patients with impaired renal function or patients who cannot tolerate cisplatin, carboplatin-based regimens, nonplatinum-based combinations, or supportive care only can be considered. For all other patients, single-agent chemotherapy and treatment with BSC are reasonable options. For patients who relapse following treatment with cisplatin, multiple agents have modest activity, including gemcitabine, vinflunine, ifosfamide, paclitaxel, docetaxel, and pemetrexed. The choice of the optimal treatment regimen is challenging and the best starting time and duration for second-line treatment is still undetermined. A choice among various second-line agents should be based on clinical factors such as the patient's performance status, symptom burden, and comorbidities and medical judgment as to the patient's ability to tolerate chemotherapy.

The prognosis of metastatic bladder cancer remains very poor. Novel therapeutic agents must be developed to improve outcomes and patients should be encouraged to participate in clinical trials whenever possible. Recent results with novel immune checkpoint blocking agents, such as atezolizumab, show promising antitumor activity with good tolerability. Additional preclinical and clinical investigations are urgently needed to improve treatment outcomes of metastatic bladder cancer.

REFERENCES

[1] Raghavan D. Chemotherapy and cystectomy for invasive transitional cell carcinoma of bladder. Urol Oncol 2003;21:468−74.

[2] Loehrer PJ, Einhorn LH, Elson PJ, et al. A randomized comparison of cisplatin alone or in combination with methotrexate, vinblastine, and doxorubicin in patients with metastatic urothelial carcinoma: a cooperative group study. J Clin Oncol 1992;10:1066−73.

[3] von der Maase H, Hansen SW, Roberts JT, et al. Gemcitabine and cisplatin versus methotrexate, vinblastine, doxorubicin, and cisplatin in advanced or metastatic bladder cancer: results of a large, randomized, multinational, multicenter, phase III study. J Clin Oncol 2000;18:3068−77.

[4] von der Maase H, Sengelov L, Roberts JT, et al. Long-term survival results of a randomized trial comparing gemcitabine plus cisplatin, with methotrexate, vinblastine, doxorubicin, plus cisplatin in patients with bladder cancer. J Clin Oncol 2005;23:4602−8.

[5] Dash A, Galsky MD, Vickers AJ, et al. Impact of renal impairment on eligibility for adjuvant cisplatin-based chemotherapy in patients with urothelial carcinoma of the bladder. Cancer 2006;107:506−13.

[6] Galsky MD, Hahn NM, Rosenberg J, et al. A consensus definition of patients with metastatic urothelial carcinoma who are unfit for cisplatin-based chemotherapy. Lancet Oncol 2011;12:211−14.

[7] Logothetis CJ, Dexeus FH, Finn L, et al. A prospective randomized trial comparing MVAC and CISCA chemotherapy for patients with metastatic urothelial tumors. J Clin Oncol 1990;8:1050−5.

[8] Sternberg CN, Yagoda A, Scher HI, et al. Methotrexate, vinblastine, doxorubicin, and cisplatin for advanced transitional cell carcinoma of the urothelium. Efficacy and patterns of response and relapse. Cancer 1989;64:2448−58.

[9] Harker WG, Meyers FJ, Freiha FS, et al. Cisplatin, methotrexate, and vinblastine (CMV): an effective chemotherapy regimen for metastatic transitional cell carcinoma of the urinary tract. A Northern California Oncology Group study. J Clin Oncol 1985;3:1463−70.

[10] Bellmunt J, von der Maase H, Mead GM, et al. Randomized phase III study comparing paclitaxel/cisplatin/gemcitabine and gemcitabine/cisplatin in patients with locally advanced or metastatic urothelial cancer without prior systemic therapy: EORTC Intergroup Study 30987. J Clin Oncol 2012;30:1107−13.

[11] Sternberg CN, de Mulder PH, Schornagel JH, et al. Randomized phase III trial of high-dose-intensity methotrexate, vinblastine, doxorubicin, and cisplatin (MVAC) chemotherapy and recombinant human granulocyte colony-stimulating factor versus classic MVAC in advanced urothelial tract tumors: European Organization for Research and Treatment of Cancer Protocol no. 30924. J Clin Oncol 2001;19:2638−46.

[12] Sternberg CN, de Mulder P, Schornagel JH, et al. Seven year update of an EORTC phase III trial of high-dose intensity M-VAC chemotherapy and G-CSF versus classic M-VAC in advanced urothelial tract tumours. Eur J Cancer Oxf Engl 1990 2006;42:50−4.

[13] Tannock I, Gospodarowicz M, Connolly J, et al. M-VAC (methotrexate, vinblastine, doxorubicin and cisplatin) chemotherapy for transitional cell carcinoma: the Princess Margaret Hospital experience. J Urol 1989;142:289−92.

[14] Gabrilove JL, Jakubowski A, Scher H, et al. Effect of granulocyte colony-stimulating factor on neutropenia and associated morbidity due to chemotherapy for transitional-cell carcinoma of the urothelium. N Engl J Med 1988;318:1414−22.

[15] Moore MJ, Iscoe N, Tannock IF. A phase II study of methotrexate, vinblastine, doxorubicin and cisplatin plus recombinant human granulocyte-macrophage colony stimulating factors in patients with advanced transitional cell carcinoma. J Urol 1993;150:1131−4.

[16] von der Maase H, Andersen L, Crinò L, et al. Weekly gemcitabine and cisplatin combination therapy in patients with transitional cell carcinoma of the urothelium: a phase II clinical trial. Ann Oncol 1999;10:1461−5.

[17] Kaufman D, Raghavan D, Carducci M, et al. Phase II trial of gemcitabine plus cisplatin in patients with metastatic urothelial cancer. J Clin Oncol 2000;18:1921−7.

[18] Adamo V, Magno C, Spitaleri G, et al. Phase II study of gemcitabine and cisplatin in patients with advanced or metastatic bladder cancer: long-term follow-up of a 3-week regimen. Oncology 2005;69:391−8.

[19] Soto Parra H, Cavina R, Latteri F, et al. Three-week versus four-week schedule of cisplatin and gemcitabine: results of a randomized phase II study. Ann Oncol 2002;13:1080−6.

[20] De Santis M, Bellmunt J, Mead G, et al. Randomized phase II/III trial assessing gemcitabine/carboplatin and methotrexate/carboplatin/vinblastine in patients with advanced urothelial cancer who are unfit for cisplatin-based chemotherapy: EORTC study 30986. J Clin Oncol 2012;30:191−9.

[21] Li J, Juliar B, Yiannoutsos C, et al. Weekly paclitaxel and gemcitabine in advanced transitional-cell carcinoma of the urothelium: a phase II Hoosier Oncology Group study. J Clin Oncol 2005;23:1185−91.

[22] Meluch AA, Greco FA, Burris HA, et al. Paclitaxel and gemcitabine chemotherapy for advanced transitional-cell carcinoma of the urothelial tract: a phase II trial of the Minnie pearl cancer research network. J Clin Oncol 2001;19:3018−24.

[23] Bellmunt J, Choueiri TK, Schutz FaB, et al. Randomized phase III trials of second-line chemotherapy in patients with advanced bladder cancer: progress and pitfalls. Ann Oncol 2011;22:245−7.

[24] Oing C, Rink M, Oechsle K, et al. Second line chemotherapy for advanced and metastatic urothelial carcinoma: vinflunine and beyond-a comprehensive review of the current literature. J Urol 2016;195:254−63.

[25] Bellmunt J, Théodore C, Demkov T, et al. Phase III trial of vinflunine plus best supportive care compared with best supportive care alone after a platinum-containing regimen in patients with advanced transitional cell carcinoma of the urothelial tract. J Clin Oncol 2009;27:4454−61.

[26] Han KS, Joung JY, Kim TS, et al. Methotrexate, vinblastine, doxorubicin and cisplatin combination regimen as salvage chemotherapy for patients with advanced or metastatic transitional cell carcinoma after failure of gemcitabine and cisplatin chemotherapy. Br J Cancer 2008;98:86−90.

[27] Kim KH, Hong SJ, Han KS. Predicting the response of patients with advanced urothelial cancer to methotrexate, vinblastine, adriamycin, and cisplatin (MVAC) after the failure of gemcitabine and platinum (GP). BMC Cancer 2015;15:812.

[28] Dreicer R. Second-line chemotherapy for advanced urothelial cancer: because we should or because we can? J Clin Oncol 2009;27:4444−5.

[29] Culine S, Theodore C, De Santis M, et al. A phase II study of vinflunine in bladder cancer patients progressing after first-line platinum-containing regimen. Br J Cancer 2006;94:1395−401.

[30] Sweeney CJ, Roth BJ, Kabbinavar FF, et al. Phase II study of pemetrexed for second-line treatment of transitional cell cancer of the urothelium. J Clin Oncol 2006;24:3451−7.

[31] Galsky MD, Mironov S, Iasonos A, et al. Phase II trial of pemetrexed as second-line therapy in patients with metastatic urothelial carcinoma. Invest New Drugs 2007;25:265—70.

[32] Vaughn DJ, Broome CM, Hussain M, et al. Phase II trial of weekly paclitaxel in patients with previously treated advanced urothelial cancer. J Clin Oncol 2002;20:937—40.

[33] Papamichael D, Gallagher CJ, Oliver RT, et al. Phase II study of paclitaxel in pretreated patients with locally advanced/metastatic cancer of the bladder and ureter. Br J Cancer 1997;75:606—7.

[34] Vaughn DJ, Srinivas S, Stadler WM, et al. Vinflunine in platinum-pretreated patients with locally advanced or metastatic urothelial carcinoma: results of a large phase 2 study. Cancer 2009;115:4110—17.

[35] McCaffrey JA, Hilton S, Mazumdar M, et al. Phase II trial of docetaxel in patients with advanced or metastatic transitional-cell carcinoma. J Clin Oncol 1997;15:1853—7.

[36] Albers P, Siener R, Härtlein M, et al. Gemcitabine monotherapy as second-line treatment in cisplatin-refractory transitional cell carcinoma—prognostic factors for response and improvement of quality of life. Onkologie 2002;25:47—52.

[37] Akaza H, Naito S, Usami M, et al. Efficacy and safety of gemcitabine monotherapy in patients with transitional cell carcinoma after Cisplatin-containing therapy: a Japanese experience. Jpn J Clin Oncol 2007;37:201—6.

[38] Witte RS, Elson P, Bono B, et al. Eastern cooperative oncology group phase II trial of ifosfamide in the treatment of previously treated advanced urothelial carcinoma. J Clin Oncol 1997;15:589—93.

[39] Cancer Genome Atlas Research Network. Comprehensive molecular characterization of urothelial bladder carcinoma. Nature 2014;507:315—22.

[40] Powles T, Eder JP, Fine GD, et al. MPDL3280A (anti-PD-L1) treatment leads to clinical activity in metastatic bladder cancer. Nature 2014;515:558—62.

[41] Rosenberg JE, Hoffman-Censits J, Powles T, et al. Atezolizumab in patients with locally advanced and metastatic urothelial carcinoma who have progressed following treatment with platinum-based chemotherapy: a single-arm, multicentre, phase 2 trial. Lancet Lond Engl 2016;387:1909—20.

[42] Dahm P, Gschwend JE. Malignant non-urothelial neoplasms of the urinary bladder: a review. Eur Urol 2003;44:672—81.

[43] Galsky MD, Iasonos A, Mironov S, et al. Prospective trial of ifosfamide, paclitaxel, and cisplatin in patients with advanced non-transitional cell carcinoma of the urothelial tract. Urology 2007;69:255—9.

Section VII

Follow-Up (Surveillance)

Chapter 29

Surveillance for Non-Muscle-Invasive Bladder Cancer

Ji Sung Shim and Sung Gu Kang
Korea University College of Medicine, Seoul, South Korea

Chapter Outline

INTRODUCTION

Most new cases of urothelial cancer (UC) of the bladder are Ta, T1, or carcinoma in situ (CIS). These are often grouped as non-muscle-invasive bladder cancer (NMIBC) formerly known as "superficial" bladder cancer [1]. Initial management is complete endoscopic resection. Initial staging is critical for management decisions. After the initial surgery, the urologist should consider a repeat resection or perioperative and/or adjuvant intravesical therapy depending on tumor grade, stage, and multiplicity. The high recurrence rates of Ta low grade (LG) with low progression rates demand risk-adapted treatment and surveillance to provide thorough care while minimizing treatment-related burden. However, the propensity of high-grade (HG) Ta, T1, and CIS to progress demands intense care and timely consideration of radical cystectomy to provide oncologic safety [2].

During surveillance such as for initial diagnosis, hematuria is the most common finding and notable sign. Lower urinary tract symptoms also demand attention from clinicians because sometimes they may reveal a CIS. Cystourethroscopy is the cornerstone of diagnosis. Follow-up of lower urinary tract disease including malignant neoplasms of the bladder is needed. Although time-consuming and invasive, cystoscopies are essential. However, how often and how long they should be performed remains

Bladder Cancer. DOI: http://dx.doi.org/10.1016/B978-0-12-809939-1.00029-1

unclear. Surveillance strategies for UC recurrence have historically relied on diagnostic combination of cystoscopy and urinary cytology. Although the accuracy of both tests relies on subjective and operator-dependent interpretation of visible findings, they have been widely accepted as the gold standard [3].

CYSTOSCOPIC SURVEILLANCE

1. Role of cystoscopy

   Rod-lens cystoscopy has an important role in the diagnosis and follow-up of bladder tumor patients, although it has some drawbacks such as difficulties in identifying flat lesions without diagnostic value for upper urinary tract disease. Office-based cystoscopy offers rapid and relatively painless visual access to the urothelium. Papillary tumors arising from the smooth bladder surface can be readily identified. CIS can present as a velvet-like reddish area that is indistinguishable from inflammation. It might be invisible at all. The endoscopic appearance cannot reliably predict tumor stage or grade, although sessile morphology and/or the presence of necrosis suggests that HG disease is likely to be invasive. Nevertheless, for office-based diagnosis, cystoscopy allows for the identification of the site and overall characteristics of most tumors.

2. Flexible cystoscopy

   Although rod-lens cystoscopy has an important role in the diagnosis and follow-up of bladder tumor patients, it is difficult to evaluate the whole bladder, including tumors that are located near the bladder neck in male patients. This situation is further aggravated when the patient has benign prostatic hyperplasia, a severely elevated bladder neck, or even relatively large genitalia.

   To avoid missing bladder tumors located near the bladder neck, flexible cystoscopy can be considered in male patients [4]. Even if there are some difficulties in orienting the bladder anatomy, with "J" maneuver, this fiberscope can be used to visualize bladder tumors or the degree of prostate cancer infiltration at the bladder neck (Fig. 29.1A and B). With the development of high-resolution imaging, flexible scope has essentially replaced rigid cystoscopy for surveillance in men.

3. Relieving discomfort

   The majority of both men and women tolerate office-based cystoscopy with minimal discomfort. Intra-urethral injection of local anesthetics is almost universally used by urologists despite a paucity of data to support such practice [5–7].

   Use of a video monitor allows the patient to see and understand the findings, theoretically distracting them from any discomfort. Men who are able to do so can tolerate the procedure with approximately 50% less pain (visual analog scale: 2.21 vs 1.31, $P < 0.01$) than those who cannot see their findings on the monitor [8]. Recently, several studies have shown

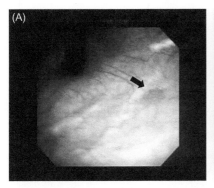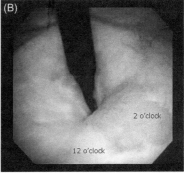

FIGURE 29.1 Flexible cystoscopy finding. Bladder tumors (A, B) were just adjacent to the bladder neck. They were diagnosed as urothelial cell carcinoma after transurethral resection. (A) Black arrow: tiny papillary tumor.

that listening to music can decrease anxiety and pain during outpatient-based cystoscopy [9−11].

4. Fluorescence cystoscopy (FC)

There is increasing consensus about the possibility that early recurrence may in fact arise from residual tumor left behind at resection or from the growth of previously undetected microscopic lesions [12−14]. Visual inspection of the bladder with white light is relatively reliable for the detection of papillary tumors. However, flat carcinomas (particularly CIS), dysplasia, multifocal growth, and microscopic lesions can be overlooked or inadequately resected. Illumination with blue-violet light (380−440 nm) produces a clearly demarcated red fluorescence from malignant tissue.

The beneficial effect of hexaminolevulinate (HAL) or 5-aminolaevulinic acid FC on recurrence rates in patients with transurethral resection of bladder tumor (TURBT) have shown controversial results [15−19]. However, a meta-analysis has reported an increase in detection of tumor lesions in HAL arms across all risk groups with an absolute reduction of <10% in recurrence rates within 12 months [20]. In that study, the benefit of HAL cystoscopy is particularly high in CIS patients, independent of the level of risk. However, despite the value of FC improves the outcome of progression rate, survival and clinical management benefits remain to be demonstrated.

5. Narrow-band imaging (NBI)

Initial studies have demonstrated that NBI-guided biopsies and resection can improve cancer detection [21,22] (Fig. 29.2A and B). Although the suggested reduction of recurrence rate when NBI is used for TURBT has not been fully confirmed yet, a recent meta-analysis has shown that NBI is an effective method for the identification of abnormal lesions (including CIS) and that NBI can provide a high diagnostic precision method to white-light imaging cystoscopy [22]. However, more prospective studies are needed to determine whether the visual advantages of NBI can bring real therapeutic benefit for individual patients.

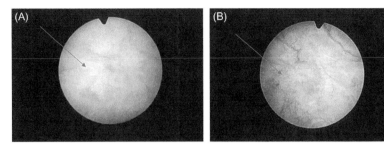

FIGURE 29.2 Images by white-light cystoscopy (WLC) and by NBI cystoscopy. (A) WLI image of CIS, (B) Enhanced visualization of CIS with NBI. (A) red arrow: grossly non visible bladder tumor; (B) red arrow: green colored area which is diagnosed in tumor in histologic examination.

URINE CYTOLOGY

The examination of voided urine or bladder-washing specimens for exfoliated cancer cells has high sensitivity for G3 tumors and CIS, with sensitivities exceeding 90%. However, it has low sensitivity for G1 tumors. The sensitivity of cytology for CIS detection is 28%−100% [23]. Positive voided urinary cytology indicates urothelial tumor anywhere in the urinary tract. A negative cytology, however, does not exclude the presence of a tumor. Cytologic interpretation is user dependent [24]. Even if an evaluation is hampered by low cellular yield, urinary tract infections, stones, or intravesical instillations, the specificity is known to exceed 90% in experienced hands [25].

URINE-BASED MARKERS

Although the diagnosis and surveillance of patients with NMIBC can rely on cystoscopy, cytology, and biopsy when necessary, there has been an intense search for noninvasive adjunctive urine-based markers to improve or perhaps replace cytology and cystoscopy in recent years. Driven by the low sensitivity of urine cytology, extensive laboratory research studies have been conducted to develop numerous urinary tests for bladder cancer detection [25−27]. These tests usually have higher sensitivity but lower specificity than urinary cytology [28].

One potential role of using urinary markers is reducing the frequency of cystoscopy during surveillance. While most protein-based urinary markers such as nuclear matrix protein (NMP) 22 are affected by tumor volume, recurrent LG UCs often are small. Hence, urinary markers may only have a role in low-intensity surveillance programs to monitor larger recurrent Ta LG UC of bladder during the cystoscopy intervals.

Several markers may aid in the surveillance of patients with NMIBCs. Currently available and Food and Drug Administration—approved tests include bladder tumor antigen STAT test (Bard Diagnostics, Redmond, WA, USA), BTA TRAK test (Poly Med Co., Cortlandt Manor, NY, USA), NMP 22 and NMP22 BladderChek assays (Matritech, Newton, MA, USA), ImmunoCyt test (Diagnocure Inc., Quebec City, Quebec, Canada), and fluorescence in situ hybridization (FISH) analysis (UroVysion Systems Vysis, Abbott Laboratories, Abbott Park, IL, USA). Other recently investigated tests and identified markers include Quanticyt (Gentian Scientific, Niawer, the Netherlands), BLCA-4, hyaluronic acid, telomerase, Lewis^X blood group antigens, microsatellite polymorphism analysis, cytokeratins, and survival [29,30]. Despite their present and future potentials, critical evaluation and comparison of urine-based markers are beyond the scope of the current guideline involving the management of NMIBC.

EXTRAVESICAL SURVEILLANCE

The likelihood of patients developing upper tract CIS or invasive UC after the diagnosis and treatment of NMIBC has been reported to be 0.002—2.4% over surveillance intervals of 5—13 years [31—33], although the risk is increasing substantially over time to as high as 18% in very high-risk populations [34]. Risk factors for the development of upper tract tumors in patients with NMIBC are tumor multiplicity, tumor in the trigone, bladder CIS, tumor grade, stage, and vesicoureteral reflux [35,36]. In the Surveillance, Epidemiology, and End Results (SEER) database, only 0.8% of bladder cancer patients developed subsequent upper tract tumors. Therefore, surveillance is of limited value unless the patient has hematuria or a HG tumor, especially if it is near the ureteral orifice [36]. The risk of tumor recurrence as an upper urinary tract tumor during follow-up increases in multiple and high-risk tumors [35].

Most reviews have concluded that patients who have HG or multiple tumors should undergo upper tract imaging based on the risk of upper tract disease. However, those with LG tumors probably do not benefit from imaging unless they have hematuria [17,35—37]. In addition, many guidelines do not support surveillance upper tract imaging, urinary cytology, or any other urinary biomarker for low-risk bladder cancer patients. This is supported by patient registry data of 99,338 bladder cancer patients with only 0.7% of LG bladder cancer patients who developed upper tract tumor at a median duration of 33 months [36].

The proper study to evaluate the upper tract is debatable. Intravenous urography (IVU) is a traditional choice for upper tract imaging. However, it gives limited information about renal parenchyma. In addition, it can miss small tumors. Transabdominal ultrasound permits the characterization of renal masses, detection of hydronephrosis, and visualization of intraluminal masses in the bladder. However, like IVU, it cannot exclude the presence of upper tract tumors. In addition, it has low sensitivity in detecting small bladder tumors [38]. CT urography is a promising technology. It has been used as an alternative to conventional IVU despite a larger radiation exposure [39]. An alternative is MRI urography. However, CIS cannot be diagnosed with imaging methods [40,41].

Selective cytology of the upper tract may increase the yield. However, in the presence of a bladder tumor, selective upper tract cytology may be false positive. Therefore, it is not recommended for most patients [32]. Bilateral ureteroscopy is often employed. However, data on its yield are lacking. Nevertheless, patients with positive cytology but negative cystoscopic and radiographic evaluation may warrant bilateral flexible ureteroscopy. Although selective collection of tumor markers is logical, there is no evidence to date to support this practice.

SURVEILLANCE SCHEDULE

The intent of NMIBC management is to control recurrence and progression and identify invasive tumors at the earliest stage possible. Due to the risk of recurrence and progression, patients with NMIBC need to be followed up. However, the frequency and duration of cystoscopy and imaging should reflect the individual patient's degree of risk. The European Association of Urology has supported recent efforts in the development of risk stratification schemes and included them in the guidelines for NMIBC [28]. Using risk stratification tables (Tables 29.1 and 29.2), the follow-up schedule can be adapted to patients accordingly [43]. The recommendation is similar to that provided by the International Bladder Cancer Group [44].

TABLE 29.1 Risk Group Stratification (EAU, 2016 [28])

Risk	Tumor Status
Low-risk tumors	Primary, solitary, Ta, LG/G1, <3 cm, no CIS
Intermediate-risk tumors	All tumors not defined in the two adjacent categories (between the category of low and high risk)
High-risk tumors	Any of the following: • T1 tumor • HG/G3 tumor • CIS • Multiple and recurrent and large (>3 cm) Ta, G1, G2 tumors (all conditions must be presented in this point)

EAU: European Association of Urology.

TABLE 29.2 Suggested Surveillance Strategies According to Risk

Risk	Cystoscopy Schedule	Urine Cytology and Markers[a]	Upper Tract Imaging
Low-risk tumors	Should undergo at 3 months If negative, subsequent cystoscopy is advised 9 months later Then, yearly for 5 years	Cytology: low sensitivity for LG recurrences Markers: better than cytology but still do not detect half of the LG tumor identified by cystoscopy	Not necessary unless hematuria present
Intermediate-risk tumors	Adapted according to personal and subjective factors Lifelong follow-up is recommended [42]		Imaging recommended for every 2 years [42] Imaging for recurrence or hematuria present
High-risk tumors	Should undergo both at 3 months If negative, both should be repeated every 3 months for a period of 2 years, and every 6 months thereafter until 5 years, and then yearly resetting the clock with each newly identified tumor Lifelong follow-up is recommended [42]		Regular yearly upper tract imaging is recommended

[a]According to current knowledge, no urinary marker can replace cystoscopy during follow-up or help lower cystoscopic frequency in a routine fashion.

Clinical follow-up involves appropriate patient history including voiding symptoms and hematuria, urinalysis, cystoscopy, and urine cytology. Among them, the first cystoscopy after complete TURBT of the NMIBC is of great importance as it has prognostic value [43,45–48]. At the present time, the use of urine-based molecular markers in the follow-up of patients remains uncertain. Surveillance often includes periodic upper tract imaging, especially for high-risk patients [49]. When planning the follow-up schedule and methods, the following aspects should be considered:

- The follow-up of NMIBC is based on regular cystoscopy.
- The first cystoscopy after TURBT at 3 months is a very important prognostic indicator for recurrence and progression [47,50]. Therefore, the initial cystoscopy should always be performed at 3 months after TURBT in all patients with Ta, T1 tumors, and CIS.

- The prompt detection of muscle-invasive and HG/G3 non-muscle-invasive recurrence is important because a delay in diagnosis and therapy can be fatal.
- Endoscopic procedure under anesthesia and bladder biopsies should be performed when cystoscopic finding shows suspicious lesion or if cytology is positive. Bladder biopsy is unnecessary after initial BCG with erythematous findings if urine cytology is normal [42].
- The follow-up strategy should reflect the risk of extravesical recurrence (prostatic urethra in men and upper urinary tract).

Currently there is no evidence that intensive cystoscopic surveillance in low-risk NMIBC will actually improve the overall survival. In addition, cystoscopy is not without morbidity. Up to 5.5% of patients can develop urinary tract infection. In addition, a long surveillance protocol has significant healthcare cost implications [51,52].

No noninvasive method has been proposed to be able to replace endoscopy. Therefore, follow-up is based on regular cystoscopy. Randomized studies to investigate the possibility of safely reducing the frequency of follow-up cystoscopy are lacking. As CIS is often invisible, multiple biopsies may be necessary in selected cases to confirm the efficacy of intravesical treatment in patients treated for CIS [53]. General guidelines for bladder cancer surveillance are shown in Table 29.2.

REFERENCES

[1] Soloway MS. It is time to abandon the "superficial" in bladder cancer. Eur Urol 2007;52:1564—5.

[2] Burger M, Oosterlinck W, Konety B, Chang S, Gudjonsson S, Pruthi R, et al. ICUD-EAU International Consultation on Bladder Cancer 2012: non-muscle-invasive urothelial carcinoma of the bladder. Eur Urol 2013;63:36—44.

[3] Brown FM. Urine cytology. It is still the gold standard for screening? Urol Clin N Am 2000;27:25—37.

[4] Aaronson DS, Walsh TJ, Smith JF, Davies BJ, Hsieh MH, Konety BR. Meta-analysis: does lidocaine gel before flexible cystoscopy provide pain relief? BJU Int 2009;104:506—9, discussion 9—10.

[5] GoldFischer Evan R, Cromie WJ, Karrison Theodore G, Gerber Glenn S. Randomized, prospective, double blind study of the effects on pain perception of lidocaine jelly versus plain lubricant during outpatient rigid cystoscopy. J Urol 1997;157:90—4.

[6] Harry W, Herr MS. Outpatient flexible cystoscopy in men: a randomized study of patient tolerance. J Urol 2001;165:1971—2.

[7] Patel AR, Jones JS, Babineau D. Lidocaine 2% gel versus plain lubricating gel for pain reduction during flexible cystoscopy: a meta-analysis of prospective, randomized, controlled trials. J Urol 2008;179:986—90.

[8] Patel AR, Jones JS, Angie S, Babineau D. Office based flexible cystoscopy may be less painful for men allowed to view the procedure. J Urol 2007;177:1843—5.

[9]   Raheem OA, Mirheydar HS, Lee HJ, Patel ND, Godebu E, Sakamoto K. Does listening to music during office-based flexible cystoscopy decrease anxiety in patients: a prospective randomized trial. J Endourol 2015;29:791−6.

[10] Yeo JK, Cho DY, Oh MM, Park SS, Park MG. Listening to music during cystoscopy decreases anxiety, pain, and dissatisfaction in patients: a pilot randomized controlled trial. J Endourol 2013;27:459−62.

[11] Zhang ZS, Wang XL, Xu CL, Zhang C, Cao Z, Xu WD, et al. Music reduces panic: an initial study of listening to preferred music improves male patient discomfort and anxiety during flexible cystoscopy. J Endourol 2014;28:739−44.

[12] Jakse G, Algaba F, Malmstrom PU, Oosterlinck W. A second-look TUR in T1 transitional cell carcinoma: why?. Eur Urol 2004;45:539−46, discussion 46.

[13] Jocham D, Witjes F, Wagner S, Zeylemaker B, van Moorselaar J, Grimm MO, et al. Improved detection and treatment of bladder cancer using hexaminolevulinate imaging: a prospective, phase III multicenter study. J Urol 2005;174:862−6, discussion 6.

[14] Mostafid H, Brausi M. Measuring and improving the quality of transurethral resection for bladder tumour (TURBT). BJU Int 2012;109:1579−82.

[15] Kausch I, Sommerauer M, Montorsi F, Stenzl A, Jacqmin D, Jichlinski P, et al. Photodynamic diagnosis in non-muscle-invasive bladder cancer: a systematic review and cumulative analysis of prospective studies. Eur Urol 2010;57:595−606.

[16] Mowatt G, N'Dow J, Vale L, Nabi G, Boachie C, Cook JA, et al. Photodynamic diagnosis of bladder cancer compared with white light cystoscopy: Systematic review and meta-analysis. Int J Technol Assess Health Care 2011;27:3−10.

[17] Schumacher MC, Holmang S, Davidsson T, Friedrich B, Pedersen J, Wiklund NP. Transurethral resection of non-muscle-invasive bladder transitional cell cancers with or without 5-aminolevulinic Acid under visible and fluorescent light: results of a prospective, randomised, multicentre study. Eur Urol 2010;57:293−9.

[18] Stenzl A, Penkoff H, Dajc-Sommerer E, Zumbraegel A, Hoeltl L, Scholz M, et al. Detection and clinical outcome of urinary bladder cancer with 5-aminolevulinic acid-induced fluorescence cystoscopy: a multicenter randomized, double-blind, placebo-controlled trial. Cancer 2011;117:938−47.

[19] Draga RO, Grimbergen MC, Kok ET, Jonges TN, van Swol CF, Bosch JL. Photodynamic diagnosis (5-aminolevulinic acid) of transitional cell carcinoma after bacillus Calmette-Guerin immunotherapy and mitomycin C intravesical therapy. Eur Urol 2010;57:655−60.

[20] Burger M, Grossman HB, Droller M, Schmidbauer J, Hermann G, Dragoescu O, et al. Photodynamic diagnosis of non-muscle-invasive bladder cancer with hexaminolevulinate cystoscopy: a meta-analysis of detection and recurrence based on raw data. Eur Urol 2013;64:846−54.

[21] Cauberg EC, Kloen S, Visser M, de la Rosette JJ, Babjuk M, Soukup V, et al. Narrow band imaging cystoscopy improves the detection of non-muscle-invasive bladder cancer. Urology 2010;76:658−63.

[22] Zheng C, Lv Y, Zhong Q, Wang R, Jiang Q. Narrow band imaging diagnosis of bladder cancer: systematic review and meta-analysis. BJU Int 2012;110:E680−7.

[23] Tetu B. Diagnosis of urothelial carcinoma from urine. Mod Pathol 2009;22(Suppl 2): S53−9.

[24] Raitanen MP, Aine R, Rintala E, Kallio J, Rajala P, Juusela H, et al. Differences between local and review urinary cytology in diagnosis of bladder cancer. An interobserver multi-center analysis. Eur Urol 2002;41:284−9.

[25] Lokeshwar VB, Habuchi T, Grossman HB, Murphy WM, Hautmann SH, Hemstreet GP, et al. Bladder tumor markers beyond cytology: International Consensus Panel on bladder tumor markers. Urology 2005;66:35–63.

[26] van Rhijn BW, van der Poel HG, van der Kwast TH. Urine markers for bladder cancer surveillance: a systematic review. Eur Urol 2005;47:736–48.

[27] Vrooman OP, Witjes JA. Urinary markers in bladder cancer. Eur Urol 2008;53:909–16.

[28] Babjuk M, Böhle A, Burger M, Capoun O, Cohen D, Compérat EM, et al. EAU guidelines on non-muscle-invasive urothelial carcinoma of the bladder: update 2016. Eur Urol 2017;71(3):447–61.

[29] Gaston KE, Pruthi RS. Value of urinary cytology in the diagnosis and management of urinary tract malignancies. Urology 2004;63:1009–16.

[30] Konety BR. Molecular markers in bladder cancer: a critical appraisal. Urol Oncol 2006;24:326–37.

[31] Holmang S, Hedelin H, Anderstrom C, Johansson SL. The relationship among multiple recurrences, progression and prognosis of patients with stages Ta and T1 transitional cell cancer of the bladder followed for at least 20 years. J Urol 1995;153:1823–6, discussion 6–7.

[32] Sadek S, Soloway MS, Hook S, Civantos F. The value of upper tract cytology after transurethral resection of bladder tumor in patients with bladder transitional cell cancer. J Urol 1999;161:77–9, discussion 9–80.

[33] Shinka T, Uekado Y, Aoshi H, Hirano A, Ohkawa T. Occurrence of uroepithelial tumors of the upper urinary tract after the initial diagnosis of bladder cancer. J Urol 1988;140:745–8.

[34] Herr HW, Cookson MS, Soloway SM. Upper tract tumors in patients with primary bladder cancer followed for 15 years. J Urol 1996;156:1286–7.

[35] Millan-Rodriguez F, Chechile-Toniolo G, Salvador-Bayarri J, Huguet-Perez J, Vicente-Rodriguez J. Upper urinary tract tumors after primary superficial bladder tumors: prognostic factors and risk groups. J Urol 2000;164:1183–7.

[36] Wright JL, Hotaling J, Porter MP. Predictors of upper tract urothelial cell carcinoma after primary bladder cancer: a population based analysis. J Urol 2009;181:1035–9, discussion 9.

[37] Tan WS, Rodney S, Lamb B, Feneley M, Kelly J. Management of non-muscle invasive bladder cancer: A comprehensive analysis of guidelines from the United States, Europe and Asia. Cancer Treat Rev 2016;47:22–31.

[38] Cohan RH, Caoili EM, Cowan NC, Weizer AZ, Ellis JH. MDCT Urography: Exploring a new paradigm for imaging of bladder cancer. AJR Am J Roentgenol 2009;192:1501–8.

[39] Roupret M, Zigeuner R, Palou J, Boehle A, Kaasinen E, Sylvester R, et al. European guidelines for the diagnosis and management of upper urinary tract urothelial cell carcinomas: 2011 update. Eur Urol 2011;59:584–94.

[40] Herts BR. Imaging for renal tumors. Curr Opin Urol 2003;13:181–6.

[41] Davis R, Jones JS, Barocas DA, Castle EP, Lang EK, Leveille RJ, et al. Diagnosis, evaluation and follow-up of asymptomatic microhematuria (AMH) in adults: AUA guideline. J Urol 2012;188:2473–81.

[42] Soukup V, Babjuk M, Bellmunt J, Dalbagni G, Giannarini G, Hakenberg OW, et al. Follow-up after surgical treatment of bladder cancer: a critical analysis of the literature. Eur Urol 2012;62:290–302.

[43] Sylvester RJ, van der Meijden AP, Oosterlinck W, Witjes JA, Bouffioux C, Denis L, et al. Predicting recurrence and progression in individual patients with stage Ta T1 bladder

cancer using EORTC risk tables: a combined analysis of 2596 patients from seven EORTC trials. Eur Urol 2006;49, 466-5; discussion 75−7.

[44]   Brausi M, Witjes JA, Lamm D, Persad R, Palou J, Colombel M, et al. A review of current guidelines and best practice recommendations for the management of nonmuscle invasive bladder cancer by the International Bladder Cancer Group. J Urol 2011;186:2158−67.

[45]   Fernandez-Gomez J, Solsona E, Unda M, Martinez-Pineiro L, Gonzalez M, Hernandez R, et al. Prognostic factors in patients with non-muscle-invasive bladder cancer treated with bacillus Calmette-Guerin: multivariate analysis of data from four randomized CUETO trials. Eur Urol 2008;53:992−1001.

[46]   Holmang S, Johansson SL. Stage Ta-T1 bladder cancer: the relationship between findings at first followup cystoscopy and subsequent recurrence and progression. J Urol 2002;167:1634−7.

[47]   Palou J, Rodriguez-Rubio F, Millan F, Algaba F, Rodriguez-Faba O, Huguet J, et al. Recurrence at three months and high-grade recurrence as prognostic factor of progression in multivariate analysis of T1G2 bladder tumors. Urology 2009;73:1313−17.

[48]   Brausi M, Collette L, Kurth K, van der Meijden AP, Oosterlinck W, Witjes JA, et al. Variability in the recurrence rate at first follow-up cystoscopy after TUR in stage Ta T1 transitional cell carcinoma of the bladder: a combined analysis of seven EORTC studies. Eur Urol 2002;41:523−31.

[49]   Smith H, Weaver D, Barjenbruch O, Weinstein S, Ross Jr. G. Routine excretory urography in follow-up of superficial transitional cell carcinoma of bladder. Urology 1989; 34:193−6.

[50]   Mariappan P, Smith G. A surveillance schedule for G1Ta bladder cancer allowing efficient use of check cystoscopy and safe discharge at 5 years based on a 25-year prospective database. J Urol 2005;173:1108−11.

[51]   Botteman MF, Pashos CL, Redaelli A, Laskin B, Hauser R. The health economics of bladder cancer: a comprehensive review of the published literature. PharmacoEconomics 2003;21:1315−30.

[52]   Burke DM, Shackley DC, O'Reilly PH. The community-based morbidity of flexible cystoscopy. BJU Int 2002;89:347−9.

[53]   Kurth KH, Schellhammer PF, Okajima E. Current methods of assessing and treating carcinoma in situ of the bladder with or without involvement of the prostatic urethra. Int J Urol 1995;2(Suppl 2):8−22.

Chapter 30

The Surveillance for Muscle-Invasive Bladder Cancer (MIBC)

Yun-Sok Ha and Tae-Hwan Kim
Kyungpook National University, Daegu, South Korea

Chapter Outline

INTRODUCTION

The follow-up of patients treated for muscle-invasive bladder cancer (MIBC) is of great importance because of the high incidence of local recurrence and distant metastasis after both radical cystectomy (RC) and bladder preservation [1,2]. However, the schedule and method of follow-up should reflect the individual's clinical situation. In this chapter, we aim to evaluate the follow-up results including oncological and functional outcomes as well as the existing evidence for the duration and extent of surveillance in patients after treatment for MIBC, and to provide recommendations to practicing physicians based on the conclusions of the evaluation.

Bladder Cancer. DOI: http://dx.doi.org/10.1016/B978-0-12-809939-1.00030-8

FOLLOW-UP FOR MIBC AFTER RC

The Rationale

The goal of all the follow-up strategies is to detect systemic metastases as early as possible to gain time for adequate systemic treatment with or without removal of metastatic lesions, which is beneficial in terms of progression-free and cancer-specific survival (CSS). In order to design an individualized follow-up scheme, the natural timing, and probability of recurrence, functional deteriorations at particular sites and the treatment options available for the recurrence should be considered [3]. The commonly used surveillance protocols are built on the recurrence patterns that were observed in retrospective RC series. Data from prospective trials demonstrating the effectiveness of follow-up after RC, with a particular emphasis on its impact on survival, are lacking.

Estimation of the Risk of Recurrence

Recently, a nomogram was created based on data from 728 patients who underwent cystectomy. Standard predictors for the risk of recurrence were the pathological stage of the primary tumor (pT) and nodal status (pN). The predictive capacity of the nomogram for recurrent disease improved by 3.2% when the nomogram included the age, lymphovascular invasion (LVI), carcinoma in situ (CIS), neoadjuvant chemotherapy, adjuvant chemotherapy, and adjuvant radiation therapy (RT) [4]. This nomogram could be used to predict the individual risk of systemic relapse and to develop a risk-adapted follow-up protocol. Similar results were obtained with The International Bladder Cancer Nomogram, which is based on the information on 9000 bladder cancer (BC) patients from 12 institutes worldwide [5].

Site of Recurrence

Local Recurrence

Local recurrence takes place at the original surgical site in soft tissues or at the lymph nodes in the area of lymph node dissection. Lymph node involvement above the aortic bifurcation can be considered as metastatic recurrence [6]. Contemporary cystectomy carries a 5%−15% probability of pelvic recurrence. Most of the recurrences manifest during the first 24 months, usually within 6−18 months after the surgery. However, late recurrence can occur up to 5 years after cystectomy. Up to 70% of patients with local recurrence will also have distant metastases [7]. Pathological stage and lymph node status as well as positive margins, extent of lymph node dissection, and peri-operative chemotherapy are predictors of pelvic recurrence [8]. Patients with pelvic recurrence have poor prognoses. Even after treatment, approximately 80% of the patients die of disease within 1 year, and only 3.5% of the patients show a survival of 5 years [9]. Definitive therapy can prolong survival; however, it mostly serves as palliative therapy. The treatment strategies used are systemic chemotherapy, local surgery, or RT [7].

Distant Metastasis

Recently the long-term oncological outcome of RC was analyzed in a contemporary series of 2287 patients who underwent RC between 1998 and 2008 [10]. The mean and median follow-up durations were 35 and 29 months, respectively. The 5-year overall, recurrence-free, and CSS rates were 57%, 48%, and 67%, respectively, with distant metastasis rates of 37%. In a series of 212 patients with a mean follow-up duration of 28 months, Canter et al. [11] reported 5-year recurrence-free and CSS rates of 56.5% and 59.5%, respectively. The majority of the patients in this series developed distant metastases as well.

Distant metastases have been observed in up to 50% of patients treated with cystectomy. Most of the recurrences have been observed during the first 24 months after treatment; however, disease progression has been observed after more than 10 years [6,12−14]. The most likely sites for distant metastases are the lungs, liver, and the bones [15]. Treatment of metastatic disease using cisplatin-based combination chemotherapy with either M-VAC or gemcitabine has resulted in a mean survival time of approximately 14 months. Helical computed tomography (CT) represents the standard imaging modality used for the detection of lung metastases [16,17]. The use of reconstructed 5-mm-thick contiguous CT images enables the detection of lesions with a minimum size of 10 mm. For the detection of liver metastases, conventional CT as well as contrast-enhanced CT with nonionic, iodine-containing water-soluble contrast agents should be performed. Multidetector helical CT is currently the standard imaging modality [18,19] and 5-mm reconstructions should be used, in order to allow for the detection of lesions with a minimum size of 10 mm.

The majority of lymph node metastases originating from urogenital cancer are located in the retroperitoneum; therefore, CT scan is the imaging procedure of choice for the abdomen and the pelvis [20,21]. On these cross-sectional modalities, nodal metastases are usually suspected depending on the location and size criteria, that is, a maximum short-axis diameter ≥ 1 cm was considered malignant [20]. However, CT scans of the abdomen and pelvis might give false-negative results in up to 30% of the cases due to difficulties in the interpretation of lymph node status based on morphology and size alone [21]. Magnetic resonance tomography scans of the abdomen and pelvis do not provide additional information and should be restricted to patients with contraindications to CT [13]. To date, positron emission tomography (PET) has not been shown to improve sensitivity in patients with metastatic urogenital cancers overstaged via CT alone [22,23]. Bone scintigraphy, conventional radiographic techniques, CT, ^{18}F-fluorodeoxyglucose PET/CT, and whole body MRI represent potential imaging modalities to diagnose and to monitor skeletal metastases [24−27].

It is generally presumed that the early detection of tumor recurrence, in an asymptomatic state with good performance status, should enable treatment and might confer a survival benefit. However, the results of two recent retrospective clinical studies indicate that whether the early detection of recurrences is associated with a survival benefit when compared to recurrences that are detected owing to the development of symptoms appears to be questionable [6,13]. In the first study, 479 patients who underwent RC with adjuvant therapy were assessed by routine follow-up investigations according to a standardized follow-up protocol, to determine whether the diagnosis of asymptomatic recurrence after RC conferred a survival benefit compared to symptomatic recurrence. After a median follow-up duration of 4.3 years, 174 recurrences were detected, of which 87 were symptomatic, and 87 were asymptomatic. The 5-year cancer-specific and overall survival (OS) rates were significantly higher in the group of patients with asymptomatic metastases; therefore, the authors recommended routine cross-sectional imaging of the chest and the abdomen. On the other hand, Volkmer et al. [13] identified that 444 out of 1270 patients developed recurrences after RC, of which 154 and 290 were asymptomatic and symptomatic, respectively. The OS rates at 1, 2, and 5 years did not differ significantly between both groups. The authors concluded that symptom-guided follow-up might provide similar results to that of a strict follow-up protocol, but at a lower cost. It is important to realize that the follow-up studies conducted after RC implemented different follow-up regimens and different follow-up imaging methods. Therefore the data from these studies are not sufficient to make final recommendations.

Detection of Recurrence in the Remnant Urothelium

According to recent series, the secondary urothelial tumors account for approximately up to 20% of all recurrences after RC for MIBC [6].

Upper Urinary Tract Recurrence

Incidence and Time to Upper Urinary Tract Tumor Recurrence Upper urinary tract tumors (UUTTs) occur in 1.8%−4.8% of cases in contemporary series (Table 30.1). As opposed to local recurrence and distant metastases, metachronous UUTT recurrences after MIBC are considered late oncological events. In fact the UUTT is the most common site of late recurrence [28,31,34]. Most UUTT recurrences have been reported to occur after a median time of 24−41 months following RC [30,31,35−37]. Because of the improved survival rates in patients with MIBC, the number of patients who

TABLE 30.1 The Incidence Rates of UUTTs Following RC

Source	Year	N	UUTT Recurrence, Incidence (%)	Time to Recurrence (months)	Follow-Up Periods (months)
Huguet-Perez et al. [28]	2001	568	4.5	28.4	>60
Hautmann et al. [29]	2006	672	2	33	36
Meissner et al. [30]	2007	322	4.7	49	49
Sanderson et al. [31]	2007	1359	2.5	39.6	124
Tran et al. [32]	2008	1329	6	25.2	38
Volkmer et al. [33]	2009	1420	1.8	39	58
Umbreit et al. [34]	2010	1388	4.8	37.2	NA

UUTT, upper urinary tract tumor; NA, not applicable.

achieve long-term survival will also increase; however, these patients will remain at risk for tumor recurrence in the upper urinary tract. In numerous studies the 5-year rate of UUTT recurrences after RC has been reported as 2%−9% [6,28,31,32,35,38−42]. In a longitudinal study using a landmark time analysis of 1329 patients treated with RC, it was shown that the risk of UUTT recurrence did not decrease over time, with 3- and 5-year cumulative incidences of 4% [95% confidence interval (CI), 3%−6%] and 7% (95% CI, 5%−8%), respectively [32]. Furthermore, ureteral recurrences have been reported to occur even 9 years after curative surgery [31], which highlights the importance of the long-term surveillance of the upper urinary tract after RC.

Rationale Behind a Risk-Adapted Strategy for Follow-Up Several clinical and pathological parameters have been identified as risk factors for the recurrence of metachronous UUTT and they should be taken into consideration when addressing the patient's individual risk of recurrence. The rationale behind a risk-adapted strategy has been supported by a recently performed large retrospective analysis evaluating the long-term risk of upper tract recurrence in 1420 patients who had undergone cystectomy [33]. In this study, we showed that a number of risk factors could potentiate the risk of upper tract recurrence. Multivariate analysis revealed that patients with no risk factors (no history of CIS and recurrent BC, high-grade pTa−pT1 BC, and distal ureteral malignancy after RC) had only a 0.8% risk of developing ureteral recurrence 15 years after surgery, whereas in patients with three to four existing risk factors, the rate of recurrence increased to 13.5% [33]. Furthermore, a recent large retrospective single-center series of 174 patients with recurrence after RC showed that the rate of concomitant distant recurrences in patients with secondary urothelial carcinoma was only 11% [6].

Approximately 75% of the UUTT recurrences are discovered when patients present with symptoms, such as gross hematuria or flank pain. These symptoms are often associated with locally advanced disease and consequently are associated with poor outcomes after radical nephroureterectomy [31]. Thus new strategies should be developed for the early detection of upper tract recurrences while they are still localized, to render radical nephroureterectomy an effective local curative treatment option [31]. The assessment of the risk factors for upper tract recurrence might help in the identification of high-risk patients and thus in the tailoring of surveillance regimes according to a risk-adapted strategy, thereby reducing the need for unnecessary follow-up examinations and avoiding surveillance costs in low-risk patients.

Risk Factors for Upper Urinary Tract Tumor Recurrence

Ureteral Margin and Frozen Section Analysis. Ureteral tumor involvement was identified in 4.8%−13.0% of the patients during the final pathological analysis of the RC specimens from the examined ureters [32,35,40,43,44]. Various studies showed that tumor involvement of the distal ureter following RC is an independent risk factor for upper tract recurrence [32,33], and confers an approximately 2.6-fold increase in the relative risk of recurrence [33]. Although there is substantial evidence suggesting that intraoperative frozen section analysis is a reliable tool for detecting malignant ureteral margins after RC, its significance is still controversial [35,36,40,43,44]. In two recent studies the sensitivity and specificity of frozen section analysis were reported for the detection of malignant ureteral margins to be 74%−75% and 98%−99%, respectively, with a positive predictive value (PPV) of 94%, resulting in an overall accuracy of 98% [35,43]. On the other hand, whether a sequential resection of the malignant ureteral margins can unequivocally be advocated to reduce the risk of a malignant anastomotic margins at RC is controversial due to the heterogeneity of the available data [35,36,43]. In two recent studies the conversion rates of the initially positive ureteral margins into negative margins using a sequential resection strategy were as high as 39%−41% [35,43], whereas in another study, a conversion rate of up to 82% was reported [36]. In this study the patients with initially positive but later converted margins still had 4.4-fold increased risk of recurrence compared to those patients with initially negative margins [36]. However, this risk decreased after the conversion to a finally negative ureteral margin because the patients with positive anastomotic margins had a comparatively higher 7.4-fold increased risk of recurrence [36].

Because the incidence of malignant ureteral tumors after RC was reported to be the highest in the distal ureters [45], some authors have suggested the resection of the ureters more proximally at the crossing with the iliac vessels [40]. A retrospective series among 755 patients who underwent cystectomy showed CIS in the most proximally resected ureters in only 1.2% of the patients [40]. In this study a considerable proportion of the patients with CIS (17%) were identified in frozen section analysis to have UUTT recurrence and 80% of the patients with CIS at the ureteral margin also had CIS of the bladder. The authors suggested performing frozen section analysis only in patients with known CIS of the bladder. This might minimize the risk of ureteral strictures due to ischemia of the distal part of the ureter, and be beneficial for patients who previously underwent pelvic RT; however, this necessitates the use of an afferent tubular ileal segment for ureteral reconstruction [40].

Carcinoma In Situ of the Bladder. In patients with NMIBC (pTa, pTis, pT1) the presence of CIS of the bladder was identified as a risk factor for metachronous UUTT [43]. Conversely, in patients with MIBC, concomitant CIS was not identified to be independently associated with UUTT recurrence [31,35,38,42,46]. However, in patients with CIS-only disease at RC, a significantly higher rate of upper tract recurrences was reported [47]. This finding might be artificially skewed toward the patient cohort with low-stage disease at RC because a confounding effect of survival differences between different tumor stages has to be assumed.

Tumor Stage and Multifocality. In several studies the tumor stage was investigated as a possible risk factor for UUTT recurrence. Approximately 65%−100% of the upper tract recurrences occur in patients with organ-confined BC (pT2bpN0M0 or lower stage disease) [28,38,42,46,48]. In one study patients with pTa−pT1 BC were reported to have a 1.8−3.8-fold higher risk of UUTT recurrence compared to patients with MIBC [30]. Similar to the outcome of patients with CIS-only disease at RC, the tumor stage was not identified to be an independent risk factor for UUTT recurrence; however, it was a rather strong predictor of prolonged survival after RC. These data might be biased because the patients with high-stage disease were at a considerably higher risk for early local or systemic recurrence compared to patients with NMIBC [6,49].

In a recent study multifocality of the primary bladder tumor was identified to independently contribute to a higher risk of ureteral involvement at RC and to subsequent UUTT recurrence [35], thereby supporting the results of a previous study [50]. The data on whether the urethral tumor involvement predicts a higher likelihood for UUTT recurrence are limited [31,42]. Urethral tumor involvement in female patients has been significantly associated with a higher risk of UUTT recurrence. Likewise, in male patients, urothelial carcinoma of the prostatic ducts invading the lamina propria was associated with a higher risk of secondary ureteral tumor development; however, this was not the case for patients with a continuous expansion of urothelial carcinoma into the prostate (classified as stage pT4a) [31,42]. Most presumably, this observation might also be biased due to impaired survival in patients with pT4a urothelial carcinoma of the bladder.

Survival After Upper Urinary Tract Tumor Recurrence The 3-year survival rate for patients with UUTT recurrence was reported to be 0%−25%; however, long-term survival of more than 9 years has been reported in some series [31,46,51]. Survival after secondary UUTT recurrence is mainly predicted by tumor stage and lymph node involvement. In a single-center series it was demonstrated that in patients with stage ≥ pT3 secondary UUTTs, the median survival time was only 1.3 years, compared to the 3.4 years in patients with stage pTa−pT1 cancers [31]. Similar results were observed in another series with 85 female patients who showed a UUTT recurrence rate of 2.4%. All recurrences were muscle invasive at nephroureterectomy [48]. Data from some studies suggested that tumor location also affected survival in patients with UUTT recurrence [52]. In some series recurrence at the ureteroileal anastomosis was found in up to 40%−60% of the patients with recurrent UUTT [35,52]. Importantly, patients with anastomotic tumor recurrence had the potential to develop early progression to distant metastatic disease, whereas patients with more proximal UUTT recurrence showed improved recurrence-free survival after RC [52].

Diagnosis of Upper Urinary Tract Tumor Recurrence

Radiological Imaging. According to the studies to date, patients diagnosed with asymptomatic UUTT recurrence during routine follow-up have a significantly higher survival advantage than those with symptomatic recurrences [31]. This stresses the importance of the early detection of metachronous UUTT for a timely initiation of curative treatment.

In a recent analysis the precision of the 1064 intravenous pyelography (IVP) studies conducted in 322 patients who underwent routine follow-up of their upper tract at 1, 2, 3, 5, 7, and 10 years after RC was investigated. Of these patients, UUTT recurrence was detected in only 15 patients (4.7%); however, 8 of them had suspicious findings on IVP. The patients with positive final ureteral margins had the highest risk of recurrence. Therefore the authors concluded that routine excretory urography should be limited to patients at high risk for UUTT recurrence. Likewise, Slaton et al. [53] developed a stage-specific surveillance protocol for patients who underwent RC and suggested the use of upper tract imaging every 1−2 years after RC for all tumor stages; however, specific risk factors were not taken into consideration in that study.

Although previous studies reported similar sensitivity rates (0%−55%) for IVP and multidetector CT (MD-CT) urography for the detection of upper tract recurrence [28,38,42,46,48,53], some more recent studies have adopted MD-CT urography as the preferred diagnostic option for the detection of

UUTT compared to conventional IVP [54]. Contemporary series reporting the importance of MD-CT derive mainly from series of patients with either primary UUTTs or those who underwent upper tract imaging for a history of microscopic or gross hematuria, and they are also limited by a relatively small number of patients. In order to provide some of the recent aspects and developments associated with this diagnostic field, the results of the most recent studies will be outlined in the following sections.

In patients with primary UUTTs, MD-CT urography was reported to show significantly higher sensitivity, specificity, and test accuracy (96%, 100%, and 99%, respectively) than IVP (75%, 86%, and 85%, respectively) [54]. For MD-CT urography, the location of the primary tumor appeared to have a direct impact on the detection of accuracy. The sensitivity for the detection of the tumors in the renal pelvis was 78%−94%; however, a lower sensitivity of 19%−54% was observed for the lesions in the ureter [55]. In a retrospective series of 188 patients having histories of urothelial carcinoma (using diagnostic ureterorenoscopy as the diagnostic reference standard), MD-CT urography showed a PPV of 63%−67% for the identification of tumor lesions in the upper tract [56,57]. In both of these studies the characteristic findings indicative of UUTT on MD-CT urography were filling defects and urothelial wall thickening. Interestingly, when stratified by location, urothelial wall thickening was more predictive of tumors in the pelvicalyceal system (PPV, 88%) compared to those in the ureter (PPV, 33%). Conversely, filling defects were more predictive in the ureter (PPV, 88%) than in the pelvicalyceal system (PPV, 50%) [56]. MD-CT urography was able to correctly predict the pTNM stage in 58%−88% of the patients with upper tract malignancies [55,58]. However, even in contemporary series, the main drawback of MD-CT urography is its low PPV for small tumors or urothelial wall thickening (0%−46%) [59].

The use of a split-bolus method among 200 patients who initially presented with hematuria was prospectively estimated in a recent series [60]. The split-bolus method provides improved imaging through simultaneous nephrographic and excretory CT phase acquisition. The corresponding sensitivity, specificity, and PPV rates were 100%, 99%, and 99%, respectively [55]. Alternatively, in one study, the use of magnetic resonance urography images was investigated in 17 patients with 23 upper tract lesions. A sensitivity of 74% for the detection of small urothelial carcinomas sized ≤ 2 cm was reported [61]. Possible further technical improvements include the acquisition of diffusion-weighted MRI images in patients with upper tract obstruction due to UUTT lesions [62]; however, these techniques were still reported to have failed in the detection of flat ureteral lesions [63].

For the local staging of the primary tumor lesions and regional lymph nodes, MRI has not demonstrated diagnostic superiority over MD-CT; however, it is the preferred method in patients with contraindications (e.g., iodine allergy, renal insufficiency) for MD-CT [34,61]. MRI is contraindicated in patients with pacemakers. Gadolinium infusion must be eliminated in patients with serious renal insufficiency (creatinine clearance <30 mL/min) to prevent the possibility of subsequent nephrogenic systemic fibrosis [64].

Urinary Cytology and Molecular-Based Urinary Markers. Some authors have reported an at least annual use of urinary cytology in patients who underwent RC [6,41]. It was reported that urinary cytology could detect 36%−60% of UUTTs when used for routine postcystectomy surveillance [65,66]; however, in patients who presented with symptoms, urinary cytology could detect 80%−100% of UUTTs [33]. After urinary diversion, the detection of malignant cells in voided urine samples was significantly restricted because of the difficulty in discriminating between urothelial cancer cells from the intestinal epithelial cells [67]. Most importantly, the additional use of urinary cytology in established follow-up regimens (with radiological and clinical examinations) does not significantly improve the early detection rates of UUTT recurrences [67]. Positive cytology findings might precede a possible diagnosis of UUTT by imaging. At the time of the first positive cytology, only 9% (9/101) of the patients had a confirmed UUTT diagnosis; however, eventually 56% (57/101) of these patients developed identifiable UUTTs [68]. In this study the median recurrence-free time after positive cytology was 2.1 years. Therefore a positive cytology is highly predictive of UUTT recurrence, and cytology is recommended for assessing the upper urinary tract during follow-up. Selective ureteral urinary cytology analysis results in an improved PPV of >85% for high-grade muscle-invasive upper UUTT [69]; however, for screening purposes, invasiveness and additional costs have to be considered.

Alternatively, urine-based markers have recently become popular tools for overcoming the limitations of conventional urinary cytology. Literature evidence is mainly derived from a relatively small number of patients with primary UUTTs. In a comparative analysis of 30 patients with urothelial carcinoma of the upper tract, fluorescence in situ hybridization (FISH) showed a significantly higher rate of sensitivity compared to that of urinary cytology (77% vs 36%, respectively); however, this was not the case for specificity (95% vs 100%, respectively). These findings were confirmed in other studies [66,70]. Moreover, FISH analysis, which uses gene-labeled probes for chromosomes 3, 7, 9, and 17, is less interference-prone than urinary cytology [65]. The sensitivity of immunocytology in the detection of low grade (G1-2) tumors was reported to be 100% in a small study that included 16 patients with UUTT [71]. Generally, because of the possibility of conducting noninterference probe analysis, FISH is promising as a less invasive diagnostic tool for high-grade UUTT. Nevertheless, the evidence supporting the routine use of urinary cytology and urine-based markers alone for the follow-up of the upper urinary tracts is insufficient [72].

Ureterorenoscopy. Ureterorenoscopy with biopsy using semirigid or flexible instruments is the method of choice for the histological diagnosis of

UUTT [73]. Access to the upper tract after urinary diversion can be particularly challenging and might require the use of combined retrograde and antegrade techniques [74]. Upper tract biopsies have been reported to be less reliable in the evaluation of the local T stage, because of the limited capability of biopsy instruments to retrieve an adequate amount of tissue specimen for the evaluation of the complete pelvicalyceal or ureteral wall [38]. This fact is supported by a previous study, which demonstrated that even when lamina propria was present within the biopsy specimens, almost 50% of the tumors were initially misconstrued as superficial, and they were identified as invasive in the final nephroureterectomy [75].

Treatment of Upper Urinary Tract Tumor Recurrence

Radical Nephroureterectomy. Radical nephroureterectomy is the standard treatment for recurrence [31,41,48]. The eligibility of patients (in terms of performance status and tumor extent) for open radical nephroureterectomy is a predictive factor for improved survival. A previous study demonstrated that while the overall median survival of patients with recurrent UUTT was only 10 months, that of patients who were eligible for radical nephroureterectomy was 26 months [38]. Improved experience with laparoscopic radical nephroureterectomy suggests that this technique is oncologically equivalent to open surgery for tumors of equal grade, stage, and lymph node status [76]. A limitation of this analysis was that patients who underwent laparoscopic radical nephroureterectomy had significantly lower likelihood of lymph node involvement at the time of surgery compared to patients who underwent open surgery; this might have resulted in a biased final survival analysis. Nonetheless, given the lack of data and the challenging postoperative anatomy in the retroperitoneum and pelvis after RC and urinary diversion, laparoscopic radical nephroureterectomy for secondary UUTT has to still be regarded as an investigational treatment option with the need to enter and reconstitute the ureteroileal anastomosis.

Lymphadenectomy. The role and extent of regional lymphadenectomy at radical nephroureterectomy in patients with UUTT recurrence has not been well defined and remains controversial. Open radical nephroureterectomy was accompanied by regional lymphadenectomy only in few retrospective series [31,38,42]. In these series the rate of locally advanced disease (pT3−pT4) was 54%−66% with node-positive disease found in 32%−83% of the patients.

Similar to the increasing evidence suggesting the therapeutic benefit of extended lymphadenectomy for MIBC [77,78], recent evidence has suggested that extended lymphadenectomy for invasive UUTT is a strong predictor of improved disease-free and CSS [79]. A retrospective series of 132 patients with primary muscle-invasive UUTT showed that pathological tumor stage and lymph node involvement were independent risk factors for disease-free survival [80]. Moreover, the number of resected lymph nodes and the extent of lymphadenectomy were independent risk factors of recurrence-free and CSS and the patients who did not receive any lymphadenectomy at the time of surgery had comparable survival rates to those with pathologically confirmed node-positive disease at radical nephroureterectomy. In contrast to patients with UUTT recurrence, the rate of node-positive disease in primary UUTT was only 25% [80,81]. Furthermore, an ideal anatomic template of regional lymphadenectomy according to the primary site of recurrence has not been established, owing to the inconsistent lymphatic drainage of the retroperitoneum in urologic malignancies [82]. In conclusion, given the lack of evidence suggesting a therapeutic benefit for regional lymphadenectomy, its role in patients with recurrent UUTT remains unclear; therefore, it is presently considered as a diagnostic procedure.

Adjuvant Chemotherapy. Only a limited number of studies have addressed the role of adjuvant chemotherapy in node-positive recurrent UUTT [41]. In locally advanced UUTT, adjuvant chemotherapy is ineffective and only $\leq 5\%$ of the patients achieve long-term survival [41]. The low incidence rate of recurrent UUTT reduces the likelihood of conducting randomized prospective studies that investigate the significance of adjuvant therapy. Instead, controlled observational and registration type multiinstitutional studies that pool the data are encouraged.

Conservative Treatment for Upper Urinary Tract Tumor Recurrence. The conservative treatment options for patients that develop recurrent UUTTs after treatment for MIBC include endoscopic and percutaneous resection. The indicators of renal-sparing treatment in patients with recurrent UUTT are bilateral tumors, solitary kidney, or severe renal insufficiency; and tumor features of small size, low grade, and low stage. Studies reporting the outcomes after endoscopic treatment for UUTTs derive almost exclusively from patients with primary carcinomas who have significantly improved prognoses compared to patients with metachronous tumors. Approximately 50%−75% of the patients with recurrent UUTTs initially present with high-stage, high-grade disease compared to only about 30% of the patients with de novo UUTT [28,31,38,46,48,51,83,84]. Moreover, in patient series for whom radical nephroureterectomy and regional lymphadenectomy were performed, lymph node involvement was reported in 32%−83% of the patients [31,38,42]. These data indicated that recurrent UUTTs are more aggressive malignancies than primary urothelial cancers. The optimal indicators for conservative nephron-sparing treatment of the secondary recurrent UUTTs remain to be identified.

Urethral Recurrence

The Incidence of Urethral Recurrence After Radical Cystectomy The

recurrence rate of urethral tumors after RC was reported to be 1.5%−6.0% in men, with a mean recurrence-free interval of 13.5−39.0 months and a median survival of 28−38 months; >50% of the patients die from systemic disease (Table 30.2) [29,85−91]. Secondary urethral tumors are likely to occur 1−3 years after surgery. Prophylactic urethrectomy at RC is no longer justified in most patients. The symptoms of urethral recurrence depend on the type of urinary diversion (microhematuria and/or changes in urinary stream in patients with orthotopic neobladder, and urethral bleeding and/or induration of periurethral tissue in patients with a cutaneous diversion). Most of the urethral recurrences (57%−61%) are detected via the evaluation of symptoms, whereas 31%−39% are detected through abnormal urethral cytology [87,90]. The median time to diagnosis did not differ significantly between patients with symptomatic urethral recurrences and patients diagnosed through cytological abnormalities [90]. Urethral recurrences with superficial tumor stages (pTa, pTis) have been diagnosed by abnormal cytology in 59%−100% of the cases, as opposed to invasive tumors (pT1−pT4) that are often detected after patients have developed local symptoms (∼79%) including gross hematuria, bloody urethral discharge, palpable mass, change in voiding habits, or local pain [90,92].

Risk Factors in Male Patients The independent predictors of urethral recurrence were cystectomy for NMIBC, prostatic involvement, and a history of recurrent NMIBC [8,89−91]. In a large, retrospective single-center study conducted in 729 male patients treated with RC with a median follow-up duration of 38 months, the independent risk factors for urethral recurrence were identified to be history of NMIBC, prostatic urethral involvement, and NMIBC (pTa, pTis, pT1) at RC [90]. In this study, superficial prostatic involvement (pTa, pTis) was a stronger predictor of urethral recurrence compared to invasive prostatic involvement. Similar findings were obtained in another large, retrospective, single-center study involving 768 male patients with a longer median follow-up of 13 years; prostatic urethral involvement but not tumor multifocality or bladder CIS was an independent risk factor for urethral recurrence [88]. Inconsistent with a previous report [90], patients with invasive prostatic involvement had higher risk of urethral recurrence compared to patients with superficial prostatic urethral tumors [88].

Urinary Diversion and Urethral Recurrence Some series suggested that patients with orthotopic diversion had reduced risk for urethral recurrence compared to patients with supranational diversions [88,93,94]. However, other comparable series did not identify orthotopic diversion as a significant independent risk factor compared to cutaneous diversions [90]. Previous studies had hypothesized that continued exposure of the remnant urothelium to urine in case of orthotopic diversions might confer a protective effect against the development of urethral recurrences [95]. These conflicting results might also indicate patient selection bias, because orthotopic

TABLE 30.2 The Incidence Rate of Urethral Recurrence After RC

Source	Year	N	Urethral Recurrence, Incidence (%)	Time to Recurrence (months)	Follow-Up Periods (months)	Comment
Levinson et al. [85]	1990	124	4.8	23.5	67	—
Tongaonkar et al. [86]	1993	164	9	13.5	NA	19% with orthotopic diversion, 81% with cutaneous diversion
Clark et al. [87]	2004	1054	4.5	18.5	121	—
Stein et al. [88]	2005	768	6	24	156	51% with orthotopic diversion, 49% with cutaneous diversion
Studer et al. [89]	2006	482	5	14	32	Only orthotopic bladder substitution
Hautmann et al. [29]	2006	605	1.5	39	36	Only orthotopic bladder substitution
Huguet et al. [90]	2008	729	4.6	13.9	38	2.2% of 219 patients with orthotopic diversion, 5.6% of 510 patients with cutaneous diversion

NA, not applicable.

diversion might be a better choice of treatment in patients with lower tumor stages than for patients with locally advanced disease [90].

Preoperative Prostatic Biopsy and Frozen Section Analysis In one study preoperative prostatic urethral biopsies showed a higher negative predictive value (NPV) of 99% compared to final urethral margin status, whereas a positive finding correlated with a positive final urethral margin status in only 68% of the cases [96]. Another study involving 246 patients confirmed the relatively low PPV of the transurethral loop biopsies at the level of the verumontanum compared to the final results of cystoprostatectomy [97]. The sensitivity and specificity were reported to be only 53% and 77%, respectively, resulting in a PPV and NPV of 45% and 77%, respectively. However, in this study, the sensitivity and specificity of the frozen section analyses were both 100% [96]. A recent retrospective study conducted in 294 patients confirmed that a positive urethral margin status is the strongest independent risk factor for urethral recurrence as compared to prostatic urethral and stromal invasion [98]. This places an emphasis on the importance of achieving a tumor-free urethral margin at RC.

Risk Factors in Female Patients The risk of urethral recurrence after urethral-sparing RC in females was reported as 0.83%−4.3% [48,99,100]. In contrast to the low rate of concomitant urethral malignancies in female patients with primary BC ($\sim 2\%$) [101], a higher urethral malignancy rate of 12% was reported at RC [102]. A history of multifocal or recurrent BC was identified to contribute to an increased risk of urethral recurrence [48]. Furthermore, the risk of tumor involvement of the distal urethra at RC is significantly higher in patients with bladder neck or vaginal involvement and in patients with preoperatively enlarged inguinal lymph nodes [103−105]. A pathological reevaluation of cystectomy specimens from 67 female patients revealed that concomitant urethral tumors were exclusively located in the proximal or mid portion of the urethra. Moreover, women with urethral tumors often showed localization of the primary tumor to the bladder neck. These tumors were of higher grade and stage, and harbored a higher risk of node-positive disease [104]. Stein et al. prospectively evaluated the cystectomy specimens from 71 female patients and reported that tumor localization to the bladder neck and urethra was detected in 19% and 7%, of the patients, respectively. The presence of bladder neck tumors significantly correlated with the highest risk of concomitant urethral malignancies. Conversely, approximately 60% of the patients with malignancies at the bladder neck had no evidence of tumor involvement at the proximal urethra. In this study frozen section analysis of the distal urethral margin showed a 100% sensitivity and specificity for the detection of a positive urethral margin compared to the final pathological analysis [103]. Another study involving 85 female patients confirmed the effectiveness of frozen section analysis that showed a sensitivity of 100% for the detection of malignant urethral margins [48]. Nonetheless, it should be noted that urethral recurrences might occur even in patients with negative final urethral margins, possibly owing to the submucosal extension of the primary bladder tumor into the urethra, which shows an unaffected urothelial layer in frozen section analysis [105]. This result emphasizes the importance of an adequate full-thickness biopsy of the urethral margin for frozen section analysis [102]. In conclusion the present data highlight the importance of intraoperative frozen section analysis for the detection of urethral malignancies at RC. Furthermore, these data add to the growing frame of evidence, which suggests that patients with MIBC at the bladder neck should not be excluded from an orthotopic approach in advance unless intraoperative frozen section analysis shows evidence of malignancy at the distal urethral margins [102].

Survival After Urethral Recurrence The 5-year disease-specific and OS after urethral recurrence was reported to be only 35% and 52%, respectively, with a median OS after diagnosis of 28−54 months [87,90,98]. The comparative assessment of the impact of bladder and urethral recurrence pathologies on OS after urethral recurrence has returned heterogeneous results. While Huguet et al. [90] did not identify any differences in survival, Lin et al. [106] reported in 24 patients with urethral recurrences that bladder pathology predominantly determined survival. Conversely, Clark et al. [87] reported in 47 patients with urethral recurrences that the stage of the urethral recurrence was a better predictor of OS compared to BC pathology. Possible explanations for these contradicting observations might be the differences in patient selection criteria and the use of prophylactic urethrectomies at RC, which might have resulted in biased survival analyses for both studies. Moreover, the number of patients with stage pT0 disease after urethrectomy differed considerably between the two studies. Lin et al. [106] included nine patients (37%) with stage pT0 disease, whereas Clark et al. [87] excluded all stage pT0 disease patients from the final survival analysis. In their analysis Huguet et al. [90] did not identify any patients with stage pT0 disease at urethrectomy, and most importantly, 26% of their patients with urethral recurrence had recurrent UUTTs [90], which has the potential to be a high-stage and high-grade disease at initial diagnosis [31]. Furthermore, survival in patients with urethral recurrence and concomitant distant metastases is mainly determined by the presence of metastatic disease [6]. In conclusion, whether urethral or BC pathology is a better predictor of OS after urethral recurrence is still controversial.

Diagnosis and Staging of Urethral Recurrence Given the low rate of urethral recurrence, there are little data or agreement on the optimal follow-up of asymptomatic patients with retained urethra after RC. All patients with urethral bleeding, pain, or mass should be evaluated promptly. The follow-up regimens described in the current literature are mainly derived from different high-volume centers and are based on urinary cytology, urethral washings, urethroscopy, and the use of different imaging modalities [88,93,106−109]. In terms of the frequency of follow-up, while some authors suggested the routine use of urinary cytology, urethral washings, and urethroscopy on a quarterly basis for the first 2 years and continued semiannually afterward [93], others only conducted a clinical follow-up [90]. Therefore tailoring surveillance regimens according to the patient's individual risk profile appears to be a reasonable strategy. Urinary cytology is certainly a useful and noninvasive diagnostic tool for the detection of urethral recurrences; however, its sensitivity is considerably reduced in patients who undergo urinary diversion [67]. The prognostic advantage conferred by the routine use of urethral washings in patients with a retained urethra after cystoprostatectomy is controversial. In a study conducted among 24 patients with a median follow-up duration of 28 months after urethrectomy, a significant impact on disease-free survival was not observed between patients who routinely underwent urethral washings and those who did not [106]. Urethroscopy with biopsy is certainly the method of choice for the histological diagnosis of urethral recurrence; however, the use of urethroscopy on a regular basis has not been reported to confer any survival benefit [28,88,98,107,108]. For local staging after the detection of a urethral malignancy, increasing evidence has suggested that MRI is superior to MD-CT in patients with urethral malignancies in terms of staging accuracy [109].

Management of Urethral Recurrence

Noninvasive Urethral Tumors (pTa−pTis). In patients with noninvasive urethral recurrences, a urethra-preserving strategy can be attempted using transurethral resection (TUR) of the tumor lesion [92]. However, in a series of patients who developed high-grade pTa stage urothelial carcinoma after RC and who underwent treatment with TUR, only three out of four patients with recurrence progressed to invasive disease. After the development of recurrent disease, all patients were managed with salvage urethrectomy and they remained disease-free for a median duration of 24−44 months [110]. The authors concluded that the inclusion of adjuvant local treatment in the treatment strategy for high-grade tumors, for example, bacillus Calmette-Guerin (BCG), might have reduced the risk of further recurrence [92]. In a prospective analysis of the patients who developed CIS in the urethra after RC, the weekly use of intraurethral BCG perfusion for a period of 6 weeks achieved a complete remission rate of 80%; however, it did not achieve any therapeutic response in patients with papillary or invasive disease [107].

Invasive Urethral Tumors (pT1−pT4). Urethrectomy, as the choice of treatment in male patients who developed invasive urethral recurrences, confers a long-term survival benefit [93]. Two recent studies reported that the use of prophylactic urethrectomies in male patients with invasive prostatic tumor involvement at RC did not confer any survival benefit compared to those who underwent urethrectomy at the time of urethral recurrence [90,93]. Similar results were obtained in an investigation of the timing of urethrectomy as a possible predictor of improved survival in 2401 male patients who underwent RC for BC using the Surveillance, Epidemiology, and End Results Program (SEER) database. In total, 195 men (8.1%) developed urethral recurrences and they were treated with either concurrent or salvage urethrectomy. The use of concurrent urethrectomy at RC versus salvage urethrectomy did not confer any significant independent survival benefit (HR = 0.775, 95% CI, 0.592−1.014, $P = 0.0632$). Interestingly, in contrast to patients treated at urban nonteaching hospitals, patients treated at teaching hospitals were more likely to undergo salvage urethrectomy for recurrence than immediate urethrectomy. In this study tumor stage at RC was the only independent variable that predicted the performance of concurrent urethrectomy [108]. Furthermore, the complication rates and intraoperative blood loss did not differ significantly in patients treated with delayed or immediate urethrectomy [111]. In female patients, given the overall low rate of urethral recurrence, the use of prophylactic urethrectomy without any evidence of invasive malignancy at the urethral margin did not have a significant impact on the oncological long-term outcome after RC [101,112,113]. With regards to UUTT recurrence, administering adjuvant treatment modalities for the treatment of urethral recurrences has not yet been addressed sufficiently in the literature and prospective randomized trials should be performed to address this issue.

Follow-Up for Urinary Diversion−Related Complications

Apart from the oncological outcomes, there are also metabolic and functional aspects of urinary diversion that warrant follow-up.

Vitamin B12 Deficiency

The removal of terminal ileum for the construction of a bladder substitute might predispose patients to vitamin B12 deficiency. For patients who underwent terminal ileal resections >20 cm in length, the B12 serum levels should be measured. Lack of vitamin B12 might lead to megaloblastic anemia, which is reversible by substitution treatment and irreversible neuropathy. Once vitamin B12 deficiency has been confirmed, the patient would require lifelong supplementation [114]. Because the average body deposits of vitamin B12 are large, vitamin B12 measurements and/or substitution should be realized 3−5 years after RC and onwards.

Metabolic Acidosis

The frequency and severity of metabolic acidosis are usually related to the type and length of the intestinal segment that was used for the construction of a bladder substitute; however, symptom severity and the degree of decompensation would also depend on the age and metabolic ability of the patient to compensate. Metabolic acidosis is expected in $\leq 15\%$ of the patients with an ileal conduit and in $\leq 50\%$ of the patients with a continent diversion [115]. The highest risk of metabolic acidosis is observed during the early postoperative period, in patients having a neobladder and postvoid residual urine, in patients with urinary tract infection, and in those with reduced renal function. The clinical signs of metabolic acidosis can be nausea, lack of appetite, fatigue, weakness, and ultimately vomiting or accelerated breathing. Chronic metabolic acidosis can lead to bone demineralization; thus, attention should be given to bone metabolism in patients with even mild acidosis. Sodium bicarbonate should be given generously (2–6 g/day) from the early postoperative period onwards [115].

Because the timing and degree of metabolic acidosis might vary, no definitive guidelines for its management exist. Serum evaluation for metabolic acidosis should be performed regularly during the first 12 months after RC, and probably every 6–12 months thereafter.

Urinary Diversion—Related Complications

The risk of diversion-related complications increases with time. The most frequent complications are symptomatic urinary tract infections; urolithiasis; stenosis of the ureterointestinal anastomosis with potential loss of renal function; complications related to the stoma in conduits; and in neobladder patients, urinary retention as well as day and/or night time incontinence. In a series with ileal conduit, complications developed in 45% of patients within the first 5 years. This percentage increased to 50%, 54%, and 94% in patients who survived for 10, 15, and >15 years, respectively [116].

Conclusion

The follow-up recommendations of the current literature for MIBC are described in Table 30.3. The early detection of tumor recurrence after RC allows for early treatment. As most relapses occur within 5 years and the median time to local and distant recurrence is 12–18 months after RC, the follow-up should be intensive for the first 5 years and especially in the first 2 years. Patients with extravesical and node-positive diseases at RC have the highest risk of recurrence. Regular follow-up of the male urethra by urethral washings and urethroscopy was demonstrated to confer survival benefit in case of the early detection of the urethral before the occurrence of any symptoms. Most UUTT recurrences occur >3 years after RC, at a time when the risk of local and systemic recurrences has decreased. Lifelong yearly upper urinary tract imaging is advisable for all patients. This study also enables the early detection of urinary diversion complications. Metabolic evaluation should continue throughout the lifetime, and vitamin B12 substitution should

TABLE 30.3 The Follow-Up Recommendations for MIBC in the Literature

Diagnosis	Recommendation	Comment
Tumor Recurrence		
Local and distal recurrence	No recommended follow-up strategy	Follow-up at predetermined intervals allows for early treatment and might confer survival benefit; should be intensive during first 5 years after RC.
Urethral recurrence	No recommended follow-up strategy	All symptomatic patients should be examined with cytology by urethral washings and urethroscopy. Regular follow-up might confer survival benefit (if the urethral recurrence is diagnosed as asymptomatic).
UUTT recurrence	No recommended follow-up strategy	There is a lifelong risk of UUTT after RC for MIBC. Positive cytology is highly predictive of UUTT recurrence during follow-up.
Functional Outcomes		
Vitamin B12 deficiency	Lifelong parenteral vitamin B12 supplementation in patients with terminal ileal resections with vitamin B12 serum levels <200 pg/mL 3 years after the operation	Neuropathy due to vitamin B12 deficiency is irreversible.
Metabolic acidosis	Serum evaluation for metabolic acidosis every 3 months during the first year after RC and then every 6–12 months	Patients at risk with ileal neobladder, with reduced renal function, postvoid residual urine, and urinary tract infection
Urinary diversion–related complications	The risk of diversion-related complications increases with time; lifelong examination for lithiasis, benign stricture, or hydronephrosis is necessary	Complications developed in 45% of patients within the first 5 years; this percentage increased to 50%, 54%, and 94% in patients surviving 10, 15, and >15 years, respectively.

RC, radical cystectomy; UUTT, upper urinary tract tumor; MIBC, muscle-invasive bladder cancer.

commence 3−5 years after the surgery. In general the studies regarding the follow-up after RC are based on retrospective data and the level of evidence obtained has not been convincing. Nonetheless, reasonable recommendations can be made until further prospective randomized studies that test different follow-up schedules have been performed.

FOLLOW-UP FOR MUSCLE-INVASIVE BLADDER CANCER AFTER BLADDER PRESERVATION TREATMENT

Several bladder preservation options exist, including single-modality treatments such as TUR alone, partial cystectomy, RT, or chemotherapy alone, although the trimodal approach is the most strongly supported strategy in the literature [2]. In medically operable patients, there is abundant evidence that suggests trimodal therapy (TMT) as an acceptable treatment option for highly selected, average risk patients with MIBC. The ideal candidates for this treatment strategy have good baseline bladder function, are able to obtain a visibly complete TUR, and have small solitary tumors with limited CIS and no evidence of hydronephrosis. While outcomes are worse for medically inoperable patients, bladder preservation strategies still confer curative potential in these patients as well. However, prospective trials comparing the above regimens to RC are required to obtain a better definition of their role in the treatment of MIBC.

Nonmuscle-Invasive Bladder Cancer Recurrence

In patients with persistent or recurrent MIBC undergoing any form of bladder preservation treatment, it is recommended to proceed to RC. The data are less clear on the best course of management for recurrent NMIBC. Pieras et al. [117] evaluated a selected cohort of 51 patients who underwent bladder preservation with TUR and received carboplatin and vinblastine. Of these patients, 82% were considered as responders and elected for bladder preservation. Among these patients, 18 (43%) showed recurrence as NMIBC. The authors noted no difference in the CSS between patients with superficial recurrence and those without disease recurrence at a median follow-up duration of 44 months (94% vs 89%, respectively). They treated the recurrent NMIBC in the preserved bladder with TUR and BCG instillation. Comparably, Zietman et al. treated a series of 190 enrolled patients with TMT, and they reported a superficial recurrence rate of 26%. In addition, they did not find any significant difference in the 5-year survival rates of patients with recurrent NMIBC and those that remained disease-free [118]. However, importantly, after 8 years of follow-up, in patients who had intact bladders, the survival rates of patients who did not develop any recurrences and those who developed recurrent NMIBCs were 61% and 35%, respectively. There is supporting evidence for long-term surveillance with cystoscopy, with or without imaging studies, urine cytology, or bimanual examinations. However, existing data are not sufficient to make definitive recommendations on the optimal surveillance regimens. However, it can be extrapolated from all of the preceding studies that lifelong cystoscopic evaluation is reasonable and that although recurrent NMIBC is not statistically indicative of decreased survival, it is probably associated with a poorer prognosis than no recurrence.

The Follow-Up Results of Various Treatments

Transurethral Resection Monotherapy

According to the long-term, single institution experiences reported by Solsona and Herr, TUR monotherapy is expected to produce oncological outcomes equivalent to those of RC in appropriately selected patients [119]. Bladder preservation rates have been high in individuals who had small tumors that were completely resected with negative follow-up biopsies.

Partial Cystectomy

Partial cystectomy is an alternative form of therapy for muscle-invasive disease that might only be used in a highly selected patient cohort [3]. There are no prospective phase II studies on partial cystectomy and there are no prospective comparisons or randomized trials assessing the relative efficacy of partial cystectomy versus RC or radical TUR for MIBC.

In the MD Anderson series, 37 patients underwent partial cystectomy for curative intent between 1982 and 2003 [120]. All patients had stage pT2 or pT3 disease and 14% had nodal metastases. Long-term cancer control was achieved in 65% of the patients with an intact bladder over a median follow-up duration of 53 months. NMIBC recurrences occurred in nine (24%) patients and all patients were treated successfully. On multivariate analysis, the only factor associated with recurrence-free survival was the pathologic tumor stage. Smaldone et al. [121] reported a single surgeon series of 25 patients who underwent surgery over a 10-year period. The treatment protocol included 25 Gy of preoperative RT delivered to the abdominal wall in five fractionated doses, intraoperative intravesical thiotepa, and postoperative intravesical BCG for a period of 6 weeks. Preoperative RT and/or intraoperative intravesical chemotherapy have been reported in many series in an effort to minimize the risk of wound implantation; however, there is no evidence supporting their routine use.

Partial cystectomy has been incorporated into bladder-sparing treatment protocols after initial neoadjuvant multiagent chemotherapy in highly selected patients with localized tumors. Sternberg et al. [122] reported partial cystectomy in 13 patients out of the 104 treated with a bladder-sparing approach in mind. The 5-year survival for this selected patient cohort was 69%. Therefore partial cystectomy could be an alternative to RC following chemoradiation therapy [123].

Bladder Sparing With Trimodal Therapy

A TMT approach, including maximal TUR followed by concurrent radiosensitizing chemotherapy and RT, is the most studied bladder-sparing strategy. Fig. 30.1 shows the current schema for the trimodal treatment for MIBC with selective bladder preservation.

Follow-Up Oncological Results

In Medically Inoperable Patients Bladder preservation has been assessed in different cohorts of inoperable patients including patients with prohibitive medical comorbidities contraindicating radical surgery and patients with surgically unresectable disease (Tables 30.4 and 30.5) [128,147−149]. In studies that only included patients who had surgically unresectable disease, the OS after a 4-year follow-up was poor (30%−42%) [148−150]. It should be noted that these patients were not considered to have received TMT with curative intent, and were excluded from the analyses of TMT outcomes.

In the SWOG 9312 trial Hussain et al. [147] classified patients into two categories (surgical vs medical reasons) and highlighted that this factor was

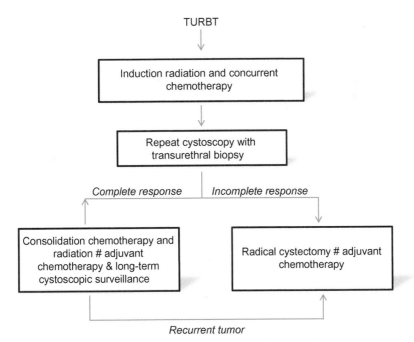

FIGURE 30.1 Algorithm for the treatment of MIBC with selective bladder preservation.

TABLE 30.4 Published Series of TMT for Bladder Preservation: Homogeneous Treatment Regimens

Study	Design and Follow-Up	Stage	No. of Patients	Concomitant Chemotherapy	RT	CR Rate	Salvage Cystectomy Rate	CSS	OS
Large Sample Size (>50 patients) Series									
Prospective Phase 3 Studies									
James et al. [124][a]	Continuous Phase 3 (second arm: RT alone) 69.9 months	T2–T4a N0	182	5-FU, MMC × 2 (neoadjuvant chemotherapy: n = 57)	55 Gy or 64 Gy	—	11.4% (at 2 years)	—	5 years: 48
Tunio et al. [125]	Continuous Phase 3 5 years	T2–T4 N0/Nx	200	Cisplatin weekly	65 Gy ST	93%	—	—	5 years: 52
Shipley et al. [126][a]	Split Phase 3 (second arm: chemotherapy-RT with neoadjuvant chemotherapy) 60.0 months	T2–T4a N0/Nx	62	Cisplatin × 3	64.8 Gy ST	60%	25.80%	—	5 years: 49
Housset et al. [127][b]	Split Phase 3 27 months	T2–T4 N0/N1: n = 4	54	Cisplatin + 5-FU × 4	44 Gy BID	74%	N/A[b]	3 years: 62	3 years: 59

Phase 2 or Retrospective Studies

Lagrange et al. [128]	Split Phase 2 8 years	T2–T4a N0/Nx	51	Cisplatin + 5-FU × 3	63 Gy ST	–	33.30%	–	8 years: 36
Gogna et al. [129]	Continuous Phase 2 23 months	T2–T4a N0/Nx <10 cmT1	113	Cisplatin weekly	63–64 Gy ST	70%	15%	5 years: 50	–
Kragelj et al. [130]	Continuous Phase 2 10.3 years	T2–T4a N0/Nx T1	84	Vinblastine weekly	63.8–64 Gy ST	78%	8.3%c	9 years: 51	9 years: 25
Weiss et al. [131]	Continuous Retrospective 27 months	T2–T4a N0/N1: n = 58 T1: n = 54	112	Cisplatin + 5-FU × 2	55.8–59.4 GyST	88%	17%	5 years: 82 (for T2–4: 73)	5 years: 74 (for T2–4: 63)

Small Size (<50 Patients) Series

Zapatero et al. [132]	Split Retrospective 60 months	T2–T4a N0	39	Cisplatin weekly (paclitaxel: n = 5)	64.8 Gy ST BID: n = 24	80%	33%	5 years: 82	5 years: 73
Choudhury et al. [133]	Continuous Phase 2 36 months	T2–T3 N0/Nx	50	Gemcitabine weekly	52.5 Gy in 20	82% (88%d)	14%	3 years: 82 5 years: 78	3 years: 75 5 years: 65

(Continued)

TABLE 30.4 (Continued)

Study	Design and Follow-Up	Stage	No. of Patients	Concomitant Chemotherapy	RT	CR Rate	Salvage Cystectomy Rate	CSS	OS
Aboziada et al. [134]	Split Retrospective 18 months	T2–T3b N0	50	Cisplatin weekly	66 Gy ST	60%	28%	1.5 years: 84	1.5 years: 100
Peyromaure et al. [135]	Split Retrospective 36.3 months	T2N0/Nx	43	Cisplatin + 5-FU × 2	24 Gy in 8 BID	74.40%	25.60%	3 years: 75 5 years: 60	–
Hussain et al. [136]	Continuous Phase 1/2 50.7 months	T2–T4a N0/Nx	41	MMC + 5-FU × 2	55 Gy in 20	71%	19,50%	2 years: 68	2 years: 49 5 years: 36
Kaufman et al. [137]	Split Phase 1/2 29 months	T2–T4a N0/Nx	34	Cisplatin + 5-FU × 4	44 Gy BID	67%	29.40%	3 years: 83	–
Varveris et al. [138]	Continuous Phase 2 32 months	T1–T4 N0/Nx	42	Cisplatin + docetaxel	68–74 Gy ST	54.70%	–	–	–
Tester et al. [139]	Split Phase 2 36 months	T2–T4a N0–N2/ Nx	48	Cisplatin × 3	64 Gy ST	66%	20.80%	–	3 years: 64

Study	Treatment	Patients	Stage	Chemotherapy	RT dose				Survival
Rotman et al. [140]	Continuous Phase 2 38 months	20	T1–T4 N0/N1 M0/M1	5-FU (+MMC in five patients)	60–65 Gy ST	74%	—	—	5 years: 54
Russell et al. [141]	Split Phase 2 18 months	34	T1–T4 N0/N1	5-FU	60 Gy ST	81%	29.40%	—	4 years: 64

5-FU, 5-fluorouracil; MMC, mitomycin C; BID, twice daily; CR, complete response; CSS, cancer-specific survival; OS, overall survival; NA, not applicable; RC, radical cystectomy; RCT, randomized controlled trial; RT = radiation therapy.

[a]Phase 3 RCT. CR is evaluated after induction (split course) or completion (continuous course) of chemotherapy-RT.

[b]Eighteen patients were treated by primary RC after CR to induction treatment; only 22 patients received full chemotherapy-RT treatment.

[c]17% of the patients with indications for salvage cystectomy did not undergo surgery because of locally advanced, inoperable tumors and/or poor performance status.

[d]Defined by pT0, pTis, or pT1 after cystoscopic assessment.

TABLE 30.5 Published Series of TMT for Bladder Preservation: Heterogeneous Cohorts Comprised of Patients Receiving Various Chemotherapy and RT Regimens

Study	Design and Follow-Up	Stage	No. of Patients	Neoadjuvant or Adjuvant Chemotherapy	Concomitant Chemotherapy	RT	CR Rate	Salvage Cystectomy Rate	CSS	OS
Efstathiou et al. [142][a]	Split Retrospective 7.7 years	T2–T4a N0/Nx	348	Various	Various	Various	78%	29%	5 years: 64 10 years: 59 15 years: 57	5 years: 52 10 years: 35 15 years: 22
Krause et al. [143]	Split Retrospective 71.5 months	T2–T4a N0/Nx	473	No	Various RT alone: n = 142	Various	70.40%	–	–	5 years: 49 10 years: 30
Chung et al. [144]	Continuous Retrospective 7.9 years	T1–T4 N0/N1: n = 44	340	Neoadjuvant Chemotherapy + RT: n = 57	Cisplatin RT alone: n = 247	Various	63.5% (79% if chemotherapy-RT)	17.40%	10 years: 35	10 years: 19
Rodel et al. [145][b]	Continuous Retrospective 60.0 months	T1: n = 89 T2–T4a N0/N1: n = 326	415	No	Various RT alone: n = 126	Various Mean 54 Gy (45–69.4) + 45 Gy para-aortic if LNI	72%	20%	5 years: 56 10 years: 42	5 years: 51 10 years: 31

BID, twice daily; CR, complete response; CSS, cancer-specific survival; LNI, lymph node involvement; OS, overall survival; RT, radiation therapy.

[a]Update of Shipley et al. [146].

[b]Update of Sauer et al., 1998 (subset of Krause et al. [143]). CR is evaluated after induction (split course) or completion (continuous course of chemotherapy-RT).

a predictor of OS. The criterion "unfit for surgery," defined by medical comorbidities contraindicating general anesthesia or surgery, has been associated with poorer OS [128,147].

Given these different patient profiles, most phase II/III trials—specifically, the Radiation Therapy Oncology Group (RTOG) trial protocols—included patients who were fit for surgery (no medical contraindications) and had resectable disease but were motivated to pursue bladder preservation.

Medically Operable Patients The overall mean response rate after TMT was 73% (Tables 30.4 and 30.5). In most series complete response (CR) was defined by the absence of a visible tumor, the absence of persistent pathologically proven bladder tumor on biopsy, and the absence of tumor cells in the urine cytology. Patients who showed CR to treatment induction had significantly better (by one-third) survival rates than those who failed to achieve CR [142,145,151]. The "real" pathologic response expected after TMT induction is unclear. In a small study by Housset et al. [127], 45% of the complete responders who had elected for RC treatment instead of the completion of a TMT protocol were identified to have stage pT0 disease. In contrast the Memorial Sloan-Kettering Cancer Center experience demonstrated that 30% of the patients who received chemotherapy alone showed residual muscle-invasive disease on cystectomy, which was not detected on the preoperative TUR [152].

Survival CSS rates reported in the literature are shown in Tables 30.1 and 30.2 [124−141]. Overall, the reported 5-year CSS was 50%−82%. In a study pooling various protocols over time, the 5-year CSS rate was approximately 60%−65% [142,146].

The 5-year OS was approximately 50%, and was reported to be in the 36%−74% range (Table 30.1). Discrepancies in CSS and OS might be explained by the inclusion period, patient selection, accurate staging, follow-up duration, differences in chemotherapy and radiation regimens, and the use of neoadjuvant or adjuvant chemotherapy.

Comparison With Radical Cystectomy Any direct comparison between bladder preservation modalities and RC is difficult because of the lack of randomized controlled trials. Nevertheless, in appropriately selected patients, the data suggest that TMT with prompt salvage cystectomy if required could achieve a 5-year OS rate of 48%−60% [142,153,154]. However, when evaluating the outcomes of cystectomy series from centers of excellence, the OS rate reached 62%−68% after a 5-year follow-up duration [155]. Similarly, in a cohort of 1100 patients, Hautmann et al. [156] recently reported the long-term oncological outcomes after RC, showing a 10-year CSS rate of 67%, for all pT stages. In a recent study by the University of Texas MD Anderson Cancer Center and the University of Southern California that examined patients with MIBC (cT2) without high-risk features (hydronephrosis, palpable mass, invasion into adjacent organs, LVI) who were treated with RC alone, the outcomes were excellent, with a 5-year CSS rate of 83.5% [157]. This outcome in cystectomy series appeared to be slightly higher compared to that of the selected TMT series (Tables 30.1 and 30.2) [158]. Furthermore, although one has to be careful when comparing the two approaches in subset analyses, the recent update of the Medical Research Council neoadjuvant trial, which randomized patients into groups that received neoadjuvant chemotherapy and who did not, followed by either RC or RT (alone or with TMT), revealed that the OS rate of patients in the cystectomy arm was higher than that of the patients in the radiation arm [159]; however, the authors recognized that the randomization was for the neoadjuvant chemotherapy and that there was a selection bias in the subsequent local therapy choice.

Unfortunately, clinicopathologic stage discordance and inclusion biases limit the validity of any comparisons between the two procedures. Patients fit for surgery and treated by bladder preservation are rigorously selected, with exclusion criteria including hydronephrosis, CIS, or inability to perform a maximally safe TUR, and they might not be comparable to all patients undergoing primary RC. Conversely, potential discordance between the clinical and pathological staging has also been suggested to introduce an outcome bias favoring the cystectomy series when oncological outcomes are stratified according to the pathological stage [160]. Nevertheless, it is worth noting that the downstaging rate between TUR and cystectomy series was 17%−30%, and presumed cT2 tumors treated by chemotherapy-RT might persist as pT0/pT1 tumors after TUR [10,157,160].

Predictors of Good Response MIBC constitutes a heterogeneous group of tumors. Thus selection criteria are required to determine the ideal candidates for receiving TMT. It would be relevant to identify the subgroup of MIBC types that would not respond to TMT, as the 5-year CSS rate was lower in nonresponders (range, 20%−40%) compared to the responders [10,126,128−132,134−136,138−142,144−149,151−177].

Historical series of RT alone have suggested that flat lesions such as CIS, incomplete resection, locally advanced stage disease (T4), and the presence of ureteral obstruction were associated with poorer response to RT [178]. The impact of several pretreatment variables on oncological outcomes has been assessed [126,132,135,142−145,148,179−188].

Hydronephrosis has also been suggested as a poor prognostic factor and several studies used it as part of the study exclusion criteria [132,137,163,189−191]. In fact, the RTOG protocols after 1993 have excluded patients with tumor-related hydronephrosis. Hydronephrosis that occurred in about 10%−35% of eligible patients was significantly linked to poorer outcomes, specifically in terms of response rates. The response rate was improved by at least 1.5-fold in the absence of ureteral obstruction [146,191].

Although multiplicity (defined in studies as more than one tumor) has been identified as a predictive factor for relapse in two studies [145,164], no significant association was found between multiplicity and CR rate or survival. However, studies did not include patients with diffuse multifocal disease, and TMT is not advocated in this subgroup of patients.

Maximal TUR before bladder preservation is a strong predictive factor of oncological control. This advantage might be explained by the extent of the tumor and by the completeness of the resection. Complete TUR led to a 20% improvement in CR and bladder preservation [142]. The role of re-TUR would be to decrease residual tumor volume and to optimize radiation treatment. The absence of complete TUR was also part of the exclusion criteria in some TMT series [132,135,190]. Most series have significantly linked incomplete TUR to poorer response rates and survival outcomes. Its independent predictive impact requires further evaluation, as incomplete TUR might be considered as a surrogate for the pT stage [142]. Pathologic prognostic factors such as high clinical stage, high tumor grade, lymph node involvement, and LVI indicate aggressive disease and, as in the RC series, have been associated with poorer outcomes in patients treated with TMT [192,193].

The presence of CIS has been correlated with higher local recurrence rates in pure RT series [194]; however, the impact of CIS on response rate after TMT has not been thoroughly studied. Although univariate analysis identified CIS as a prognostic factor, multivariate analysis performed in other series did not indicate CIS as a prognostic factor [132,145,151]. Therefore the association between CIS and response rate requires further evaluation.

Pooled together, all of these factors highlighted that a limited number of patients with MIBC meet the criteria as "ideal patients for bladder preservation." In a recent review of the current literature, Smith et al. [195] estimated that 10%−15% of medically operable patients were good candidates for bladder preservation. The recent International Consultation on Urological Diseases−European Association of Urology International Consultation on Bladder Cancer stated that the best patients eligible for bladder preservation are those having early-stage T2 disease, no hydronephrosis, no extensive CIS, and no tumor invasion into the stroma of the prostate [196]. Nevertheless, there is no clear evidence on the factors that determine TMT eligibility. Moreover, TMT remains an alternative to RC in "not ideal" candidates if they refuse surgery, and plays a more important role in patients who are unfit for surgery.

Surveillance

Good responders with intact bladders have to be followed closely by cystoscopy and CT or MRI surveillance, with prompt salvage RC in cases of invasive recurrence. Authors also suggest systematic tumor-site rebiopsy and bimanual examination under general anesthesia after the completion of therapy, because on rare occasions, patients might have a negative cystoscopy but still have tumor growth underneath the TUR scar. Additional biopsies might be performed as appropriate. Although most trials advocate and support rebiopsy following TMT, some coauthors advocate a routine resection (rather than a cold-cup biopsy) of the tumor scar at the first assessment following TMT. If the biopsied tissue and cytology do not show cancer (CR), the subsequent two to three cystoscopic evaluations over the next 9–12 months might include routine cold-cup biopsies. Nevertheless, a recommendation based on strong evidence could not be made concerning this follow-up interval subsequent to the initial assessment. Voided urine cytology is obtained before each evaluation. Ideally, the same urologist should perform both the initial maximal TUR of the bladder tumor and the post-TMT evaluations. In addition to the bladder, it is recommended that the urologist performs a risk-adapted surveillance for distant metastasis and the upper tract.

Bladder preservation studies that offer long-term follow-up and address the risk of late metastatic or muscle-invasive bladder failure suggested a decrease in the cancer-specific events and a flattening of the CSS curve beyond the first 5 years after TMT, similar to follow-up after cystectomy [142]. Other series reported that some patients might develop late recurrences beyond the first 5-year follow-up [118,197,198]. Because of the potential risk of delayed recurrences, lifelong follow-up of patients with cystoscopy is recommended.

Conclusion

In selected patients with MIBC, bladder-preserving therapy with cystectomy reserved for tumor recurrence represents a safe and effective alternative to immediate RC. Cumulative published data of more than 1000 patients in single institution and multiinstitution cooperative group trials demonstrated that TMT results in excellent local control in 70% of the patients with MIBC while preserving a native functional bladder without compromising long-term survival. The 10-year OS and disease-specific survival rates in the bladder-sparing protocols are comparable to the overall results reported with contemporary RC. Moreover, the 15-year results indicate a plateau in disease-specific survival, suggesting no evidence of increased recurrence rates with longer follow-up periods. Lifelong bladder surveillance is essential. Prompt cystectomy for tumor recurrence is necessary to prevent tumor dissemination. Thus bladder-preserving therapy is a bona fide option and a valid alternative to RC in selected patients. This approach should be discussed along with all of the other treatment options during overall initial treatment planning. This approach contributes significantly to the patient quality of life and represents a unique opportunity for the urologic surgeons, radiation oncologists, and medical oncologists to work hand-in-hand in a joint effort to provide patients with the best treatment option for this disease.

CONCLUSION

The follow-up of patients with MIBC is required for the detection of recurrences and disease progression as well as for evaluating complications after radical treatment. In case of bladder preservation treatment for MIBC, early endoscopy and imaging reassessment is required. Oncological follow-up of MIBC is adapted according to tumor stage and grade, location, and treatment modality; thus defining the risk of recurrence over time. Since randomized studies investigating the most appropriate follow-up schedule are lacking, most recommendations are based only on the results of the retrospective studies. Nonetheless, reasonable recommendations can be made based on these results, until further prospective randomized studies testing the effectiveness of different follow-up schedules have been performed.

REFERENCES

[1] Stenzl A, Cowan NC, De Santis M, Kuczyk MA, Merseburger AS, Ribal MJ, et al. Treatment of muscle-invasive and metastatic bladder cancer: update of the EAU guidelines. Eur Urol 2011;59:1009–18.

[2] Ploussard G, Daneshmand S, Efstathiou JA, Herr HW, James ND, Rödel CM, et al. Critical analysis of bladder sparing with trimodal therapy in muscle-invasive bladder cancer: a systematic review. Eur Urol 2014;66:120–37.

[3] Malkowicz SB, van Poppel H, Mickisch G, Pansadoro V, Thüroff J, Soloway MS, et al. Muscle-invasive urothelial carcinoma of the bladder. Urology 2007;69:3–16.

[4] Karakiewicz PI, Shariat SF, Palapattu GS, Gilad AE, Lotan Y, Rogers CG, et al. Nomogram for predicting disease recurrence after radical cystectomy for transitional cell carcinoma of the bladder. J Urol 2006;176:1354–61, discussion 1361-1352.

[5] Bochner BH, Kattan MW, Vora KC. Postoperative nomogram predicting risk of recurrence after radical cystectomy for bladder cancer. J Clin Oncol 2006;24:3967–72.

[6] Giannarini G, Kessler TM, Thoeny HC, Nguyen DP, Meissner C, Studer UE. Do patients benefit from routine follow-up to detect recurrences after radical cystectomy and ileal orthotopic bladder substitution? Eur Urol 2010;58:486–94.

[7] Soukup V, Babjuk M, Bellmunt J, Dalbagni G, Giannarini G, Hakenberg OW, et al. Follow-up after surgical treatment of bladder cancer: a critical analysis of the literature. Eur Urol 2012;62:290–302.

[8] Huguet J. Follow-up after radical cystectomy based on patterns of tumour recurrence and its risk factors. Actas Urol Esp 2013;37:376–82.

[9] Vrooman OP, Witjes JA. Follow-up of patients after curative bladder cancer treatment: guidelines vs. practice. Curr Opin Urol 2010;20:437–42.

[10] Yafi FA, Aprikian AG, Chin JL, Fradet Y, Izawa J, Estey E, et al. Contemporary outcomes of 2287 patients with bladder cancer who were treated with radical cystectomy: a Canadian multicentre experience. BJU Int 2011;108:539–45.

[11] Canter D, Long C, Kutikov A, Plimack E, Saad I, Oblaczynski M, et al. Clinicopathological outcomes after radical cystectomy for clinical T2 urothelial carcinoma: further evidence to support the use of neoadjuvant chemotherapy. BJU Int 2011;107:58−62.

[12] Mathers MJ, Zumbe J, Wyler S, Roth S, Gerken M, Hofstädter F, et al. Is there evidence for a multidisciplinary follow-up after urological cancer? An evaluation of subsequent cancers. World J Urol 2008;26:251−6.

[13] Volkmer BG, Kuefer R, Bartsch Jr. GC, Gust K, Hautmann RE. Oncological followup after radical cystectomy for bladder cancer-is there any benefit?. J Urol 2009;181:1587−93, discussion 1593.

[14] Bochner BH, Montie JE, Lee CT. Follow-up strategies and management of recurrence in urologic oncology bladder cancer: invasive bladder cancer. Urol Clin North Am 2003;30:777−89.

[15] Heidenreich A, Albers P, Classen J, Graefen M, Gschwend J, Kotzerke J, et al. Imaging studies in metastatic urogenital cancer patients undergoing systemic therapy: recommendations of a multidisciplinary consensus meeting of the Association of Urological Oncology of the German Cancer Society. Urol Int 2010;85:1−10.

[16] Winer-Muram HT. The solitary pulmonary nodule. Radiology 2006;239:34−49.

[17] Wormanns D, Ludwig K, Beyer F, Heindel W, Diederich S. Detection of pulmonary nodules at multirow-detector CT: effectiveness of double reading to improve sensitivity at standard-dose and low-dose chest CT. Eur Radiol 2005;15:14−22.

[18] Kanematsu M, Kondo H, Goshima S, Kato H, Tsuge U, Hirose Y, et al. Imaging liver metastases: review and update. Eur J Radiol 2006;58:217−28.

[19] Ariff B, Lloyd CR, Khan S, Shariff M, Thillainayagam AV, Bansi DS, et al. Imaging of liver cancer. World J Gastroenterol 2009;15:1289−300.

[20] Barrett T, Choyke PL, Kobayashi H. Imaging of the lymphatic system: new horizons. Contrast Media Mol Imaging 2006;1:230−45.

[21] Morisawa N, Koyama T, Togashi K. Metastatic lymph nodes in urogenital cancers: contribution of imaging findings. Abdom Imaging 2006;31:620−9.

[22] Powles T, Murray I, Brock C, Oliver T, Avril N. Molecular positron emission tomography and PET/CT imaging in urological malignancies. Eur Urol 2007;51:1511−20, discussion 1520-1511.

[23] Kibel AS, Dehdashti F, Katz MD, Klim AP, Grubb RL, Humphrey PA, et al. Prospective study of [18F]fluorodeoxyglucose positron emission tomography/computed tomography for staging of muscle-invasive bladder carcinoma. J Clin Oncol 2009;27:4314−20.

[24] Pollen JJ, Gerber K, Ashburn WL, Schmidt JD. The value of nuclear bone imaging in advanced prostatic cancer. J Urol 1981;125:222−3.

[25] Ghanem N, Uhl M, Brink I, Schäfer O, Kelly T, Moser E, et al. Diagnostic value of MRI in comparison to scintigraphy, PET, MS-CT and PET/CT for the detection of metastases of bone. Eur J Radiol 2005;55:41−55.

[26] Nakanishi K, Kobayashi M, Nakaguchi K, Kyakuno M, Hashimoto N, Onishi H, et al. Whole-body MRI for detecting metastatic bone tumor: diagnostic value of diffusion-weighted images. Magn Reson Med Sci 2007;6:147−55.

[27] Schlemmer HP, Schafer J, Pfannenberg C, Radny P, Korchidi S, Müller-Horvat C, et al. Fast whole-body assessment of metastatic disease using a novel magnetic resonance imaging system: initial experiences. Invest Radiol 2005;40:64−71.

[28] Huguet-Perez J, Palou J, Millan-Rodriguez F, Salvador-Bayarri J, Villavicencio-Mavrich H, Vicente-Rodriguez J. Upper tract transitional cell carcinoma following cystectomy for bladder cancer. Eur Urol 2001;40:318−23.

[29] Hautmann RE, Volkmer BG, Schumacher MC, Gschwend JE, Studer UE. Long-term results of standard procedures in urology: the ileal neobladder. World J Urol 2006;24:305—14.

[30] Meissner C, Giannarini G, Schumacher MC, Thoeny H, Studer UE, Burkhard FC. The efficiency of excretory urography to detect upper urinary tract tumors after cystectomy for urothelial cancer. J Urol 2007;178:2287—90.

[31] Sanderson KM, Cai J, Miranda G, Skinner DG, Stein JP. Upper tract urothelial recurrence following radical cystectomy for transitional cell carcinoma of the bladder: an analysis of 1,069 patients with 10-year followup. J Urol 2007;177:2088—94.

[32] Tran W, Serio AM, Raj GV, Dalbagni G, Vickers AJ, Bochner BH, et al. Longitudinal risk of upper tract recurrence following radical cystectomy for urothelial cancer and the potential implications for long-term surveillance. J Urol 2008;179:96—100.

[33] Volkmer BG, Schnoeller T, Kuefer R, Gust K, Finter F, Hautmann RE. Upper urinary tract recurrence after radical cystectomy for bladder cancer—who is at risk? J Urol 2009;182:2632—7.

[34] Umbreit EC, Crispen PL, Shimko MS, Farmer SA, Blute ML, Frank I. Multifactorial, site-specific recurrence model after radical cystectomy for urothelial carcinoma. Cancer 2010;116:3399—407.

[35] Gakis G, Schilling D, Perner S, Schwentner C, Sievert KD, Stenzl A. Sequential resection of malignant ureteral margins at radical cystectomy: a critical assessment of the value of frozen section analysis. World J Urol 2011;29:451—6.

[36] Tollefson MK, Blute ML, Farmer SA, Frank I. Significance of distal ureteral margin at radical cystectomy for urothelial carcinoma. J Urol 2010;183:81—6.

[37] Schoenberg MP, Carter HB, Epstein JI. Ureteral frozen section analysis during cystectomy: a reassessment. J Urol 1996;155:1218—20.

[38] Balaji KC, McGuire M, Grotas J, Grimaldi G, Russo P. Upper tract recurrences following radical cystectomy: an analysis of prognostic factors, recurrence pattern and stage at presentation. J Urol 1999;162:1603—6.

[39] Janardhan S, Pandiaraja P, Pandey V, Karande A, Kaliraj P. Development and characterization of monoclonal antibodies against WbSXP-1 for the detection of circulating filarial antigens. J Helminthol 2011;85:1—6.

[40] Schumacher MC, Scholz M, Weise ES, Fleischmann A, Thalmann GN, Studer UE. Is there an indication for frozen section examination of the ureteral margins during cystectomy for transitional cell carcinoma of the bladder? J Urol 2006;176:2409—13, discussion 2413.

[41] Solsona E, Iborra I, Rubio J, Casanova J, Dumont R, Monros JL. Late oncological occurrences following radical cystectomy in patients with bladder cancer. Eur Urol 2003;43:489—94.

[42] Sved PD, Gomez P, Nieder AM, Manoharan M, Kim SS, Soloway MS. Upper tract tumour after radical cystectomy for transitional cell carcinoma of the bladder: incidence and risk factors. BJU Int 2004;94:785—9.

[43] Raj GV, Tal R, Vickers A, Bochner BH, Serio A, Donat SM, et al. Significance of intraoperative ureteral evaluation at radical cystectomy for urothelial cancer. Cancer 2006;107:2167—72.

[44] Osman Y, El-Tabey N, Abdel-Latif M, Mosbah A, Moustafa N, Shaaban A. The value of frozen-section analysis of ureteric margins on surgical decision-making in patients undergoing radical cystectomy for bladder cancer. BJU Int 2007;99:81—4.

[45] Herr HW, Whitmore Jr. WF. Ureteral carcinoma in situ after successful intravesical therapy for superficial bladder tumors: incidence, possible pathogenesis and management. J Urol 1987;138:292—4.

[46] Kenworthy P, Tanguay S, Dinney CP. The risk of upper tract recurrence following cystectomy in patients with transitional cell carcinoma involving the distal ureter. J Urol 1996;155:501–3.

[47] Solsona E, Iborra I, Ricos JV, Dumont R, Casanova JL, Calabuig C. Upper urinary tract involvement in patients with bladder carcinoma in situ (Tis): its impact on management. Urology 1997;49:347–52.

[48] Akkad T, Gozzi C, Deibl M, Müller T, Pelzer AE, Pinggera GM, et al. Tumor recurrence in the remnant urothelium of females undergoing radical cystectomy for transitional cell carcinoma of the bladder: long-term results from a single center. J Urol 2006;175:1268–71.

[49] Stein JP, Lieskovsky G, Cote R, Groshen S, Feng AC, Boyd S, et al. Radical cystectomy in the treatment of invasive bladder cancer: long-term results in 1,054 patients. J Clin Oncol 2001;19:666–75.

[50] Sharma TC, Melamed MR, Whitmore Jr. WF. Carcinoma in-situ of the ureter in patients with bladder carcinoma treated by cystectomy. Cancer 1970;26:583–7.

[51] Malkowicz SB, Skinner DG. Development of upper tract carcinoma after cystectomy for bladder carcinoma. Urology 1990;36:20–2.

[52] Yossepowitch O, Dalbagni G, Golijanin D, Donat SM, Bochner BH, Herr HW, et al. Orthotopic urinary diversion after cystectomy for bladder cancer: implications for cancer control and patterns of disease recurrence. J Urol 2003;169:177–81.

[53] Slaton JW, Swanson DA, Grossman HB, Dinney CP. A stage specific approach to tumor surveillance after radical cystectomy for transitional cell carcinoma of the bladder. J Urol 1999;162:710–14.

[54] Wang LJ, Wong YC, Huang CC, Wu CH, Hung SC, Chen HW. Multidetector computerized tomography urography is more accurate than excretory urography for diagnosing transitional cell carcinoma of the upper urinary tract in adults with hematuria. J Urol 2010;183:48–55.

[55] Scolieri MJ, Paik ML, Brown SL, Resnick MI. Limitations of computed tomography in the preoperative staging of upper tract urothelial carcinoma. Urology 2000;56:930–4.

[56] Xu AD, Ng CS, Kamat A, Grossman HB, Dinney C, Sandler CM. Significance of upper urinary tract urothelial thickening and filling defect seen on MDCT urography in patients with a history of urothelial neoplasms. Am J Roentgenol 2010;195:959–65.

[57] Caoili EM, Cohan RH, Inampudi P, Ellis JH, Shah RB, Faerber GJ, et al. MDCT urography of upper tract urothelial neoplasms. Am J Roentgenol 2005;184:1873–81.

[58] Fritz GA, Schoellnast H, Deutschmann HA, Quehenberger F, Tillich M. Multiphasic multidetector-row CT (MDCT) in detection and staging of transitional cell carcinomas of the upper urinary tract. Eur Radiol 2006;16:1244–52.

[59] Sadow CA, Wheeler SC, Kim J, Ohno-Machado L, Silverman SG. Positive predictive value of CT urography in the evaluation of upper tract urothelial cancer. Am J Roentgenol 2010;195:W337–343.

[60] Maheshwari E, O'Malley ME, Ghai S, Staunton M, Massey C. Split-bolus MDCT urography: upper tract opacification and performance for upper tract tumors in patients with hematuria. Am J Roentgenol 2010;194:453–8.

[61] Takahashi N, Kawashima A, Glockner JF, Hartman RP, Leibovich BC, Brau AC, et al. Small (<2-cm) upper-tract urothelial carcinoma: evaluation with gadolinium-enhanced three-dimensional spoiled gradient-recalled echo MR urography. Radiology 2008;247:451–7.

[62] Takeuchi M, Matsuzaki K, Kubo H, Nishitani H. Diffusion-weighted magnetic resonance imaging of urinary epithelial cancer with upper urinary tract obstruction: preliminary results. Acta Radiol 2008;49:1195–9.

[63]   Nishizawa S, Imai S, Okaneya T, Nakayama T, Kamigaito T, Minagawa T. Diffusion weighted imaging in the detection of upper urinary tract urothelial tumors. Int Braz J Urol 2010;36:18−28.

[64]   Kim KH, Fonda JR, Lawler EV, Gagnon D, Kaufman JS. Change in use of gadolinium-enhanced magnetic resonance studies in kidney disease patients after US Food and Drug Administration warnings: a cross-sectional study of Veterans Affairs Health Care System data from 2005-2008. Am J Kidney Dis 2010;56:458−67.

[65]   Akkad T, Brunner A, Pallwein L, et al. Fluorescence in situ hybridization for detecting upper urinary tract tumors—a preliminary report. Urology 2007;70:753−7.

[66]   Marin-Aguilera M, Mengual L, Ribal MJ, Gozzi C, Bartsch G, Mikuz G, et al. Utility of fluorescence in situ hybridization as a non-invasive technique in the diagnosis of upper urinary tract urothelial carcinoma. Eur Urol 2007;51:409−15, discussion 415.

[67]   Yoshimine S, Kikuchi E, Matsumoto K, Ide H, Miyajima A, Nakagawa K, et al. The clinical significance of urine cytology after a radical cystectomy for urothelial cancer. Int J Urol 2010;17:527−32.

[68]   Raj GV, Bochner BH, Serio AM, Vickers A, Donat SM, Herr H, et al. Natural history of positive urinary cytology after radical cystectomy. J Urol 2006;176:2000−5.

[69]   Messer J, Shariat SF, Brien JC, Herman MP, Ng CK, Scherr DS, et al. Urinary cytology has a poor performance for predicting invasive or high-grade upper-tract urothelial carcinoma. BJU Int 2011;108:701−5.

[70]   Shan Z, Wu P, Zheng S, Tan W, Zhou H, Zuo Y, et al. Evaluation of upper urinary tract tumors by FISH in Chinese patients. Cancer Genet Cytogenet 2010;203:238−46.

[71]   Lodde M, Mian C, Wiener H, Haitel A, Pycha A, Marberger M. Detection of upper urinary tract transitional cell carcinoma with ImmunoCyt: a preliminary report. Urology 2001;58:362−6.

[72]   Johannes JR, Nelson E, Bibbo M, Bagley DH. Voided urine fluorescence in situ hybridization testing for upper tract urothelial carcinoma surveillance. J Urol 2010;184:879−82.

[73]   Brien JC, Shariat SF, Herman MP, Ng CK, Scherr DS, Scoll B, et al. Preoperative hydronephrosis, ureteroscopic biopsy grade and urinary cytology can improve prediction of advanced upper tract urothelial carcinoma. J Urol 2010;184:69−73.

[74]   Sanderson KM, Roupret M. Upper urinary tract tumour after radical cystectomy for transitional cell carcinoma of the bladder: an update on the risk factors, surveillance regimens and treatments. BJU Int 2007;100:11−16.

[75]   Lee BR, Jabbour ME, Marshall FF, Smith AD, Jarrett TW. 13-Year survival comparison of percutaneous and open nephroureterectomy approaches for management of transitional cell carcinoma of renal collecting system: equivalent outcomes. J Endourol 1999;13:289−94.

[76]   Lee JN, Kim BS, Kim HT, Kim TH, Yoo ES, Choi GS, et al. Oncologic outcomes of laparoscopic nephroureterectomy for pT3 upper urinary tract urothelial carcinoma. Minerva Urol Nefrol 2014;66:157−64.

[77]   Dhar NB, Klein EA, Reuther AM, Thalmann GN, Madersbacher S, Studer UE. Outcome after radical cystectomy with limited or extended pelvic lymph node dissection. J Urol 2008;179:873−8, discussion 878.

[78]   Dhar NB, Campbell SC, Zippe CD, Derweesh IH, Reuther AM, Fergany A, et al. Outcomes in patients with urothelial carcinoma of the bladder with limited pelvic lymph node dissection. BJU Int 2006;98:1172−5.

[79]   Kondo T, Hashimoto Y, Kobayashi H, Iizuka J, Nakazawa H, Ito F, et al. Template-based lymphadenectomy in urothelial carcinoma of the upper urinary tract: impact on patient survival. Int J Urol 2010;17:848−54.

[80] Roscigno M, Shariat SF, Freschi M, Margulis V, Karakiewizc P, Suardi N, et al. Assessment of the minimum number of lymph nodes needed to detect lymph node invasion at radical nephroureterectomy in patients with upper tract urothelial cancer. Urology 2009;74:1070−4.

[81] Roscigno M, Shariat SF, Margulis V, Karakiewicz P, Remzi M, Kikuchi E, et al. The extent of lymphadenectomy seems to be associated with better survival in patients with nonmetastatic upper-tract urothelial carcinoma: how many lymph nodes should be removed? Eur Urol 2009;56:512−18.

[82] Pano B, Sebastia C, Bunesch L, Mestres J, Salvador R, Macías NG, et al. Pathways of lymphatic spread in male urogenital pelvic malignancies. Radiographics 2011;31:135−60.

[83] Roupret M, Hupertan V, Traxer O, Loison G, Chartier-Kastler E, Conort P, et al. Comparison of open nephroureterectomy and ureteroscopic and percutaneous management of upper urinary tract transitional cell carcinoma. Urology 2006;67:1181−7.

[84] Guarnizo E, Pavlovich CP, Seiba M, Carlson DL, Vaughan Jr. ED, Sosa RE. Ureteroscopic biopsy of upper tract urothelial carcinoma: improved diagnostic accuracy and histopathological considerations using a multi-biopsy approach. J Urol 2000;163:52−5.

[85] Levinson AK, Johnson DE, Wishnow KI. Indications for urethrectomy in an era of continent urinary diversion. J Urol 1990;144:73−5.

[86] Tongaonkar HB, Dalal AV, Kulkarni JN, Kamat MR. Urethral recurrences following radical cystectomy for invasive transitional cell carcinoma of the bladder. Br J Urol 1993;72:910−14.

[87] Clark PE, Stein JP, Groshen SG, Miranda G, Cai J, Lieskovsky G, et al. The management of urethral transitional cell carcinoma after radical cystectomy for invasive bladder cancer. J Urol 2004;172:1342−7.

[88] Stein JP, Clark P, Miranda G, Cai J, Groshen S, Skinner DG. Urethral tumor recurrence following cystectomy and urinary diversion: clinical and pathological characteristics in 768 male patients. J Urol 2005;173:1163−8.

[89] Studer UE, Burkhard FC, Schumacher M, Kessler TM, Thoeny H, Fleischmann A, et al. Twenty years experience with an ileal orthotopic low pressure bladder substitute—lessons to be learned. J Urol 2006;176:161−6.

[90] Huguet J, Monllau V, Sabate S, Rodriguez-Faba O, Algaba F, Palou J, et al. Diagnosis, risk factors, and outcome of urethral recurrences following radical cystectomy for bladder cancer in 729 male patients. Eur Urol 2008;53:785−92, discussion 792-783.

[91] Sherwood JB, Sagalowsky AI. The diagnosis and treatment of urethral recurrence after radical cystectomy. Urol Oncol 2006;24:356−61.

[92] Yoshida K, Nishiyama H, Kinoshita H, Matsuda T, Ogawa O. Surgical treatment for urethral recurrence after ileal neobladder reconstruction in patients with bladder cancer. BJU Int 2006;98:1008−11.

[93] Nieder AM, Sved PD, Gomez P, Kim SS, Manoharan M, Soloway MS. Urethral recurrence after cystoprostatectomy: implications for urinary diversion and monitoring. Urology 2004;64:950−4.

[94] Hassan JM, Cookson MS, Smith Jr. JA, Chang SS. Urethral recurrence in patients following orthotopic urinary diversion. J Urol 2004;172:1338−41.

[95] Freeman JA, Tarter TA, Esrig D, Stein JP, Elmajian DA, Chen SC, et al. Urethral recurrence in patients with orthotopic ileal neobladders. J Urol 1996;156:1615−19.

[96] Kassouf W, Spiess PE, Brown GA, Liu P, Grossman HB, Dinney CP, et al. Prostatic urethral biopsy has limited usefulness in counseling patients regarding final urethral margin status during orthotopic neobladder reconstruction. J Urol 2008;180:164−7, discussion 167.

[97]   Donat SM, Wei DC, McGuire MS, Herr HW. The efficacy of transurethral biopsy for predicting the long-term clinical impact of prostatic invasive bladder cancer. J Urol 2001;165:1580−4.

[98]   Cho KS, Seo JW, Park SJ, Lee YH, Choi YD, Cho NH, et al. The risk factor for urethral recurrence after radical cystectomy in patients with transitional cell carcinoma of the bladder. Urol Int 2009;82:306−11.

[99]   Ali-el-Dein B, Abdel-Latif M, Ashamallah A, Abdel-Rahim M, Ghoneim M. Local urethral recurrence after radical cystectomy and orthotopic bladder substitution in women: a prospective study. J Urol 2004;171:275−8.

[100]   Stein JP, Penson DF, Lee C, Cai J, Miranda G, Skinner DG. Long-term oncological outcomes in women undergoing radical cystectomy and orthotopic diversion for bladder cancer. J Urol 2009;181:2052−8, discussion 2058-2059.

[101]   Stenzl A, Draxl H, Posch B, Colleselli K, Falk M, Bartsch G. The risk of urethral tumors in female bladder cancer: can the urethra be used for orthotopic reconstruction of the lower urinary tract? J Urol 1995;153:950−5.

[102]   Stein JP, Penson DF, Wu SD, Skinner DG. Pathological guidelines for orthotopic urinary diversion in women with bladder cancer: a review of the literature. J Urol 2007;178: 756−60.

[103]   Stein JP, Esrig D, Freeman JA, Grossfeld GD, Ginsberg DA, Cote RJ, et al. Prospective pathologic analysis of female cystectomy specimens: risk factors for orthotopic diversion in women. Urology 1998;51:951−5.

[104]   Stein JP, Cote RJ, Freeman JA, Esrig D, Elmajian DA, Groshen S, et al. Indications for lower urinary tract reconstruction in women after cystectomy for bladder cancer: a pathological review of female cystectomy specimens. J Urol 1995;154:1329−33.

[105]   Maralani S, Wood Jr. DP, Grignon D, Banerjee M, Sakr W, Pontes JE. Incidence of urethral involvement in female bladder cancer: an anatomic pathologic study. Urology 1997;50:537−41.

[106]   Lin DW, Herr HW, Dalbagni G. Value of urethral wash cytology in the retained male urethra after radical cystoprostatectomy. J Urol 2003;169:961−3.

[107]   Varol C, Thalmann GN, Burkhard FC, Studer UE. Treatment of urethral recurrence following radical cystectomy and ileal bladder substitution. J Urol 2004;172:937−42.

[108]   Nelles JL, Konety BR, Saigal C, Pace J, Lai J. Urethrectomy following cystectomy for bladder cancer in men: practice patterns and impact on survival. J Urol 2008;180: 1933−6, discussion 1936-1937.

[109]   Stewart SB, Leder RA, Inman BA. Imaging tumors of the penis and urethra. Urol Clin North Am 2010;37:353−67.

[110]   Nagata H, Ochiai K, Aotani Y, Ando K, Yoshida M, Takahashi I, et al. Lymphostin (LK6-A), a novel immunosuppressant from *Streptomyces* sp. KY11783: taxonomy of the producing organism, fermentation, isolation and biological activities. J Antibiot (Tokyo) 1997;50:537−42.

[111]   Spiess PE, Kassouf W, Brown G, Highshaw R, Wang X, Do KA, et al. Immediate versus staged urethrectomy in patients at high risk of urethral recurrence: is there a benefit to either approach? Urology 2006;67:466−71.

[112]   Stenzl A, Colleselli K, Poisel S, Feichtinger H, Pontasch H, Bartsch G. Rationale and technique of nerve sparing radical cystectomy before an orthotopic neobladder procedure in women. J Urol 1995;154:2044−9.

[113]   Stenzl A, Jarolim L, Coloby P, Golia S, Bartsch G, Babjuk M, et al. Urethra-sparing cystectomy and orthotopic urinary diversion in women with malignant pelvic tumors. Cancer 2001;92:1864−71.

[114] Duerksen DR, Fallows G, Bernstein CN. Vitamin B12 malabsorption in patients with limited ileal resection. Nutrition 2006;22:1210–13.

[115] Mills RD, Studer UE. Metabolic consequences of continent urinary diversion. J Urol 1999;161:1057–66.

[116] Madersbacher S, Schmidt J, Eberle JM, Golia S, Bartsch G, Babjuk M, et al. Long-term outcome of ileal conduit diversion. J Urol 2003;169:985–90.

[117] Pieras E, Palou J, Salvador J, Rosales A, Marcuello E, Villavicencio H. Management and prognosis of transitional cell carcinoma superficial recurrence in muscle-invasive bladder cancer after bladder preservation. Eur Urol 2003;44:222–5, discussoion 225.

[118] Zietman AL, Grocela J, Zehr E, Kaufman DS, Young RH, Althausen AF, et al. Selective bladder conservation using transurethral resection, chemotherapy, and radiation: management and consequences of Ta, T1, and Tis recurrence within the retained bladder. Urology 2001;58:380–5.

[119] Solsona E, Iborra I, Ricos JV, Monros JL, Casanova J, Calabuig C. Feasibility of transurethral resection for muscle infiltrating carcinoma of the bladder: long-term followup of a prospective study. J Urol 1998;159:95–8, discussion 98-99.

[120] Kassouf W, Swanson D, Kamat AM, Leibovici D, Siefker-Radtke A, Munsell MF, et al. Partial cystectomy for muscle invasive urothelial carcinoma of the bladder: a contemporary review of the M. D. Anderson Cancer Center experience. J Urol 2006;175:2058–62.

[121] Smaldone MC, Jacobs BL, Smaldone AM, Hrebinko Jr. RL. Long-term results of selective partial cystectomy for invasive urothelial bladder carcinoma. Urology 2008;72:613–16.

[122] Sternberg CN, Pansadoro V, Calabro F, Schnetzer S, Giannarelli D, Emiliozzi P, et al. Can patient selection for bladder preservation be based on response to chemotherapy? Cancer 2003;97:1644–52.

[123] Koga F, Kihara K, Fujii Y, Saito K, Masuda H, Kageyama Y, et al. Favourable outcomes of patients with clinical stage T3N0M0 bladder cancer treated with induction low-dose chemo-radiotherapy plus partial or radical cystectomy vs immediate radical cystectomy: a single-institutional retrospective comparative study. BJU Int 2009;104:189–94.

[124] James ND, Hussain SA, Hall E, Jenkins P, Tremlett J, Rawlings C, et al. Radiotherapy with or without chemotherapy in muscle-invasive bladder cancer. N Engl J Med 2012;366:1477–88.

[125] Tunio MA, Hashmi A, Qayyum A, Mohsin R, Zaeem A. Whole-pelvis or bladder-only chemoradiation for lymph node-negative invasive bladder cancer: single-institution experience. Int J Radiat Oncol Biol Phys 2012;82:e457–462.

[126] Shipley WU, Winter KA, Kaufman DS, Lee WR, Heney NM, Tester WR, et al. Phase III trial of neoadjuvant chemotherapy in patients with invasive bladder cancer treated with selective bladder preservation by combined radiation therapy and chemotherapy: initial results of Radiation Therapy Oncology Group 89-03. J Clin Oncol 1998;16:3576–83.

[127] Housset M, Maulard C, Chretien Y, Dufour B, Delanian S, Huart J, et al. Combined radiation and chemotherapy for invasive transitional-cell carcinoma of the bladder: a prospective study. J Clin Oncol 1993;11:2150–7.

[128] Lagrange JL, Bascoul-Mollevi C, Geoffrois L, Beckendorf V, Ferrero JM, Joly F, et al. Quality of life assessment after concurrent chemoradiation for invasive bladder cancer: results of a multicenter prospective study (GETUG 97-015). Int J Radiat Oncol Biol Phys 2011;79:172–8.

[129] Gogna NK, Matthews JH, Turner SL, Mameghan H, Duchesne GM, Spry N, et al. Efficacy and tolerability of concurrent weekly low dose cisplatin during radiation treatment of localised muscle invasive bladder transitional cell carcinoma: a report of two

sequential Phase II studies from the Trans Tasman Radiation Oncology Group. Radiother Oncol 2006;81:9−17.

[130] Kragelj B, Zaletel-Kragelj L, Sedmak B, Cufer T, Cervek J. Phase II study of radiochemotherapy with vinblastine in invasive bladder cancer. Radiother Oncol 2005;75:44−7.

[131] Weiss C, Engehausen DG, Krause FS, Papadopoulos T, Dunst J, Sauer R, et al. Radiochemotherapy with cisplatin and 5-fluorouracil after transurethral surgery in patients with bladder cancer. Int J Radiat Oncol Biol Phys 2007;68:1072−80.

[132] Zapatero A, Martin De Vidales C, Arellano R, Ibañez Y, Bocardo G, Perez M, et al. Long-term results of two prospective bladder-sparing trimodality approaches for invasive bladder cancer: neoadjuvant chemotherapy and concurrent radio-chemotherapy. Urology 2012;80:1056−62.

[133] Choudhury A, Swindell R, Logue JP, Elliott PA, Livsey JE, Wise M, et al. Phase II study of conformal hypofractionated radiotherapy with concurrent gemcitabine in muscle-invasive bladder cancer. J Clin Oncol 2011;29:733−8.

[134] Aboziada MA, Hamza HM, Abdlrahem AM. Initial results of bladder preserving approach by chemo-radiotherapy in patients with muscle invading transitional cell carcinoma. J Egypt Natl Canc Inst 2009;21:167−74.

[135] Peyromaure M, Slama J, Beuzeboc P, Ponvert D, Debre B, Zerbib M. Concurrent chemoradiotherapy for clinical stage T2 bladder cancer: report of a single institution. Urology 2004;63:73−7.

[136] Hussain SA, Stocken DD, Peake DR, Glaholm JG, Zarkar A, Wallace DM, et al. Long-term results of a phase II study of synchronous chemoradiotherapy in advanced muscle invasive bladder cancer. Br J Cancer 2004;90:2106−11.

[137] Kaufman DS, Winter KA, Shipley WU, Heney NM, Chetner MP, Souhami L, et al. The initial results in muscle-invading bladder cancer of RTOG 95-06: phase I/II trial of transurethral surgery plus radiation therapy with concurrent cisplatin and 5-fluorouracil followed by selective bladder preservation or cystectomy depending on the initial response. Oncologist 2000;5:471−6.

[138] Varveris H, Delakas D, Anezinis P, Haldeopoulos D, Mazonakis M, Damilakis J, et al. Concurrent platinum and docetaxel chemotherapy and external radical radiotherapy in patients with invasive transitional cell bladder carcinoma. A preliminary report of tolerance and local control. Anticancer Res 1997;17:4771−80.

[139] Tester W, Porter A, Asbell S, Coughlin C, Heaney J, Krall J, et al. Combined modality program with possible organ preservation for invasive bladder carcinoma: results of RTOG protocol 85-12. Int J Radiat Oncol Biol Phys 1993;25:783−90.

[140] Rotman M, Aziz H, Porrazzo M, Choi KN, Silverstein M, Rosenthal J, et al. Treatment of advanced transitional cell carcinoma of the bladder with irradiation and concomitant 5-fluorouracil infusion. Int J Radiat Oncol Biol Phys 1990;18:1131−7.

[141] Russell KJ, Boileau MA, Higano C, Collins C, Russell AH, Koh W, et al. Combined 5-fluorouracil and irradiation for transitional cell carcinoma of the urinary bladder. Int J Radiat Oncol Biol Phys 1990;19:693−9.

[142] Efstathiou JA, Spiegel DY, Shipley WU, Heney NM, Kaufman DS, Niemierko A, et al. Long-term outcomes of selective bladder preservation by combined-modality therapy for invasive bladder cancer: the MGH experience. Eur Urol 2012;61:705−11.

[143] Krause FS, Walter B, Ott OJ, Häberle L, Weiss C, Rödel C, et al. 15-Year survival rates after transurethral resection and radiochemotherapy or radiation in bladder cancer treatment. Anticancer Res 2011;31:985−90.

[144] Chung PW, Bristow RG, Milosevic MF, Yi QL, Jewett MA, Warde PR, et al. Long-term outcome of radiation-based conservation therapy for invasive bladder cancer. Urol Oncol 2007;25:303−9.

[145] Rodel C, Grabenbauer GG, Kuhn R, Papadopoulos T, Dunst J, Meyer M, et al. Combined-modality treatment and selective organ preservation in invasive bladder cancer: long-term results. J Clin Oncol 2002;20:3061−71.

[146] Shipley WU, Kaufman DS, Zehr E, Heney NM, Lane SC, Thakral HK, et al. Selective bladder preservation by combined modality protocol treatment: long-term outcomes of 190 patients with invasive bladder cancer. Urology 2002;60:62−7, discussion 67-68.

[147] Hussain MH, Glass TR, Forman J, Sakr W, Smith DC, Al-Sarraf M, et al. Combination cisplatin, 5-fluorouracil and radiation therapy for locally advanced unresectable or medically unfit bladder cancer cases: a Southwest Oncology Group Study. J Urol 2001;165:56−60, discussion 60-51.

[148] Chauvet B, Brewer Y, Felix-Faure C, Davin JL, Choquenet C, Reboul F. Concurrent cisplatin and radiotherapy for patients with muscle invasive bladder cancer who are not candidates for radical cystectomy. J Urol 1996;156:1258−62.

[149] Einstein Jr. AB, Wolf M, Halliday KR, Miller GJ, Hafermann M, Lowe BA, et al. Combination transurethral resection, systemic chemotherapy, and pelvic radiotherapy for invasive (T2-T4) bladder cancer unsuitable for cystectomy: a phase I/II Southwestern Oncology Group study. Urology 1996;47:652−7.

[150] Shipley WU, Prout Jr. GR, Einstein AB, Coombs LJ, Wajsman Z, Soloway MS, et al. Treatment of invasive bladder cancer by cisplatin and radiation in patients unsuited for surgery. JAMA 1987;258:931−5.

[151] Koga F, Numao N, Saito K, Masuda H, Fujii Y, Kawakami S, et al. Sensitivity to chemoradiation predicts development of metastasis in muscle-invasive bladder cancer patients. Urol Oncol 2013;31:1270−5.

[152] Donat SM, Herr HW, Bajorin DF, Fair WR, Sogani PC, Russo P, et al. Methotrexate, vinblastine, doxorubicin and cisplatin chemotherapy and cystectomy for unresectable bladder cancer. J Urol 1996;156:368−71.

[153] Mitin T, Hunt D, Shipley WU, Kaufman DS, Uzzo R, Wu CL, et al. Transurethral surgery and twice-daily radiation plus paclitaxel-cisplatin or fluorouracil-cisplatin with selective bladder preservation and adjuvant chemotherapy for patients with muscle invasive bladder cancer (RTOG 0233): a randomised multicentre phase 2 trial. Lancet Oncol 2013;14:863−72.

[154] Kotwal S, Choudhury A, Johnston C, Paul AB, Whelan P, Kiltie AE. Similar treatment outcomes for radical cystectomy and radical radiotherapy in invasive bladder cancer treated at a United Kingdom specialist treatment center. Int J Radiat Oncol Biol Phys 2008;70:456−63.

[155] Madersbacher S, Hochreiter W, Burkhard F, Thalmann GN, Danuser H, Markwalder R, et al. Radical cystectomy for bladder cancer today—a homogeneous series without neoadjuvant therapy. J Clin Oncol 2003;21:690−6.

[156] Hautmann RE, de Petriconi RC, Pfeiffer C, Volkmer BG. Radical cystectomy for urothelial carcinoma of the bladder without neoadjuvant or adjuvant therapy: long-term results in 1100 patients. Eur Urol 2012;61:1039−47.

[157] Culp SH, Dickstein RJ, Grossman HB, et al. Refining patient selection for neoadjuvant chemotherapy before radical cystectomy. J Urol 2014;191:40−7.

[158] Bekelman JE, Handorf EA, Guzzo T, Pretzsch SM, Porten S, Daneshmand S, et al. Radical cystectomy versus bladder-preserving therapy for muscle-invasive urothelial

carcinoma: examining confounding and misclassification biasin cancer observational comparative effectiveness research. Value Health 2013;16:610−18.

[159]   Griffiths G, Hall R, Sylvester R, Raghavan D, Parmar MK. International phase III trial assessing neoadjuvant cisplatin, methotrexate, and vinblastine chemotherapy for muscle-invasive bladder cancer: long-term results of the BA06 30894 trial. J Clin Oncol 2011;29:2171−7.

[160]   Svatek RS, Shariat SF, Novara G, Skinner EC, Fradet Y, Bastian PJ, et al. Discrepancy between clinical and pathological stage: external validation of the impact on prognosis in an international radical cystectomy cohort. BJU Int 2011;107:898−904.

[161]   Danesi DT, Arcangeli G, Cruciani E, Mecozzi A, Saracino B, Giacobini S, et al. Combined treatment of invasive bladder carcinoma with transurethral resection, induction chemotherapy, and radical radiotherapy plus concomitant protracted infusion of cisplatin and 5-fluorouracil: a phase I study. Cancer 1997;80:1464−71.

[162]   Nichols Jr. RC, Sweetser MG, Mahmood SK, Malamud FC, Dunn NP, Adams JP, et al. Radiation therapy and concomitant paclitaxel/carboplatin chemotherapy for muscle invasive transitional cell carcinoma of the bladder: a well-tolerated combination. Int J Cancer 2000;90:281−6.

[163]   Kaufman DS, Winter KA, Shipley WU, Heney NM, Wallace III HJ, Toonkel LM, et al. Phase I-II RTOG study (99-06) of patients with muscle-invasive bladder cancer undergoing transurethral surgery, paclitaxel, cisplatin, and twice-daily radiotherapy followed by selective bladder preservation or radical cystectomy and adjuvant chemotherapy. Urology 2009;73:833−7.

[164]   Onozawa M, Miyanaga N, Hinotsu S, Miyazaki J, Oikawa T, Kimura T, et al. Analysis of intravesical recurrence after bladder-preserving therapy for muscle-invasive bladder cancer. Jpn J Clin Oncol 2012;42:825−30.

[165]   Eapen L, Stewart D, Collins J, Peterson R. Effective bladder sparing therapy with intra-arterial cisplatin and radiotherapy for localized bladder cancer. J Urol 2004;172:1276−80.

[166]   Wittlinger M, Rodel CM, Weiss C, Krause SF, Kühn R, Fietkau R, et al. Quadrimodal treatment of high-risk T1 and T2 bladder cancer: transurethral tumor resection followed by concurrent radiochemotherapy and regional deep hyperthermia. Radiother Oncol 2009;93:358−63.

[167]   Epidermoid anal cancer: results from the UKCCCR randomised trial of radiotherapy alone versus radiotherapy, 5-fluorouracil, and mitomycin. UKCCCR Anal Cancer Trial Working Party. UK Co-ordinating Committee on Cancer Research. Lancet 1996;348:1049−54.

[168]   Caffo O, Fellin G, Graffer U, Valduga F, Bolner A, Luciani L, et al. Phase I study of gemcitabine and radiotherapy plus cisplatin after transurethral resection as conservative treatment for infiltrating bladder cancer. Int J Radiat Oncol Biol Phys 2003;57:1310−16.

[169]   Oh KS, Soto DE, Smith DC, Montie JE, Lee CT, Sandler HM. Combined-modality therapy with gemcitabine and radiation therapy as a bladder preservation strategy: long-term results of a phase I trial. Int J Radiat Oncol Biol Phys 2009;74:511−17.

[170]   Hoskin PJ, Rojas AM, Bentzen SM, Saunders MI. Radiotherapy with concurrent carbogen and nicotinamide in bladder carcinoma. J Clin Oncol 2010;28:4912−18.

[171]   Pollack A, Zagars GK, Swanson DA. Muscle-invasive bladder cancer treated with external beam radiotherapy: prognostic factors. Int J Radiat Oncol Biol Phys 1994;30:267−77.

[172]   Leibovici D, Kassouf W, Pisters LL, Pettaway CA, Wu X, Dinney CP, et al. Organ preservation for muscle-invasive bladder cancer by transurethral resection. Urology 2007;70:473−6.

[173] Herr HW. Transurethral resection of muscle-invasive bladder cancer: 10-year outcome. J Clin Oncol 2001;19:89−93.

[174] Solsona E, Iborra I, Collado A, Rubio-Briones J, Casanova J, Calatrava A. Feasibility of radical transurethral resection as monotherapy for selected patients with muscle invasive bladder cancer. J Urol 2010;184:475−80.

[175] Herr HW. Outcome of patients who refuse cystectomy after receiving neoadjuvant chemotherapy for muscle-invasive bladder cancer. Eur Urol 2008;54:126−32.

[176] Solsona E, Climent MA, Iborra I, Collado A, Rubio J, Ricós JV, et al. Bladder preservation in selected patients with muscle-invasive bladder cancer by complete transurethral resection of the bladder plus systemic chemotherapy: long-term follow-up of a phase 2 nonrandomized comparative trial with radical cystectomy. Eur Urol 2009;55:911−19.

[177] Grossman HB, Natale RB, Tangen CM, Speights VO, Vogelzang NJ, Trump DL, et al. Neoadjuvant chemotherapy plus cystectomy compared with cystectomy alone for locally advanced bladder cancer. N Engl J Med 2003;349:859−66.

[178] Shipley WU, Rose MA, Perrone TL, Mannix CM, Heney NM, Prout Jr. GR. Full-dose irradiation for patients with invasive bladder carcinoma: clinical and histological factors prognostic of improved survival. J Urol 1985;134:679−83.

[179] Hagan MP, Winter KA, Kaufman DS, Wajsman Z, Zietman AL, Heney NM, et al. RTOG 97-06: initial report of a phase I-II trial of selective bladder conservation using TURBT, twice-daily accelerated irradiation sensitized with cisplatin, and adjuvant MCV combination chemotherapy. Int J Radiat Oncol Biol Phys 2003;57:665−72.

[180] Coen JJ, Paly JJ, Niemierko A, Kaufman DS, Heney NM, Spiegel DY, et al. Nomograms predicting response to therapy and outcomes after bladder-preserving trimodality therapy for muscle-invasive bladder cancer. Int J Radiat Oncol Biol Phys 2013;86:311−16.

[181] Fung CY, Shipley WU, Young RH, Griffin PP, Convery KM, Kaufman DS, et al. Prognostic factors in invasive bladder carcinoma in a prospective trial of preoperative adjuvant chemotherapy and radiotherapy. J Clin Oncol 1991;9:1533−42.

[182] Tester W, Caplan R, Heaney J, Venner P, Whittington R, Byhardt R, et al. Neoadjuvant combined modality program with selective organ preservation for invasive bladder cancer: results of Radiation Therapy Oncology Group phase II trial 8802. J Clin Oncol 1996;14:119−26.

[183] Danesi DT, Arcangeli G, Cruciani E, Altavista P, Mecozzi A, Saracino B, et al. Conservative treatment of invasive bladder carcinoma by transurethral resection, protracted intravenous infusion chemotherapy, and hyperfractionated radiotherapy: long term results. Cancer 2004;101:2540−8.

[184] Arias F, Dominguez MA, Martinez E, Illarramendi JJ, Miquelez S, Pascual I, et al. Chemoradiotherapy for muscle invading bladder carcinoma. Final report of a single institutional organ-sparing program. Int J Radiat Oncol Biol Phys 2000;47:373−8.

[185] Perdona S, Autorino R, Damiano R, De Sio M, Morrica B, Gallo L, et al. Bladder-sparing, combined-modality approach for muscle-invasive bladder cancer: a multi-institutional, long-term experience. Cancer 2008;112:75−83.

[186] Sabaa MA, El-Gamal OM, Abo-Elenen M, Khanam A. Combined modality treatment with bladder preservation for muscle invasive bladder cancer. Urol Oncol 2010;28:14−20.

[187] May M, Bastian PJ, Brookman-May S, Fritsche HM, Tilki D, Otto W, et al. Gender-specific differences in cancer-specific survival after radical cystectomy for patients with urothelial carcinoma of the urinary bladder in pathologic tumor stage T4a. Urol Oncol 2013;31:1141−7.

[188] Keck B, Ott OJ, Haberle L, Kunath F, Weiss C, Rödel C, et al. Female sex is an independent risk factor for reduced overall survival in bladder cancer patients treated by transurethral resection and radio- or radiochemotherapy. World J Urol 2013;31:1023−8.

[189] Zietman AL, Shipley WU, Kaufman DS, Zehr EM, Heney NM, Althausen AF, et al. A phase I/II trial of transurethral surgery combined with concurrent cisplatin, 5-fluorouracil and twice daily radiation followed by selective bladder preservation in operable patients with muscle invading bladder cancer. J Urol 1998;160:1673−7.

[190] Lin CC, Hsu CH, Cheng JC, Huang CY, Tsai YC, Hsu FM, et al. Induction cisplatin and fluorouracil-based chemotherapy followed by concurrent chemoradiation for muscle-invasive bladder cancer. Int J Radiat Oncol Biol Phys 2009;75:442−8.

[191] Kachnic LA, Kaufman DS, Heney NM, Althausen AF, Griffin PP, Zietman AL, et al. Bladder preservation by combined modality therapy for invasive bladder cancer. J Clin Oncol 1997;15:1022−9.

[192] Tilki D, Shariat SF, Lotan Y, Rink M, Karakiewicz PI, Schoenberg MP, et al. Lymphovascular invasion is independently associated with bladder cancer recurrence and survival in patients with final stage T1 disease and negative lymph nodes after radical cystectomy. BJU Int 2013;111:1215−21.

[193] Watts KL, Ristau BT, Yamase HT, Taylor III JA. Prognostic implications of lymph node involvement in bladder cancer: are we understaging using current methods? BJU Int 2011;108:484−92.

[194] Gospodarowicz MK, Hawkins NV, Rawlings GA, Connolly JG, Jewett MA, Thomas GM, et al. Radical radiotherapy for muscle invasive transitional cell carcinoma of the bladder: failure analysis. J Urol 1989;142:1448−53, discussion 1453-1444.

[195] Smith ZL, Christodouleas JP, Keefe SM, Malkowicz SB, Guzzo TJ. Bladder preservation in the treatment of muscle-invasive bladder cancer (MIBC): a review of the literature and a practical approach to therapy. BJU Int 2013;112:13−25.

[196] Gakis G, Efstathiou J, Lerner SP, Cookson MS, Keegan KA, Guru KA, et al. ICUD-EAU International Consultation on Bladder Cancer 2012: radical cystectomy and bladder preservation for muscle-invasive urothelial carcinoma of the bladder. Eur Urol 2013;63:45−57.

[197] Weiss C, Wittlinger M, Engehausen DG, Krause FS, Ott OJ, Dunst J, et al. Management of superficial recurrences in an irradiated bladder after combined-modality organ-preserving therapy. Int J Radiat Oncol Biol Phys 2008;70:1502−6.

[198] Herr HW. Tumour progression and survival in patients with T1G3 bladder tumours: 15-year outcome. Br J Urol 1997;80:762−5.

Chapter 31

Novel and Emerging Surveillance Markers for Bladder Cancer

Yang Hyun Cho, Seung Il Jung and Eu Chang Hwang
Chonnam National University Medical School, Gwangju, South Korea

Chapter Outline

INTRODUCTION

Bladder cancer is one of the most common malignancies of the urinary tract. It is the fourth most common cancer in men and the ninth most common cancer in women, which results in significant morbidity and mortality [1]. Approximately 70% of the patients have bladder cancers confined to the epithelium or subepithelial connective tissue, but it does not invade the muscle of the bladder and has not spread to lymph nodes at initial diagnosis. However, the recurrence rate for these tumors ranges from 50% to 70%, and 10%−15% progress to muscle invasion over a 5-year period and rarely in the upper urinary tract even after several years. Therefore, bladder cancer tends to require lifelong surveillance in many patients [2]. Diagnosis and surveillance of bladder cancer consists of cystoscopy and cytology. Current

Bladder Cancer. DOI: http://dx.doi.org/10.1016/B978-0-12-809939-1.00031-X

follow-up protocols after the initial presentation typically include flexible cystoscopy and urine cytology every 3 months for 1−3 years, every 6 months for an additional 2−3 years, and then annually, assuming no recurrence. However, both small papillary tumors and almost 33% more cases of carcinoma in situ (CIS) overlooked by cystoscopy were identified [3,4]. Urine cytology has a high sensitivity and specificity for the detection of high-grade urothelial carcinoma, but it lacks the sensitivity to detect low-grade tumors from 4% to 31% [5]. These factors necessitate the development of relatively noninvasive, cost-effective tests with equivalent or improved sensitivity and specificity compared to the current tools. The ultimate goal of these novel tests would be to aid in the risk stratification of patients and serve as prognostic indicators for individual patients. Based on the limitations of cytology, several biomarkers have been developed for diagnosis or surveillance (Table 31.1). But, numerous potential markers have been described and are under investigation, though relatively few have been validated to be clinically useful. The FDA has approved bladder tumor antigen (BTA) Stat, BTA TRAK, nuclear matrix protein (NMP22)/BladderChek, and UroVysion for diagnosis and follow-up, while ImmunoCyt/UCyt has been approved for follow-up. Other promising markers include BLCA-4, CYFRA 21-1, Survivin, UBC, and DD23. Among these, only UroVysion is a frequently used tool because it has been shown to be more sensitive than urinary cytology by detecting aneuploidy in chromosomes 3, 7, 17, and 9p21 through fluorescence in situ hybridization (FISH) analysis.

URINE MARKERS (COMMERCIALLY AVAILABLE URINE MARKERS)

Although the ideal use of a urine-based marker for the diagnosis of bladder cancer has not been determined, several tests have been approved for use by the US Food and Drug Administration (FDA). These include the BTA, the BTA Stat (Polymedco Inc., Cortlandt Manor, NY, USA), NMP22 (Matritech Inc., Newton, MA, USA), and UroVysion (Abbott Molecular/Abbott Laboratories Inc., Des Plaines, IL, USA).

BTA Stat/BTA TRAK

BTA Stat/BTA TRAK test is an in vitro immunoassay that detects the presence of human complement factor H-related protein (hCFHrp) in the urine of patients with bladder cancer [6]. BTA Stat (Polymedco Inc., Cortlandt Manor, NY, USA) is a qualitative bedside point-of-care immunochromatographic assay approved by the FDA as an adjunct to cystoscopy for monitoring bladder cancer recurrence, while BTA TRAK (Polymedco Inc., Cortlandt Manor, NY, USA) is a quantitative enzyme-linked immunosorbent assay (ELISA) assay requiring trained personnel and a reference laboratory. In a

TABLE 31.1 Characteristics of Urine-Based Bladder Tumor Marker

Test	Marker Detected	Assay Type	Testing Situation	Sensitivity[a] (%)	Specificity[a] (%)
BTA Stat	Complement factor H-related protein	Colorimetric Ag-Ab reaction	Point of care	57–83	68–72
BTA TRAK	Complement factor H	Sandwich immunoassay	Specialized laboratory	66–72	51–75
NMP22 (nuclear matrix protein)	Nuclear mitotic apparatus	Sandwich immunoassay	Specialized laboratory	47–100	60–70
UroVysion test	Aneuploidy chromosome 3, 7, and 17 and loss of 9p21 locus	Multitarget FISH	Specialized laboratory	51–92	55–95
ImmunoCyt test	Mucins, high-molecular-weight CEA	Immunofluoroscence, cytology	Specialized laboratory	55–90	33–87
CYFRA 21-2 (cytokeratins)	Detection of cytokeratins in bladder cancer	RT-PCR	Specialized laboratory	43–79.3	68–84
Telomerase	Human telomerase messenger RNA	PCR	Specialized laboratory	62–81	80–96
BLCA-1 and BLCA-4	BLCA-1 and BLCA-4 transcription factor	ELISA	Specialized laboratory	89–96	100
AURKA	Overexpression of AURKA	Multitarget FISH	Specialized laboratory	84–87	65

(Continued)

TABLE 31.1 (Continued)

Test	Marker Detected	Assay Type	Testing Situation	Sensitivity[a] (%)	Specificity[a] (%)
Survivin	Survivin antiapoptotic proteins	BioDot system	Specialized laboratory	64–100	87–93
Microsatellite detection	Highly polymorphic DNA repeats	PCR	Specialized laboratory	72–97	80–100
HA, hyaluronidase	HA, hyaluronidase	Immunoassay	Specialized laboratory	92–100	89–93
miRNAs	Detection of noncoding RNAs that posttranscriptionally regulate gene expression	RT-PCR	Specialized laboratory	71–94	51–100

[a]Vary between low-grade and high-grade urothelial carcinoma.

side-by-side comparison of tumor markers, BTA Stat was found to have a much higher sensitivity for high-grade tumors (74%) than for low-grade tumors (25%). Its specificity was 77% [7]. Sensitivity of BTA Stat ranges from 57% to 82% and its specificity ranges from 68% to 93% [8−11]. BTA TRAK has a range of sensitivity from 66% to 77% and specificity range from 50% to 75 [11−13]. These tests are more sensitive than cytology, but they can be falsely positive in patients with benign prostatic hyperplasia, hematuria, urinary tract infections, and urolithiasis, in patients taking caffeine, nicotine, acetaminophen, or acetyl salicylic acid, or in patients with hematuria [14,15]. These tests have been approved by the FDA only for monitoring bladder cancer recurrence in combination with cystoscopy.

NUCLEAR MATRIX PROTEIN 22

The NMP22 BladderChek Test is based on the detection of nuclear matrix protein 22, part of the nuclear mitotic apparatus protein that is responsible for the distribution of chromatin to daughter cells during mitosis. This protein is elevated in bladder cancer but is also released from the dead and dying urothelial cells. The NMP22 tests come as a quantitative ELISA or a quantitative point-of-care test known as BladderChek (Matritech Inc.). The sensitivity ranges from 68.5% to 88.5% and specificity from 65.2% to 91.3% [15]. Gutierrez Banos et al. and Ponsky et al. compared the sensitivity of NMP22 according to the tumor grade, and the test has lower sensitivity to detect low-grade tumors [16,17]. However, in most studies, the sensitivity of the NMP22 test for detecting intermediate- and high-grade tumors varies between 50% and 70%, and 70% and 100%, respectively. Unfortunately, false-positive results with NMP22 are common in patients with benign bladder conditions such as stones, infection, inflammation, hematuria, and cystoscopy can cause a false-positive reading. Therefore, there is a decrease in its potential as a screening biomarker for incidental bladder tumors. However, NMP22 has been approved by the FDA for both detection and monitoring of patients with known bladder cancer. A multi-institutional trial revealed that addition of the NMP22 BladderChek test to cystoscopy improves the detection rate of recurrent bladder cancer in patients with a history of bladder cancer [18].

UroVysion TEST

UroVysion (Abbott Molecular, Chicago, IL, USA) is a composite of labeled DNA probes or "labels" specific to certain chromosomal foci. Use of FISH for alterations in chromosomes 3, 7, 17, and 9p21 locus identified in a given cell has been approved by the FDA for the detection of bladder cancer using voided urine. The cells are observed under a fluorescence microscope. The criteria set for detecting bladder cancer by the UroVysion test are 4 or more cells with gains of 2 or more chromosomes, 10 or more cells with a gain of a single chromosome or 10 or more cells with tetrasomic signal patterns (i.e., 4 copies for each of the 4 probes), homozygous deletion of the 9p21 locus in 20% or more cells [19,20]. The sensitivity of UroVysion ranges from 69% to 74% and its specificity ranges from 65% to 95% [21–24]. Cumulative data from comparative studies show a sensitivity of 19% vs 58% for Grade 1, 50% vs 77% for Grade 2, and 71% vs 96% for Grade 3 for cytology compared to FISH. Similar findings occurred by stage, where the sensitivity for cytology compared to FISH was 35% vs 64% for Ta, 66% vs 83% for T1, and 76% vs 94% for muscle-invasive carcinoma [25]. Also, the test has excellent sensitivity to detect CIS and high-grade tumors (range 83%–100%). It is useful as an adjunct to cytology because it maintains the specificity but increases the sensitivity (45.8% vs 72.22%) [26,27]. Also, it is not affected by hematuria, inflammation, or other factors that can cause false-positive readings with some tumor markers, so it appears to be useful as a marker of CIS in response to bacillus Calmette–Guerin [28]. However, it is important to note that a positive UroVysion result is not specific for urothelial carcinoma. Other primary tumors of the renal pelvic system or ureteral transitional cell carcinoma, prostatic carcinoma with urethral invasion, renal cell carcinoma, or metastatic cancer involving the genitourinary tract are occasionally the cause of a positive urine FISH result. This assay is intended for detecting the tumor and it does not provide information on the tumor stage.

INVESTIGATION OF THE PROMISE OF NOVEL MOLECULAR MARKERS

ImmunoCyt Test

ImmunoCyt/UCytt (DiagnoCure Inc., Québec, Canada) has been developed by Fradet et al., and it was aimed at improving the low sensitivity of cytology [29]. The ImmunoCyt test is based on the visualization of carcinoembryonic antigen (CEA) and sulfated mucin glycoproteins on bladder cancer cells using immunofluorescent-labeled antibodies. This fluorescence test combines three monoclonal antibodies. M344 and LDQ10, labeled with fluorescein, a green fluorescence, have been raised against mucin-like antigens. M344 is expressed by 71% of Ta-T1 tumors. 19A211, labeled with Texas Red, recognizes a high molecular form of CEA and is expressed by 90% of Ta-T1 tumors [30,31]. The sensitivity of ImmunoCyt varies among studies, ranging between 60% and 100%; specificity ranges from 75% to 84%, and it is superior to conventional urine cytology and is clearly one of the most promising diagnostic markers for bladder cancer [30–35]. ImmunoCyt has been shown to be significantly affected by urinary tract infection, urolithiasis, and benign prostatic hyperplasia. The adoption of ImmunoCyt has been limited because the interpretation is complex, and it currently requires a highly trained laboratory technician [36,37]. ImmunoCyt has been approved by the FDA to aid in the management of bladder cancer in conjunction with cytology and cystoscopy.

CYTOKERATINS

Cytokeratins (CK) are differentiation intermediate filament proteins; their main function is to enable cells to withstand mechanical stress. In humans, 20 different cytokeratin isotypes have been identified. CK 8, 18, 19, and 20 have been associated with bladder cancer [38]. IDL Biotech AB (Bromma, Sweden) developed the urinary bladder cancer (UBC) test, a point-of-care qualitative assay, and the UBC ELISA, a quantitative assay that measures CK 8 and 18 in the urine [39,40]. The sensitivity of the UBC test varies from 35% to 79% and depends on the tumor grade and stage, but UBC tests were inferior to voided cytology in test quality [20,41]. For CIS, UBC had a higher sensitivity (100%) compared with cytology (67%) and BTA (0%). The overall performance of the UBC test is not superior to cytology or other current biomarkers [42].

TELOMERASE

Telomeres are repetitive sequences at the end of the chromosomes that protect genetic stability during DNA replication. There is loss of telomeres during each cell division, which causes chromosomal instability and cellular senescence. Bladder cancer cells express telomerase, an enzyme that regenerates telomeres at the end of each DNA replication and therefore sets the cellular clock to immortality. Determination of telomerase activity requires a PCR-based technology, and it must be performed in specialized laboratories. Overall, sensitivity and specificity of the telomerase assay, as reported by Lokeshwar et al., were between 70% and 100% and 60% and 70%, respectively [20]. A systematic review showed that telomerase had the best sensitivity (75%) compared with the other markers, including cytology. However, the specificity of telomeres was lower than that of cytology [43].

BLCA-1 AND BLCA-4

BLCA-1 and BLCA-4 are nuclear transcription factors present in bladder cancer. BLCA-1 is not expressed in nonmalignant urothelium [44], whereas BLCA-4 is expressed in both the tumor and adjacent benign areas of the bladder but not in nonmalignant bladders [45]. BLCA-4 is measured in the urine using an ELISA; its reported sensitivity is between 89% and 96.4%, and specificity is between 95% and 100% [45,46]. BLCA-4 seems to be a promising marker for bladder cancer, with a high sensitivity and specificity, but a larger trial is needed to confirm this observation.

AURORA KINASE A

The Aurora kinase A (AURKA) gene encodes a serine/threonine kinase associated with aneuploidy and chromosomal instability. This gene has been explored in urine sediment by FISH. A training set was used to establish test conditions. In a case–control study, involving bladder cancer, normal individuals, and patients with benign conditions, they reported 96.6% specificity and 87% sensitivity for AURKA-FISH test to detect bladder cancer. The AURKA-FISH assay was more effective than cytology in detecting bladder cancer, and this marker holds promise for the future [47].

SURVIVIN

Survivin is a novel member of the inhibitor-of-apoptosis gene family. Survivin mRNA is overexpressed in human cancers and can be detected in urine using a bio-dot immunoassay incorporating a rabbit polyclonal anti-Survivin antibody. Horstmann et al. showed that Survivin is a reliable biomarker for high-grade urothelial bladder cancer (sensitivity 83%) but not for low-grade (sensitivity 35%) urothelial bladder cancer with a high specificity (88%) [48]. Although the results are promising, the lack of assay standardization and cut-off value has to be resolved before clinical use [49].

MICROSATELLITE DETECTION

Microsatellites are polymorphic repeating units of 1–6 base pairs in length, found in human DNA. Microsatellites can be amplified for identification by PCR and can be used as molecular markers. Microsatellite analysis (MSA) is a PCR analysis of DNA in exfoliated urine cells. One of the most common genetic changes in bladder cancer is loss of heterogeneity in chromosome 9 [50]. Chromosomes 4p, 8p, 9p, 11p, and 17p also often display loss of heterogeneity in patients with bladder cancer. The overall sensitivity from these studies ranged from 72% to 97%, and the overall specificity ranged from 80% to 100% [51,52]. Despite early promising results in the detection of recurrence or progression of bladder cancer, the MSA markers need to be standardized for this clinical setting.

HYALURONIC ACID AND HYALURONIDASE

Hyaluronidase (HAase), an endoglycosidase, degrades hyaluronic acid (HA) into small fragments that promote angiogenesis [53]. Urine HA, a non-sulfated glycosaminoglycan, has been shown to yield 92% sensitivity and 93% specificity for bladder cancer detection [54]. Further refinement of the assay and evaluation in larger clinical trials would help define the clinical applicability of this marker.

MicroRNAs

MicroRNAs (miRNAs) are small, non-protein-coding RNAs that function as negative gene regulators controlling hundreds of gene targets. Neely et al. studied miRNAs in bladder tumors and identified a miR-21:miR-205 expression ratio that has the ability to distinguish between invasive and noninvasive bladder tumors with the potential to identify superficial lesions at high risk for progression [55]. Recently, urinary miRNA expression was reported and the upregulation of miRs-126/182/199a was found to discriminate bladder cancer patients from disease-free controls, and it was observed that the ratio of miRNA-126:miRNA-152 has 72% sensitivity and 82% specificity to detect bladder cancer [56]. Larger clinical trials are necessary to further define these markers.

CARCINOEMBRYONIC ANTIGEN—RELATED CELL ADHESION MOLECULE 1

Bladder tumor growth and progression depend on angiogenesis. Human carcinoembryonic antigen—related cell adhesion molecule (CEACAM)1 is a cell adhesion molecule with proangiogenic activity. CEACAM1 is ubiquitously expressed in the luminal surface of normal bladder urothelium and downregulated in bladder cancer cells, whereas it is concurrently upregulated in endothelial cells of adjacent blood vessels. CEACAM1 was detectable in urine and its levels could help differentiate bladder cancer patients from healthy subjects. Higher urinary levels of CEACAM1 were associated with bladder cancer presence and advanced stage. Within bladder cancer patients, higher CEACAM1 levels were associated with invasive tumor stage [57]. Many studies are needed to determine the potential role of urinary CEACAM1 in the management of patients who are at risk for bladder cancer.

EPIGENETIC URINARY MARKERS

Analysis of gene methylation has been shown to be feasible from voided urine. In urine, hypermethylation of DAPK, RARbeta, E-cadherin, and p16 has been shown to have a high sensitivity and specificity for bladder cancer detection. Renard et al. initially unveiled candidate methylated genes using DNA extracted from noncancerous and bladder cancer tissue and subsequently analyzed the genes of interest in urine. They identified WIST1 and NID2 to be frequently methylated in urine samples collected from bladder cancer patients with sensitivity and specificity of a two-gene panel >90% [58,59]. More studies are necessary to validate these findings.

FIBROBLAST GROWTH FACTOR RECEPTOR 3 MUTATIONS

Mutations in the fibroblast growth factor receptor (FGFR) 3 occur in 50% of primary bladder tumors and might be associated with good prognosis and especially prevalent in low-grade/stage tumors, with pTa tumors harboring mutations in 85% of the cases [60]. Zuiverloon et al. evaluated FGFR3 mutation in voided urine to detect recurrences during surveillance in patients with low-grade non-muscle-invasive bladder cancer (NMIBC) with an FGFR3-mutant tumor, and sensitivity (58%) of the assay for detection of recurrences was higher than urinary cytology only but still far from perfect [61].

CONCLUSION

Early diagnosis of bladder cancer and careful follow-up for detection of recurrences after initial treatment are main tasks of current urological research. The high rate of recurrences and the prolonged follow-up by cystoscopy and cytology make bladder cancer the most expensive cancer to treat overall. However, by utilizing noninvasive urinary markers, it may be possible to improve the diagnosis of new cancers as well as to improve the management of NMIBC. NMP22, UroVysion, and ImmunoCyt are well-examined urinary markers. NMP22 and UroVysion are both FDA-approved tests for the initial diagnosis of bladder cancer in patients with a suspicion of bladder cancer and for surveillance of bladder cancer. However, ImmunoCyt is only approved for the surveillance of bladder cancer in conjunction with urinary cytology and cystoscopy. Detecting bladder cancer using diagnostic or surveillance markers remains a challenge, as none of the currently approved markers can replace cystoscopy or prolong the time between cystoscopies. For most of the investigated urine markers, equal or higher sensitivities for bladder cancer detection have been reported than for cytology, certainly for low-grade disease. None of these tests, however, meet the criteria of an ideal urine marker and thus can facilitate reliable bladder cancer detection. If fully tested and optimized, multiplex diagnostic assays may enter the clinical setting to augment, or eventually even replace, cystoscopy and/or cytology for diagnosis and recurrence monitoring. With more research, the role for bladder cancer markers will be further defined. Until then, cystoscopy and urinary cytology still represent the gold standard for diagnosis of bladder cancer.

REFERENCES

[1] Jemal A, Siegel R, Xu J, Ward E. Cancer statistics, 2010. CA Cancer J Clin 2010;60:227–300.

[2] Witjes JA, Hendricksen K. Intravesical pharmacotherapy for non–muscle-invasive bladder cancer: a critical analysis of currently available drugs, treatment schedules, and long-term results. Eur Urol 2008;53:45–52.

[3] Schmidbauer J, Witjes F, Schmeller N, Donat R, Susani M, Marberger M, et al. Improved detection of urothelial carcinoma in situ with hexaminolevulinate fluorescence cystoscopy. J Urol 2004;171:135–8.

[4] Jichlinski P, Guillou L, Karlsen SJ, Malmström PU, Jocham D, Brennhovd B, et al. Hexyl aminolevulinate fluorescence cystoscopy: new diagnostic tool for photodiagnosis of super-ficial bladder cancer—a multicenter study. J Urol 2003;170:226–9.

[5] Lotan Y, Roehrborn CG. Sensitivity and specificity of commonly available bladder tumor markers versus cytology: results of a comprehensive literature review and meta-analyses. Urology 2003;61:109–18.

[6] Kinders R, Jones T, Root R, Bruce C, Murchison H, Corey M, et al. Complement factor H or a related protein is a marker for transitional cell cancer of the bladder. Clin Cancer Res 1998;4:2511–20.

[7] Lokeshwar VB, Schroeder GL, Selzer MG, Hautmann SH, Posey JT, Duncan RC, et al. Bladder tumor markers for monitoring recurrence and screening comparison of hyaluronic acid-hyaluronidase and BTA-Stat tests. Cancer 2002;95:61–72.

[8] Wiener HG, Mian C, Haitel A, Pycha A, Schatzl G, Marberger M. Can urine bound diagnos-tic tests replace cystoscopy in the management of bladder cancer? J Urol 1998;159:1876–80.

[9] Sarosdy MF, Hudson MA, Ellis WJ, Soloway MS, deVere White R, Sheinfeld J, et al. Improved detection of recurrent bladder cancer using the bard BTA Stat test. Urology 1997;50:349–53.

[10] Heicappell R, Muller M, Fimmers R, Miller K. Qualitative determination of urinary human complement factor H-related protein (hcfHrp) in patients with bladder cancer, healthy controls, and patients with benign urologic disease. Urol Int 2000;65(4):181–4.

[11] Pode D, Shapiro A, Wald M, Nativ O, Laufer M, Kaver I. Noninvasive detection of blad-der cancer with the BTA Stat test. J Urol 1999;161:443–6.

[12] Ellis WJ, Blumenstein BA, Ishak LM, Enfield DL. Clinical evaluation of the BTA TRAK assay and comparison to voided urine cytology and the Bard BTA test in patients with recurrent bladder tumors. Urology 1997;50(6):882–7.

[13] Thomas L, Leyh H, Marberger M, Bombardieri E, Bassi P, Pagano F, et al. Multicenter trial of the quantitative BTA TRAK assay in the detection of bladder cancer. Clin Chem 1999;45:472–7.

[14] Irani J, Desgrandchamps F, Millet C, Toubert ME, Bon D, Aubert J, et al. BTA Stat and BTA TRAK: a comparative evaluation of urine testing for the diagnosis of transitional cell carcinoma of the bladder. Eur Urol 1999;35:89–92.

[15] Liou LS. Urothelial cancer biomarkers for detection and surveillance. Urology 2006;67:25–33.

[16] Gutiérrez Baños JL, del Henar Rebollo Rodrigo M, Antolín Juárez FM, García BM. Usefulness of the BTA STAT test for the diagnosis of bladder cancer. Urology 2001;57:685–9.

[17] Ponsky LE, Sharma S, Pandrangi L, Kedia S, Nelson D, Agarwal A, et al. Screening and monitoring for bladder cancer: refining the use of NMP22. J Urol 2001;166:75–8.

[18] Grossman HB, Soloway M, Messing E, Katz G, Stein B, Kassabian V, et al. Surveillance for recurrent bladder cancer using a point-of-care proteomic assay. JAMA 2006; 295:299–305.

[19] Lokeshwar VB, Civantos F. Tumor markers: current status. In: Droller MJ, editor. American Cancer Society Atlas of Clinical Oncology: bladder cancer. Hamilton, ON, Canada: BC Decker Inc.; 2004. p. 160–205.

[20] Lokeshwar VB, Habuchi T, Grossman B. Bladder tumor markers beyond cytology: International consensus on bladder tumor markers. Urology 2005;66:35–63.

[21] Yoder BJ, Skacel M, Hedgepeth R, Babineau D, Ulchaker JC, Liou LS, et al. Reflex UroVysion testing of bladder cancer surveillance patients with equivocal or negative urine cytology: a prospective study with focus on the natural history of anticipatory positive findings. Am J Clin Pathol 2007;127:295–301.

[22] Sarosdy MF, Schellhammer P, Bokinsky G, Kahn P, Chao R, Yore L, et al. Clinical evaluation of a multi-target fluorescent in situ hybridization assay for detection of bladder cancer. J Urol 2002;168:1950–4.

[23] Friedrich MG, Toma AH, Pantel K, Weisenberger DJ, Noldus J, Huland H. Comparison of multitarget fluorescence in situ hybridization in urine with other noninvasive tests for detecting bladder cancer. BJU Int 2003;92:911–14.

[24] Laudadio J, Keane TE, Reeves HM, Savage SJ, Hoda RS, Lage JM, et al. Fluorescence in situ hybridization for detecting transitional cell carcinoma: implications for clinical practice. BJU Int 2005;96:1280–5.

[25] Jones JS, Patel A, Angie M, Kitay R, Sanders S. Office cystoscopy more tolerated with patient visualized real-time video monitoring. Abstract#: 94765, Presented at the AUA Annual Meeting, Atlanta, GA, May 20 2006.

[26] Halling KC, King W, Sokolova IA, Meyer RG, Burkhardt HM, Halling AC, et al. A comparison of cytology and fluorescence in situ hybridization for the detection of urothelial carcinoma. J Urol 2000;164:1768–75.

[27] Sokolova IA, Halling KC, Jenkins RB, Burkhardt HM, Meyer RG, Seelig SA, et al. The development of a multitarget, multicolor fluorescence in situ hybridization assay for the detection of urothelial carcinoma in urine. J Mol Diagn 2000;2:116–23.

[28] Highsaw RA, Tanaka ST, Evans CP, deVere White RW. Is bladder biopsy necessary at three or six months post BCG therapy? Urol Oncol 2003;21:207–9.

[29] Fradet Y, Lockhart C. The Immunocyt trialists. Performance characteristics of a new monoclonal antibody test for bladder cancer: ImmunoCyt. Can J Urol 1997;4:400–5.

[30] Mian C, Pycha A, Wiener H, Haitel A, Lodde M, Marberger M. Immunocyt: a new tool for detecting transitional cell cancer of the urinary tract. J Urol 1999;161:1486–9.

[31] Allard P, Fradet Y, Têtu B, Bernard P. Tumor-associated antigens as prognostic factors for recurrence in 382 patients with primary transitional cell carcinoma of the bladder. Clin Cancer Res 1995;1:1195–202.

[32] Lodde M, Mian C, Negri G, Berner L, Maffei N, Lusuardi L, et al. Role of uCyt+ in the detection and surveillance of urothelial carcinoma. Urology 2003;61:243–7.

[33] Pfister C, Chautard D, Devonec M, Perrin P, Chopin D, Rischmann P, et al. Immunocyt test improves the diagnostic accuracy of urinary cytology: results of a French multicenter study. J Urol 2003;169:921–4.

[34] Hautmann S, Toma M, Lorenzo Gomez MF, Friedrich MG, Jaekel T, Michl U, et al. Immunocyt and the HA-HAase urine tests for the detection of bladder cancer: a side-by-side comparison. Eur Urol 2004;46:466–71.

[35] Messing EM, Teot L, Korman H, Underhill E, Barker E, Stork B, et al. Performance of urine test in patients monitored for recurrence of bladder cancer: a multicenter study in the United States. J Urol 2005;174:1238–41.

[36] Têtu B, Tiguert R, Harel F, Fradet Y. ImmunoCyt/uCyt+ improves the sensitivity of urine cytology in patients followed for urothelial carcinoma. Mod Pathol 2005;18:83–9.

[37] Toma MI, Friedrich MG, Hautmann SH, Jäkel KT, Erbersdobler A, Hellstern A, et al. Comparison of the ImmunoCyt test and urinary cytology with other urine tests in the detection and surveillance of bladder cancer. World J Urol 2004;22:145–9.

[38] Southgate J, Harnden P, Trejdosiewicz LK. Cytokeratin expression patterns in normal and malignant urothelium: a review of the biological and diagnostic implications. Histol Histopathol 1999;14:657–64.

[39] Heicappell R, Schostak M, Muller M, Miller K. Evaluation of urinary bladder cancer antigen as a marker for diagnosis of transitional cell carcinoma of the urinary bladder. Scand J Clin Lab Invest 2000;60:275–82.

[40] Mian C, Lodde M, Haitel A, Egarter Vigl E, Marberger M, Pycha A. Comparison of two qualitative assays, the UBC rapid test and the BTA stat test, in the diagnosis of urothelial cell carcinoma of the bladder. Urology 2000;56:228–31.

[41] Hakenberg O, Fuessel S, Richter K, Froehner M, Oehlschlaeger S, Rathert P, et al. Qualitative and quantitative assessment of urinary cytokeratin 8 and 18 fragments compared with voided urine cytology in diagnosis of bladder carcinoma. Urology 2004; 64:1121–6.

[42] Tilki D, Burger M, Dalbagni G, Grossman HB, Hakenberg OW, Palou J, et al. Urine markers for detection and surveillance of non-muscle-invasive bladder cancer. Eur Urol 2011;60:484–92.

[43] Glas A, Roos D, Deutekom M, Zwinderman A, Bossuyt PM, Kurth KH. Tumor markers in the diagnosis of primary bladder cancer. A systematic review. J Urol 2003;169:1975–82.

[44] Myers-Irvin JM, Landsittel D, Getzenberg RH. Use of the novel marker BLCA-1 for the detection of bladder cancer. J Urol 2005;174:64–8.

[45] Konety BR, Nguyen TS, Dhir R, Day RS, Becich MJ, Stadler WM, et al. Detection of bladder cancer using a novel nuclear matrix protein, BLCA-4. Clin Cancer Res 2000;6:2618–25.

[46] Van Le TS, Miller R, Barder T, Babjuk M, Potter DM, Getzenberg RH. Highly specific urine-based marker of bladder cancer. Urology 2005;66:1256–60.

[47] Park HS, Park WS, Bondaruk J, Tanaka N, Katayama H, Lee S, et al. Quantitation of Aurora kinase A gene copy number in urine sediments and bladder cancer detection. J Natl Cancer Inst 2008;100:1401–11.

[48] Horstmann M, Bontrup H, Hennenlotter J, Taeger D, Weber A, Pesch B, et al. Clinical experience with survivin as a biomarker for urothelial bladder cancer. World J Urol 2010;28:399–404.

[49] Shariat SF, Casella R, Khoddami SM, Hernandez G, Sulser T, Gasser TC, et al. Urine detection of survivin is a sensitive marker for the noninvasive diagnosis of bladder cancer. J Urol 2004;171:626–30.

[50] Van Rhijn BW, Lurkin I, Kirkels WJ, van der Kwast TH, Zwarthoff EC. Microsatellite analysis—DNA test in urine competes with cystoscopy in follow-up of superficial bladder carcinoma: a phase II trial. Cancer 2001;92:768–75.

[51] Czerniak B, Chaturvedi V, Li L, Hodges S, Johnston D, Roy JY, et al. Superimposed histologic and genetic mapping of chromosome 9 in progression of human urinary bladder

neoplasia: implications for a genetic model of multistep urothelial carcinogenesis and early detection of urinary bladder cancer. Oncogene 1999;18:1185−96.

[52] Knowles MA, Elder PA, Williamson M, Cairns JP, Shaw ME, Law MG. Allelotype of human bladder cancer. Cancer Res 1994;54:531−8.

[53] Lokeshwar VB, Block NL. HA-HAase urine test. A sensitive and specific method for detecting bladder cancer and evaluating its grade. Urol Clin North Am 2000;27:53−61.

[54] Lokeshwar VB, Obek C, Soloway MS, Block NL. Tumor-associated hyaluronic acid: a new sensitive and specific urine marker for bladder cancer. Cancer Res 1997;57:773−7.

[55] Neely LA, Rieger-Christ KM, Neto BS, Eroshkin A, Garver J, Patel S, et al. A microRNA expression ratio defining the invasive phenotype in bladder tumors. Urol Oncol 2010;28:39−48.

[56] Hanke M, Hoefig K, Merz H, Feller AC, Kausch I, Jocham D, et al. A robust methodology to study urine microRNA as tumor marker: microRNA-126 and microRNA-182 are related to urinary bladder cancer. Urol Oncol 2010;28:655−61.

[57] Tilki D, Singer BB, Shariat SF, Behrend A, Fernando M, Irmak S, et al. CEACAM1: a novel urinary marker for bladder cancer detection. Eur Urol 2010;57:648−54.

[58] Yu J, Zhu T, Wang Z, Zhang H, Qian Z, Xu H, et al. A novel set of DNA methylation markers in urine sediments for sensitive/specific detection of bladder cancer. Clin Cancer Res 2007;13:7296−304.

[59] Renard I, Joniau S, van Cleynenbreugel B, Collette C, Naômé C, Vlassenbroeck I, et al. Identification and validation of the methylated TWIST1 and NID2 genes through real-time methylation-specific polymerase chain reaction assays for the noninvasive detection of primary bladder cancer in urine samples. Eur Urol 2010;58:96−104.

[60] van Oers JM, Lurkin I, van Exsel AJ, Nijsen Y, van Rhijn BW, van der Aa MN, et al. A simple and fast method for the simultaneous detection of nine fibroblast growth factor receptor 3 mutations in bladder cancer and voided urine. Clin Cancer Res 2005; 11:7743−8.

[61] Zuiverloon TC, van der Aa MN, van der Kwast TH, Steyerberg EW, Lingsma HF, Bangma CH, et al. Fibroblast growth factor receptor 3 mutation analysis on voided urine for surveillance of patients with low-grade non-muscle-invasive bladder cancer. Clin Cancer Res 2010;16:3011−18.

Future Perspective in Bladder Cancer

Chapter 32

Microbiome

Malcolm Dewar[1], Jonathan Izawa[1], Fan Li[1], Ryan M. Chanyi[1,2,3], Gregor Reid[1,2,3] and Jeremy P. Burton[1,2,3]

[1]*Schulich School of Medicine & Dentistry, London, ON, Canada,* [2]*University of Western Ontario, London, ON, Canada,* [3]*Canadian Centre for Human Microbiome and Probiotics Research, London, ON, Canada*

Chapter Outline

INTRODUCTION

In the past 10–15 years, 16S rRNA gene sequencing and expanded quantitative urine culture have led to the realization that microbes are present throughout the human body, not simply in sites exposed to the outside. Correlations between health and disease states have further indicated that microbial populations are capable of influencing many conditions. The studies showing the presence of a urinary tract microbiome proximal to the urethra [1], countered the long held belief that the bladder and kidneys are normally sterile [2,3]. The precise nature and potential role of these microbes remain under investigation, but the potential that they alter the risk of cancer [4], incontinence, urinary tract infections (UTIs), and other urological conditions is now being seriously considered.

At various sites, including the intestine, vagina, and likely the urinary tract, the microbiome has been shown to be critical in the attenuation of infection and maintaining epithelial barrier function. The disruption of the microbiota leads to clinical conditions, best illustrated in the intestinal tract where the body's largest reservoir of bacteria exists and where irritable bowel disease,

Bladder Cancer. DOI: http://dx.doi.org/10.1016/B978-0-12-809939-1.00032-1

Crohn's disease, and ulcerative colitis afflict millions of people worldwide. The bacteria present and the metabolites they produce appear to act as global modulators of inflammation. In addition, the collection of bacteria in the intestinal tract, respiratory tract, and potentially urinary tract form a barrier against toxic compounds that are ingested, inhaled, or pass through the body. Probiotics are believed to act through these and other mechanisms.

Xenobiotic metabolism—the breakdown of human-intended compounds by the microbiome—is becoming an important aspect of pharmaceutical research as it has implications for how all drugs act on an individual basis. Orally administered pharmaceutical compounds are exposed to the microbiome of the oral cavity, stomach, and the gastrointestinal tract, often for an extended period of time. This interaction is often overlooked despite the fact that many bacteria are able to metabolize a diverse range of compounds, and therefore embellish or reduce their activity and absorption into the human body.

The purpose of this chapter is to examine the role the microbiome may play in the prevention, occurrence, and treatment of bladder cancer.

THE MICROBIOME AND BLADDER

The urothelium is the membrane lining the interior of almost the entire urinary tract from kidneys to proximal urethra. The vast majority of bladder tumors arise in the urothelium. In developed countries, approximately 90% of primary bladder cancer is urothelial. An estimated 70% of patients present with non-muscle-invasive tumors that can be treated with transurethral resection, with or without subsequent intravesical therapy. Fifty to seventy percent of these tumors will recur and 10%−30% progress to invasive disease. Muscle invasive bladder cancer (MIBC) is also present in approximately 30% of primary cases. The treatment of MIBC is generally radical cystectomy with urinary diversion. Because these patients are at high risk of metastatic tumor progression and cancer-related death with 5-year overall survival of approximately 50%, neoadjuvant and adjuvant chemotherapy are utilized, but only a modest survival benefit is gained [4]. Bladder tumors are associated with changes in the microenvironment in the host. Alfano et al. [5] have provided a detailed background on the tumor extracellular matrix (ECM) in urothelial bladder cancer.

Studies on the microbiome in bladder cancer, to date, have only been performed on mid-stream urine. It is therefore impossible to say whether there are any specific localized changes in the urinary microbiome in the immediate vicinity of bladder tumors. Ablation of these tumors is also likely to alter the subsequent microenvironment and microbiome. Studies are needed to identify microbes at the site of tumor origin and clarify the effect on the ECM.

Inflammatory processes have clearly been associated with local tumor proliferation [6]. Bacterial species interact differently with the host immune system, with some sustaining their growth by breaking down host components that accentuate the problem. For example, the breakdown of host epithelial surface carbohydrates can eventually lead to disrupting epithelial cell tight junctions [7]. Lizath et al. [8] recently showed that structural constituents of lipopolysaccharide can mediate multiple aspects of the uropathogenic *Escherichia coli* (UPEC) life cycle, including the ability to acutely colonize bladders, form reservoirs, and evoke innate and adaptive immune responses. Not all pathogens that cause UTI promote inflammation, for example, enterococci can persist without symptoms and signs.

The microbiome of males significantly differs from the microbiome of females, as does the prevalence of bladder cancer. In females, it consists largely of *Lactobacillus iners* and other *Lactobacillus* species, *Gardnerella vaginalis*, and other minor constituents. *Lactobacillus iners* has also been detected in men, but the microbiome is also predominated by *Corynebacterium*, *Staphylococcus*, *Sneathia*, *Gemella*, and *Aerococcus*, bacterial types that exist in the lower genital tract and skin [9–11]. A recent Japanese study indicated that there were sex differences within the epidemiological characteristics of bladder cancer, with female patients having less favorable pathology and poorer survival compared with male patients [12]. A number of confounding factors, such as work environment and tobacco use, make it difficult to ascertain from such studies the extent to which the microbiome plays a role. In addition, it is not fully clear what constitutes a deleterious microbiome from a nondeleterious or even an advantageous one, because functionality has not yet been determined. It could be the presence of a single organism like *E. coli* causing inflammation during infection or a whole consortium of bacterial types producing damaging compounds through complex metabolic networks. All of these have the potential to damage the epithelial membrane or disrupt tight junctions. Further studies are needed before epidemiological associations with bladder cancer can be ascertained in more depth.

Current analysis of the bladder microbiome relies mainly upon sampling mid-stream urine, which is representative of what is in the bladder [13], albeit this does not rule out kidney isolates. Allowances need to be made to subtract minor background noise generated by the sample passing through the lower genital tract as this has an associated microbiome itself. Even samples collected "cleanly," free of bacteria from the lower genital tract only give a simplistic view of the bladder microenvironment. Many microorganisms in the body are not planktonic but found within biofilms associated with a surface in the host [4]. Furthermore, the bacteria in the urine could have come from parts of the bladder that are cancerous and parts that are not. The tumor in its early stages will only make up a small portion of the surface of the bladder, and determining which organisms are associated with the cancer is difficult without obtaining tissue samples for microbiome analysis. Many tumors will be ablated during treatment adding to the difficulty in determining the specific tumor microbiome.

MICROORGANISMS AND CANCER

There is a well-recognized association between schistosomiasis caused by *Schistosoma haematobium*, a trematode parasite, and the occurrence of squamous cell and urothelial carcinoma of the bladder [14]. The eggs laid in the urinary system produce irritation and tissue fibrosis that contribute to the development of cancer [15]. Under the same principle, it is possible that the continuous irritation and inflammation in patients with recurrent UTI may contribute to urinary cancers [16]. One of the most recent and detailed studies examining the relationship between UTI and bladder cancer (number, location, and treatment of UTIs) was published by Vermeulen et al. in 2015 [17]. A total of 1809 urinary bladder cancer patients and 4370 controls were compared in the Nijmegen Bladder Cancer Study. Age of cystitis onset, education, smoking, antiinflammatories, and gender were all taken into account. The findings reported that recurrent cystitis was associated with an increased incidence of bladder carcinoma, and that among patients who had received antibiotics for UTI on fewer than five occasions, there was a lower incidence of bladder cancer. This is not without precedent as an association has already been made between chronic catheter use in patients with spinal cord injury and squamous cell carcinoma of the bladder, which may well be mediated by chronic inflammation [18]. The association between diagnosis of bladder cancer and a history of recurrent UTI is in agreement with the findings from several other studies where more than three episodes of cystitis were found to be associated with an increased incidence of bladder cancer [17,19]. These small studies, however, do not adequately address the large potential risk of bias, confounding, or reverse causality. This makes it difficult to draw any firm conclusions on the matter. It is further complicated by the large numbers of asymptomatic bacteriuria cases in women.

Several mechanisms have been proposed to explain the positive correlations between bladder cancer and lower UTI. During an inflammatory response, inducible nitric oxide synthase (iNOS) is activated and produces the bioactive small molecule, nitric oxide (NO). Although NO has been demonstrated to have antitumor properties, it has also been shown to be angiogenic [20]. At low levels, NO has been shown to promote tumor growth, increase tissue invasiveness, and increase its metastatic ability [21]. N-nitrosamines, which are a downstream by-product of iNOS activation, cause damage to DNA through the deamination of bases and forming DNA crosslinks. Studies using rats showed that chronic UTIs caused by *E. coli* produced increased urinary levels of N,N-dimethylnitrosamine, and over time this correlated with hyperplasia and early neoplasia of the bladder epithelium [22]. Several studies also noted the ability of commensal bacteria and probiotics to negate this effect [23−28]. In other in vitro studies, UPEC strains have been shown to induce the methylation of CDKN2A exon 1 that may increase the risk of bladder cancer risk [29]. Interestingly, the intestinal tract is often the source of *E. coli* infection, and certain *E. coli* strains, including those with UPEC virulence factors, have been shown to induce DNA damage and other angiogenic traits. Arthur and colleagues [30] identified a genotoxic island in *E. coli* NC101 that was responsible for causing neoplastic lesions in inflammation-induced $IL10^{-/-}$ mice treated with azoxymethane. While these mechanisms are not firmly established, the close proximity of the bacterial reservoir of the rectum and the female urinary tract makes it feasible that intestinal bacteria can influence bladder carcinogenesis.

In nonsmokers, bladder cancer incidence is higher in males than females [31]; therefore, incidence of UTI is not the main driving force for the disease. One possibility is that bacterial species within the female bladder microbiota are more protective against cancer. The high prevalence of *Lactobacillus* species is one such potential organism, given not only anticancer properties attributed to some strains [32−35] but also their ability to degrade or neutralize carcinogenic compounds and modulate inflammation [28,36,37].

MICROORGANISMS, CADMIUM, AND CARCINOGENS

Many carcinogens gain access into the body through the oral and nasal routes. The first line of defense against these substances is typically the intestinal tract microbiome. This provides a protective barrier against absorption of carcinogens in the distal small intestine and colon. For example, heavy metals such as lead, cadmium, mercury, and metalloid arsenic are toxic to cells; however, the amount that reaches the circulatory system is significantly less than what was originally ingested [38]. Bacteria have many mechanisms to mediate the toxic effect of these compounds. Many compounds, like heavy metals or even pesticides, are bound to the cell surface, decreasing the amount that is able to be absorbed. Even more beneficial to the host, some bacteria can metabolize toxic compounds into less harmful by-products, such as the conversion of toxic mercury(II) $[Hg^{2+}]$ to the less toxic elemental mercury $[Hg^0]$ through the mercuric reductase enzyme [39,40]. Although the intestinal microbiome is the most abundant, there are also bacteria within the lung, nasopharynx, and other mucosal surfaces. As their numbers are significantly lower than most other sites occupied by bacteria on the human host, it may not be feasible to assume similar processes occur to the same degree. Again, this may also be the case in the sparsely inhabited bladder.

Cadmium exposure has been established as a risk factor for bladder cancer [41]. Similar with many other carcinogenic chemicals, constant low exposure is associated with work place hazardous materials [42]. Long-term low-dose occupational exposure might occur even when not working directly with concentrated cadmium sources. There are many environmental risk factors associated with cadmium exposure. To some degree, it is present in most foods, especially at the higher end of the food chain. Smoking is one of the major sources of cadmium exposure (among many other carcinogenic compounds). Compared to nonsmokers, one pack-a-day smoker will have approximately double the serum concentration of cadmium [38]. Biochemical changes induced by cadmium have the potential to play a role in most stages of tumor progression, including initiation, promotion, and advancement. Firstly, through the induction of the oxidative stress response, there is decreased DNA repair capacity that can lead to genetic mutations and premalignant lesions. This is followed by aberrant gene expression resulting in cell proliferation and E-cadherin dysfunction resulting in tumor progression [42].

Microorganisms are able to ameliorate the harmful effects of many heavy metals and other toxic compounds before they are absorbed into the body. This is known to occur in the gut but it is unknown if it occurs at other sites where bacteria are found, such as the lung and the bladder. Anionic surface groups and exopolysaccharides are found on the cell surface of some Gram-positive bacteria, such as *Bacillus subtilis, Lactobacillus rhamnosus* GG, and some *Bifidobacterium longum* strains. These negative surface constituents can bind the positively charged heavy metals, preventing their absorption into the body [32,38]. As the bacteria are naturally passed through our digestive system, they are excreted as waste, along with the heavy metals bound to them. Halttunen et al. [43] showed that commonly used probiotic strains of *Lactobacillus* and *Bifidobacterium* species can bind lead and cadmium when in solution. They observed a rapid binding phenomenon across all studied species, with most cadmium being bound within 5 minutes to 1 hour after exposure. The cadmium remained strongly sequestered by the cell and did not disassociate, even after 2 days. These are supported by experimental studies from several other groups that showed probiotic *L. rhamnosus* and other bacterial types less commonly applied in food and probiotic applications such as *Propionibacterium freudenreichii* and *Enterococcus* strains could bind and absorb cadmium and lead [44,45]. Human studies in areas endemic with heavy metal exposure showed that administering probiotics prevented further increase of heavy metal absorption, although whether such intervention would have a role in the small levels of metals and occurrence of bladder cancer is speculative [40]. The mechanisms by which cadmium induces bladder cancer are not well characterized. Regardless, many organisms have this capability to bind heavy metals and there may be some potential role for bacteria within the bladder to prevent its toxicity. It is plausible that other carcinogenic agents implicated in bladder cancer, such as aromatic amines, could also be detoxified by microorganisms. This possibility certainly warrants further investigation.

XENOBIOTIC METABOLISM OF CHEMOTHERAPEUTIC AGENTS

The genetic capacity of the gut microbiome vastly exceeds the host, and this is supposedly reflected in the biochemical abilities of these microorganisms; they are able to undertake a number of activities that the host is unable to perform. Orally ingested compounds can spend a considerable amount of time in the presence of bacteria in the gastrointestinal tract. While chemotherapy is tough on the body, it is also tough on the microbiome. In a study performed in our own laboratory, milk samples were collected from a lactating woman undergoing chemotherapy for Hodgkin's lymphoma. Bacterial populations dramatically changed; there was a depletion of *Bifidobacterium*, *Eubacterium*, *Staphylococcus*, and *Cloacibacterium*, deviating from what is believed to be a healthy microbial profile [46,47]. It has been suggested that xenobiotic metabolism will be able to modify up to 40% of all drugs being developed for the market [47]. However, the bacteria and the metabolic pathways involved remain uncharacterized. Essentially, bacteria may modify, activate, or inactivate ingested compounds before the compound is able to act upon its' intended target; this has huge implications for the host. For example, the anticancer efficacy of alkylating agents (cyclophosphamide) and platinum salts (cisplatin) is reduced in germ-free mice and animals treated with antibiotics [48]. This indicates that these drugs might require the gut microbiota to achieve full therapeutic potential. Few agents used in bladder cancer have been investigated in this regard. Doxorubicin, used in bladder cancer treatment, was initially isolated from specific strains of *Streptomyces*. As is the nature of interbacterial warfare, other strains (such as Streptomyces WAC04685) are able to inactivate it via a deglycosylation mechanism. Similarly, preliminary work has shown that *Raoultella planticola* is also able to inactivate doxorubicin [49]. Although these experiments were performed in vitro, these are normal inhabitants of the microbiome and, therefore, may carry out this function in patients receiving this treatment. Thus, depending on the microbiota composition of the target site, drugs may or may not reach efficacious levels.

BCG TREATMENT AND THE MICROBIOME

Due to the rate of recurrence of high-grade urothelial bladder cancer, intravesical instillation therapy using bacillus Calmette—Guerin (BCG) is widely used to reduce recurrence and progression of higher risk non-muscle-invasive disease [50]. BCG is instilled intravesically as a therapy for carcinoma in situ and high-grade papillary lesions of the bladder several weeks after transurethral resection. While BCG is currently considered the most effective strategy for management of recurrence and possibly progression for intermediate and high-risk superficial tumors, up to 40% of patients will not respond to treatment, and nonresponders carry an even greater risk of disease progression [51]. BCG is an attenuated strain of *Mycobacterium bovis*, primarily used as a vaccine against tuberculosis caused by *Mycobacterium tuberculosis*. The use of BCG has been associated with adverse effects, including rare cases of BCG sepsis [52]. Thus, research into alternative postoperative therapies to lower the risk of recurrence of superficial bladder cancer is warranted. BCG is believed to work by stimulating the immune response through attachment of fibronectin and integrin α5β1. BCG is able to gain access into bladder cells through macropinocytosis, instead of conventional phagocytosis. Research has shown that genetic differences in the ability to upregulate the macropinocytosis pathways in tumor cells may determine the effectiveness of BCG treatment [53,54]. There may still be avenues for improvement and even personalized approaches by using the indigenous bladder microbiome or other microorganisms to stimulate a more targeted response.

As many different bacteria are able to adhere to fibronectin, it is possible that indigenous bacteria are preoccupying binding sites used by BCG. This would decrease BCG efficacy and potentially downregulate the strong cytotoxic response needed to remove cancerous cells. Dampening of immune responses by commensal bacterial strains is common at other mucosal sites [55]. Our studies with fibronectin binding indicate that urogenitally derived predominant *L. iners* may be superior to other members of the same genera [56]. Studies using gastrointestinal or food grade lactobacilli have been undertaken in models and humans [57,58]. With human bladder cancer cells, *Lactobacillus* induced antiproliferative and cytotoxic effects and was shown to be more effective than BCG [59]. *Lactobacillus* also exhibits antibladder tumor effects in animals [24,60,61] and in clinical studies, thus reducing the rate of recurrence [60,62−64].

USE OF PROBIOTICS IN THE TREATMENT AND PREVENTION OF BLADDER CANCER

Probiotics may help in cancer patients' lives as an antidiarrheal support adjunct to medicines that may cause diarrhea [12]. Although it seems unfeasible, probiotics may also provide some benefit in the treatment of bladder cancer. In studies where participants consumed fermented milk products and probiotics, a reduction in bladder cancer incidence and recurrence was observed [65,66]. *Lactobacillus* is nonpathogenic lactic acid−producing bacterial species living in the digestive, urinary, and genital systems. They have been increasingly used in fermented foods and as supplemental probiotics found in many products, such as yogurt. Supplementing patients with lactobacilli has been shown to induce improvements of inflammatory disorders such as arthritis, Type I diabetes, inflammatory bowel disease, allergic rhinitis, and importantly here, urogenital infections [67].

Several studies first commencing in Japan in the 1980s used *Lactobacillus* [*casei*] Shirota strain in animal studies of bladder cancer [57,59,61,66,68−75]. The immune potentiating effect of Biolactis powder (BLP) was assessed in tumor-bearing BALB/c mice, and its inhibitory effect on N-butyl-N-(4-hydroxybutyl) nitrosamine-induced bladder carcinogenesis was assessed in male Wistar rats and C3H/He mice. BLP reduced the growth of secondary tumors and augmented proliferation and cytokine production by splenocytes. It also significantly inhibited bladder tumor formation in rats and mice, and the tumors developing in BLP-treated animals showed a lower grade of malignancy [24,25,36]. These studies were continued in humans using oral *L. casei* preparations to reduce the recurrence of superficial bladder cancer [57]. Unfortunately, due to the high discontinuation rates and open study design, the reliability and reproducibility of the data remain uncertain [57].

When taken together, it is compelling that *Lactobacillus* spp. may provide some beneficial role in the treatment, and possibly the prevention, of bladder cancer. Further investigation seems warranted. A thorough characterization of *Lactobacillus* activity beyond its clinical efficiency, in combination with monitoring host response to these species, will lead to a better understanding of its contribution as a bladder cancer probiotic and may reveal novel functions. While the mechanistic action of lactobacilli against cancer remains to be elucidated, reducing the generation and excretion of carcinogenic metabolites [76,77], modulating host immune responses by augmenting macrophage, T cell, and NK function [78−80], downregulating severe inflammation [81], and nonimmunologically mediated cytotoxicity [82] are possible routes. Despite that many studies have shown promising results for probiotic use, the dosing regimen (dose, time of exposure, etc.) is critical, as illustrated with *L. rhamnosus* GG in the activation of dendritic cells and neutrophils [83]. Therefore, we may be underestimating the true potential of these probiotics and how they can help to better patient lives.

CONCLUSIONS

The microbiome likely impacts bladder cancer at many different stages of its development and treatment. Until now, the potential to affect the bladder microenvironment through the use of probiotics has been limited, because of the difficulties of instilling strains directly into the bladder. However, subtle changes in the microenvironment may not require such an invasive procedure, and potentially seeding the bladder via oral intake of probiotics then ascension from the rectum and urethra, or modulation through metabolites excreted in urine from the gut microbiome, may work.

Bacteria provide the first line of defense against insults from pathogens, carcinogens, and other toxins. They can metabolize chemotherapeutic agents and manipulate how the host responds, and because of this we are likely to see significant investment in research of this area by pharmaceutical and other industries. Medicine is advancing to more personalized approaches and the rapidly emerging ability to determine then alter, the microbiome of the urinary tract has great appeal. The extent to which this truly influences bladder and other urinary cancers remains to be seen, but the next 10 years should see exciting developments in this field.

REFERENCES

[1] Thomas-White K, Brady M, Wolfe A, Mueller E. The bladder is not sterile: history and current discoveries on the urinary microbiome. Curr Bladder Dysfunct Rep 2016;18−24.

[2] Hilt E, McKinley K, Pearce M, Rosenfeld A, Zilliox M, Mueller E, et al. Urine is not sterile: use of enhanced urine culture techniques to detect resident bacterial flora in the adult female bladder. J Clin Microbiol 2014;52(3):871−6.

[3] Wolfe A, Brubaker L. "Sterile urine" and the presence of bacteria. Eur Urol 2015;68 (2):173−4.

[4] Witjes A, Lebret T, Compérat E, Cowan N, Santis M, Bruins H, et al. Updated 2016 EAU guidelines on muscle-invasive and metastatic bladder cancer. Eur Urol 2017;71 (3):462−75.

[5] Alfano M, Canducci F, Nebuloni M, Clementi M, Montorsi F, Salonia A. The interplay of extracellular matrix and microbiome in urothelial bladder cancer. Nat Rev Urol 2016;13 (2):77−90.

[6] Michaud D. Chronic inflammation and bladder cancer. Urol Oncol 2007;25(3):260−8.

[7] Wood MW, Breitschwerdt EB, Nordone SK, Linder KE, Gookin JL. Uropathogenic *E. coli* promote a paracellular urothelial barrier defect characterized by altered tight junction integrity, epithelial cell sloughing and cytokine release. J Comp Pathol 2012;147 (1):11−19.

[8] Aguiniga LM, Yaggie RE, Schaeffer AJ, Klumpp DJ. Lipopolysaccharide domains modulate urovirulence. Infect Immun 2016;84(11):3131−40.

[9] Thomas-White KJ, Kliethermes S, Rickey L, Lukacz ES, Richter HE, Moalli P, et al. Evaluation of the urinary microbiota of women with uncomplicated stress urinary incontinence. Am J Obstet Gynecol 2017;216(1):55.e1−55.e16.

[10] Nelson DE, Van Der Pol B, Dong Q, Revanna KV, Fan B, Easwaran S, et al. Characteristic male urine microbiomes associate with asymptomatic sexually transmitted infection. PLoS One 2010;5(11):e14116.

[11] Nelson DE, Dong Q, Van der Pol B, Toh E, Fan B, Katz BP, et al. Bacterial communities of the coronal sulcus and distal urethra of adolescent males. PloS one 2012;7(5):e36298.

[12] Zaitsu M, Toyokawa S, Tonooka A, Nakamura F, Takeuchi T, Homma Y, et al. Sex differences in bladder cancer pathology and survival: analysis of a population-based cancer registry. Cancer Med 2014;363−70.

[13] Brubaker L, Wolfe A. The urinary microbiota: a paradigm shift for bladder disorders? Curr Opin Obstet Gynecol 2016;28(5):407−12.

[14] Mostafa MH, Sheweita SA, O'Connor PJ. Relationship between schistosomiasis and bladder cancer. Clin Microbiol Rev 1999;12(1):97−111.

[15] Urquhart AL. Cyst formation in the ureter, associated with bilharziasis. Br J Urol 1931;3 (1):21–5.

[16] Kantor AF, Hartge P, Hoover RN, Narayana AS, Sullivan JW, Fraumeni JF. Urinary tract infection and risk of bladder cancer. Am J Epidemiol 1984;510–15.

[17] Vermeulen SH, Hanum N, Grotenhuis AJ, Castaño-Vinyals G, van der Heijden AG, Aben KK, et al. Recurrent urinary tract infection and risk of bladder cancer in the Nijmegen bladder cancer study. Br J Cancer 2015;112(3):594–600.

[18] Hess MJ, Zhan EH, Foo DK, Yalla SV. Bladder cancer in patients with spinal cord injury. J Spinal Cord Med 2003;26(4):335–8.

[19] La Vecchia C, Negri E, D'Avanzo B, Savoldelli R, Franceschi S. Genital and urinary tract diseases and bladder cancer. Cancer Res 1991;51(2):629–31.

[20] Hibbs JB, Taintor RR, Vavrin Z. Macrophage cytotoxicity: role for L-arginine deiminase and amino nitrogen oxidation to nitrite. Science 1987;235(4787):473–6.

[21] Jenkins DC, Charles IG, Thomsen LL, Moss DW, Holmes LS, Baylis SA, et al. Roles of nitric oxide in tumor growth. Proc Natl Acad Sci USA 1995;92(10):4392–6.

[22] Davis CP, Cohen MS, Hackett RL, Anderson MD, Warren MM. Urothelial hyperplasia and neoplasia. III. Detection of nitrosamine production with different bacterial genera in chronic urinary tract infections of rats. J Urol 1991;145(4):875–80.

[23] Tomita K, Akaza H, Nomoto K, Yokokura T, Matsushima H, Homma Y, et al. Influence of *Lactobacillus casei* on rat bladder carcinogenesis. Jpn J Urol 1994;655–63.

[24] Sakamoto S, Akaza H. Prophylactic effect of a *Lactobacillus casei* preparation on the recurrence of bladder cancer. Japan: Springer; 1997. p. 371–4.

[25] Haza A, Zabala A, Morales P. Protective effect and cytokine production of a *Lactobacillus plantarum* strain isolated from ewes' milk cheese. Int Dairy J 2004; 14:29–38.

[26] Kailasapathy K, Chin J. Survival and therapeutic potential of probiotic organisms with reference to *Lactobacillus acidophilus* and *Bifidobacterium* spp. Immunol Cell Biol 2000;80–8.

[27] Haza A, Zabala A, Arranz N, García A, Morales P. The inhibition of the viability of myeloma cells and the production of cytokine by two strains of *Lactobacillus sakei* from meat. Int J Food Sci Technol 2005;437–49.

[28] Nowak A, Kuberski S, Libudzisz Z. Probiotic lactic acid bacteria detoxify N-nitrosodimethylamine. Food Addit Contam Part A Chem Anal Control Expo Risk Assess 2014;31(10):1678–87.

[29] Tolg C, Sabha N, Cortese R, Panchal T, Ahsan A, Soliman A, et al. Uropathogenic E. coli infection provokes epigenetic downregulation of CDKN2A (p16INK4A) in uroepithelial cells. Lab Invest 2011;825–36.

[30] Arthur J, Perez-Chanona E, Mühlbauer M, Tomkovich S, Uronis J, Fan T-J, et al. Intestinal inflammation targets cancer-inducing activity of the microbiota. Science 2012;338(6103):p.120–3.

[31] Freedman N, Silverman D, Hollenbeck A, Schatzkin A, Abnet C. Association between smoking and risk of bladder cancer among men and women. J Am Med Assoc 2011;306 (7):737.

[32] McGroarty JA, Hawthorn LA, Reid G. Anti-tumour activity of lactobacilli in vitro. Microbios letters. Microb Lett 1988;39(155–156):105–12.

[33] Burns AJ, Rowland IR. Anti-carcinogenicity of probiotics and prebiotics. Curr Issues Intest Microbiol 2000;1(1):13–24.

[34] Perisić Z, Perisić N, Golocorbin Kon S, Vesović D, Jovanović AM, Mikov M. The influence of probiotics on the cervical malignancy diagnostics quality. Vojnosanit Pregl 2011;68(11):956−60.

[35] Tiptiri-Kourpeti A, Spyridopoulou K, Santarmaki V, Aindelis G, Tompoulidou E. *Lactobacillus casei* exerts anti-proliferative effects accompanied by apoptotic cell death and up-regulation of TRAIL in colon carcinoma cells. PLoS One 2016;11(2):e0147960.

[36] Akaza H. New strategy of bio-chemoprevention on recurrence of superficial bladder cancer based on a hypothesis of the mechanism of recurrence. Gan To Kagaku Ryoho 1997;24(Suppl 1):253−6.

[37] Fei Y, Liu D, Luo T, Chen G, Wu H, Li L, et al. Molecular characterization of *Lactobacillus plantarum* DMDL 9010, a strain with efficient nitrite degradation capacity. PLoS One 2014;9(11):e113792.

[38] Monachese M, Burton JP, Reid G. Bioremediation and tolerance of humans to heavy metals through microbial processes: a potential role for probiotics? Appl Environ Microbiol 2012;78(18):6397−404.

[39] Trinder M, Bisanz JE, Burton JP, Reid G. Probiotic lactobacilli: a potential prophylactic treatment for reducing pesticide absorption in humans and wildlife. Benef Microbes 2015;6(6):841−7.

[40] Bisanz JE, Enos MK, Mwanga JR, Changalucha J, Burton JP, Gloor GB, et al. Randomized open-label pilot study of the influence of probiotics and the gut microbiome on toxic metal levels in Tanzanian pregnant women and school children. mBio 2014;5(5): e01580−14.

[41] Kellen E, Zeegers MP, Den Hond E, Buntinx F. Blood cadmium may be associated with bladder carcinogenesis: the Belgian case−control study on bladder cancer. Cancer Detect Prev 2007;31(1):77−82.

[42] Huff J, Lunn RM, Waalkes MP, Tomatis L, Infante PF. Cadmium-induced cancers in animals and in humans. Int J Occup Environ Health 2007;13(2):202−12.

[43] Halttunen T, Salminen S, Tahvonen R. Rapid removal of lead and cadmium from water by specific lactic acid bacteria. Int J Food Microbiol 2007;114(1):30−5.

[44] Ibrahim F, Halttunen T, Tahvonen R, Salminen S. Probiotic bacteria as potential detoxification tools: assessing their heavy metal binding isotherms. Can J Microbiol 2006;52 (9):877−85.

[45] Topcu A, Bulat T. Removal of cadmium and lead from aqueous solution by Enterococcus faecium strains. J Food Sci 2010;75(1):T13−17.

[46] Urbaniak C, McMillan A, Angelini M, Gloor G, Sumarah M, Burton J, et al. Effect of chemotherapy on the microbiota and metabolome of human milk, a case report. Microbiome 2014;1−11.

[47] Taguer M, Maurice CF. The complex interplay of diet, xenobiotics, and microbial metabolism in the gut: Implications for clinical outcomes. Clin Pharmacol Ther 2016;588−99.

[48] Viaud S, Daillère R, Boneca IG, Lepage P, Langella P, Chamaillard M, et al. Gut microbiome and anticancer immune response: really hot Sh*t! Cell Death Differ 2015;199−214.

[49] Yan A. Identifying drug-microbiome interactions: the inactivation of doxorubicin by the gut bacterium *Raoultella planticola*. MSc Thesis MacMaster University, Canada 2015.

[50] Sylvester R, Meijden A, Lamm D. Intravesical Bacillus Calmette-Guerin reduces the risk of progression in patients with superficial bladder cancer: a meta-analysis of the published results of randomized clinical trials. J Urol 2002;168(5):1964−70.

[51]   Fahmy N, Lazo-Langner A, Iansavichene AE, Pautler SE. Effect of anticoagulants and antiplatelet agents on the efficacy of intravesical BCG treatment of bladder cancer: a systematic review. Can Urol Assoc J 2013;7(11−12):E740−9.

[52]   Lamm DL. Efficacy and safety of bacille Calmette-Guérin immunotherapy in superficial bladder cancer. Clin Infect Dis 2000;31(Suppl 3):S86−90.

[53]   Redelman-Sidi G, Iyer G, Solit D, Glickman M. Oncogenic activation of Pak1-dependent pathway of macropinocytosis determines BCG entry into bladder cancer cells. Cancer Res 2013;73(3):1156−67.

[54]   Redelman-Sidi G, Glickman M, Bochner B. The mechanism of action of BCG therapy for bladder cancer—a current perspective. Nat Rev Urol 2014;11(3):153−62.

[55]   Cosseau C, Devine D, Dullaghan E, Gardy J, Chikatamarla A, Gellatly S, et al. The commensal *Streptococcus salivarius* K12 downregulates the innate immune responses of human epithelial cells and promotes host-microbe homeostasis. Infect Immun 2008;76 (9):4163−75.

[56]   McMillan A, Macklaim J, Burton J, Reid G. Adhesion of *Lactobacillus iners* AB-1 to human fibronectin a key mediator for persistence in the vagina?. Reprod Sci 2013;20 (7):791−6.

[57]   O'Donnell M. Does the probiotic *L. casei* help prevent recurrence after transurethral resection for superficial bladder cancer?. Nat Clin Pract Urol 2008;5(10):526−7.

[58]   Naito S. Comment on "Does the probiotic *L. casei* help prevent recurrence after transurethral resection for superficial bladder cancer?" Nat Clin Pract Urol 2009;6(3):E5.

[59]   Seow S, Rahmat J, Mohamed A, Mahendran R, Lee Y, Boon H. *Lactobacillus* species is more cytotoxic to human bladder cancer cells than *Mycobacterium bovis* (bacillus Calmette-Guerin). J Urol 2002;2236−9.

[60]   Asano M, Karasawa E, Takayama T. Antitumor activity of *Lactobacillus casei* (LC 9018) against experimental mouse bladder tumor (MBT-2). J Urol 1986;136(3):719−21.

[61]   Takahashi T, Kushiro A, Nomoto K, Uchida K, Morotomi M, Yokokura T, et al. Antitumor effects of the intravesical instillation of heat killed cells of the *Lactobacillus casei* strain Shirota on the murine orthotopic bladder tumor MBT-2. J Urol 2002;166 (6):2506−11.

[62]   Aso Y, Akazan H. Prophylactic effect of a *Lactobacillus casei* preparation on the recurrence of superficial bladder cancer. BLP study group. Urol Int 1992;49(3):125−9.

[63]   Aso Y, Akaza H, Kotake T, Tsukamoto T, Imai K, Naito S. Preventive effect of a *Lactobacillus casei* preparation on the recurrence of superficial bladder cancer in a double-blind trial. The BLP study group. Eur Urol 1995;27(2):104−9.

[64]   Naito S, Koga H, Yamaguchi A, Fujimoto N, Hasui Y, Kuramoto H, et al. Prevention of recurrence with epirubicin and *Lactobacillus casei* after transurethral resection of bladder cancer. J Urol 2008;179(2):485−90.

[65]   Larsson SC, Andersson S-OO, Johansson J-EE, Wolk A. Cultured milk, yogurt, and dairy intake in relation to bladder cancer risk in a prospective study of Swedish women and men. Am J Clin Nutr 2008;88(4):1083−7.

[66]   Ohashi Y, Nakai S, Tsukamoto T, Masumori N, Akaza H, Miyanaga N, et al. Habitual intake of lactic acid bacteria and risk reduction of bladder cancer. Urol Int 2002;68 (4):273−80.

[67]   Reid G. Probiotic Lactobacilli for urogenital health in women. J Clin Gastroenterol 2008;42(Suppl 3 Pt 2):S234−6.

[68] Asahara T, Nomoto K, Watanuki M, Yokokura T. Antimicrobial activity of intraurethrally administered probiotic *Lactobacillus casei* in a murine model of *Escherichia coli* urinary tract infection. Antimicrob Agents Chemother 2001;1751−60.

[69] Seow S, Cai S, Rahmat J, Bay B, Lee Y, Chan Y, et al. *Lactobacillus rhamnosus* GG induces tumor regression in mice bearing orthotopic bladder tumors. Cancer Sci 2009;751−8.

[70] Brandau S, Böhle A. Re: Antitumor effects of the intravesical instillation of heat killed cells of the *Lactobacillus casei* strain Shirota on the murine orthotopic bladder tumor MBT-2. J Urol 2002;199−200, author reply 200.

[71] Nanno M, Kato I, Kobayashi T, Shida K. Biological effects of probiotics: what impact does *Lactobacillus casei* Shirota have on us? Int J Immunopathol Pharmacol 2011;45S−50S.

[72] Matsuzaki T. Immunomodulation by treatment with *Lactobacillus casei* strain Shirota. Int J Food Microbiol 1998;133−40.

[73] Moyad M. Review of lifestyle and CAM for miscellaneous urologic topics (bladder cancer, CP/CPPS, IC/PBS, kidney cancer): Part One 2014;231−247.

[74] Bruce A, Reid G. Probiotics and the urologist. Can J Urol 2003;1785−9.

[75] Kanamori Y, Iwanaka T, Sugiyama M, Komura M, Takahashi T, Yuki N, et al. Early use of probiotics is important therapy in infants with severe congenital anomaly. Pediatr Int 2010;362−7.

[76] Spanhaak S, Havenaar R, Schaafsma G. The effect of consumption of milk fermented by *Lactobacillus casei* strain Shirota on the intestinal microflora and immune parameters in humans. Eur J Clin Nutr 1999;52(12):899−907.

[77] Hayatsu H, Hayatsu T. Suppressing effect of *Lactobacillus casei* administration on the urinary mutagenicity arising from ingestion of fried ground beef in the human. Cancer Lett 1993;73(2−3):173−9.

[78] Shida K, Makino K, Morishita A, Takamizawa K, Hachimura S, Ametani A, et al. *Lactobacillus casei* inhibits antigen-induced IgE secretion through regulation of cytokine production in murine splenocyte cultures. Int Arch Allergy Immunol 1998;115 (4):278−87.

[79] Kato I, Yokokura T, Mutai M. Augmentation of mouse natural killer cell activity by *Lactobacillus casei* and its surface antigens. Microbiol Immunol 1984;28(2):209−17.

[80] Matsuzaki T, Chin J. Modulating immune responses with probiotic bacteria. Immunol Cell Biol 2000;78(1):67−73.

[81] Matsumoto S, Hara T, Nagaoka M, Mike A, Mitsuyama K, Sako T, et al. A component of polysaccharide peptidoglycan complex on *Lactobacillus* induced an improvement of murine model of inflammatory bowel disease and colitis-associated cancer. Immunology 2009;128(1 Suppl):e170−80.

[82] Fichera GA, Giese G. Non-immunologically-mediated cytotoxicity of *Lactobacillus casei* and its derivative peptidoglycan against tumor cell lines. Cancer Lett 1994;85(1):93−103.

[83] Cai S, Kandasamy M, Rahmat JN, Tham SM, Bay BH, Lee YK, et al. *Lactobacillus rhamnosus* GG activation of dendritic cells and neutrophils depends on the dose and time of exposure. J Immunol Res 2016;2016:7402760.

FURTHER READING

Whiteside SA, Razvi H, Dave S, Reid G, Burton JP. The microbiome of the urinary tract—a role beyond infection. Nat Rev Urol 2015;12(2):81−90.

Chapter 33

Genetic Testing, Genetic Variation, and Genetic Susceptibility

Evangelina López de Maturana[1,2] and Núria Malats[1,2]

[1]Spanish National Cancer Research Centre (CNIO), Madrid, Spain, [2]Centro de Investigación Biomédica en red Cáncer (CIBERONC), Madrid, Spain

Chapter Outline

ABBREVIATIONS

AUC   (area under the roc curve)
DNA   (deoxyribonucleic acid)
GWAS   (genome-wide association studies)
HG-NMIBC   (high-grade nonmuscle invasive bladder cancer)
LD   (linkage disequilibrium)
LG-NMIBC   (low-grade nonmuscle invasive bladder cancer)
MIBC   (muscle-invasive form)
NMIBC   (nonmuscle invasive bladder cancer)
OR   (odds ratio)
SNP   (single nucleotide polymorphism)
TCGA   (The Cancer Genome Atlas)
UBC   (urothelial bladder cancer)

Bladder Cancer. DOI: http://dx.doi.org/10.1016/B978-0-12-809939-1.00033-3

INTRODUCTION

Urothelial (transitional cell) bladder cancer (UBC), comprising 95% of the neoplasms raising in the bladder, is a paradigm of a complex disease with both genetic and nongenetic factors participating in its development. The best-established nongenetic UBC risk factors are cigarette smoking, occupational exposure to aromatic amines, consumption of water contaminated with arsenic, and exposure to some medications and radiation [1]. Regarding the genetic component role, probably overestimated by Lichtenstein et al. [2] as explaining up to 31% (95% CI: 0%−45%) of the disease variance, it has been reported that the risk of UBC is twofold higher in first-degree relatives of UBC cases [3], and ∼12% (95% CI: 0.086−0.160) of the phenotypic variance of the liability to UBC is explained by genome-wide common single nucleotide polymorphisms (SNPs) [4]. While familial aggregation of UBC has been described, no high-penetrance allele/gene has been identified to date explaining these familial clusters. Therefore genetic testing in this high-risk population is not possible. Nonetheless, strong evidence for the effect of common genetic variants have been established in the last years for sporadic (nonfamilial) UBC with a small effect at the individual level [odds ratios (OR) ranging 1.11−1.47] (see Fig. 33.1). Figueroa et al. [5] estimated that the proportion of familial risk explained by the variants identified in genome-wide association studies (GWAS) conducted till 2015 was 12%. This suggests that the screening of the whole population is not cost-effective, and secondary intervention (i.e., screening) has been debated for to-be-defined high-risk populations [6]. However, there is no model to identify high-risk groups at present [7].

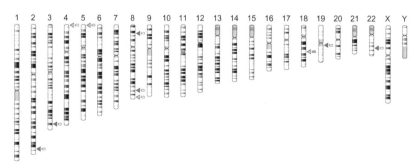

FIGURE 33.1 Genetic susceptibility genes associated with urothelial bladder cancer in the GWAS catalogue displayed according to their minor allele frequency (*x*-axis) and effect size (*y*-axis).

GENETIC SUSCEPTIBILITY TO UROTHELIAL BLADDER CARCINOMA RISK

In preparation of this review a literature search of English articles was performed using PubMed for the keywords: bladder cancer, genetic susceptibility, GWAS. No restriction of years of publication was applied. Relevant papers were selected in addition to those reported in the GWAS catalogue [8] for the bladder cancer keyword.

Whole-genome scan has represented an important approach to identify novel variants associated with a phenotype without any prior assumptions. So far, eight GWAS, which have primarily included UBC cases in European (six studies), Japanese (one study), and Chinese (one study) populations, have identified 24 loci distributed in 19 regions of 14 chromosomes, according to the GWAS catalogue [8] (see Table 33.1 for further details).

Chromosome 8 has the largest number of variants ($N = 5$, see Fig. 33.2) associated with UBC, mapping *MYC*, *PSCA*, and *N*-acetyltransferase 2 (*NAT2*) genes. The rs9642880 risk variant was first identified as associated with UBC in a GWAS [11] and confirmed by posterior GWAS, also in individuals of European descent [9,10,12]. It confers a UBC risk ranging from 1.22 to 1.24 and it is an intronic variant now mapping Cancer Susceptibility Candidate 11 (*CASC11*) located on 8q24.21 region, which is linked to a variety of cancers: prostate [19], breast [20], and colon [21]. This variant has been suggested to be associated with an increased risk of UBC in multiple racial/ethnic groups, as non-Hispanic whites and Chinese population from Shanghai [22], which risk was more pronounced among young men with low risk of progression [23]. However, its association with UBC in those populations is still not clear because the *P*-value in both studies did not reach the genome-wide significance, and the only GWAS lately conducted in a Chinese cohort [13] did not identified it. The SNP is 30 kb upstream of the v-myc myelocytomatosis viral oncogene homolog (*MYC*), a well-studied proto-oncogene that has been suggested to have a role in tumorigenesis [24] as it is one of the most frequently upregulated genes in cancer. In addition, *MYC* is involved in a large variety of biological processes, both in normal and malignant cells [25]. Although no functional analysis has been done for rs9642880, it has been hypothesized that this variant may modify *MYC* expression (Dudek et al. 2013). Interestingly, it is in moderate linkage disequilibrium (LD) ($r^2 = 0.598$) with rs10094872, another UBC risk variant (OR = 1.26) found on the same region [14].

The rs2294008 risk variant on region 8q24.3 has shown consistent association (OR = 1.3−1.15) with UBC in individuals of European descent [9,26] (Table 33.1). Its association with UBC in Chinese individuals is still controversial, the study of Wang et al. [15] suggesting an association with UBC risk while the only GWAS conducted with Chinese individuals did not find it [13]. This variant is a missense variation that alters the start codon of

TABLE 33.1 Summary of the Urothelial Bladder Cancer Variants Reported in the GWAS Catalogue

Region	Reference	Mapped Gene	Reported Gene	Strongest SNP Risk Allele	OR	P-Value
1p13.3	Rothman et al. [9]	GSTM1	GSTM1	Deletion assay	1.47	5.00E-31
2q37.1	Rothman et al. [9]	UGT1A10, UGT1A, UGT1A8	UGT1A	rs11892031-?	1.19	1.00E-07
2q37.1	Figueroa et al. [10]	UGT1A10, UGT1A, UGT1A8	UGT1A	rs11892031-A	1.17	1.00E-07
3q26.2	Figueroa et al. [10]	MYNN	ACTRT3, MYNN, TERC, LRRC34	rs10936599-C	1.18	5.00E-09
3q28	Kiemeney et al. [11]	TP63–P3H2	TP63	rs710521-A	1.19	1.00E-07
3q28	Rothman et al. [9]	TP63–P3H2	TP63	rs710521-A	1.18	2.00E-10
3q28	Kiemeney et al. [12]	TP63–P3H2	TP63	rs710521-A	1.19	6.00E-08
3q28	Figueroa et al. [10]	TP63–P3H2	TP63	rs710521-A	1.14	2.00E-11
4p16.3	Rothman et al. [9]	TACC3	TMEM129, TACC3, FGFR3	rs798766-T	1.2	4.00E-13
4p16.3	Kiemeney et al. [12]	TACC3	TMEM129, SLBP, TACC3, FGFR3	rs798766-T	1.24	1.00E-11
4p16.3	Figueroa et al. [10]	TACC3	TMEM129, TACC3, FGFR3	rs798766-T	1.22	7.00E-25
5q12.3	Wang et al. [13]	CWC27	CWC27	rs2042329-T	1.4	5.00E-11
5p15.33	Rothman et al. [9]	CLPTM1L	TERT, CLPTM1L	rs401681-C	1.11	5.00E-07

5p15.33	Figueroa et al. [10]	CLPTM1L	TERT, CLPTML	rs401681-C	1.12	4.00E-11
6p22.3	Figueroa et al. [10]	CDKAL1	NR	rs7774724-?	1.11	1.00E-06
6p22.3	Figueroa et al. [10]	CDKAL1	CDKAL1	rs4510656-C	1.12	7.00E-07
8p22	Rothman et al. [9]	NAT2–PSD3	NAT2	rs1495741-?	1.15	4.00E-11
8p22	Figueroa et al. [10]	NAT2–PSD3	NAT2	rs1495741-A	1.14	2.00E-10
8q21.13	Figueroa et al. [10]	PAG1	NR	rs5003154-?	1.11	1.00E-06
8q24.21	Kiemeney et al. [11]	CASC11	MYC, BC042052	rs9642880-T	1.22	9.00E-12
8q24.21	Rothman et al. [9]	CASC11	MYC	rs9642880-T	1.21	2.00E-18
8q24.21	Kiemeney et al. [12]	CASC11	MYC	rs9642880-T	1.21	7.00E-12
8q24.21	Figueroa et al. [10]	CASC11	Intergenic	rs9642880-T	1.24	4.00E-38
8q24.21	Rafnar et al. [14]	CASC11	MYC, POU5F1B, PVT1	rs10094872-T	1.26	2.00E-07
8q24.3	Wang et al. [15]	PSCA	PSCA	rs2294008-T	1.15	2.00E-10
8q24.3	Rothman et al. [9]	PSCA	PSCA	rs2294008-T	1.13	4.00E-11
8q24.3	Figueroa et al. [10]	PSCA	PSCA	rs2294008-T	1.13	3.00E-15
11p15.5	Figueroa et al. [10]	LOC107984299–LSP1	LSP1	rs907611-A	1.15	4.00E-08
13q34	Figueroa et al. [10]	MCF2L, LOC107984591	NR	rs4907479-?	1.13	3.00E-06
15q24.1	Matsuda et al. [16]	CLK3	CLK3, CYP1A2	rs11543198-G	1.41	4.00E-09
18q12.3	Rafnar et al. [17]	SLC14A1, LOC105372093	SLC14A1	rs17674580-T	1.17	8.00E-11
18q12.3	Garcia-Closas et al. [18]	LOC105372093, SLC14A1	SLC14A1	rs7238033-?	1.2	9.00E-09

(Continued)

TABLE 33.1 (Continued)

Region	Reference	Mapped Gene	Reported Gene	Strongest SNP Risk Allele	OR	P-Value
18q12.3	Figueroa et al. [10]	LOC105372093, SLC14A1	SLC14A2	rs10775480-T	1.13	6.00E-08
19q12	Rothman et al. [9]	LOC107985345–CCNE1	CCNE1	rs8102137-C	1.13	2.00E-11
19q12	Figueroa et al. [10]	LOC107985345–CCNE1	CCNE1	rs8102137-C	1.13	1.00E-11
20p12.2	Rafnar et al. [14]	C20orf187	JAG1	rs62185668-A	1.19	2.00E-11
20p12.2	Figueroa et al. [10]	C20orf187	C20orf187, LOC339593	rs6104690-A	1.12	7.00E-07
22q13.1	Rothman et al. [9]	LOC105373032–APOBEC3A	CBX6, APOBEC3A	rs1014971-?	1.18	8.00E-12
22q13.1	Figueroa et al. [10]	LOC105373032–APOBEC3A	CBX6, APOBEC3A	rs1014971-T	1.13	1.00E-11

OR, odds ratio.

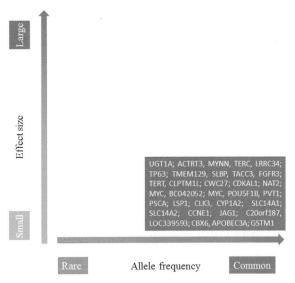

FIGURE 33.2 Ideogram localizing the GWAS identified common genetic susceptibility variants in the chromosome bands. *From the Phenotype-Genotype Integrator (PheGenI) after searching for urinary bladder neoplasm.*

PSCA gene, which encodes the glycosylphosphatidylinositol-anchored cell surface protein that belongs to the *Thy-1/Ly-6* family. *PSCA* is found to be expressed in several normal tissues (prostate, placenta, kidney, colon, and stomach), in addition to bladder, although at low levels. This gene is highly overexpressed in the majority of UBC, including both nonmuscle invasive bladder cancer (NMIBC) and muscle-invasive bladder cancer (MIBC) [27]. *PSCA* function is unknown, although it was chosen as a target for immunotherapy [28,29]. The SNP rs2294008 is on region 8q24 independent from the previously described variant rs9642880, from which is ∼15 mb distant.

Regions 8p22 and 8q21 also harbor UBC risk variants. In particular, 8p22 contains the SNP rs1495741 in the *NAT2* associated with UBC (OR = 1.14−1.15) (Table 33.1, Fig. 33.2). *NAT2* is a carcinogen-metabolizing gene that participates in the detoxification of bladder carcinogens such as aromatic amines from tobacco smoke, among other sources. This variant is one of the best-known susceptibility locus associated with UBC risk, confirmed by candidate-gene studies [30] previously to GWAS [9,10]. Region 8q21 harbors rs5003154 variant, recently suggested as associated with UBC (OR = 1.11), although it did not reach the GWAS significance (P-value = 10^{-6}) [10].

Chromosome 18 is the second chromosome with more risk variants ($N = 3$) associated with UBC (Fig. 33.2). All of them [rs17674580 (OR = 1.17), rs7238033 (OR = 1.2), and rs10775480 (OR = 1.13)] are on region 18q12, which harbors *SLC14A1* and *SLC14A2* genes pertaining to the solute carrier family 14 and separated by approximately 50 kb [10,17,18]. These genes are members of *SLC14* family of urea transporters, which are crucial to the kidney's ability to concentrate urine. In particular, *SLC14A1* gene regulates urine volume and concentration in kidney, whereas in erythrocytes it determines the Kidd blood group. Two missense variants, rs1058396 and rs11877062, also in *SLC14A1* and highly correlated ($r^2 = 0.88$), almost reached the GWAS significance level in Ref. [17]. There is no evidence for functionality of rs17674580 or markers in strong LD. Rafnar et al. did not find associations between any of these variants and serum urea levels. It has been hypothesized that the association with UBC is indirect through urine concentration, which might be related to the fact that amount of daily fluid intake and urinary frequency may affect UBC risk [31,32].

Chromosome 3 harbors two susceptibility variants associated with UBC: rs710521 (OR = 1.14−1.19) [9−12] and rs10936599 (OR = 1.18) [10]. rs710521 on 3q28 region is located in an LD block that overlaps the tumor protein 63 (*TP63*), which has strong homology with the tumor suppressor gene *TP53* and with the *TP73*. It is involved in apoptosis and regulates cell-cycle arrest. It has been suggested that *TP63* may have a critical role in the progression of UBC and the expression of this protein is often lost in UBC. However, the functional role of rs710521 variant is not clear, as Kiemeney et al. [11] did not find any significant correlation between *TP63* mRNA expression and the number of copies of the risk allele. rs10936599, on 3q26.2, maps to a multigenic region including *TERC*, *ACTRT3*, *MYNN*, and *LRRC34*, although its functional role in the development of UBC is undetermined.

Region 20p12.2 is a multisignal locus, with two UBC genetic associations: one marked by rs6104690 (OR = 1.12) and a second by rs62185668 (OR = 1.19) [10,14], and rs6108803 (OR = 1.18), the latter almost reaching the GWAS *P*-value threshold [5]. Figueroa et al. [5] found the most significant association with UBC risk for a haplotype of the risk alleles of rs6104690 and rs6108803 (OR = 1.21, $P = 2 \times 10^{-7}$). These markers map to a gene desert area and, although this region showed enrichment of multiple functional signals close to rs6104690, no specific risk patterns were found [5].

Region 6p22.3 also harbors two variants, rs7747724 (OR = 1.11) and rs4510656 (OR = 1.12) associated with UBC, tagging *CDAKL1* [10]. Their functional role is not clear as *CDKAL1* expression levels did not show significant differences according to rs4510656 genotypes.

Another important variant that has been associated with UBC risk is rs798766 (OR = 1.20−1.24) on region 4p16.3 [9,10,12]. SNP rs798766 is an intronic variant in transforming acidic coiled-coil containing protein 3 (*TACC3*). It is ~60 kb away from *FGFR3* gene, which encodes fibroblast growth factor receptor 3 and harbors activating mutations in low-grade,

NMIBC. This SNP strongly correlates with 20 other SNPs in the region (HapMap CEU), although none of them showed a stronger association with UBC risk.

CLPTM1L and *TERT* (Telomerase Reverse Transcriptase) genes on region 5p15.33 have been associated with multiple cancers [33−37], besides UBC [9,10] (Table 33.1). From the two SNPs associated with UBC risk (rs401681 and rs2736098), only rs401681 reached genome-wide significance (OR = 1.11−1.12). Rafnar et al. [35] found that the UBC risk allele of rs2736098 correlated with a shorter length of telomeres in blood of old women. Both SNPs have been reported to be associated with increased risk of basal cell carcinoma, lung cancer, and cervical cancer, too [38]. The role of rs401681 in the development of UBC has not been thoroughly studied. In lung tissue, its risk allele has been associated with increased levels of DNA adduct accumulation [38].

The rs8102137 UBC susceptibility SNP (OR = 1.13) on 19q12 was firstly reported by Rothman et al. [9]. This association was later on confirmed by Figueroa et al. [10]. The variant tags *CCNE1*, a key member of the cyclin-dependent kinase-retinoblastoma protein pathway, which determines the rate of cell-cycle transition from the G1 to the S phase. This gene has been found commonly altered in UBC tumors [39].

The intronic variant rs11892031 is on region 2q37.1 and was firstly reported to be associated with UBC (OR = 1.19) by Rothman et al. [9], and later on Figueroa et al. [10] confirmed that association (OR = 1.17). This variant maps uridine 5′ diphosphoglucuronosyltransferase 1A (*UGT1A*), a carcinogen-metabolizing gene encoding UGT1A family of proteins that has been functionally characterized [38]. The variant is synonymous and located in the long isoforms of *UGT1A6*. Tang et al. hypothesized that it can modify the UGT1A6.1 expression level in an allele-specific manner. The protective allele was found to be correlated with increased expression of UGT1A6.1, which can lead to enhanced removal of carcinogens dissociated from glucuronid from bladder tissue into the urine, reducing UBC risk [40].

SNP rs907611 found to be associated with UBC (OR = 1.15) by Figueroa et al. [10] is located on region 11p15, 130 bp upstream of the transcription start site for the longer transcript of *LSP1*, an intracellular F-actin−binding protein, important for regulation of leukocyte recruitment to inflamed sites [41]. This finding might partially explain the importance of chronic information with UBC initiation and development.

GSTM1 deletion in chromosome 1 is the only copy number variant associated with UBC risk (OR = 1.7), the association being firstly confirmed by Garcia-Closas et al. [30] through a metaanalysis of candidate-gene studies and confirmed by Rothman et al. [9] in a GWAS (OR = 1.47).

The UBC susceptibility variant rs4907479 (OR = 1.13) is on 13q34 region [5,42]. A fine mapping of the region showed that the signal detected for that variant can be captured by at least 29 highly correlated variants, all located within the first two introns of *MCF2L*, a gene encoding a guanine nucleotide exchange factor that interacts specifically with the GTP-bound Rac1 and plays a role in the Rho/Rac signaling pathways. Figueroa et al. [5] performed an in silico annotation using ENCODE. They indicated that 13q34 region contains two regions showing deoxyribonuclease hypersensivity sites and enrichment of multiple functional marks suggestive of regulatory functions that are close to SNPs in high LD with rs4907479. However, rs4907479 did not show associations with mRNA expression of *MCF2L* overall survival or bladder cancer using The Cancer Genome Atlas (TCGA) bladder cancer dataset, and their functional role remains unclear.

There are other SNPs in intergenic regions that have been associated with UBC risk. Variant rs1014971 with OR ranging from 1.13 to 1.18 [9,10] is located on region 22q13 and ∼16 kb away from apolipoprotein B mRNA editing enzyme catalytic subunit 3A (*APOBEC3A*), which can play a role in the initiation of tumorigenesis by deamination of cytosine to uracil [43] and ∼75 kb from chromobox6 (*CBX6*), involved in transcriptional repression. Moreover, Middlebrooks et al. [44] recently suggested that the increased UBC risk observed in carriers of risk allele of rs1014971 could be due to its association with increased expression of APOBEC3B and generation of *APOBEC*-signature mutations in bladder tissue showing allele-specific protein binding in bladder cancer cell types.

All the variants described earlier have been associated in GWAS conducted in individuals of European descent. The variants rs17674580, rs1014971, rs2294008, and rs9642880 were also reported as associated with UBC risk in Japanese populations [16]. Since the remaining GWAS loci were not replicated, genetic heterogeneity between European and Asian populations has been suggested. Besides, this GWAS found rs11543198 as a new UBC susceptibility variant (OR = 1.41) on region 15q24.1 in Japanese population. It is located within the *CLK3* gene encoding a serine/threonine protein kinase and regulates localization of SR family of splicing factors. This SNP does not affect aminoacid sequence of catalytic domain, which might suggest that it is not the causal variant. Matsuda et al. [16] performed an imputation analysis and reported that a SNP close to *CYP1A2* might be the causative mutation, because of its stronger association with UBC risk. *CYP1A2* metabolizes heterocyclic aromatic amines contained in tobacco smoke [45], generates carcinogenic intermediates [46], and has been associated with regular coffee drinkers [47–49].

Only one variant (rs2042329) was found to be specifically associated with UBC risk in the Chinese GWAS (OR = 1.4) [13]. Its risk allele was associated with an increase of the expression levels of *CWC27* mRNA and protein in UBC tissues from Chinese patients. Although the complete biological mechanism of this variant remains unclear, Wang et al. found that its function might include chromatin binding and driving allele-specific regulation of *RFX5*. They also suggested an oncogenic role of *CWC27* by inducing cell proliferation and suppressing apoptosis. The fact that this variant was not reported to be associated with UBC risk in individuals of European descent and that variants previously associated with UBC risk in European and Japanese populations did not reach the genome-wide statistical significance in the Chinese cohort supports the hypothesis of a heterogeneous genetic susceptibility to UBC across populations. More GWAS/whole-genome sequencing studies should be conducted worldwide to confirm this hypothesis.

GWAS confirmed two variants previously identified by candidate-gene studies with the largest effect increasing UBC risk (although modestly): *GSTM1*-null and the slow acetylator phenotype conferred SNPs of *NAT2* [30]. Additional hypothesis-driven candidate-gene studies reported many other genetic variants and pathways associated with UBC, the sounder being those belonging to NER and BER DNA repair pathways [50,51]. However, the majority of results were not reproduced in GWAS. Whether the restrictive *P*-value threshold applied in GWAS explains this lack of replication should be elucidated.

Recently, by applying for the first time a multimarker approach that is expected to capture genetic variants with very small effect by imitating the complexity of genetics of UBC, López de Maturana et al. [52] found associations tagging the inflammatory genes *IL6R*, *TBK1*, *IL21R*, *MAP3K3*, *IL17A*, *FADD*, and *TLR2*, which were validated in an independent population.

UBC a Genetically Heterogeneous Disease

UBC is also a heterogeneous disease. At least, three forms of UBC are considered by uropathologists: low-grade nonmuscle invasive bladder cancer (LG-NMIBC), high-grade nonmuscle invasive bladder cancer (HG-NMIBC), and MIBC. A preliminary stratified exploration taking into account the pathological UBC subclassification identified SNPs differentially associated with UBC subphenotypes (i.e., rs6463524 in *PMS2* and rs3213427 in *CD4*), while the established variants did not [53]. Some loci discovered through GWAS have been reported to be differentially associated according to stage and grade. Kiemeney et al. and Rothman et al. found that loci on 8q24.21 (*MYC*), 4p16.3 (*TMEM129*, *TACC3-FGFR3*), and 5p15.33 (*TERT-CLPTM1L*) were more associated with LG-NMIBC, whereas 22q13.1 and 19.12 (*CCNE1*) regions were mainly associated with risk of HG-NMIBC [9,11,12].

SNPs rs6108803 and rs62185668 on 20p12.2 were reported as stronger associated with MIBC (T2−T4 stages) compared with NMIBC (stages Ta and T1), although not with the grading classification [5].

Gene–Environment Interaction

As mentioned earlier, bladder cancer is a multifactorial disease with genetic and nongenetic factors contributing to its development by interacting among them. Some studies have assessed gene–environment interactions.

Smoking

Cigarette smoking is the best-established risk factor for UBC [1]. However, its effect is not as strong as lung cancers, which may suggest a role of gene–smoking interactions, among other explanations. This hypothesis has been explored through family history, candidate-gene studies, and GWAS approaches. Lin et al. [54] suggested that a positive family history of bladder cancer may have interacted with smoking habits to increase the risk of UBC. Both candidate-gene and GWAS studies have shown that *NAT2* slow acetylation genotype moderately increases UBC risk among smokers while it does not in nonsmokers [30].

Figueroa et al. [10] performed the first genome-wide interaction study and found 10 SNPs showing a consistent evidence of both multiplicative and additive interactions with tobacco use (P-value $= 5 \times 10^{-5}$). In particular, tests for multiplicative interactions showed that rs1711973 (*FOXF2*), rs2969540 (*HTR5A*, *PAXIP1*, *INSIG1*), rs3752645 (*PRKARB2*), and rs2411843 (*HDAC4*) were associated with UBC risk in never smokers, whereas in the subgroup of smokers, rs3752645 (*PRKARB2*) showed an inverse association with UBC risk (especially among current smokers). *PRKARB2* encodes for a regulatory subunit for cyclic adenosine $3',5'$-monophosphate kinase and knockout studies in mice suggest that this subunit may play an important role in regulating energy balance and adiposity. Tests for additive interactions showed that rs1495741 tagging *NAT2* acetylation status, rs12216499, rs948798, rs9502305, rs846906, rs1258767, rs2380945, and rs1258767 variants (all mapping *RSPH3-TAGAP-EZR*) were inversely associated with UBC risk only among ever smokers.

Alcohol

Few candidate-gene studies have investigated the role of alcohol-metabolizing enzymes and UBC risk. The polymorphic enzyme alcohol dehydrogenase (ADH) catalyzes the conversion of ethanol into the carcinogenic metabolite acetaldehyde, which is partly excreted into the urine. A recent study [55] found that *ALDH2* and *ADH1B* functional polymorphisms are associated with UBC risk according to drinking status: *ALDH2* Glu/Lys genotype exacerbates UBC risk associated with alcohol drinking (OR $= 2.03$, P-value $= 0.017$), although no significant elevation of risk was found among never drinkers. In addition, individuals with *ALDH2* Glu/Lys and *ADH1B* Arg + (slow *ADH1B* genotype) are at the highest risk of UBC compared with *ALDH2* Glu/Glu and *ADH1B* His/His (OR = 4.00, *P*-value = 0.001). A kind of contradictory result regarding the effect of *ADH1C* (previously known as *ADH3*) was found in the study of van Dijk et al. [56]: moderate drinkers with the "high-risk" (gamma1gamma1) *ADH1C* genotype had a threefold higher UBC risk than the moderate drinkers with a "low-risk" (gamma1-gamma2/gamma2gamma2) genotype, although no gene−environment interaction was indicated.

Drinking Water Arsenic Exposure

The study by Andrew et al. [57] supports the hypothesis that genetic variation in DNA repair genes can modify the arsenic−cancer relationship, possibly because arsenic impairs DNA repair capacity. Gene−environment interaction with arsenic exposure was reported in relation to UBC risk for a variant allele of the double-strand break repair gene *XRCC3*, although this interaction has not been replicated.

UBC Risk Prediction

As it was commented previously, UBC is a complex disease also at the genetic level. The effect of genetic variants detected by GWAS has been estimated to be small, with individual OR ranging 1.11−1.47. Therefore they are not medically actionable at the individual level. Considering risk factors in isolation when complex traits are analyzed could ignore relevant genetic signal and would lead to a low predictive accuracy. López de Maturana et al. [58] attempted, for the first time to build a predictive model for UBC risk combining both genomic and nongenomic data, using a multimarker model. Importantly, this model does not need a precise biological understanding of genetic or genomic associations and can also handle a huge number of variants, often exceeding the number of individuals. The authors of this study showed that in terms of classification performance, the model including smoking status performed the best (area under the roc curve, AUC = 0.62). This value is low being tobacco consumption the main UBC risk factor and thus pointing to the multifactorial nature of UBC. The genomic model, including almost ∼500,000 SNPs, had a poorer classification performance (AUC = 0.53). Adding them to the tobacco model did not increase its predictive ability. The poor performance of genome-wide common variants in predicting UBC risk is in agreement with those obtained in studies predicting risk for other cancers, such as breast or colorectal. López de Maturana et al. [58] showed that, by further refining the definition of phenotypes of UBC on the basis of a theoretically stronger genetic susceptibility, the prediction with whole-genome data increased (AUC = 0.61).

GENETICS UNDERLYING UBC PROGNOSIS

UBC outcomes are tumor recurrence and progression for NMIBC and progression and death for MIBC. Based on tumor characteristics, mainly stage and grade, NMIBC are subsequently classified as "low risk" and "high risk" of progression. So far, clinicians use nomograms that incorporate multiple clinico-pathological variables [59]. However, their predictive ability is not completely satisfactory due to the large variability in the clinical course of these patients and therefore more objective biomarkers are needed.

Most of the attempts to identify prognostic and treatment response biomarkers are conducted at the tumor level or using urine tumor exfoliated cells. Germline genetic variants such as SNPs or copy number variants (CNVs) have been less studied. Candidate-genes and pathways analyses have been conducted to identify genetic variants associated with prognosis in NMIBC patients, although results have not been validated in independent studies. No genetic variant is reported in the GWAS catalogue [8] as associated with UBC prognosis. This may probably due to the limited sample sizes and the heterogeneity in methods applied in the follow-up studies, which makes it difficult to detect small-effect associations at the genome-wide statistical level with the classical single marker approach.

Grotenhuis et al. [60] studied the prognostic relevance of UBC susceptibility loci and reported that none of the genetic variants studied, GWAS hits for UBC risk, showed an association with disease recurrence. The variant rs9642880 at the *MYC* locus on 8q24 showed the most statistically significant association with risk of progression (P-value $= 2.6 \times 10^{-3}$). The authors also investigated the role of smoking status as a modifier of the prognostic effect of the GWAS loci, and reported that locus rs798766 on 4p16.3 region (*TACC3-FGFR3*) was likely associated with risk of recurrence specially among never smokers (P-value $= 2.7 \times 10^{-5}$).

Suggestive associations with UBC prognosis have been reported in carcinogenesis-related processes (*TP53* and *MDM2*), DNA repair pathways (*ERCC6, XPD, XPF, XPG, XRCC1*, and *MSH6*), growth factor signaling processes (*EGFR, TGB1*, and *TGFBR*), cell signaling pathways (*PI3K-AKT-mTOR*), Sonic hedgehog pathway, genes involved in cell cycle, cell adhesion and hypoxia (*CDKN2A, E-cadherin*, and *HIF-1α*), and inflammation-related pathways (*IL6, PPARG*, and *NFKB1*). However, there is a lack of validation of these associations that recommends caution in interpretation.

Recently, Masson-Lecomte et al. [61] explored the joint effect of multiple SNPs tagging genes involved in inflammation processes in the prognosis of patients with NMIBC, identifying variants individually conferring a small risk of NMIBC recurrence or progression. rs6523 (*JAK3*) and rs7104333 (*CD5*) were already identified as associated with UBC risk in a previous candidate-gene association study [52]. Noteworthy, most of the reported variants are placed in genes involved in immune tolerance processes (e.g., *JAK3*, *CD5*, *AIRE*, and *CARD4/NOD1*). Their results also suggested that different inflammatory genes trigger distinct NMIBC outcomes and supported the hypothesis that genetic susceptibility may partially explain the variability in the clinical course of these patients (polymorphisms in inflammatory genes were differently associated with time to progression in patients at HG-NMIBC versus LG-NMIBC).

A few number of association studies have been conducted to identify associations between genetic variants and prognosis of patients with MIBC. None of the 12 genetic variants found in GWAS [9,11,12,17,26,35] showed any association with overall death [60]. Candidate-gene/pathway studies have suggested associations between survival in patients with MIBC and genes in carcinogenesis-related processes (*MDM2*), DNA repair pathway (*XPD* and *XRCC1*), cell signaling pathways (*PI3K*, *AKT*, and *RAPTOR*), or inflammation pathway (*IL6*) that need to be confirmed in larger studies.

Genetic Prediction of UBC Prognosis

The major goal on managing NMIBC patients is to prevent tumor relapse by tailoring the treatments according to the aggressiveness of the disease as much as possible. To this end, building accurate prognostic models for these patients is crucial. However, there is no clinically implemented prognostic biomarkers for NMIBC patients at present and urologists base their treatment decisions on risk models including only clinic-pathological variables [62].

Recently, by applying multimarker approaches for the first time to the prognosis field, López de Maturana et al. [63] showed that genome-wide common SNPs had limited role in the prediction of risk of recurrence and progression of NMIBC. SNP classification performance was poor and similar for risks of first recurrence and progression independently of whether patients had high-risk or low-risk tumors (AUCs ranging 0.55−0.58). Unexpectedly, no improvement in terms of classification was observed when SNPs were added to the classical clinical factors. In terms of percentage of explained variance, they showed that SNPs increased the proportion explained by classical clinical factors for first recurrence risk (from 3.1% to 4%), and that for progression in individuals at high risk (from 15.1% to 15.4%).

The limited role of genetics on prognosis prediction of NMIBC patients is indirectly supported by Egbers et al. [64], who showed that family history did not aid in prediction of NMIBC recurrence or progression. Up to date, the role of genetic variants when predicting prognosis in patients with MIBC has not been studied yet.

CONCLUSION

UBC is a multifactorial disease with a genetic component. However, the lack of high-penetrance mutations explaining family aggregation of this cancer impedes the possibility of genetic testing. In addition, there is a limited number of genetic variants associated with UBC risk, in comparison to other cancers as breast, prostate, or colon.

Defining UBC subphenotypes at the molecular level provides potential for identifying more risk variants, although larger studies are required. Exploring gene−gene and gene−environment interactions may also help to identify and understand biological mechanisms underlying UBC initiation, but again larger samples sizes are needed for this purpose.

UBC progression also involves a complex network of genes and pathways. Although the evidences on the effect of SNPs in the prognostic field are promising, the evidences are still inconclusive, and larger and more homogeneous studies are needed to comprehensively explore the field.

ACKNOWLEDGMENTS

The work was partially supported by Red Temática de Investigación Cooperativa en Cáncer, Instituto de Salud Carlos III-FEDER, Spain (#RD12/0036/0050) and Asociación Española Contra el Cáncer (#GE2014).

REFERENCES

[1] Malats N, Real FX. Epidemiology of bladder cancer. Hematol Oncol Clin North Am 2015. Available from: http://dx.doi.org/10.1016/j.hoc.2014.10.001.

[2] Lichtenstein P, Holm NV, Verkasalo PK, Iliadou A, Kaprio J, Koskenvuo M, et al. Environmental & heritable factors in the causation of cancer. N Engl J Med 2000;343 (2):78−85. Available from: http://dx.doi.org/10.1056/NEJM200007133430201.

[3] Murta-Nascimento C, Schmitz-Dräger BJ, Zeegers MP, Steineck G, Kogevinas M, Real FX, et al. Epidemiology of urinary bladder cancer: from tumor development to patient's death. World J Urol 2007;25:285. Available from: http://dx.doi.org/10.1007/s00345-007-0168-5.

[4] Sampson JN, Wheeler WA, Yeager M, Panagiotou O, Wang Z, Berndt SI, et al. Analysis of heritability and shared heritability based on genome-wide association studies for thirteen cancer types. J Natl Cancer Inst 2016;107(12):1−11. Available from: http://dx.doi.org/10.1093/jnci/djv279.

[5] Figueroa JD, Middlebrooks CD, Banday AR, Ye Y, Garcia-Closas M, Chatterjee N, et al. Identification of a novel susceptibility locus at 13q34 and refinement of the 20p12.2 region as a multi-signal locus associated with bladder cancer risk in individuals of european ancestry. Hum Mol Genet 2016;25(6):1203−14. Available from: http://dx.doi.org/10.1093/hmg/ddv492.

[6] Zlotta AR, Roumeguere T, Kuk C, Alkhateeb S, Rorive S, Lemy A, et al. Select screening in a specific high-risk population of patients suggests a stage migration toward detection of non-muscle-invasive bladder cancer. Eur Urol 2011;59(6):1026−31. Available from: http://dx.doi.org/10.1016/j.eururo.2011.03.027.

[7]   Lotan Y, Svatek RS, Malats N. Screening for bladder cancer: a perspective. World J Urol 2008. Available from: http://dx.doi.org/10.1007/s00345-007-0223-2.

[8]   Welter D, MacArthur J, Morales J, Burdett T, Hall P, Junkins H, et al. The NHGRI GWAS Catalog, a curated resource of SNP-trait associations. Nucleic Acids Res 2014;42 (D1). Available from: http://dx.doi.org/10.1093/nar/gkt1229.

[9]   Rothman N, Garcia-Closas M, Chatterjee N, Malats N, Wu X, Figueroa JD, et al. A multi-stage genome-wide association study of bladder cancer identifies multiple suscepti-bility loci. Nat Genet 2010;42(11):978−84. Available from: http://dx.doi.org/10.1038/ ng.687.

[10] Figueroa JD, Han SS, Garcia-Closas M, Baris D, Jacobs EJ, Kogevinas M, et al. Genome-wide interaction study of smoking and bladder cancer risk. Carcinogenesis 2014;35 (8):1737−44. Available from: http://dx.doi.org/10.1093/carcin/bgu064.

[11] Kiemeney LA, Thorlacius S, Sulem P, Geller F, Aben KKH, Stacey SN, et al. Sequence variant on 8q24 confers susceptibility to urinary bladder cancer. Nat Genet 2008;40 (11):1307−12. Available from: http://dx.doi.org/10.1038/ng.229.

[12] Kiemeney LA, Sulem P, Besenbacher S, Vermeulen SH, Sigurdsson A, Thorleifsson G, et al. A sequence variant at 4p16. 3 confers susceptibility to urinary bladder cancer. Nat Genet 2010;42(5):415−19. Available from: http://dx.doi.org/10.1038/ng.558.A.

[13] Wang M, Li Z, Chu H, Lv Q, Ye D, Ding Q, et al. Genome-wide association study of bladder cancer in a Chinese cohort reveals a new susceptibility locus at 5q12.3. Cancer Res 2016;76(11):3277−84. Available from: http://dx.doi.org/10.1158/0008-5472.CAN-15- 2564.

[14] Rafnar T, Sulem P, Thorleifsson G, Vermeulen SH, Helgason H, Saemundsdottir J, et al. Genome-wide association study yields variants at 20p12.2 that associate with urinary blad-der cancer. Hum Mol Genet 2014;23(20):5545−57. Available from: http://dx.doi.org/ 10.1093/hmg/ddu264.

[15] Wang S, Tang J, Wang M, Yuan L, Zhang Z. Genetic variation in PSCA and bladder can-cer susceptibility in a Chinese population. Carcinogenesis 2010;31(4):621−4. Available from: http://dx.doi.org/10.1093/carcin/bgp323.

[16] Matsuda K, Takahashi A, Middlebrooks CD, Obara W, Nasu Y, Inoue K, et al. Genome-wide association study identified SNP on 15q24 associated with bladder cancer risk in Japanese population. Hum Mol Genet 2015;24(4):1177−84. Available from: http://dx.doi. org/10.1093/hmg/ddu512.

[17] Rafnar T, Vermeulen SH, Sulem P, Thorleifsson G, Aben KK, Witjes JA, et al. European genome-wide association study identifies SLC14A1 as a new urinary bladder cancer sus-ceptibility gene. Hum Mol Genet 2011;20(21):4268−81. Available from: http://dx.doi.org/ 10.1093/hmg/ddr303.

[18] Garcia-Closas M, Ye Y, Rothman N, Figueroa JD, Malats N, Dinney CP, et al. A genome-wide association study of bladder cancer identifies a new susceptibility locus within SLC14A1, a urea transporter gene on chromosome 18q12.3. Hum Mol Genet 2011;20(21):4282−9. Available from: http://dx.doi.org/10.1093/hmg/ddr342.

[19] Al Olama AA, Kote-Jarai Z, Giles GG, Guy M, Morrison J, Severi G, et al. Multiple loci on 8q24 associated with prostate cancer susceptibility. Nat Genet 2009;41(10):1058−60. Available from: http://dx.doi.org/10.1038/ng.452.

[20] Easton DF, Pooley KA, Dunning AM, Pharoah PDP, Thompson D, Ballinger DG, et al. Genome-wide association study identifies novel breast cancer susceptibility loci. Nature 2007;447(7148):1087−93. Available from: http://dx.doi.org/10.1038/nature05887.

[21] Montazeri Z, Theodoratou E, Nyiraneza C, Timofeeva M, Chen W, Svinti V, et al. Systematic meta-analyses and field synopsis of genetic association studies in colorectal adenomas. Int J Epidemiol 2016;45(1):186–205. Available from: http://dx.doi.org/10.1093/ije/dyv185.

[22] Cortessis VK, Yuan JM, Van Den Berg D, Jiang X, Gago-Dominguez M, Stern MC, et al. Risk of urinary bladder cancer is associated with 8q24 variant rs9642880[T] in multiple racial/ethnic groups: results from the Los Angeles-Shanghai case-control study. Cancer Epidemiol Biomarkers Prevent 2010;19(12):3150–6. Available from: http://dx.doi.org/10.1158/1055-9965.EPI-10-0763.

[23] Wang M, Wang M, Zhang W, Yuan L, Fu G, Wei Q, et al. Common genetic variants on 8q24 contribute to susceptibility to bladder cancer in a Chinese population. Carcinogenesis 2009;30(6):991–6. Available from: http://dx.doi.org/10.1093/carcin/bgp091.

[24] Nilsson JA, Cleveland JL. Myc pathways provoking cell suicide and cancer. Oncogene 2003;22(56):9007–21. Available from: http://dx.doi.org/10.1038/sj.onc.1207261.

[25] Eilers M, Eisenman RN. Myc's broad reach. Genes Develop 2008. Available from: http://dx.doi.org/10.1101/gad.1712408.

[26] Wu X, Ye Y, Kiemeney LA, Sulem P, Rafnar T, Matullo G, et al. Genetic variation in the prostate stem cell antigen gene PSCA confers susceptibility to urinary bladder cancer. Nat Genet 2009;41(9):991–5. Available from: http://dx.doi.org/10.1038/ng1009-1156a.

[27] Amara N, Palapattu GS, Schrage M, Gu Z, Thomas GV, Dorey F, et al. Prostate stem cell antigen is overexpressed in human transitional cell carcinoma. Cancer Res 2001;61 (12):4660–5.

[28] Kohaar I, Porter-Gill P, Lenz P, Fu YP, Mumy A, Tang W, et al. Genetic variant as a selection marker for anti-prostate stem cell antigen immunotherapy of bladder cancer. J Natl Cancer Inst 2013;105(1):69–73. Available from: http://dx.doi.org/10.1093/jnci/djs458.

[29] Saffran DC, Raitano AB, Hubert RS, Witte ON, Reiter RE, Jakobovits A. Anti-PSCA mAbs inhibit tumor growth and metastasis formation and prolong the survival of mice bearing human prostate cancer xenografts. Proc Natl Acad Sci USA 2001;98(5):2658–63. Available from: http://dx.doi.org/10.1073/pnas.051624698.

[30] García-Closas M, Malats N, Silverman D, Dosemeci M, Kogevinas M, Hein DW, et al. NAT2 slow acetylation, GSTM1 null genotype, and risk of bladder cancer: results from the Spanish Bladder Cancer Study and meta-analyses. Lancet 2005;366(9486):649–59. doi:10.1016/S0140-6736(05)67137-1.

[31] Michaud DS, Kogevinas M, Cantor KP, Villanueva CM, Garcia-Closas M, Rothman N, et al. Total fluid and water consumption and the joint effect of exposure to disinfection by-products on risk of bladder cancer. Environ Health Perspect 2007;115(11):1569–72. Available from: http://dx.doi.org/10.1289/ehp.10281.

[32] Silverman DT, Alguacil J, Rothman N, Real FX, Garcia-Closas M, Cantor KP, et al. Does increased urination frequency protect against bladder cancer? Int J Cancer 2008;123 (7):1644–8. Available from: http://dx.doi.org/10.1002/ijc.23572.

[33] Landi MT, Chatterjee N, Yu K, Goldin LR, Goldstein AM, Rotunno M, et al. A genome-wide association study of lung cancer identifies a region of chromosome 5p15 associated with risk for adenocarcinoma. Am J Hum Genet 2009;85(5):679–91. Available from: http://dx.doi.org/10.1016/j.ajhg.2009.09.012.

[34] Petersen GM, Amundadottir L, Fuchs CS, Kraft P, Stolzenberg-Solomon RZ, Jacobs KB, et al. A genome-wide association study identifies pancreatic cancer susceptibility loci on

chromosomes 13q22.1, 1q32.1 and 5p15.33. Nat Genet 2010;42(3):224—8. Available from: http://dx.doi.org/10.1038/ng.522.

[35]   Rafnar T, Sulem P, Stacey SN, Geller F, Gudmundsson J, Sigurdsson A, et al. Sequence variants at the TERT-CLPTM1L locus associate with many cancer types. Nat Genet 2009;41(2):221—7. Available from: http://dx.doi.org/10.1038/ng.296.

[36]   Shete S, Hosking FJ, Robertson LB, Dobbins SE, Sanson M, Malmer B, et al. Genome-wide association study identifies five susceptibility loci for glioma. Nat Genet 2009;41(8):899—904. Available from: http://dx.doi.org/10.1038/ng.407.

[37]   Stacey SN, Sulem P, Masson G, Gudjonsson SA, Thorleifsson G, Jakobsdottir M, et al. New common variants affecting susceptibility to basal cell carcinoma. Nat Genet 2009;41(8):909—14. Available from: http://dx.doi.org/10.1038/ng.412.

[38]   Dudek AM, Grotenhuis AJ, Vermeulen SH, Kiemeney LALM, Verhaegh GW. Urinary bladder cancer susceptibility markers. What do we know about functional mechanisms? Int J Molec Sci 2013. Available from: http://dx.doi.org/10.3390/ijms140612346.

[39]   Lindgren D, Sjödahl G, Lauss M, Staaf J, Chebil G, Lövgren K, et al. Integrated genomic and gene expression profiling identifies two major genomic circuits in urothelial carcinoma. PLoS One 2012;7(6). Available from: http://dx.doi.org/10.1371/journal.pone.0038863.

[40]   Tang W, Fu YP, Figueroa JD, Malats N, Garcia-Closas M, Chatterjee N, et al. Mapping of the UGT1A locus identifies an uncommon coding variant that affects mRNA expression and protects from bladder cancer. Hum Mol Genet 2012;21(8):1918—30. Available from: http://dx.doi.org/10.1093/hmg/ddr619.

[41]   Jongstra-Bilen J, Jongstra J. Leukocyte-specific protein 1 (LSP1): a regulator of leukocyte emigration in inflammation. Immunol Res 2006;35(1—2):65—74. Available from: http://dx.doi.org/10.1385/IR:35:1:65.

[42]   Figueroa JD, Ye Y, Siddiq A, Garcia-Closas M, Chatterjee N, Prokunina-olsson L, et al. Genome-wide association study identifies multiple loci associated with bladder cancer risk. Hum Mol Genet 2014;23(5). Available from: http://dx.doi.org/10.1093/hmg/ddt519.

[43]   Conticello SG. The AID/APOBEC family of nucleic acid mutators. Genome Biol 2008;9(6):229. Available from: http://dx.doi.org/10.1186/gb-2008-9-6-229.

[44]   Middlebrooks CD, Banday AR, Matsuda K, Udquim K-I, Onabajo OO, Paquin A, et al. Association of germline variants in the APOBEC3 region with cancer risk and enrichment with APOBEC-signature mutations in tumors. Nat Genet 2016;48(11). Available from: http://dx.doi.org/10.1038/ng.3670.

[45]   Wogan GN, Hecht SS, Felton JS, Conney AH, Loeb LA. Environmental and chemical carcinogenesis. Semin Cancer Biol 2004. Available from: http://dx.doi.org/10.1016/j.semcancer.2004.06.010.

[46]   Boobis AR, Lynch AM, Murray S, de la Torre R, Solans A, Farre M, et al. CYP1A2-catalyzed conversion of dietary heterocyclic amines to their proximate carcinogens is their major route of metabolism in humans. Cancer Res 1994;54(1):89—94.

[47]   Amin N, Byrne E, Johnson J, Chenevix-Trench G, Walter S, Nolte IM, et al. Genome-wide association analysis of coffee drinking suggests association with CYP1A1/CYP1A2 and NRCAM. Mol Psychiatry 2012;17(11):1116—29. Available from: http://dx.doi.org/10.1038/mp.2011.101.

[48]   Cornelis MC, Byrne EM, Esko T, Nalls MA, Ganna A, Paynter N, et al. Genome-wide meta-analysis identifies six novel loci associated with habitual coffee consumption. Mol Psychiatry 2015;20(5):647—56. Available from: http://dx.doi.org/10.1038/mp.2014.107.

[49]   Cornelis MC, Monda KL, Yu K, Paynter N, Azzato EM, Bennett SN, et al. Genome-wide meta-analysis identifies regions on 7p21 (AHR) and 15q24 (CYP1A2) as determinants of

habitual caffeine consumption. PLoS Genet 2011;7(4). Available from: http://dx.doi.org/10.1371/journal.pgen.1002033.

[50] Figueroa JD, Malats N, Real FX, Silverman D, Kogevinas M, Chanock S, et al. Genetic variation in the base excision repair pathway and bladder cancer risk. Hum Genet 2007;121(2):233–42. Available from: http://dx.doi.org/10.1007/s00439-006-0294-y.

[51] García-Closas M, Malats N, Real FX, Welch R, Kogevinas M, Chatterjee N, et al. Genetic variation in the nucleotide excision repair pathway and bladder cancer risk. Cancer Epidemiol Biomark Prevent: Public Am Assoc Cancer Res Cosponsor Am Soc Prevent Oncol 2006;15(3):536–42. Available from: http://dx.doi.org/10.1158/1055-9965. EPI-05-0749.

[52] López de Maturana E, Ye Y, Calle ML, Rothman N, Urrea V, Kogevinas M, et al. Application of multi-SNP approaches Bayesian LASSO and AUC-RF to detect main effects of inflammatory-gene variants associated with bladder cancer risk. PLoS One 2013;8(12):e83745. Available from: http://dx.doi.org/10.1371/journal.pone.0083745.

[53] Guey LT, García-Closas M, Murta-Nascimento C, Lloreta J, Palencia L, Kogevinas M, et al. Genetic susceptibility to distinct bladder cancer subphenotypes. Eur Urol 2010;57 (2):283–92. Available from: http://dx.doi.org/10.1016/j.eururo.2009.08.001.

[54] Lin J, Spitz MR, Dinney CP, Etzel CJ, Grossman HB, Wu X. Bladder cancer risk as modified by family history and smoking. Cancer 2006;107(4):705–11. Available from: http://dx.doi.org/10.1002/cncr.22071.

[55] Masaoka H, Ito H, Soga N, Hosono S, Oze I, Watanabe M, et al. Aldehyde dehydrogenase 2 (ALDH2) and alcohol dehydrogenase 1B (ADH1B) polymorphisms exacerbate bladder cancer risk associated with alcohol drinking: gene–environment interaction. Carcinogenesis 2016;37(6):583–8. Available from: http://dx.doi.org/10.1093/carcin/bgw033.

[56] van Dijk B, van Houwelingen KP, Witjes JA, Schalken JA, Kiemeney LA. Alcohol dehydrogenase type 3 (ADH3) and the risk of bladder cancer. Eur Urol 2001;40(5):509–14.

[57] Andrew AS, Mason RA, Kelsey KT, Schned AR, Marsit CJ, Nelson HH, et al. DNA repair genotype interacts with arsenic exposure to increase bladder cancer risk. Toxicol Lett 2009;187(1):10–14. Available from: http://dx.doi.org/10.1016/j.toxlet.2009.01.013.

[58] López de Maturana EL, Chanok SJ, Picornell AC, Rothman N, Herranz J, Calle ML, et al. Whole genome prediction of bladder cancer risk with the Bayesian LASSO. Genet Epidemiol 2014;38(5):467–76. Available from: http://dx.doi.org/10.1002/gepi.21809.

[59] Sylvester RJ, Van Der Meijden APM, Oosterlinck W, Witjes JA, Bouffioux C, Denis L, et al. Predicting recurrence and progression in individual patients with stage Ta T1 bladder cancer using EORTC risk tables: a combined analysis of 2596 patients from seven EORTC trials. Eur Urol 2006;49(3):466–75. Available from: http://dx.doi.org/10.1016/j.eururo.2005.12.031.

[60] Grotenhuis AJ, Dudek AM, Verhaegh GW, Witjes JA, Aben KK, Van Der Marel SL, et al. Prognostic relevance of urinary bladder cancer susceptibility loci. PLoS One 2014;9 (2). Available from: http://dx.doi.org/10.1371/journal.pone.0089164.

[61] Masson-Lecomte A, López de Maturana E, Goddard ME, Picornell AC, Rava M, González-Neira A, et al. Inflammatory-related genetic variants in non–muscle-invasive bladder cancer prognosis: a multimarker Bayesian assessment. Cancer Epidemiol Biomarkers Prev 2016;25(7):1144–50.

[62] Sylvester RJ. How well can you actually predict which non-muscle-invasive bladder cancer patients will progress?. Eur Urol 2011;60(3):431–3. Available from: http://dx.doi.org/10.1016/j.eururo.2011.06.001.

[63] Lopez de Maturana E, Picornell A, Masson-Lecomte A, Kogevinas M, Marquez M, Carrato A, et al. Prediction of non-muscle invasive bladder cancer outcomes assessed by innovative multimarker prognostic models. BMC Cancer 2016;16(1):351. Available from: http://dx.doi.org/10.1186/s12885-016-2361-7.

[64] Egbers L, Grotenhuis AJ, Aben KK, Alfred Witjes J, Kiemeney LA, Vermeulen SH. The prognostic value of family history among patients with urinary bladder cancer. Int J Cancer 2015;136(5):1117—24. Available from: http://dx.doi.org/10.1002/ijc.29062.

Chapter 34

CRISPR-Genome Editing

Yuchen Liu
Shenzhen Second People's Hospital, The First Affiliated Hospital of Shenzhen University, Shenzhen, P.R. China

Chapter Outline

INTRODUCTION TO CRISPR TECHNOLOGY

CRISPR/Cas is a kind of adaptive immune defense system used by bacteria and archaea during the long-term evolution [1]. In *Streptococcus pyogenes*, CRISPR/9 (Cas-associated protein 9, Cas9), a component of CRISPR/Cas II, is the only enzyme that is required for the function of CRISPR/Cas II. The short-guide RNA (sgRNA) and the Protospacer Adjacent Motif (PAM) module codetermine the DNA specificity of Cas9 [1,2]. The Cas9 protein cleaves the double-stranded DNA at the target site of the gRNA leader sequence and induces nonhomologous end joining or homologous recombination, causing DNA insertion or deletion to the cleavage site and leading to inactivation of the target gene [3]. The mutant Cas9 (deactivated Cas9, dCas9), which losses the nuclease activity, binds to the DNA target site and functions as an RNA-mediated artificial transcription factor for regulating gene expression [4,5]. dCas9 protein can also be fused to other functional domains to induce point mutation, single-base modification and gene editing [6−9].

Bladder Cancer. DOI: http://dx.doi.org/10.1016/B978-0-12-809939-1.00034-5

REPURPOSED CRISPRs FOR TREATING BLADDER CANCER

There are many oncogenes and tumor suppressor genes in human bladder cancer that have undergone genetic and epigenetic changes [10−12]. They can effectively manipulate the malignant biological behavior of cancer cells and will be helpful for cancer research and biotherapy. The CRISPR-Cas9-based applications will lead to a technological change in the field of cancer research and treatment. The technology can quickly simulate the genetic events in cancer and establish cancer models to help understand the mechanism of tumor development and metastasis [13,14]. This gene-editing technology can also be used to reconstruct immune cells for cancer immunotherapy [15,16].

In order to apply the repurposed CRISPR technology to identify and treat bladder cancer, our team has also done the following works:

Logic AND Gates for Identifying Bladder Cancers and Suppressing Malignant Phenotypes

Many years of clinical practices found that traditional treatments for bladder cancer, such as radiotherapy, chemotherapy, and surgical treatment, usually lack specificity and efficiency. Therefore there are many defects in the clinical applications, although some new targeted therapy-based drugs have been developed during recent years. These current therapies cannot meet the huge demand for treatment of many patients with bladder cancer. The previous works have explored a large number of genetic targets that have potential application values in the diagnosis or control of bladder cancer. On the basis of these biological targets, we set out to use the CRISPR-tools to build novel artificial biological devices that target a combination of cancer-related genes, thus improving the identification and control of bladder cancer. One latest work of our group has used CRISPR-Cas9 to construct a logical "AND" gate circuit [17] that can recognize and kill bladder cancer cells in vitro (Fig. 34.1).

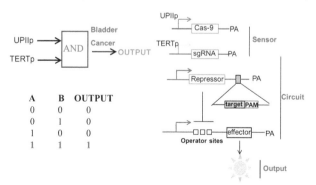

FIGURE 34.1   Logic AND gates for identifying and killing bladder cancer. The AND gate circuit based on CRISPR−Cas9 system integrates cellular information from two promoters as inputs and activates the output gene only when both inputs are active in the bladder cancer cells.

The construct utilizes a bladder cell-specific promoter (UPIIp) and a tumor cell-specific promoter (TERTp) as the sensors that response to various endogenous transcriptional signals. In principle, only in the bladder cancer cells, the two input promoters can be activated at the same time and effectively drive the expression of the downstream effector gene (output). Other tissue-derived cells or normal cells cannot be influenced. Using the luciferase reporter as the output gene, we demonstrated that this construct can specifically recognize the differences between bladder cancer cells and other types of cells, such as cervical cancer cell HeLa, lung cancer cell A549, prostate cancer cell PC3, normal spermatogenic cell GC-1, and normal fibroblast epithelial cells, and significantly increased luciferase expression. By using other cell functional genes including hBAX, p21, and E-cadherin as the outputs, this construct can effectively slow down the growth rate of bladder cancer cells, induce it to enter the suicide program, and decrease its migration ability. This method provides a CRISPR platform for targeting and controlling bladder cancer cells in vitro. In the future, we will try to use this construct for in vivo treatment of mice suffering from bladder cancer, and further test and optimize its specific killing ability.

CRISPR Signal Conductors for Reprogramming Bladder Cancer Cells

Our group has developed another tool for directing cancer signals based on CRISPR-dCas9 [18], which enables directional control of different proteins and complex molecular networks. By integrating the riboswitch from the bacterial metabolic control system into the sgRNA, the leader sequence of the recombinant sgRNA binds to the aptamer stem in the absence of a specific signal, resulting in the sgRNA being at the close state. When there is a cancer signal within the cell, the sgRNA structure changes and then the closed state is released—the sgRNA leader sequence pairs with its target DNA, and exerts transcriptional activation and suppression activities (Fig. 34.2).

In the specific anticancer studies, our team modified the RNA component of the CRISPR-Cas9 system and activated it by a signal NPM that normally promotes bladder tumor growth. The activated CRISPR-Cas9 system then introduced the transcription activator VP64 into the promoter regions of the two tumor suppressor genes p21 and p53, which consistently induce cell growth arrest. Using the same strategy the transcription factor Ets-1, which promotes the migration of bladder tumor cells, has been used to "unlock" sgRNA, and then the transcription of the tumor migration suppressor gene E-cadherin was activated by VP64 to inhibit the migration of bladder cancer cells.

In another case, we reprogramed the tumor cells to respond to the expression of NF-κB and β-catenin: activating Bax and inhibiting Bcl2 expression

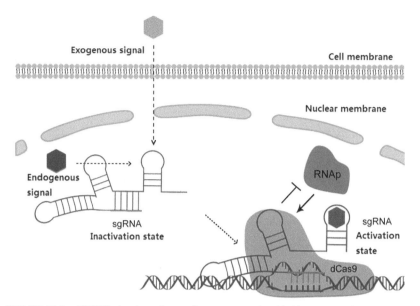

FIGURE 34.2   CRISPR signal conductors for reprogramming bladder cancer cells. By extending sgRNAs to include modified riboswitches that recognize specific signals, the CRISPR—cas9-based "signal conductors" regulate transcription of endogenous genes in response to external or internal signals of interest.

to promote programmed cell death. It was found that nude mice bearing these reprogrammed cells had much smaller tumors than those in the control group. Since normal cells do not have cancer cell-specific signaling molecules NF-κB and β-catenin, so they are almost unaffected. CRISPR technology has achieved significant results in identifying and interfering with tumors, demonstrating their potential useful applications, providing a powerful gene-editing tool for bladder cancer diagnosis and treatment.

An Efficient Light-Inducible P53 Expression System for Inhibiting Bladder Cancer

The light-controlled Cas9 expression device [19] mainly includes gene anchoring element (dCas9-CIB1 fusion protein), transcriptional activation element (CRY2-AD fusion protein), sgRNA vector, and reporter/effect gene vector (Fig. 34.3). In the dark the gene anchoring element is bound to the target sequence (gene promoter sequence) under the guidance of the sgRNA, while the transcriptional activator is dispersed across the nucleus; when the blue light is irradiated, CRY2 and CIBI are bound together, and the transcriptional activation domain is recruited near the target sequence (promoter) to activate the expression of the downstream gene.

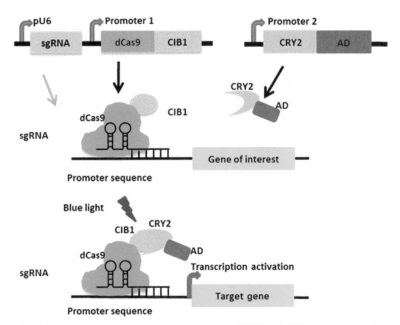

FIGURE 34.3 Cas9-based light-inducible P53 system. CRY2 and CIBI are bound together and the transcriptional activation domain is recruited near the target sequence (promoter) to activate the expression of the downstream gene only when the blue light is irradiated.

Further studies showed that the device cannot only control the reporter gene in bladder cancer cells, but also drive the effector gene in bladder cancer cells. The expression of reporter gene and effector gene is also increased with the enhancement of light dose. The light can significantly increase the expression of P53 protein in bladder cancer cells and upregulate the downstream P21 gene, which means that light-induced P53 can play a corresponding function.

We used CCK-8 and EDU assays to study the effect of light-controlled P53 expression system on the growth of bladder cancer cells. The results showed that this device could significantly inhibit the growth of bladder cancer cells 5637 and UMUC-3.

FUTURE PERSPECTIVES

CRISPR-Cas9 still cannot be used directly in clinical research and treatment due to the lack of a compact expression system. Traditional CRISPR-Cas9 gene-editing system uses the lentiviral vector, which causes random integration of the genome and has low biosafety [20]. In contrast the adeno-associated virus (AAV) is not integrated into the genome. It cannot cause the side effects on human body and can regulate the long-term stable expression of the genes [21]. It is the preferred choice for bladder cancer treatment.

However, the length of the Cas9 coding gene and its expression control sequence is too large and the DNA load capacity of AAV virus is limited (typically less than 4.7 kb). Some studies have attempted to use the "intein" to break down the Cas9 protein into multiple components [22−24], each of which is carried by the AAV vector. But this greatly reduces the expression stability of the Cas9−sgRNA complex within the cells. How to "reduce" the CRISPR-Cas9 expression system and overcome the limitation of AAV loading capacity is an urgent problem to be solved in Cas9−sgRNA system.

At present, many teams have also prepared to create CRISPR/Cas9-mediated PD-1 gene knockout T cells for clinical trials [25]. However, these T cells should be in a state of continuous activation through this way and continuously secret many lymphatic factors, thus causing a lot of toxic side effects. So the specificity and safety of this technology need to be further improved. Conditional control of PD-1 expression may be an effective way to solve the above problems. Therefore how to design intelligent T cells which dynamically respond to tumor environment and quantitatively regulate PD-1 expression will be the key scientific issue in future cancer cell therapy.

REFERENCES

[1] Jinek M, et al. A programmable dual-RNA—guided DNA endonuclease in adaptive bacterial immunity. Science 2012;337:816−22.

[2] Fu Y, Sander JD, Reyon D, Cascio VM, Joung JK. Improving CRISPR-Cas nuclease specificity using truncated guide RNAs. Nat Biotechnol 2014;32:279−84.

[3] Cong L, et al. Multiplex genome engineering using CRISPR/Cas systems. Science 2013;339:819−23.

[4] Tanenbaum ME, Gilbert LA, Qi LS, Weissman JS, Vale RD. A protein-tagging system for signal amplification in gene expression and fluorescence imaging. Cell 2014;159:635−46.

[5] Chavez A, et al. Highly efficient Cas9-mediated transcriptional programming. Nat Methods 2015;12:326−8.

[6] Hilton IB, et al. Epigenome editing by a CRISPR-Cas9-based acetyltransferase activates genes from promoters and enhancers. Nat Biotechnol 2015;33:510−17.

[7] Ma Y, et al. Targeted AID-mediated mutagenesis (TAM) enables efficient genomic diversification in mammalian cells. Nat Methods 2016;13:1029−35.

[8] Guilinger JP, Thompson DB, Liu DR. Fusion of catalytically inactive Cas9 to FokI nuclease improves the specificity of genome modification. Nat Biotechnol 2014;32:577−82.

[9] Komor AC, Kim YB, Packer MS, Zuris JA, Liu DR. Programmable editing of a target base in genomic DNA without double-stranded DNA cleavage. Nature 2016;533:420−4.

[10] Dong L, Lin F, Wu W, et al. Transcriptional cofactor Mask2 is required for YAP-induced cell growth and migration in bladder cancer cell. J Cancer 2016;7:2132.

[11] Liu L, Liu Y, Zhang X, et al. Inhibiting cell migration and cell invasion by silencing the transcription factor ETS-1 in human bladder cancer. Oncotarget 2016;7:25125.

[12] Zhan Y, Liu Y, Lin J, et al. Synthetic Tet-inducible artificial microRNAs targeting β-catenin or HIF-1α inhibit malignant phenotypes of bladder cancer cells T24 and 5637. Sci Reports 2015;5:16177.

[13]   Xue W, Chen S, Yin H, et al. CRISPR-mediated direct mutation of cancer genes in the mouse liver. Nature 2014;514:380−4.

[14]   Chen S, Sanjana NE, Zheng K, et al. Genome-wide CRISPR screen in a mouse model of tumor growth and metastasis. Cell 2015;160:1246−60.

[15]   Osborn MJ, Webber BR, Knipping F, et al. Evaluation of TCR gene editing achieved by TALENs, CRISPR/Cas9, and megaTAL nucleases. Mol Ther 2016;24:570−81.

[16]   Chen YY. Efficient gene editing in primary human T cells. Trends Immunol 2015; 36:667−9.

[17]   Liu Y, Zeng Y, Liu L, et al. Synthesizing AND gate genetic circuits based on CRISPR-Cas9 for identification of bladder cancer cells. Nat Commun 2014;5:5393.

[18]   Liu Y, Zhan Y, Chen Z, et al. Directing cellular information flow via CRISPR signal conductors. Nat Methods 2016;13:938−44.

[19]   Lin F, Dong L, Wang W, et al. An efficient light-inducible P53 expression system for inhibiting proliferation of bladder cancer cell. Int J Biol Sci 2016;12:1273.

[20]   Schambach A, Zychlinski D, Ehrnstroem B, Baum C. Biosafety features of lentiviral vectors. Hum Gene Ther 2013;24:132−42.

[21]   Balakrishnan B, Jayandharan GR. Basic biology of adeno-associated virus (AAV) vectors used in gene therapy. Curr Gene Ther 2014;14:86−100.

[22]   Ma D, Peng S, Xie Z. Integration and exchange of split dCas9 domains for transcriptional controls in mammalian cells. Nat Commun 2016;7:100084.

[23]   Chew WL, et al. A multifunctional AAV−CRISPR−Cas9 and its host response. Nat Methods 2016;13:868−74.

[24]   Zetsche B, Volz SE, Zhang F. A split-Cas9 architecture for inducible genome editing and transcription modulation. Nat Biotechnol 2015;33:9−11.

[25]   Cyranoski D. Chinese scientists to pioneer first human CRISPR trial. Nature 2016; 535:476−7.

Chapter 35

Personalized Medicine

Garrett M. Dancik[1] and Dan Theodorescu[2]
[1]*Eastern Connecticut State University, Willimantic, CT, United States,* [2]*University of Colorado, Aurora, CO, United States*

Chapter Outline

INTRODUCTION

Personalized medicine in cancer is based on our understanding of cancer as a genomic disease driven by somatic DNA mutations [1]. Unlike current standard of care treatments guided primarily by considering clinicopathological features, personalized medicine in cancer involves developing and tailoring treatments based on the genomic alterations that drive and maintain tumor growth (Table 35.1). As a result, personalized medicine will optimize treatment efficacy while minimizing excess risk, treatment toxicities, and unnecessary medical costs. The promise of personalized medicine is to improve healthcare by reliably determining the following: whether a particular individual has an elevated risk of developing cancer, and whether aggressive prevention or detection strategies are warranted (see Section "Diagnosis" in Chapter 8: Bladder Cancer: Imaging); what primary treatment would be most appropriate for a cancer patient; whether a cancer patient would benefit by adjuvant treatments; and if adjuvant treatment is warranted, what regimen and dosage are most appropriate.

Bladder Cancer. DOI: http://dx.doi.org/10.1016/B978-0-12-809939-1.00035-7

TABLE 35.1 Paradigms in Personalized Medicine

Paradigm	Example
Rational drug development	The identification of a BCR-ABL fusion protein in patients with CML led to the screening of inhibitors for this alteration and the subsequent development of the kinase inhibitor imatinib mesylate (Gleevec) [2].
Personalized treatment based on biomarkers of prognosis and response to therapy	For patients with node-negative, estrogen-receptor-positive breast cancer, *Oncotype* DX calculates the likelihood of recurrence as well as the likely benefit from chemotherapy, informing treatment for these patients [3].
Personalized treatment using targeted therapies	For patients with nonsmall-cell lung cancer harboring epidermal growth factor receptor (EGFR) mutations, recommended first-line therapies include tyrosine kinase inhibitors such as gefitinib that target EGFR. Notably, the effectiveness of gefitinib was realized only after identifying EGFR as a predictive biomarker and selecting patients on the basis of EGFR mutation status [4].

Treatments targeted at specific molecular lesions in cancer are a foundation of the personalized medicine paradigm. Emblematic of this is the rational development of imatinib mesylate (Gleevec) for patients with chronic myeloid leukemia (CML). The development of this highly effective therapy began with the identification of the genomic driver of CML, the "Philadelphia chromosome" containing a BCR-ABL gene fusion [5,6]. A chemical screen for compounds that inhibited BCR-ABL led to the development of the kinase inhibitor imatinib mesylate. When evaluated in a phase III clinical trial, CML patients treated with imatinib mesylate had an 89% 5-year survival rate, demonstrating the high efficacy of the drug [2]. The rational development of this targeted therapy serves as a model for personalized medicine in other cancer types, though the success of imatinib mesylate in CML patients can be attributed, in part, to the fact that approximately 95% of CML patients have a BCR-ABL fusion protein. The personalized treatment of bladder cancer, like CML and other cancers, will be rooted in our understanding of its genomic basis. However, the genomic landscape and hence the genetic drivers of bladder cancer are more complex (see next section) making personalized medicine for this disease more difficult.

BLADDER CANCER IS A GENOMIC DISEASE

Technological advances within the past ∼20 years have led to the development of high-throughput technologies for genome-wide profiling of samples at the genomic, transcriptomic, proteomic, and epigenetic levels. As a result, bladder and other cancers have been characterized based on these molecular profiles. Each technology has its own set of strengths and limitations [7]. Gene expression microarrays can simultaneously measure the mRNA or miRNA expression of large numbers of genes, but can only detect molecules whose sequences are known, and can only differentiate between molecules at the nucleotide sequence level. Protein microarrays, in comparison, can detect phosphorylation and other posttranslational modifications, but require antibodies for proteins of interest and are not robust against the large dynamic range of protein concentrations found in the cell. Next-generation sequencing (NGS) methods use sequencing-by-synthesis approaches to sequence DNA or RNA. RNA-seq uses NGS to measure the amount of RNA in a sample. Although NGS technologies were once cost-prohibitive, costing $100 million to sequence a genome in 2001, the decrease in sequencing costs has far outpaced Moore's Law, with the cost to sequence a single genome hovering slightly above $1000 at the time of this writing [8]. Compared with microarrays, RNA-seq is better able to detect low abundant transcripts and can detect important variants [9]. However, microarrays are less costly and will continue to be used as long as their costs relative to RNA-seq technologies remain low.

The comprehensive molecular profiling of bladder tumors is the basis for the identification of prognostic biomarkers, predictive biomarkers, and molecular targets for personalized treatment, which are discussed in the remaining sections. To aid in biomarker discovery and evaluation, molecular profiles of bladder and other cancer types are publicly available. The Cancer Genome Atlas (TCGA; http://cancergenome.nih.gov) is a database of "omic" (genomic, transcriptomic, proteomic, and epigenomic) profiles for a large number of cancer types (currently 33). The Gene Expression Omnibus (GEO; http://www.ncbi.nlm.nih.gov/geo/) is a repository of gene expression studies involving patients, cell lines, and mice with >12,000 containing the keyword "cancer." The public availability of molecular cancer profiles aids in the discovery of cancer biomarkers and the advancement of personalized medicine.

For example, molecular profiling informs us that nonmuscle invasive (NMI) and muscle-invasive (MI) bladder tumors have unique mutational profiles [10], with *TP53* mutations found in approximately 50% of high-grade MI tumors [11], and *FGFR3* mutations found in ∼70% of low-grade NMI tumors [12]. The histone demethylase *KDM6A* is also more frequently mutated in NMI tumors [13]. The genomic landscape of bladder cancer is complex. An analysis of 131 chemotherapy-naïve bladder cancer patients with high-grade MI tumors found that each patient had, on average, 302 exonic mutations and 22 genomic rearrangements. Overall, recurrent somatic mutations were found in 32 genes [11]. In a separate whole genome analysis of 99 patients, investigators identified 37 significantly mutated genes [13], suggesting that bladder cancer has a large number of driver mutations. Significantly mutated genes include *TP53, KDM6A, ARID1A, EP300, HRAS, RB1, MLL2, PIK3CA,* and *STAG2,* among others. The large number of possible genomic drivers in bladder cancer has important implications for personalized treatment, since unlike targeted treatment of CML, a single-targeted therapy is unlikely to improve disease outcome for a majority of patients. Instead, drug cocktails will likely be needed in the personalized treatment of bladder cancer.

MOLECULAR BIOMARKERS PREDICT PATIENT PROGNOSIS AND INFORM TREATMENT NECESSITY

Molecular biomarkers (DNA, RNA, protein, metabolic, etc.) can stratify patients into low- and high-risk groups based on disease outcome in the absence of systemic treatment. Such biomarkers identify patients likely to benefit from aggressive therapy so that low-risk patients can be spared from the burden of unnecessary treatments. For example, *Oncotype* DX is a commercially available prognostic tool for breast cancer patients that identifies patients at high-risk of recurrence based on the gene expression of 21 genes, and helps inform patients about the appropriateness of chemotherapy [3]. Standard of care treatments in bladder cancer is based predominantly on whether the tumor is NMI or MI (see Chapter 4: Symptoms, and Chapter 5: Physical Examination). But treatment strategies could be better tailored to individual patients by identifying patients with NMI tumors that have a high-risk of progression and patients with MI tumors that have a high-risk of metastasis. Although patients with NMI tumors generally have >90% 5-year survival rates, progression to MI disease occurs in ~20% of these patients leading to 5-year survival rates of ~43% [14]. Not surprisingly, this is similar to that of patients initially diagnosed with MI tumors [15].

Early attention focused on identifying individual prognostic biomarkers. Examples include high EGFR expression and the accumulation of nuclear p53, both associated with progression [16,17]. COX-2 positive immunohistochemical staining is associated with the extent of lymph node involvement in patients with MI tumors. However, COX-2 was not significantly associated with outcome in these patients [18]. For cell-cycle−related biomarkers such as p53 and RB1, it is now appreciated that multigene biomarkers perform better than individual ones [19]. The Bladder Cancer Biomarker Evaluation

Tool (*BC-BET*) and the cBioPortal for Cancer Genomics are complementary tools for the rapid evaluation of individual candidate prognostic biomarkers in bladder cancer. Both tools integrate molecular and clinical data from genomic resources so that users can quickly analyze a gene of interest across multiple bladder cancer patient cohorts. *BC-BET* evaluates whether the expression of a selected gene is significantly associated with outcome (as well as stage, grade, and cancer) [20], while the cBioPortal evaluates whether mutation status or copy number is associated with outcome in multiple cancer types including bladder cancer [21].

Although multigene prognostic biomarkers have been identified from high-throughput gene expression profiling studies, the identification of robust and clinically useful multigene biomarkers (gene signatures) has remained elusive. Notably, a validation study found that of six published survival signatures, none performed better than chance when evaluated in independent datasets [22]. However, a more recent analysis found that cell-cycle–related genes are consistently associated with outcome in bladder cancer and that a specific 31-gene cell cycle proliferation (CCP) signature was predictive of progression and survival in all bladder cancer cohorts analyzed [23]. To have clinical utility, however, molecular biomarkers must be prognostic in multivariate analyses that include readily available clinicopathological variables such as stage and grade. The identification of such biomarkers has proved difficult. The CCP signature, for example, is not prognostic in patients with high-grade MI tumors [24]. However, CCP alone may be a better predictor of outcome than stage or grade, raising the intriguing concept of staging and grading cancers based on their molecular pathology [23]. Other promising signatures include a 20-gene signature that predicts nodal involvement in patients at cystectomy [25], and a (separate) 20-gene signature that predicts recurrence free survival in MI patients, and improves the predictive accuracy of a postradical cystectomy nomogram that includes stage and grade [26]. In MI bladder cancer, the identification of basal and luminal molecular subtypes that resemble their breast cancer counterparts, and that are associated with disease outcome, has important implications for personalized treatment [27,28]. However, for all published gene signatures so far, prospective validation in multivariate analyses to assess clinical utility is required.

MOLECULAR BIOMARKERS PREDICT PATIENT RESPONSE TO SYSTEMIC THERAPY AND INFORM TREATMENT SELECTION

Cisplatinum-based combination neoadjuvant chemotherapy is recommended for patients with MI disease, based on a clinical trial finding a complete response rate of ~38% [29] and a meta-analysis finding an absolute disease-free survival benefit of 9% at 5 years in these patients [30]. However, the proportion of patients who receive neoadjuvant chemotherapy is <16% [31,32]. This limited use of neoadjuvant chemotherapy can be partly attributed to the ineligibility of patients with poor renal function [33], but also the reluctance of clinicians to administer chemotherapy in patients, most of which (91%) will likely not benefit. The standard treatment for metastatic bladder cancer is cisplatinum-based combination chemotherapy with close to a 50% response rate [34]. In addition, a meta-analysis involving 945 patients across 9 clinical trials found that adjuvant chemotherapy is associated with higher overall and disease-specific survival rates [35]. In all three settings, predictive biomarkers would identify patients most likely to respond to specific treatments and nonresponders for which novel treatments may be more appropriate.

The number of promising single-gene predictive biomarkers in bladder cancer is limited. Perhaps the most promising biomarker is p53, an appealing chemotherapy biomarker because of its role in DNA repair, cell cycle regulation, and apoptosis [36]. However, a phase III trial evaluating the predictive ability of p53 expression in patients randomized to receive either methotrexate, vinblastine, doxorubicin (Adriamycin), and cisplatinum (MVAC) adjuvant chemotherapy or observation did not find a statistically significant difference in disease-specific survival rates between the two arms [37]. However, several limitations of this trial have been acknowledged, including a high refusal rate for randomization, a lower than expected event rate, failure to complete treatment, and a higher number of p53-positive patients than expected, likely due to changes in immunohistochemistry technology during the trial [37,38]. Although no other predictive biomarkers have been prospectively evaluated, several other candidates have been identified. One candidate is multidrug resistance gene-1 (*MDR1*), which is an efflux pump that can export chemicals such as methotrexate across the cell membrane. A retrospective analysis of 108 patients with advanced bladder cancer that were enrolled in a phase III clinical trial (AUO-AB 05/95) found that high *MDR1* expression was significantly associated with poor survival in patients randomized to either adjuvant cisplatin + methotrexate (CM) or methotrexate, vinblastine, epirubicin, and cisplatin chemotherapy [39].

Similar to prognostic markers, panels of predictive biomarkers have been developed. The most common approach to identify multigene predictive biomarkers is by analyzing gene expression profiles of patients, and identifying genes (signatures) that are differentially expressed between responders and nonresponders to treatment. One promising multigene signature has been identified [40]. Gene expression profiles across ~27,000 genes were obtained from 27 patients with MI tumors who received neoadjuvant MVAC chemotherapy. A 14-gene signature was then identified that discriminated responders (downstaging to ≤pT1) and nonresponders (no downstaging; ≥pT2). When evaluated on an independent set of 22 patients, the signature correctly identified 100% of the responders and 73% of nonresponders, with all predicted responders surviving >2 years after MVAC treatment, compared to <50% of predicted nonresponders [41]. Although promising, this multigene MVAC signature still awaits prospective evaluation.

An appealing strategy for predictive biomarker identification and drug discovery involves the use of in vitro cell line models. Unlike studies involving human subjects, cell line models provide a cost-effective way of investigating newly discovered drugs and novel combination therapies, as well as monotherapies. Public resources of in vitro drug sensitivity data can be harnessed, such as the National Cancer Institute (NCI)-60 cell line screen that contains drug sensitivity data for more than 45,000 compounds, including 93 FDA-approved anticancer agents [42]. For these data, the COMPARE algorithm was developed to identify compounds having drug sensitivity associated with a compound or biomarker of interest. Another tool, the connectivity map (CMAP), extends this concept by identifying compounds associated with multigene biomarkers, based on perturbations of human cell lines [43]. Both tools are valuable resources for personalized medicine. An initial COMPARE analysis found that the compound bortezomib had a unique mechanism of action (which turned out to be protease inhibition), prompting additional investigation. Bortezomib was later FDA-approved to treat patients with multiple myeloma [44]. A CMAP analysis of glucocorticoid dexamethasone resistance biomarkers in acute lymphoblastic leukemia patients identified the FDA-approved mTOR inhibitor sirolimus, which follow-up studies found induce glucocorticoid sensitivity in malignant lymphoid cell lines [45].

Despite the advantages of in vitro models, cell lines may lack clinical utility as they are not always predictive of human therapeutic responses [46]. In order to address this limitation, an innovative strategy named COXEN (coexpression extrapolation) was devised (Fig. 35.1). COXEN first identifies predictive biomarkers from cell line models, then leverages patient gene expression data to identify those predictive biomarkers that are concordantly expressed between cell lines and patients. As a result, COXEN functions as a "Rosetta Stone" for translating drug activity from cell lines to drug activity in patient tumors. In initial studies, COXEN identified biomarkers of docetaxel and tamoxifen response in breast cancer, based on the NCI-60 drug sensitivity data. COXEN was also used in a discovery pipeline, which identified the agent C1311 as a potent inhibitor of bladder cancer cell lines [47]. Subsequent studies using COXEN identified a multigene signature that predicted response to neoadjuvant MVAC therapy in the cohort (described in references [40,41]) and response to MVAC therapy in 14 additional patients with locally advanced or metastatic disease. A national clinical trial in the United States is ongoing to prospectively evaluate a COXEN-derived biomarker signature as a tool for distinguishing responders from nonresponders following neoadjuvant treatment with dose-dense methotrexate, vinblastin, doxorubicin, and cisplatin (DDMVAC) and gemcitabine + cisplatin (GC) therapies (NCT02177695).

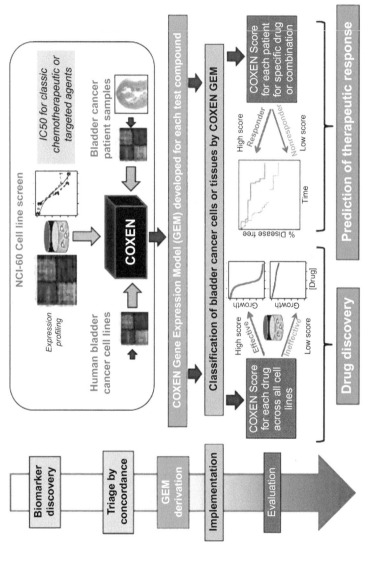

FIGURE 35.1 **The COXEN system for drug discovery and predictive biomarker identification.** Predictive biomarkers of therapeutic response are first identified from molecular profiles (e.g., gene expression) and in vitro drug sensitivity (e.g., from NCI-60) for a compound of interest. The list of predictive bio-markers is then refined, including only those biomarkers that are concordantly expressed between cell lines and patients. The list of concordant biomarkers is then used to classify patient or cell line samples as responders or nonresponders. COXEN scores for multiple compounds can be combined to predict responses to combination therapies. For drug discovery, COXEN scores can be calculated quickly for a large number of compounds, and compounds ranked by their predicted efficacy can be prioritized for further investigation. *From Smith SC, Baras AS, Lee JK, et al. Cancer Res 2010;70:1753−8.*

TARGETED THERAPIES IN BLADDER CANCER

A targeted therapy is a drug that suppresses tumor growth through recognition of a genomic alteration or dependency. Because the treatment specifically targets tumor cells, toxicity in the patient is minimized as normal cells are spared. The targeted therapy paradigm follows directly from our understanding of cancer as a genomic disease, where genomic alterations cause cancer cells to acquire "hallmark" characteristics such as sustained proliferative signaling and replicative immortality [48]. Currently, a large number of therapies targeting these cancer hallmarks are Food and Drug Administration (FDA)-approved or are being actively investigated [49]. Examples of approved targeted therapies include the aforementioned imatinib mesylate that targets BCR-ABL tyrosine kinase, the tyrosine kinase inhibitor gefitinib that targets EGFR mutations in nonsmall-cell lung and other cancers, the monoclonal antibody trastuzumab (Herceptin), which targets the HER-2 protein that is overexpressed in up to 25% of patients with invasive breast cancer [50], and vemurafenib (Zelboraf), which inhibits a specific BRAF mutant present in ~50% of melanoma patients [51].

The majority of bladder cancer patients have tumors with molecular targets that could potentially be inhibited by known therapies. Among the 131 patients with MI tumors described previously, therapeutic targets were identified in 69% of patients [11]. Of these patients, 42% had targets in the phosphoinositol 3-kinase/AKT/mechanistic target of rapamycin (PI3K/AKT/mTOR) pathway and 45% had targets in the receptor tyrosine kinase/mapkinase (RTK/MAPK) pathway. Specifically, patients with alterations in *PIK3CA* (17% of patients), *TSC1* or *TSC2* (9% of patients), and *AKT3* (10% of patients) would potentially respond to treatment by PI-3 kinase inhibitors, mTOR inhibitors, and AKT inhibitors, respectively. Similarly, patients with alterations in *FGFR3* (17% of patients), *EGFR* (9% of patients), *ERBB3* (6% of patients), and *ERBB2* (9% of patients) would potentially respond to treatments that inhibit their respective proteins. For patients with low-grade, NMI tumors, *FGFR3* and *RAS* alterations occur in approximately 30% to 40% and 70% of patients, respectively [10], and these patients would potentially respond to therapies that target the RTK-Ras pathway. In addition the recent finding that mutations in chromatin remodeling genes such as *KDM6A*, *ARID4A*, and *MLL* are common in bladder cancer [13] suggest that epigenetic alterations could be targeted.

The effectiveness of a targeted therapy across multiple tumor types has been evaluated in so-called "basket" studies that enroll patients with specific genomic alterations. One notable basket study evaluated vemurafenib in nonmelanoma patients with tumors harboring a *BRAF* V600 mutation. The study enrolled 122 patients and had 9 "baskets" for patients with nonsmall-cell lung cancer, ovarian cancer, colorectal cancer, cholangiocarcinoma, and others, as well as an "all others" category. The study found that in patients with this BRAF mutation, vemurafenib was effective in some but not all tumors. Notably, response rates were >40% in the 19 patients with nonsmall-cell lung cancer, and the 14 patients with Erdheim–Chester disease or Langerhans' cell histiocytosis, but was lower in other cancers, including colorectal cancers where none of the patients receiving vemurafenib monotherapy responded [52]. This study highlights an important challenge in the evaluation of targeted therapies, since their efficacy can depend on tissue type in addition to whether or not the molecular target is present.

The nature of clinical trials is such that promising drugs may be abandoned if a study-wide endpoint is not obtained, even if several individuals in the study have durable responses. However, the molecular characterization of tumors from patients enrolled in clinical trials may lead to the identification of predictive biomarkers for patients likely to respond. The identification of predictive biomarkers is necessary to ensure that the "right treatment" is given to the "right patient." An example in bladder cancer demonstrates the importance of molecular profiling in conjunction with drug evaluation. By conventional standards, a phase II clinical trial evaluating the mTOR inhibitor everolimus in patients with metastatic bladder cancer failed, as the trial did not reach its primary progression-free survival endpoint. However, one patient achieved a complete response and was investigated further. Whole genome sequencing of this patient found mutations in the mTOR pathway genes *TSC1* and *NF2*, suggesting that these genes were biomarkers of everolimus sensitivity. Subsequent genomic evaluation of 13 patients from the same clinical trial found that progression-free survival was higher in patients with *TSC1* mutations than those who were wild-type [53], and prospective evaluation of everolimus treatment in patients with *TSC1* mutations is now ongoing.

One of the most interesting and important developments in bladder cancer management is the resurgence of immunotherapy. The interaction between the bladder tumor and the immune response is complex and provides several potential therapeutic options such as immune checkpoint inhibitors. Immune checkpoints are molecules involved in the suppression of the immune response, and involve T-cell receptors such as cytotoxic T-lymphocyte-associated antigen 4 (CTL-4) and programmed death 1 (PD-1), and molecules such as PD-1 ligand (PD-L1), which can be expressed by tumors [54]. A clinical trial with ipilimumab, a monoclonal antibody that targets CTLA-4, was the first randomized trial to show a survival benefit in patients with advanced melanoma, where 60% of patients receiving ipilimumab sustained an objective response for at least 2 years, with an overall 2-year survival rate of 23.5% compared to 13.7% in patients not receiving ipilimumab [55]. In bladder cancer, PD-1 is overexpressed in tumor samples [56], and PD-L1 overexpression is associated with poor outcome [57], suggesting that immunotherapies targeting these proteins may be effective. Recently the PD-L1 inhibitor atezolizumab (Tecentriq) became the first

FDA-approved PD-L1 inhibitor, for patients with locally advanced or metastatic bladder cancer, following a clinical trial finding an objective response rate of 26% for patients with $\geq$5% of PD-L1 positive immune cells in the tumor microenvironment, and a response rate of 15% across all patients [58].

CONCLUSIONS AND CHALLENGES FOR PERSONALIZED MEDICINE IN BLADDER CANCER

We are moving toward a more personalized approach to bladder cancer treatment. Perhaps most promising, a large number of the genomic alterations that drive bladder cancer can be targeted by FDA-approved therapies, though it remains to be seen whether existing targeted therapies can be repositioned for the treatment of bladder cancer patients. Basket trials will partially answer this question. For targeted therapies, appropriate patient selection will be critical.

The identification of predictive biomarkers allows for the selection of patients likely to respond, and the identification of drugs that are efficacious in these enriched patient populations but would otherwise elicit poor responses in unselected populations. However, the identification of predictive biomarkers to cisplatinum-based chemotherapy may be more challenging. The difficulty in predicting response to chemotherapies has been acknowledged through classification studies carried out by the Microarray Quality Control Consortium, which found that for breast cancer patients, response to chemotherapy was more difficult to predict than other outcomes including sex, estrogen-receptor status, and survival [59], and that predictive biomarkers are less informative (i.e., have lower fold changes) than biomarkers for other endpoints [60]. In general, drug response may be difficult to predict due to the multiple mechanisms of drug resistance that exist, including those relating to drug transport, metabolism, and targeting [61].

The personalized treatment of bladder cancer will likely lead to better patient outcomes; however, few targeted therapies in use today result in lifetime remission of disease. Important challenges remain. Tumor heterogeneity and genomic instability are both hallmarks of cancer and contribute to drug resistance. Heterogeneous populations of tumor cells may include subclonal resistant populations that become dominant following treatment, though resistant cells can potentially be identified prior to treatment through single-cell—sequencing technologies [62]. Genomic instability allows tumor cells to become resistant following treatment by acquiring mutations that confer resistance. Combination therapies may be an effective strategy for preventing drug resistance from developing, as has been the case in the treatment of human immunodeficiency virus [63]. In addition, immunotherapy either alone or in combination with targeted agents may provide a significant therapeutic advance. The identification of appropriate combination therapies in bladder cancer will be a major challenge as personalized medicine in bladder cancer is realized.

REFERENCES

[1] Stratton MR, Campbell PJ, Futreal PA. The cancer genome. Nature 2009;458 (7239):719−24.

[2] Druker BJ, Guilhot F, O'Brien SG, Gathmann I, Kantarjian H, Gattermann N, et al. Five-year follow-up of patients receiving imatinib for chronic myeloid leukemia. N Engl J Med 2006;355(23):2408−17.

[3] Allison M. Is personalized medicine finally arriving? Nat Biotechnol 2008;26(5):509−17.

[4] Chan BA, Hughes BGM. Targeted therapy for non-small cell lung cancer: current standards and the promise of the future. Transl Lung Cancer Res 2015;4(1):36−54.

[5] Rowley JD. A new consistent chromosomal abnormality in chronic myelogenous leukaemia identified by quinacrine fluorescence and giemsa staining. Nature 1973;243 (5405):290−3.

[6] Shtivelman E, Lifshitz B, Gale RP, Canaani E. Fused transcript of ABL and BCR genes in chronic myelogenous leukaemia. Nature 1985;315(6020):550−4.

[7] Dancik GM, Theodorescu D. New approaches to personalized medicine and targeted drug discovery. In: Tan D, Lynch HT, editors. Principles of molecular diagnostics and personalized cancer medicine. Philadelphia, PA: Lippincott Williams & Wilkins; 2012.

[8] Wetterstrand KA. DNA sequencing costs: data from the NHGRI Genome Sequencing Program (GSP) [Internet], <www.genome.gov/sequencingcostsdata>; 2016 [accessed 02.06.16].

[9] Zhao S, Fung-Leung W-P, Bittner A, Ngo K, Liu X. Comparison of RNA-Seq and microarray in transcriptome profiling of activated T cells. PLoS One 2014;9(1):e78644.

[10] Wu X-R. Urothelial tumorigenesis: a tale of divergent pathways. Nat Rev Cancer 2005;5 (9):713−25.

[11] The Cancer Genome Atlas Research Network. Comprehensive molecular characterization of urothelial bladder carcinoma. Nature 2014;507(7492):315−22.

[12] van Rhijn BWG, van der Kwast TH, Vis AN, Kirkels WJ, Boevé ER, Jöbsis AC, et al. FGFR3 and P53 characterize alternative genetic pathways in the pathogenesis of urothelial cell carcinoma. Cancer Res 2004;64(6):1911−14.

[13] Guo G, Sun X, Chen C, Wu S, Huang P, Li Z, et al. Whole-genome and whole-exome sequencing of bladder cancer identifies frequent alterations in genes involved in sister chromatid cohesion and segregation. Nat Genet 2013;45(12):1459−63.

[14] Türkölmez K, Tokgöz H, Reşorlu B, Köse K, Bedük Y. Muscle-invasive bladder cancer: predictive factors and prognostic difference between primary and progressive tumors. Urology 2007;70(3):477−81.

[15] Siegel R, Naishadham D, Jemal A. Cancer statistics, 2013. CA Cancer J Clin 2013;63 (1):11−30.

[16] Lipponen P, Eskelinen M. Expression of epidermal growth factor receptor in bladder cancer as related to established prognostic factors, oncoprotein (c-erbB-2, p53) expression and long-term prognosis. Br J Cancer 1994;69(6):1120−5.

[17] Esrig D, Elmajian D, Groshen S, Freeman JA, Stein JP, Chen SC, et al. Accumulation of nuclear p53 and tumor progression in bladder cancer. N Engl J Med 1994;331 (19):1259−64.

[18] Naruse K, Yamada Y, Nakamura K, Aoki S, Taki T, Zennami K, et al. Potential of molecular targeted therapy of HER-2 and Cox-2 for invasive transitional cell carcinoma of the urinary bladder. Oncol Rep 2010;23(6):1577−83.

[19] Mitra AP, Hansel DE, Cote RJ. Prognostic value of cell-cycle regulation biomarkers in bladder cancer. Semin Oncol 2012;39(5):524−33.

[20] Dancik GM. An online tool for evaluating diagnostic and prognostic gene expression biomarkers in bladder cancer. BMC Urol 2015;15:59.

[21] Cerami E, Gao J, Dogrusoz U, Gross BE, Sumer SO, Aksoy BA, et al. The cBio cancer genomics portal: an open platform for exploring multidimensional cancer genomics data. Cancer Discov 2012;2(5):401−4.

[22] Lauss M, Ringnér M, Höglund M. Prediction of stage, grade, and survival in bladder cancer using genome-wide expression data: a validation study. Clin Cancer Res Off J Am Assoc Cancer Res 2010;16(17):4421−33.

[23] Dancik GM, Theodorescu D. Robust prognostic gene expression signatures in bladder cancer and lung adenocarcinoma depend on cell cycle related genes. PLoS One 2014;9(1): e85249.

[24] Dancik GM, Theodorescu D. The prognostic value of cell cycle gene expression signatures in muscle invasive, high-grade bladder cancer. Bladder Cancer 2015;1(1):45−63.

[25] Smith SC, Baras AS, Dancik G, Ru Y, Ding K-F, Moskaluk CA, et al. A 20-gene model for molecular nodal staging of bladder cancer: development and prospective assessment. Lancet Oncol 2011;12(2):137−43.

[26] Riester M, Taylor JM, Feifer A, Koppie T, Rosenberg JE, Downey RJ, et al. Combination of a novel gene expression signature with a clinical nomogram improves the prediction of survival in high-risk bladder cancer. Clin Cancer Res Off J Am Assoc Cancer Res 2012;18(5):1323−33.

[27] Choi W, Porten S, Kim S, Willis D, Plimack ER, Hoffman-Censits J, et al. Identification of distinct basal and luminal subtypes of muscle-invasive bladder cancer with different sensitivities to frontline chemotherapy. Cancer Cell 2014;25(2):152−65.

[28] Damrauer JS, Hoadley KA, Chism DD, Fan C, Tiganelli CJ, Wobker SE, et al. Intrinsic subtypes of high-grade bladder cancer reflect the hallmarks of breast cancer biology. Proc Natl Acad Sci 2014;111(8):3110−15.

[29] Grossman HB, Natale RB, Tangen CM, Speights VO, Vogelzang NJ, Trump DL, et al. Neoadjuvant chemotherapy plus cystectomy compared with cystectomy alone for locally advanced bladder cancer. N Engl J Med 2003;349(9):859−66.

[30] Advanced Bladder Cancer (ABC) Meta-analysis Collaboration. Neoadjuvant chemotherapy in invasive bladder cancer: update of a systematic review and meta-analysis of individual patient data advanced bladder cancer (ABC) meta-analysis collaboration. Eur Urol 2005;48(2):202-205-206.

[31] David KA, Milowsky MI, Ritchey J, Carroll PR, Nanus DM. Low incidence of perioperative chemotherapy for stage III bladder cancer 1998 to 2003: a report from the National Cancer Data Base. J Urol 2007;178(2):451−4.

[32] Johar RS, Hayn MH, Stegemann AP, Ahmed K, Agarwal P, Balbay MD, et al. Complications after robot-assisted radical cystectomy: results from the International Robotic Cystectomy Consortium. Eur Urol 2013;64(1):52−7.

[33] Canter D, Viterbo R, Kutikov A, Wong Y-N, Plimack E, Zhu F, et al. Baseline renal function status limits patient eligibility to receive perioperative chemotherapy for invasive bladder cancer and is minimally affected by radical cystectomy. Urology 2011;77 (1):160–5.

[34] von der Maase H, Hansen SW, Roberts JT, Dogliotti L, Oliver T, Moore MJ, et al. Gemcitabine and cisplatin versus methotrexate, vinblastine, doxorubicin, and cisplatin in advanced or metastatic bladder cancer: results of a large, randomized, multinational, multicenter, phase III study. J Clin Oncol Off J Am Soc Clin Oncol 2000;18(17):3068–77.

[35] Leow JJ, Martin-Doyle W, Rajagopal PS, Patel CG, Anderson EM, Rothman AT, et al. Adjuvant chemotherapy for invasive bladder cancer: a 2013 updated systematic review and meta-analysis of randomized trials. Eur Urol 2014;66(1):42–54.

[36] Ferreira CG, Tolis C, Giaccone G. p53 and chemosensitivity. Ann Oncol Off J Eur Soc Med Oncol 1999;10(9):1011–21.

[37] Stadler WM, Lerner SP, Groshen S, Stein JP, Shi S-R, Raghavan D, et al. Phase III study of molecularly targeted adjuvant therapy in locally advanced urothelial cancer of the bladder based on p53 status. J Clin Oncol Off J Am Soc Clin Oncol 2011;29(25):3443–9.

[38] Hilton WM, Svatek RS. Words of wisdom. Re: phase III study of molecularly targeted adjuvant therapy in locally advanced urothelial cancer of the bladder based on p53 status. Eur Urol 2012;61(5):1062–3.

[39] Hoffmann A-C, Wild P, Leicht C, Bertz S, Danenberg KD, Danenberg PV, et al. MDR1 and ERCC1 expression predict outcome of patients with locally advanced bladder cancer receiving adjuvant chemotherapy. Neoplasia 2010;12(8):628–36.

[40] Takata R, Katagiri T, Kanehira M, Tsunoda T, Shuin T, Miki T, et al. Predicting response to methotrexate, vinblastine, doxorubicin, and cisplatin neoadjuvant chemotherapy for bladder cancers through genome-wide gene expression profiling. Clin Cancer Res Off J Am Assoc Cancer Res 2005;11(7):2625–36.

[41] Takata R, Katagiri T, Kanehira M, Shuin T, Miki T, Namiki M, et al. Validation study of the prediction system for clinical response of M-VAC neoadjuvant chemotherapy. Cancer Sci 2007;98(1):113–17.

[42] Shoemaker RH. The NCI60 human tumour cell line anticancer drug screen. Nat Rev Cancer 2006;6(10):813–23.

[43] Lamb J, Crawford ED, Peck D, Modell JW, Blat IC, Wrobel MJ, et al. The Connectivity Map: using gene-expression signatures to connect small molecules, genes, and disease. Science 2006;313(5795):1929–35.

[44] Bai RL, Paull KD, Herald CL, Malspeis L, Pettit GR, Hamel E. Halichondrin B and homohalichondrin B, marine natural products binding in the vinca domain of tubulin. Discovery of tubulin-based mechanism of action by analysis of differential cytotoxicity data. J Biol Chem 1991;266(24):15882–9.

[45] Wei G, Twomey D, Lamb J, Schlis K, Agarwal J, Stam RW, et al. Gene expression-based chemical genomics identifies rapamycin as a modulator of MCL1 and glucocorticoid resistance. Cancer Cell 2006;10(4):331–42.

[46] Voskoglou-Nomikos T, Pater JL, Seymour L. Clinical predictive value of the in vitro cell line, human xenograft, and mouse allograft preclinical cancer models. Clin Cancer Res Off J Am Assoc Cancer Res 2003;9(11):4227–39.

[47] Lee JK, Havaleshko DM, Cho H, Weinstein JN, Kaldjian EP, Karpovich J, et al. A strategy for predicting the chemosensitivity of human cancers and its application to drug discovery. Proc Natl Acad Sci 2007;104(32):13086–91.

[48] Hanahan D, Weinberg RA. Hallmarks of cancer: the next generation. Cell 2011;144 (5):646–74.

[49] Overview of FDA-approved anti cancer drugs used for targeted therapy [Internet], World Cancer Research Journal, <http://www.wcrj.net/article/553>; 2015 [accessed 08.06.16].

[50] Ménard S, Casalini P, Campiglio M, Pupa S, Agresti R, Tagliabue E. HER2 overexpression in various tumor types, focussing on its relationship to the development of invasive breast cancer. Ann Oncol 2001;12(suppl 1):S15–19.

[51] Chapman PB, Hauschild A, Robert C, Haanen JB, Ascierto P, Larkin J, et al. Improved survival with vemurafenib in melanoma with BRAF V600E mutation. N Engl J Med 2011;364(26):2507–16.

[52] Hyman DM, Puzanov I, Subbiah V, Faris JE, Chau I, Blay J-Y, et al. Vemurafenib in multiple nonmelanoma cancers with BRAF V600 mutations. N Engl J Med 2015;373 (8):726–36.

[53] Iyer G, Hanrahan AJ, Milowsky MI, Al-Ahmadie H, Scott SN, Janakiraman M, et al. Genome sequencing identifies a basis for everolimus sensitivity. Science 2012;338 (6104):221.

[54] Mellman I, Coukos G, Dranoff G. Cancer immunotherapy comes of age. Nature 2011;480 (7378):480–9.

[55] Hodi FS, O'Day SJ, McDermott DF, Weber RW, Sosman JA, Haanen JB, et al. Improved survival with ipilimumab in patients with metastatic melanoma. N Engl J Med 2010;363 (8):711–23.

[56] Xylinas E, Robinson BD, Kluth LA, Volkmer BG, Hautmann R, Küfer R, et al. Association of T-cell co-regulatory protein expression with clinical outcomes following radical cystectomy for urothelial carcinoma of the bladder. Eur J Surg Oncol J Eur Soc Surg Oncol Br Assoc Surg Oncol 2014;40(1):121–7.

[57] Nakanishi J, Wada Y, Matsumoto K, Azuma M, Kikuchi K, Ueda S. Overexpression of B7-H1 (PD-L1) significantly associates with tumor grade and postoperative prognosis in human urothelial cancers. Cancer Immunol Immunother 2006;56(8):1173–82.

[58] Rosenberg JE, Hoffman-Censits J, Powles T, van der Heijden MS, Balar AV, Necchi A, et al. Atezolizumab in patients with locally advanced and metastatic urothelial carcinoma who have progressed following treatment with platinum-based chemotherapy: a single-arm, multicentre, phase 2 trial. Lancet Lond Engl 2016;387(10031):1909–20.

[59] Shi L, Campbell G, Jones WD, Campagne F, Wen Z, Walker SJ, et al. The MicroArray Quality Control (MAQC)-II study of common practices for the development and validation of microarray-based predictive models. Nat Biotechnol 2010;28(8):827–38.

[60] Hess KR, Wei C, Qi Y, Iwamoto T, Symmans WF, Pusztai L. Lack of sufficiently strong informative features limits the potential of gene expression analysis as predictive tool for many clinical classification problems. BMC Bioinform 2011;12:463.

[61] Luqmani YA. Mechanisms of drug resistance in cancer chemotherapy. Med Princ Pract Int J Kuwait Univ Health Sci Cent 2005;14(Suppl 1):35–48.

[62] Bose S, Wan Z, Carr A, Rizvi AH, Vieira G, Pe'er D, et al. Scalable microfluidics for single-cell RNA printing and sequencing. Genome Biol 2015;16:120.

[63] Deeks SG, Lewin SR, Havlir DV. The end of AIDS: HIV infection as a chronic disease. Lancet Lond Engl 2013;382(9903):1525–33.

Index